D0533368

DISPOSED OF BY CTM
LIBRARY SERVICES
2022
NEWER INFORMATION
MAY BE AVAILABLE

PC00006403

Evidence-Based OBSTETRICS

Edited by

David K James MA, MD, FRCOG, DCH

Kassam Mahomed MBChB, FRCOG, MD, FRANZCOG

Peter Stone MBChB, MD, FRCOG, FRANZCOG, DDU, CMEM

Willem van Wijngaarden MD, DM, MRCOG, DGO

Lyndon M Hill MD, FACOG

SAUNDERS
An Imprint of Elsevier Science

SAUNDERS
An Imprint of Elsevier Science

First published 2003

ISBN 0 7020 2547 X

British Library Cataloguing in Publication Data
A catalogue record for this book is available from the British Library

Library of Congress Cataloging in Publication Data
A catalog record for this book is available from the Library of Congress

Note
Medical knowledge is constantly changing. As new information becomes available, changes in treatment, procedures, equipment and the use of drugs become necessary. The authors and the publishers have taken care to ensure that the information given in this text is accurate and up to date. However, readers are strongly advised to confirm that the information, especially with regard to drug usage, complies with the latest legislation and standards of practice.

Existing UK drug nomenclature is changing to the system of Recommended International Nonproprietary Names (rINNs). Until the UK names are no longer in use, these more familiar names are used in this book in preference to rINNs, details of which may be obtained from the British National Formulary.

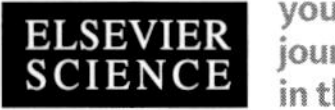

your source for books, journals and multimedia in the health sciences

www.elsevierhealth.com

The Publisher's policy is to use **paper manufactured from sustainable forests**

Printed in China by RDC Group Limited

Commissioning Editor: **Judy Fletcher**
Associate Editor: **Paul Fam**
Project Development Manager: **Shuet-Kei Cheung**
Project Manager: **Susan Skinner**
Design Manager: **Jayne Jones**

Contents

MATERNAL PROBLEMS

POSTNATAL

Contributors

Paul Adinkra MBBS
Registrar in Obstetrics and Gynaecology, Northwick Park Hospital, Middlesex

Janet R Ashworth BM BS BMed Sci (Hons) DM MRCOG
Sub-Specialty Trainee in Fetomaternal Medicine, Birmingham Women's Hospital, Birmingham

Paul Ayuk BSc (Hons) MBBS PhD MRCOG
Clinical Lecturer in Obstetrics and Gynaecology, John Radcliffe Hospital, Headington, Oxford

Bryan Beattie MD FRCOG
Consultant in Fetal Medicine, Department of Obstetrics and Gynaecology, University Hospital of Wales, Cardiff

Karen Brackley MD MRCOG
Consultant in Fetomaternal Medicine, Department of Fetal Medicine, Princess Anne Hospital, Southampton

Doris M Campbell MD FRCOG
Reader, Department of Obstetrics and Gynaecology, University of Aberdeen, Aberdeen

Stephen Carroll MD MRCPI MRCOG
Consultant in Obstetrics and Gynaecology, National Maternity Hospital, Dublin, Ireland

David Churchill MB ChB MD MRCOG
Consultant Obstetrician, Department of Obstetrics and Gynaecology, Good Hope Hospital, Sutton Coldfield, Birmingham

Janet L Cresswell MBChB MRCOG MFFP
Consultant Obstetrician and Gynaecologist, Chesterfield and North Derbyshire Royal Hospital, Calow, Chesterfield

Andrew Dawson MD FRCOG
Consultant Obstetrician and Gynaecologist, Nevill Hall Hospital, Abergavenny

A Petra Deering MBBS
Senior House Officer, Queen's Medical Centre, University Hospital NHS Trust, Nottingham

Jim C Dornan MD FRCOG
Director of Fetal Medicine, Royal Maternity Hospital, Belfast

Diana C Dunlop MA MBBS MD MRCOG
Consultant Obstetrician and Gynaecologist, Royal United Hospital, Bath

Hazeem El-Refaey MD MRCOG
Consultant and Senior Lecturer in Obstetrics and Gynaecology, Chelsea and Westminster Hospital, London

Fiona Fairlie MD MRCOG
Consultant Obstetrician and Gynaecologist, The Jessop Wing, Sheffield

Roy G Farquharson MBChB FRCOG
Consultant in Obstetrics and Gynaecology, Liverpool Women's Hospital, Liverpool

Diana Fothergill MBChB FRCOG DipEd
Consultant Obstetrician and Gynaecologist, The Jessop Wing, Sheffield

Robert B Fraser MBChB MD FRCOG DCH
Reader in Obstetrics and Gynaecology, The Jessop Wing, Sheffield

Helena Gardiner MD PhD FRCP DCH FRCPCH
Senior Lecturer and Hon Consultant in Perinatal Cardiology, Royal Brompton Hospital, London

Harry Gee MD FRCOG
Consultant Obstetrician and Medical Director, Director of Postgraduate Education, Department of Fetal Medicine, Birmingham Women's Hospital, Edgbaston, Birmingham

Jane Gould MD
Consultant Haematologist, Queen's Medical Centre, University Hospital NHS Trust, Nottingham

Simon R Grant DM MRCOG
Consultant Obstetrician and Gynaecologist, Princess Alexandra Maternity Wing, Treliske Hospital, Truro

Marion Hall MD FRCOG
Consultant Obstetrician and Gynaecologist, Aberdeen Maternity Hospital, Aberdeen

Lyndon Hill MD FACOG
Professor of Obstetrics and Gynecology, Ultrasound Division, Magee Women's Hospital, Pittsburgh, Pennsylvania

Sharon Hodgkiss RN RM DipNurs BSc(Hons)
West Midlands Regional Co-ordinator, Antenatal Screening, West Midlands Perinatal Institute, Birmingham

Ed Howarth MBCHB MRCOG
Consultant in Maternal and Fetal Medicine, University Hospitals of Leicester NHS Trust, Leicester

David T Howe DM FRCOG FRCS(Ed)
Consultant in Fetomaternal Medicine, Wessex Fetal Medicine Unit, Princess Anne Hospital, Southampton

David K James MA MD FRCOG DCH
Professor of Fetomaternal Medicine, Department of Obstetrics and Gynaecology, Queen's Medical Centre, University Hospital NHS Trust, Nottingham

Tracey A Johnston MD MRCOG
Consultant in Fetal–Maternal Medicine, St Mary's Hospital for Women and Children, Manchester

Lucy Kean DM MA MRCOG
Consultant Obstetrician (Subspecialist in Maternal and Fetal Medicine), City Hospital, Nottingham

Tony Kelly MBBS MRCOG
Specialist Registrar, Department of Obstetrics and Gynaecology, St Michael's Hospital, Bristol

Ellen M Knox BSc MBCHB MRCOG
Obstetric Research Fellow, West Midlands Perinatal Institute, Birmingham

Aneesa Lala MBChB
Specialist Registrar in Obstetrics and Gynaecology, Derby City General Hospital, Derby

Ronnie F Lamont BSc MD FRCOG
Consultant Obstetrician and Gynaecologist, Northwick Park Hospital, Middlesex

Christianne Lok MD
Vliehors 4, Graan voor Visch 16212, 2134 XN Hoofddorp, Netherlands

Mike Lumb MA MRCOG
Consultant in Obstetrics and Gynaecology, Maternity Unit, Peterborough District Hospital, Peterborough

Peter McParland MD FRCPI FRCOG
Director of Fetal Medicine, National Maternity Hospital, Dublin, Ireland

Ian W Mahady MBChB FRCOG
Consultant Obstetrician, Burnley Health Care NHS Trust, Burnley

Kassam Mahomed MBChB FRCOG MD FRANZCOG
Associate Professor, Departement of Obstetrics and Gynecology, University of Adelaide, Port Pirie, South Australia

Michael Maresh MD FRCOG
Consultant Obstetrician, St Mary's Hospital for Women and Children, Manchester

Michelle Mohajer MD FRCOG
Consultant in Fetomaternal Medicine, Royal Shrewsbury Hospital, Shrewsbury, Shropshire

Etelka Moll MD
Department of Obstetrics and Gynecology, University of Amsterdam, Amsterdam, Netherlands

Catherine Nelson-Piercy MA FRCP
Consultant Obstetric Physician, Guy's Hospital St Thomas' Hospital Trust, London

Sandra M Newbold MD MRCOG
Consultant in Obstetrics and Gynaecology, Ashford and St Peters Hospital, Surrey

Katinka Overmars MD
Academic Medical Center, University of Amsterdam, Amsterdam, Netherlands

Tim Overton BSc MD MRCGP MRCOG
Consultant Obstetrician and Gynaecologist, Norfolk & Norwich University Hospital, Norwich

Philip Owen MD MRCOG
Consultant Obstetrician and Gynaecologist, Princess Royal Maternity Unit, Glasgow

David Penman MD MRCOG
Consultant in Maternal and Fetal Medicine, Medway Maritime Hospital, Gillingham, Kent

Margaret Ramsay MA MD MRCP MRCOG
Fetomaternal Medicine Fellow, Queen's Medical Centre, University Hospital NHS Trust, Nottingham

Janet M Rennie MA MD FRCP DCH
Consultant and Senior Lecturer in Neonatal Medicine, King's College Hospital, London

Jane Rutherford DM MRCOG
Subspecialty Trainee in Fetomaternal Medicine, Obstetrics and Gynaecology, Queen's Medical Centre, University Hospital NHS Trust, Nottingham

Ian Scudamore MD MRCOG
Consultant, Department of Obstetrics and Gynaecology, Leceister General Hospital, Leicester

Mark Selinger BMed Sci BMBS FRCOG DM
Director of Obstetrics, Royal Berkshire Hospital, Reading

Sunita Sharma MRCOG
Clinical Research Fellow, Academic Department of Obstetrics and Gynaecology, Chelsea and Westminster Hospital, London

Farah Siddiqui MD MRCOG
Senior House Officer, Department of Obstetrics and Gynaecology, Queen's Medical Centre, University Hospital NHS Trust, Nottingham

Peter Stone MBChB MD FRCOG FRANZCOG DDU CMEM
School of Medicine and Health Sciences, University of Auckland, National Women's Hospital, Epsom, Auckland, New Zealand

Jane Thomas MD MRCOG
Director CESU, Royal College of Obstetricians and Gynaecologists, London

Clare Tower MBChB
Clinical Research Fellow, Queen's Medical Centre, University Hospital NHS Trust, Nottingham

Shantala Vadeyar MD MRCOG
Consultant in Fetal and Maternal Medicine, Queen's Medical Centre, University Hospital NHS Trust, Nottingham

Jeroen E van de Riet MD BSc
Registrar in Obstetrics and Gynecology, Academic Medical Center, University of Amsterdam, Amsterdam, Netherlands

Rajesh Varma MRCOG
Specialist Registrar in Obstetrics and Gynaecology, Bedford Hospitals NHS Trust, Bedford

Willem van Wijngaarden MD DM MRCOG DGO
Lecturer, Academic Medical Center, University of Amsterdam, Amsterdam, Netherlands

David J Williams MD MBBS MRCP
Senior Lecturer and Honorary Consultant in Maternal Medicine, Department of Academic Obstetrics and Gynaecology, Imperial College Science, Technology & Medicine, London

John Williams MD FRCOG
Consultant Obstetrician and Gynaecologist, Countess of Chester Hospital, Chester

Michael P Wyldes MD FRCOG
Consultant Obstetrician and Gynaecologist, Princess of Wales Women's Unit, Birmingham Heartlands Hospital, Birmingham

Foreword

Eccentricity was once a prized attribute of famous clinicians. 'Characters' were part of the Medical School mythology, and stories of peculiar clinical practice were embellished during their telling and retelling by generations of students. However, aberrations in obstetrics such as the generation of several million children with genital tract abnormalities resulting from the use of diethyl stilbestrol to treat threatened miscarriage (despite trials showing no benefit) and the use of thalidomide resulting in tens of thousands of children with phocomelia have led to widespread reluctance on the part of patients (or clients or consumers, depending on viewpoint) to accept bland reassurances that 'the doctor knows best'. In these days of ready access to the Internet, one needs to justify one's choice of management. Maverick practitioners are no longer seen as 'stimulating' or 'original' but as dangerous and a liability to themselves, the medical defense organizations and society. But where to get the evidence on which to base one's management? The burgeoning literature (for example, an explosive growth in papers on preeclampsia on Medline from 17 per year in 1966 to 567 in 2001) makes it impossible for a single practitioner to acquire, assess and summarize the information available across the whole range of obstetrics. Fortunately, help is at hand. David James and his colleagues have done a superb job in persuading top-class clinicians and researchers to summarize for us topics in which they have specific expertise. Based on the best-selling *High Risk Pregnancy – Management Options*, this book is a collection and expansion of the very popular management options summary boxes. For each topic, the management options, quality of evidence and strength of recommendation are graded, and the key references are appended (with summaries) to inform the reader, guide practice and be available as a summary for the questioning patient. For anyone involved in preparing clinical guidelines for their own unit, this book will be a godsend and an essential starting point from which recommendations can be tailored to meet local needs. No antenatal clinic, labor ward or individual pocket will be complete without a copy. Our patients deserve it.

Philip Steer, Bernie Gonik, Carl Weiner

June 2002

Preface

Evidence-based medicine is a 'growth industry' with an exponentially rising number of articles, journals, books and websites on the topic. There are two main reasons for this expanding interest in the evidence basis for medical management. First, doctors wish to maintain a critical approach to their practice. They need to understand the strength of the evidence supporting any treatment they advise, although it has to be admitted that the supporting evidence for the management of some medical problems is either weak or non-existent. Second, patients want to evaluate for themselves the value of any suggested treatment rather than taking the advice on trust.

Evidence-Based Obstetrics is the latest addition to the evidence based publishing literature. Its origins, however, are not new, in that it is the second 'spin-off' publication from the very successful postgraduate textbook *High Risk Pregnancy – Management Options*, soon to appear in its third edition. That book has a very stylized but detailed approach to the management of problems in pregnancy including the compilation of the management options at the end of each topic in a 'Summary of Management Options' (SOMO) box. This feature proved popular in reader feedback. Thus, we decided to produce a separate collection of the SOMO boxes for problems in pregnancy but with the evidence basis for the management strategies summarized and scored.

The approach we used was as follows:

- The SOMO box for the given topic from the second edition of *High Risk Pregnancy – Management Options* was used as the starting point.
- A reviewer/contributor, not the author of the original chapter, was asked to critically examine the evidence for each management strategy proposed in the SOMO box using:
  - The references provided by the author(s) in the chapter
  - Extra references (some only published after the chapter was written) to allow a more comprehensive and up-to-date evidence review
  - In a few cases (e.g. the management of a breech presentation) this new evidence meant that the management options had to be rewritten .
- Each supporting reference was summarized and scored by the reviewer/contributor. The evidence scoring system used is shown in the Key on page xvi.

Because the aim was to produce a pocket-sized book that was significantly smaller than *High Risk Pregnancy – Management Options*, it meant that we had to limit the number of references included and exclude those that were poor-quality and 'low-scoring'. For some treatments, especially in the maternal problems section, there may be high-quality evidence of the value of a given approach outside pregnancy but an absence of such studies in pregnant women. We have tried to identify clearly where this occurs. It was also clear that no supporting evidence exists for many management strategies and yet many of them are reasonable approaches. Such examples have been given a 'good practice point' rating.

We feel that this critical approach to the management of problems in pregnancy is very important. It is the format we will be using in the SOMO boxes in the third edition of *High Risk Pregnancy – Management Options*.

The steps to follow when using the book are:

1. Find the problem/topic for which you need a SOMO.
2. In the SOMO box you will find a score for the quality of evidence that supports a given management strategy and hence the strength of recommendation for that approach.
3. For each Quality of Evidence score at least one summarized reference is provided.

The production of the book has been very hard work and I am very grateful to the reviewers/contributors and the editors for all their efforts.

Finally, we would welcome your comments for improvement to incorporate in the next edition of *Evidence-Based Obstetrics*.

David James
2002

Key

Rating system:

Quality of evidence:

Ia	Evidence obtained from meta-analysis of randomized controlled trials
Ib	Evidence obtained from at least one randomized controlled trial
IIa	Evidence obtained from at least one well designed controlled study without randomization
IIb	Evidence obtained from at least one other type of well-designed quasi-experimental study
III	Evidence obtained from well-designed non-experimental descriptive studies, such as comparative studies, correlation studies and case studies
IV	Evidence obtained from expert committee reports or opinions and/or clinical experience of respected authorities

Strength of recommendation:

A	At least one randomized controlled trial as part of a body of literature of overall good quality and consistency addressing the specific recommendation (Evidence levels Ia, Ib)
B	Well-controlled clinical studies available but no randomized clinical trials on the topic of recommendations (Evidence levels IIa, IIb, III)
C	Evidence obtained from expert committee reports or opinions and/or clinical experiences of respected authorities. Indicates an absence of directly applicable clinical studies of good quality (Evidence level IV)
✔	Good practice point: recommended best practice based on the clinical experience of the guideline development group

PREPREGNANCY

Chapter 1

Prepregnancy education

1.1 Nutritional preparation for pregnancy *Jeroen van de Riet*

Management option	Quality of evidence	Strength of recommendation	References
Advise healthy balanced diet for all	IV	C	1
Periconceptual folic acid supplementation for all	Ia	A	2
Avoid undercooked meats and eggs, soft cheeses, shellfish and raw fish and unpasteurized milk	IV	C	3
Low maternal body mass is associated with low birthweight and may have a negative effect on birth outcome	III	B	4–7
Advise iron supplements	Ib	A	8
In ethnic groups lacking sunlight: advise extra vitamin D	IV	C	9
Avoid certain herbal teas	IV	C	10

References

1 Public Health Commission (1995) *Food and nutrition guidelines for New Zealand adults*. Wellington, New Zealand: Public Health Commission. Government recommendations based on a consensus of opinion with regards to diet, food handling and preparation concerning pregnant women. **IV C**

2 Lumley J, Watson L, Watson M *et al.* (2000) Periconceptional supplementation with folate and/or multivitamins for preventing neural tube defects (Cochrane Review). In: *The Cochrane library*, issue 2. Oxford: Update Software. Four randomized or quasi-randomized trials involving 6425 women were assessed in this meta-analysis. Periconceptional folate supplementation reduced the incidence of neural tube defects (OR 0.28, 95% CI 0.15–0.53). **Ia A**

3 Centers for Disease Control (1992) Update: foodborne listeriosis – United States, 1988–1990. *Morb Mortal Wkly Rep 41 41*, 251–258. Consensus of opinion with regards to ideas for dietary strategies to avoid exposure to *Listeria monocytogenes*. **IV C**

4 Ogunyemi D, Hullett S, Leeper J *et al.* (1998) Prepregnancy body mass index, weight gain during pregnancy, and perinatal outcome in a rural black population. *J Maternal Fetal Med* **7**, 190–193. Retrospective study on 582 consecutive term deliveries with 13% of women with a prepregnancy body mass index (BMI) less than 20. Multivariate analysis showed that the prepregnancy BMI was a significant predictor of low birth weight. **III B**

5 Rantakallio P, Laara E, Koiranen M *et al.* (1995) Maternal build and pregnancy outcome. *J Clin Epidemiol* **48**, 199–207. Retrospective study on 10969 and 9128 women in two birth cohorts in northern Finland with 13% and 24% of women with a body mass index (BMI) below 20. Logistic regression analysis did not show a better outcome for a child with a mother with a BMI between 20 and 25 compared to a mother with a BMI below 20. **III B**

6 Rasmussen KL, Borup K (1992) Prepregnancy low body mass index is not a predictor of labor complications. *Gynecol Obstet Invest* **34**, 79–81. Retrospective study on mode of delivery and fetal outcome in 149 pregnancies comparing women with a prepregnancy body mass index (BMI) below 20 to those with a prepregnancy BMI of 20–25. None were undernourished. Suspected intrauterine asphyxia was more common in those with a prepregnancy BMI below 18. There was a trend of fewer babies with a birthweight above 4000g in the low-BMI group. **III B**

7 Mavalankar DV, Trivedi CC, Gray RH (1994) Maternal weight, height and risk of poor pregnancy outcome in Ahmedabad, India. *Indian Pediatr* **31**, 1205–1212. Retrospective case-control study of low birthweight and perinatal mortality in Ahmedabad, India. Maternal height and weight was compared between mothers of 611 perinatal deaths, 644 preterm–low-birthweight and 1465 normal-birthweight controls as well as 617 small-for-gestational-age (SGA) and

1851 appropriate-for-gestational-age births. Weight and height were much lower in this population compared to Western standards. Low weight was significantly associated with an increased risk of perinatal death, prematurity and SGA. **III B**

8 De Leeuw NKM, Lowenstein L, Hsieh YS (1966) Iron deficiency and hydremia in normal pregnancy. *Medicine* **45**, 291–315. Randomized controlled trial in which pregnant women were given adequate iron supplements, either as parenteral or oral iron, or no iron therapy. During the last trimester, iron treatment was associated with a higher hemoglobin, red cell mass and serum iron concentration, whereas plasma volume changes were the same in both groups. **Ib A**

9 Hytten F (1966) Nutritional requirements in pregnancy: what should the pregnant woman be eating? *Midwifery* **6**, 93–98. Asian women who customarily spend most of their time indoors and whose calcium absorption may be impaired by an excess of wholemeal cereals in the diet should have extra vitamin D supplements during pregnancy. There is no particular evidence of the need for extra vitamin supplements in a well nourished community. **IV C**

10 Allen JR, Thompson S, Jeffs D *et al.* (1989) Are herbal teas safe for infants and children? *Aust Fam Physician* **18**, 1017–1019. Review on herbal teas. The authors feel that the potential hazards associated with herbal teas need to be exposed. **IV C**

1.2 Exercise

Jeroen van de Riet

Management option	Quality of evidence	Strength of recommendation	References
Avoid hyperthermia	III	B	1,2
Avoid dehydration	III	B	2
Exercise is associated with a higher self-esteem and confidence	III	B	3
Moderate exercise apparently carries no harm to mother or fetus	III	B	4–8

References

1 Smith DW, Clarren SK, Harvey MA (1978) Hyperthermia as a possible teratogenic agent. *J Pediatr* **92**, 878–883. Case reports on pregnancy outcomes complicated by fever over 38.9°C. In 8 cases, in which fever occurred at 4–6 weeks gestation, severe neurological problems, hypotonia, microphthalmia, midface hypoplasia and mild impairment of distal limb development were described. In 5 patients exposed to hyperthermia at 7–16 weeks gestation, the predominant features were hypotonia, neurogenic arthrogryphosis and central nervous system dysgenesis. No apparent serious problem in morphogenesis was found following hyperthermia during the latter half of pregnancy. **III B**

2 Miller P, Smith DW, Shepard TH (1978) Maternal hyperthermia as a possible cause of anencephaly. *Lancet* **1**, 519–521. Case-control study of 127 women. In 11% of 63 cases of anencephaly, a history of maternal hyperthermia (febrile illness or sauna bathing) near the presumed time of anterior neural-groove closure (gestational age of 4–7 weeks) was reported. The frequency of hyperthermia among the 64 healthy controls was 0.1%. **III B**

3 Wallace AM, Boyer DB, Dan A *et al.* (1986) Aerobic exercise, maternal self esteem and physical discomforts during pregnancy. *J Nurse Midwifery* **31**, 255–262. Case-control study of 53 pregnant women, of whom 31 participated in an aerobic exercise program, and 22 controls who did not. There was a significant inverse relationship between amount of exercise and reported discomforts (shortness of breath, backache, headache, fatigue and hot flushes) during pregnancy ($p < 0.01$). It seems that exercise during pregnancy is associated with higher self-esteem and lower physical discomfort. **III B**

4 Spinnewijn WEM, Lotgering FK, Struijk PC *et al.* (1996) Fetal heart rate and uterine contractility during maternal exercise at term. *Am J Obstet Gynecol* **174**, 43–48. Observational study of 26 term pregnant women with artificial rupture of the membranes. Moderately strenuous exercise on a cycle ergometer did not cause fetal distress; however, uterine activity increased 5.5-fold after exercise. **III B**

5 Lotgering FK, van Doom MB, Struijk PC *et al.* (1991) Maximal aerobic exercise in pregnant women: heart rate, oxygen consumption, CO_2 production and ventilation. *J Appl Physiol* **70**, 1016–1023. Observational study of 33 women on the effect of pregnancy on maximal aerobic power. The authors concluded that pregnancy did not markedly affect maximal heart rate and maximal oxygen uptake. **III B**

6 Pommerance JJ, Gluck L, Lynch VA *et al.* (1974) Physical fitness in pregnancy: its effect on pregnancy outcome. *Am J Obstet Gynecol* **119**, 867–876. Observational study of 41 pregnant women at 35–37 weeks gestation. A physical fitness score was assessed using a bicycle ergometer. Adverse fetal outcome was not correlated with the level of maternal physical fitness. **III B**

7 Hauth JC, Gilstrap LC III, Widmer K (1982) Fetal heart rate reactivity before and after maternal jogging during the third trimester. *Am J Obstet Gynecol* **145**, 545–547. Observational study of seven third-trimester pregnant women. Fetal heart rate increased significantly after jogging for 1.5 miles. It took nearly 30min before fetal heart rate returned to the normal baseline. **III B**

8 Collings CA, Curet LB, Mullin JP (1983) Maternal and fetal response to maternal aerobic exercise program. *Am J Obstet Gynecol* **145**, 702–707. Pregnant women who participated in an aerobic exercise program during the second and third trimester showed an increase in aerobic capacity compared to women who did not exercise regularly. Fetal outcome did not differ between groups. **III B**

1.3 Work

Jeroen van de Riet

Management option	Quality of evidence	Strength of recommendation	References
Avoid adverse factors: ❑ Smoke-filled environments ❑ Work with glazing ❑ Dry cleaning and laundry ❑ Operating theaters	III	B	1,2
Avoid long hours of standing and walking	III	B	3
Avoid excess lifting/exercise	III	B	4–6
Continue with work if the woman wishes this and is not unduly tired	III	B	7
No evidence that visual display units (VDUs) are associated with adverse pregnancy outcome	IIa	B	8,9

References

1 Peters TJ, Adelstein P, Golding J *et al.* (1984) The effects of work in pregnancy: short- and long-term associations. In: Chamberlain, G (ed.) *Pregnant women at work*. London: Royal Society of Medicine, 87–105. The 1958 British Perinatal Mortality Survey revealed an increase in stillbirth, neonatal death and congenital malformations among pregnant women working in the chemical industry, glass and pottery, laundry and dry cleaning, hairdressers and hospital workers. The reported death rates varied between 48.6 and 52.3/1000 total births. **III B**

2 Tomlin PJ (1979) Health problems of anaesthesists and their families in the West Midlands. *Br Med J* **1**, 779–784. Retrospective case-control study among anesthetists in England. Of the 277 children born to anesthetists, 26 (9.3%) had congenital abnormalities (central nervous system or musculoskeletal system) or developmental problems. The control group consisted of 92 infants born before one of their parents took up anesthetics or after 1 year or more away from the operating theater. 4 of the 92 infants in the control group (4.3%) had congenital or developmental problems. **III B**

3 Fenster L, Hubbard AE, Windham GC *et al.* (1997) A prospective study of work related physiological exertion and spontaneous abortion. *Epidemiology* **8**, 66–74. This prospective cohort study of 5144 pregnant women shows that none of their exertion measures at work was associated with an increased risk of spontaneous abortion. For 19 women with a history of two or more spontaneous abortions (≤20 weeks of gestation), standing at work for more than 7h per day was associated with a higher rate of abortion (OR 4.3,95% CI 1.6–11.7). **III B**

4 Spinillo A, Capuzzo E, Baltaro F *et al.* (1996) The effect of work activity in pregnancy on the risk of fetal growth retardation. *Acta Obstet Gynecol Scand* **75**, 531–536. Retrospective case-control study of 349 patients with ultrasonographically confirmed fetal growth retardation and 698 control pregnancies. The risk of fetal growth retardation was significantly higher (OR 2.4, 95% CI 1.36–4.21) among women reporting moderate-to-heavy effort as compared to women reporting light physical effort at work. **III B**

5 Brett KM, Strogatzz DS, Savitz DA (1997) Employment, job strain and preterm delivery among women in North Carolina. *Am J Pub Health* **87**, 188–204. A prospective population-based case-control study with 412 preterm deliveries and 612 term deliveries as controls. Women who worked at high-strain full-time jobs (i.e. high demand and low control) had an increased risk of preterm delivery (OR 1.4, 95% CI 0.9–2.0). Women who worked at a high-strain job for more than 30 weeks of pregnancy also had an increased risk of preterm delivery (OR 1.4, 95% CI 1.0–2.2). **III B**

6 Spinillo A, Capuzzo E, Stronati M *et al.* (1995) The effect of work activity in pregnancy on the risk of preeclampsia. *Aust N Z Obst Gynecol* **35**, 380–385. Retrospective case-control study of 160 severely preeclamptic nulliparous women and 320 normotensive nulliparous pregnant women. Moderate and high physical activity at work was associated with a twofold increase in the risk of severe preeclampsia (OR 2.08, 95% CI 1.11–3.88). **III B**

7 Luke B, Mamelle N, Keith L *et al.* (1995) The association between occupational factors and preterm birth: a United States nurses' study. Research Committee of the Association of Women's Health, Obstetric, and Neonatal Nurses. *Am J Obstet Gynecol* **173**, 849–862. Retrospective case-control study of 210 nurses who delivered prematurely and 1260 nurses whose infants were delivered at term. Preterm delivery may be related to hours worked per day (OR 1.6, 95% CI 1.1–2.2) and to occupational fatigue (OR 1.4, 95% CI 1.1–1.9). **III B**

8 Roman E, Beral V, Pelerin M *et al.* (1992) Spontaneous abortion and work with visual display units. *Br J Ind Med* **49**, 507–512. Case-control study of 150 nulliparous women working with a visual display unit and a clinically diagnosed spontaneous abortion. 297 nulliparous working women served as controls. No increased risk of spontaneous abortion was found in women who used a visual display unit at work compared with women who did not (OR 0.9, 95%CI 0.6–1.4). **IIa B**

9 McDonald AD, Cherry NM, Delorme C *et al.* (1986) Visual display units and pregnancy: evidence from the Montreal survey. *J Occup Med* **28**, 1226–1231. Retrospective study on 56 012 current and 48 608 previous pregnancies. In 17 632 pregnancies in occupations with substantial use of visual display units (VDUs), users and nonusers had similar rates of congenital defects and of abortions in both current and previous pregnancies, irrespective of the amount of VDU use. **III B**

Chapter 2

Organization of prenatal care

2.1 Organization of prenatal care and identification of risk *Marion H Hall*

Management option	Quality of evidence	Strength of recommendation	References
Aims of antenatal care:			
Identification of maternal and fetal risk: Use of risk scoring systems in pregnancy predict the likelihood of adverse outcomes but with little evidence of a reduction in these	IV	C	1,2
Intervene in at-risk pregnancies to prevent or lessen the impact of adverse outcome: There is no proof that prenatal care *per se* improves neonatal outcome	III	B	3
Intervene in at-risk pregnancies to prevent or lessen the impact of adverse outcome: Specific interventions proven to be effective for specific risks can reduce mortality and morbidity	III	B	4
Establish what constitutes routine/normal prenatal care for a given population – this is based on available resources:			
The relative role of obstetricians, family doctors (general practitioners) and individuals in the delivery of prenatal care varies between countries	III	B	5,6
Determine who will see pregnant women, when they will be seen and what will be done when they attend:			
There is no evidence that doctors need to be the medical professionals involved in the prenatal care of every pregnancy	Ib	A	7–10
For specific problems, especially social ones, midwives or general practitioners may actually offer more benefit than specialist care	Ia	A	9
Incorporating different (para-)medical professionals into one shared antenatal care program can be effective in providing appropriate care for pregnant women	Ia	A	10
A physician-based prenatal care model appears to be more expensive without actually improving pregnancy outcome	Ia	A	9,10
Frequency of prenatal visits can safely be reduced in low-risk pregnancies	Ia	A	7,10,11
Socio-demographic factors and poor utilization of prenatal care are correlated	III	B	5, 12

References

1 Alexander S, Keirse MNJC (1990) Formal risk scoring during pregnancy. In: Chalmers I, Enkin M, Keirse MJNC (eds) *Effective care in pregnancy and childbirth.* Oxford: Oxford University Press, 345–365. Extensive review of risk assessment and outcome. The authors emphasize that imprecise scoring for potential risk results in an increase of unproven interventions without an improvement in outcome. Improvements in outcome are more pronounced in low-risk pregnancies than in high-risk pregnancies and are associated more with a lower prevalence of risk markers than with an improved detection of those risk markers. Further, it is stated that risk scores behave differently in different populations. The authors conclude by not recommending formal risk scoring outside the context of trials. **IV C**

2 Hall MH (1990) Identification of high risk and low risk. *Clin Obstet Gynecol* **4**, 65–76. Review considering longitudinal data in assessing the risks associated with previous obstetric history and acknowledges the poor specificity of low-risk ascertainment. **IV C**

3 Fiscella K (1995) Does prenatal care improve birth outcomes? A critical review. *Obstet Gynecol* **85**, 468–479. Systematic review of 130 studies assessing whether they satisfy published guidelines for evaluating the evidence for causality between prenatal care and birth outcome. The issue of whether it is the screening or the interventions that are deficient is not addressed and the conclusion that outcome for the baby is not improved does not exclude the possibility that some specific components are effective for specific risk. **III B**

4 Carroli G, Rooney C, Villar J (2001) How effective is antenatal care in preventing maternal mortality and serious morbidity? An overview of the evidence. *Paediatr Perinat Epidemiol* **15**, 1–42 Overview of RCTs on the effectiveness of antenatal care in relation to maternal mortality and serious morbidity, in particular in developing countries. It looks at interventions aimed at prevention, detection and treatment. Antenatal interventions that have been shown to be effective in conditions that can lead to maternal mortality or serious morbidity are evaluated and presented. **III B**

5 Buekens P (1990) Variations in provision and uptake of antenatal care. *Clin Obstet Gynecol* **4**, 187–205. Review of the utilization of care, of barriers to care and of how barriers may be overcome. Also deals with overprovision of care, but this material is superseded by recent trials. **IV C**

6 Piaggio G, Ba'aqueel H, Bergsjo P *et al.* (1998) The practice of antenatal care: comparing four study sites in different parts of the world participating in the WHO Antenatal Care Trial Randomized Controlled Trial. *Paediatr Perinat Epidemiol* **12**(Suppl 2), 116–141. Essential background survey to the World Health Organization RCT on antenatal care in 53 clinics in differents parts of the world, describing an unjustified variation in services provided. **III B**

7 Villar J, Ba'aqeel H, Piaggio G *et al.* (2001) WHO Antenatal Care Trial Research Group. WHO antenatal care randomised trial for the evaluation of a new model of routine antenatal care. *Lancet* **357**, 1551–1564. Multicenter RCT in 53 clinics in Argentina, Cuba, Saudi Arabia and Thailand, comparing two models of antenatal care on maternal and neonatal outcomes. Women (n = 12 568) in the new model had a median of five visits compared with 11 958 women in the standard model who had a median of eight visits. More women in the new model than in the standard model were referred to higher levels of care (13.4% vs 7.3%), but rates of hospital admission, diagnosis and length of stay were similar. Outcomes (low birthweight, postpartum anemia, urinary-tract infection and preeclampsia/eclampsia) were similar between the groups. There was no cost increase and in some settings the new model decreased cost. **Ib A**

8 Keirse MJNC (1990) Interaction between primary and secondary care during pregnancy and childbirth. In: Chalmers I, Enkin M, Keirse MJNC (eds) *Effective care in pregnancy and childbirth.* Oxford: Oxford University Press, 197–201. Data-free modeling of possible interactions between primary and secondary care, powerfully argued. **IV C**

9 Blondel B, Breart G (1995) Home visits during pregnancy: consequences on pregnancy outcome, use of health services and women's situations. *Semin Perinatol* **19**, 263–271. Meta-analysis of eight RCTs of home visits for complicated pregnancy or for social support, showing no improvement in outcome (preterm delivery, decrease the rate of hospital admission for women with complications) but possible benefits from the women's perspective. Need for more research is highlighted. **Ia A**

10 Khan-Neelofur D, Gulmezoglu M, Villar J (1998) Who should provide routine antenatal care for low-risk women, and how often? A systematic review of randomised controlled trials. WHO Antenatal Care Trial Research Group. *Paediatr Perinat Epidemiol* **12**, 7–26. Systematic review of five RCTs conducted to evaluate the effectiveness of antenatal care programs for low-risk women. The available data demonstrate no significant differences in selected perinatal outcomes for low-risk women receiving care according to a reduced frequency (approximately two visits fewer) of prenatal visits versus those following the existing practice. However, there are differences in satisfaction with the prenatal care provider and the prenatal care system. A midwife's clinic for provision of antenatal care for low-risk pregnancies was found to be feasible and therapy reduction in costs achievable. **Ia A**

11 Carroli G, Villar J, Piaggio G *et al.* (2001) WHO Antenatal Care Trial Research Group. WHO systematic review of randomised controlled trials of routine antenatal care. *Lancet* **357**, 1565–1570. Systematic review of seven RCTs (n = 57 418) on the effectiveness of different models of antenatal care. No change was found in the rates of preeclampsia, urinary-tract infection, postpartum anemia, maternal mortality, low birthweight and perinatal mortality

with a reduction of clinic visits. Some dissatisfaction with care, particularly among women in more Western countries, was observed with fewer visits. Costs were the same or less. **Ia A**

12 Elam-Evans LD, Adams MM, Garguillo PM *et al.* (1996) Trends in the percentage of women who received no prenatal care in the United States 1980–94: contribution of the demographic and risk effects. *Obstet Gynecol* **87**, 575–580. Large study over a 12-year period showing that, in the USA, lack of improvement in the percentage of women receiving no prenatal care was due to more women falling into the demographic groups at high risk. Research is relevant to social policy. **III B**

Chapter 3

Genetic counseling

3.1 Genetic counseling

David James

Management option		Quality of evidence	Strength of recommendation	References
Prepregnancy, prenatal and postnatal	Adequate time should be made available in a setting that is free from disturbance	IIa	B	1
	Both partners should be seen together whenever possible	IIb	B	2
	Obtain accurate and comprehensive information to make a secure diagnosis, including the taking of a family pedigree	IIa	B	1
	Counseling should always be 'nondirective' and supportive	III	B	3–5
	Ensure risks given are accurate and up-to-date	IIa	B	1
	What constitutes an 'acceptable' risk depends on the probability of its occurrence and the condition's impact	III	B	4–9
	Consider referring complex cases to a clinical geneticist	III	B	3

Summary of counseling points for common conditions

Mendelian inheritance	Chromosome abnormalities	Specific syndromes	Organ/system abnormalities
High recurrence risks Establish accurate diagnosis and mode of inheritance before counseling Seek latest information about carrier detection tests Plan invasive procedures requiring DNA methods with laboratory	Refer families with translocations to a clinical geneticist; perform family studies to identify risk of unbalanced karyotype (miscarriage or child with abnormalities)	Ensure accuracy of diagnosis and risks	For many conditions, information should be obtained from clinical geneticist
Autosomal dominant conditions	With unexpected structural chromosome abnormality, examine parents' chromosomes	Empiric risk figures are available for some conditions	Empiric risk figures are available for some
50% risk to offspring of affected parent Potential pitfalls in conditions with variable expression	Duplication of deletion of chromosomal material can result in congenital malformation and/or mental retardation	Prenatal diagnosis available for some with a biochemical basis, where gene has been found or where due to a microdeletion or duplication If doubt about diagnosis or risks, refer to clinical geneticist	

Mendelian inheritance	Chromosome abnormalities	Specific syndromes	Organ/system abnormalities
Autosomal recessive conditions	Predicting the effects of mosaicism is difficult; karyotype other cell lines		
25% risk of affected child where both parents are carriers Prenatal diagnosis possible for some Donor gametes might be an acceptable therapeutic option for some	*De novo* chromosomal disorders have low risk of recurrence; offer fetal karyotyping for reassurance		
X-linked recessive conditions	Check karyotype reports with laboratory if doubt of meaning		
Male-to-male transmission never occurs	Make clear whether risks relate to 'at amniocentesis' or 'at delivery'		
Daughters of an affected male will be carriers			
Unaffected males never transmit the disease			
For female carriers: each son has a 1 in 2 risk of being affected, each daughter has a 1 in 2 risk of being a carrier, affected homozygous females are rare			

References

1 Marteau TM, Kidd J, Michie S *et al.* (1993) Anxiety, knowledge and satisfaction in women receiving false positive results on routine prenatal screening: a randomized controlled trial. *J Psychosom Obstet Gynecol* **14**, 185–196. Two methods of preparing women undergoing prenatal screening (serum alpha-fetoprotein testing) were compared: provision of detailed written information and anxiety management training. There was some evidence that completing the study questionnaires had an anxiety-reducing effect. There was no evidence that receipt of an abnormal alpha-fetoprotein result resulted in raised anxiety. Neither of the interventions, alone or in combination, had an effect upon anxiety following an abnormal alpha-fetoprotein result. Receipt of detailed written information, however, led to women having more knowledge and being more satisfied with the amount of information that they had. Although the interventions did not reduce anxiety in this study, the authors argue there were other reasons for considering their incorporation into routine clinical practice. **IIa B** – though RCT poor design and power

2 Hall S, Bobrow M, Marteau TM (2000) Psychological consequences for parents of false negative results on prenatal screening for Down's syndrome: retrospective interview study. *Br Med J* **320**, 407–412. Comparative study of the adjustment of parents (anxiety, depression, parenting stress, attitudes towards the child and attributions of blame for the birth of the affected child) of children with Down syndrome who received a false negative result with that of parents not offered a test and those who declined a test. Overall, 179 parent pairs were studied. A false-negative result in prenatal screening had a small adverse effect on parental adjustment (more difficult adjustment and apportioning blame) 2–6 years after the birth of an affected child. **IIb B**

3 Michie S, Bron F, Bobrow *et al.* (1997) Nondirectiveness in genetic counseling: an empirical study. *Am J Hum Genet* **60**, 40–47. Observational study of the directiveness of genetic counseling, using ratings from transcripts of 131 consultations and comparing these with counselor-reported and counselee-reported directiveness. The results showed that genetic counseling was not characterized as uniformly nondirective by counselors, counselees or a standardized rating scale. **III B**

4 Marteau T, Drake H, Bobrow M (1994) Counselling following diagnosis of a fetal abnormality: the differing approaches of obstetricians, clinical geneticists, and genetic nurses. *J Med Genet* **31**, 864–867. Observational study to document how genetic nurses, geneticists and obstetricians describe their own counseling of women

following the diagnosis of specific fetal abnormalities. Obstetricians reported counseling in a significantly more directive fashion than did geneticists, who in turn reported counseling in a more directive way than genetic nurses. The extent to which the groups differed in their reported approaches varied across conditions. Future research needs to focus on what these different groups see as the objectives of counseling in this situation, how they actually counsel and with what effects. **III B**

5 Marteau T, Drake H, Reid M *et al.* (1994) Counselling following diagnosis of fetal abnormality: a comparison between German, Portuguese and UK geneticists. *Eur J Hum Genet* **2**, 96–102. Observational study of how geneticists in three European countries, Germany, Portugal and the UK, report counseling women at risk for having children with a range of conditions. While geneticists in all three countries reported counseling in a largely non-directive style, this varied both across genetic conditions and between countries. There was no strong consensus on approaches to counseling for any of the genetic conditions, defined as agreement between 70% of all three groups of geneticists. Despite strong professional codes of non-directiveness, geneticists report being somewhat directive in some counseling situations. **III B**

6 Michie S, French D, Allanson A *et al.* (1997) Information recall in genetic counseling: a pilot study of its assessment. *Patient Educ Couns* **32**, 93–100. Observational study of 35 consultations documenting what counselors remembered telling patients and included in a follow-up letter, what was actually covered (transcripts of tape recordings) and the patients' recall 1 month later. Over 95% of the information that counselors identified as important had been given during the consultation. Patients rated this information as important. Patients more frequently judged information about family implications to be important than did counselors. Counselors more frequently judged information about test, diagnosis and prognosis to be important than did patients. These results suggest that counselors' summary letters are a valid baseline against which to measure patient recall. This measure will not, however, capture all the information that patients consider important. **III B**

7 Michie S, McDonald V, Marteau TM *et al.* (1997) Genetic counseling: information given, recall and satisfaction. *Patient Educ Couns* **32**, 101–106. Observational questionnaire-based study of the key points given in genetic counseling, assess the amount and type of information recalled, and examine the relationships between counselees' (n = 32) knowledge, satisfaction with information received, the meeting of expectations, concern and anxiety. The mean percentage of key points recalled correctly was 76% (SD 17%) with 100% recall for family issues and 68–78% recall for genetic or medical information. Knowledge was not associated with satisfaction with information received nor with level of concern or anxiety following genetic counseling. **III B**

8 Michie S, Marteau TM, Bobrow *et al.* (1997) Genetic counseling: the psychological impact of meeting patients' expectations. *J Med Genet* **34**, 237–241. Observational study of 131 consultations of patients referred to a regional genetics center, and documents their expectations, the extent to which these are met, and the predictors and consequences of expectations being met. The outcomes assessed were state anxiety, concern about the problem for which the patient was referred, and satisfaction with information given. The majority got what they were expecting: 74% had their expectation for information met, 56% had their expectation for explanation met, 60% had their expectation for reassurance met, 61% had their expectation for advice met, and 73% had their expectation for help with making decisions met. When patients' expectations for reassurance and advice were met, patients were less concerned and their anxiety level was more reduced than when such expectations were not met. **IIIB**

9 Drake H, Reid M, Marteau T (1996) Attitudes towards termination for fetal abnormality: comparisons in three European countries. *Clin Genet* **49**, 134–140. Attitudes towards termination for a range of genetic conditions were studied in over 1700 health professionals (geneticists and obstetricians) and lay people (male and female) in three European countries: Germany, Portugal and the UK. Health professionals were more likely than lay-persons to report that they would opt for termination following diagnosis of a fetal abnormality. Differences were found between countries and study groups. Further studies are needed to determine whether differences between health professionals and lay samples reflect differences in perception of disability, and whether such differences result in health professionals presenting termination of pregnancy in a way that is not concordant with patients' values and wishes. **III B**

Chapter 4

Sociodemographic factors

4.1 Pregnancy in adolescence

Jeroen van de Riet

Management option		Quality of evidence	Strength of recommendations	References
Prepregnancy	Education and advertising directed toward sexual behavior and family planning	IIa	B	1
	Emphasize self-referral for care when pregnant	–	✔	–
Prenatal	Encouragement of early referral for prenatal care and regular attendance	III	B	2, 3
	Confirm gestation with early ultrasonography	III	B	2
	Stress advice about diet and adverse habits (e.g. smoking)	III	B	4
	Mobilize social support	III	B	5
	Extra advice and education about pregnancy and child-rearing	III	B	6
Labor/delivery	Ensure adequate psychological support	–	✔	–
	Delivery in a specialist unit if dystocia is an anticipated problem	III	B	7
Postnatal	Advice and support for infant feeding and care	III	B	8
	General social and financial support, especially if secondary education is to be continued	III	B	9
	Discussion about contraception	III	B	10

References

1 Mitchell-DiCenso A, Thomas BH, Devlin MC *et al.* (1997) Evaluation of an educational program to prevent adolescent pregnancy. *Health Educ Behavior* **24**, 300–312. Controlled trial in 21 schools evaluating the effectiveness of a school-based sex education program compared to conventional didactic sex education in under-16-year-olds. There were no significant differences between the groups in time of first sexual activity for males or females and time of first pregnancy. More males in the study group reported always using birth control (difference 8.9%, 95% CI = 0.4–17.4). **IIa B**

2 Fraser AM, Brockert JE, Ward RH (1995) Association of young maternal age with adverse reproductive outcomes. *N Engl J Med* **332**, 1113–1117. Retrospective cohort study of 134088 women, aged 13–24, who delivered singleton first-born children. The younger teenage mothers (13–17 years) had a higher risk than mothers who were 20–24 years of age of delivering an infant with a low birthweight (RR 1.7, 95% CI 1.5–2.0), that was small for gestational age (RR 1.3, 95% CI 1.2–1.4) or delivered prematurely (RR 1.9, 95% CI 1.7–2.1; $p < 0.001$). **III B**

3 Orvos H, Nyirati I, Hajdu J *et al.* (1999) Is adolescent pregnancy associated with adverse perinatal outcome? *J Perinat Med* **27**, 199–203. Retrospective study of the outcomes in 207 adolescent pregnancies compared to the national data. Gestational diabetes and preeclampsia occurred more frequently in pregnant adolescents than in the

general pregnant population (11.1% vs 2.7% and 11.6% vs 3.7% respectively, $p < 0.05$). No difference was found in mode of delivery. Intrauterine growth restriction and perinatal death occurred more often in the adolescent population (16.3% vs 8.6% and 4.3% vs 1.1% respectively, $p < 0.05$). **III B**

4 Archie CL, Anderson MM, Gruber EL (1997) Positive smoking history as a preliminary screening device for substance use in pregnant adolescents. *J Pediatr Adolesc Gynecol* **10**, 13–17. Retrospective study on 1640 live births in adolescents between 15 and 19 years old. 35% of all pregnant adolescents reported a positive history of tobacco use, 32% had consumed alcohol, 9% had consumed marijuana and 1.5% had reported the use of cocaine or crack. 53% of all admitted users of alcohol or cocaine smoked cigarettes. Smokers used alcohol or cocaine four times more often than nonsmokers. **III B**

5 Quinlivan JA, Peterson RW, Gurrin LC *et al.* (1999) Adolescent pregnancy: psychopathology missed. *Aust N Z J Psychiatry* **33**, 864–868. Prospective case-control study on major psychosocial problems that interfere with the ability to carry out acts of daily living in 100 consecutive adolescent patients and 60 controls. It was concluded that failure to identify psychosocial problems and drug abuse during the antenatal period will result in missed opportunities for positive intervention. **III B**

6 Koniak-Griffin D, Mathenge C, Anderson NL *et al.* (1999) An early intervention program for adolescent mothers: a nursing demonstration project. *J Obstet Gynecol Neonat Nurs* **28**, 51–59. Retrospective study on the effects of an intensive early intervention program ($n = 63$) compared with traditional public health nursing care ($n = 58$) in adolescents and their children. Both addressed health issues, sexuality and family planning, life skills, the maternal role and social support systems. As compared to national data, both traditional and intensive public health nurse care significantly improved perinatal outcomes. As compared to traditional care, the early intervention care significantly reduced the number of infant hospitalization days after delivery. **III B**

7 Van Eyk N, Allen LM, Sermer M *et al.* (2000) Obstetric outcome of adolescent pregnancies. *J Pediatr Adolesc Gynecol* **13**, 96. Retrospective study on the obstetrical outcome in 209 patients under 19 years compared with a general obstetrical population ($n = 13557$). Labor was induced in 25.5% versus 21.8% ($p = 0.20$). Epidural anesthesia was received by 63.5% versus 53% ($p < 0.05$). The incidence of preterm delivery (< 37 weeks) was 13.5% versus 8.1% ($p < 0.05$), low-birthweight babies (< 2500 g) 13.4% versus 8.6% ($p < 0.05$) and small-for-gestational-age babies (< 2 SD) 1.9%. The incidence of post-term delivery (> 41 weeks) was 12.5% versus 4.3% ($p < 0.001$), macrosomia (> 4000 g) 1.9% versus 9.2% ($p < 0.001$) and large-for-gestational-age babies (> 2 SD) 0.5%. Instrumental delivery occurred in 19.7% versus 19.9% ($p = 0.94$) and cesarean section in 6.2% versus 20.1% ($p < 0.001$). Apgar scores less than 7 at 5 min were found in 2.4% versus 3.1% ($p = 0.60$). It was concluded that preterm deliveries and low-birthweight babies occur more frequently in the adolescent. Post-term delivery was more common, yet macrosomia occurred less frequently. **III B**

8 Wiemann CM, DuBois JC, Berenson AB (1998) Strategies to promote breast-feeding among adolescent mothers. *Arch Pediatr Adolesc Med* **152**, 862–869. Prospective descriptive study on factors associated with the decision to breastfeed in 693 adolescents 18 years old or younger (mean age 16.7 years). It was concluded that a subgroup of adolescent mothers who had considered breastfeeding but ultimately chose to bottlefeed may be identified in the late stages of gestation by collecting information on financial status, family support, perceived barriers to breastfeeding (school or working), timing of the feeding decision, breastfeeding role models and encouragement to breastfeed. The promotion of breastfeeding should focus on role modeling and facilitation. **III B**

9 Flanagan P Coll CG, Andreozzi L *et al.* (1995) Predicting maltreatment of children of teenage mothers. *Arch Pediatr Adolesc Med* **149**, 451–455. Observational cohort study of 45 teenage mother–infant pairs. Maltreatment of the infant in its first 2 years of age occurred in 15 of the 45 families. Living apart from related adults was the strongest risk factor associated with maltreatment. **III B**

10 Blumenthal PD, Wilson LE, Remsburg RE *et al.* (1994) Contraceptive outcomes among post-partum and post-abortal adolescents. *Contraception* **50**, 451–460. Prospective observational study of 280 teenagers (13–18 years) who either delivered a baby or terminated the pregnancy. Of these, 92 chose to use Norplant implants, 188 chose another method for contraception, including 'no' method. After 1 year, 47% of the oral contraceptive users had discontinued the method compared to 16% of Norplant implant users ($p < 0.03$). Among the oral contraceptive users, 25% of the adolescents had experienced a subsequent unplanned pregnancy compared to 0% of the Norplant implant group ($p < 0.01$). **III B**

4.2 Advanced maternal age and pregnancy

Jeroen van de Riet

Management option		Quality of evidence	Strength of recommendations	References
Prepregnancy	Discussion of risks with main aim to put these risks into perspective	III	B	1,2
	In practice, management in pregnancy is not altered in the woman of advanced age apart from discussion about prenatal diagnosis of chromosomal abnormalities; thus the other risks are considered to be of relatively low importance	III	B	3
Prenatal	Discussion of prenatal diagnosis of chromosomal abnormalities, serum marker screening, chorion villus sampling or amniocentesis if requested	III Ia	B A	3,4 5
Labor/delivery	Optional: delivery in a specialist unit because of the theoretical risk of dystocia and other labor problems	III	B	6
Postnatal	Discussion of long-term contraception	–	✔	–

References

1 Fretts RC, Usher RH (1997) Causes of fetal death in women of advanced maternal age. *Obstet Gynecol* **89**, 40–45. Retrospective study on the causes of 715 stillbirths and 822 neonatal deaths in 101 640 births between 1961 and 1995. From 1978–95, women over 35 years of age had an increased risk of unexplained fetal death (OR 2.2, 95% CI 1.3–3.8). **III B**

2 Tan KT, Tan KH (1994) Pregnancy and delivery in primigravidae aged 35 and over. *Singapore Med J* **35**, 495–501. Retrospective study on the risks involved with advanced maternal age in 111 primigravidas aged 35 or more delivered between 1990 and 1991 and 10 189 controls. Preeclampsia occurred in 17.1% versus 10.8%, preterm labor in 16.2% versus 6.3%, diabetes mellitus (including impaired glucose tolerance test) in 16.2% versus 2.8%, instrumental delivery in 31.5% versus 7.3%, cesarean section in 32.4% versus 16%. The perinatal mortality rate of the study group was similar to that of the control group. There were no maternal deaths. **III B**

3 Hook EB (1981) Rates of chromosome abnormalities at different maternal ages. *Obstet Gynecol* **58**, 282–285. Compilation of available data pertinent to the rates of prevalence of Down syndrome correlated to maternal age. The prevalence of Down syndrome rises from about 2/1000 at the youngest maternal age to about 2.6/1000 at age 30, 5.6/1000 at age 35, 15.8/1000 at age 40 and 53.7/1000 at age 45. **III B**

4 Conde-Agudelo A, Kafury-Goeta AC (1998) Triple-marker test as screening for Down syndrome: a meta-analysis. *Obstet Gynecol Surv* **53**, 369–376. Meta-analysis on 194 326 patients evaluating the detection of Down syndrome by use of the triple-marker test between 15 and 22 weeks gestation. The best cut-off value for predicting Down syndrome in patients of 35 years or older is 1/190 with a sensitivity of 89% (78–100%), false-positive rate of 25% (20–29%) and a screen-positive rate of 25% (20.6–29.9%). **III B**

5 Alfirevic A, Gosden CM, Neilson JP *et al.* (2000) Chorion villus sampling versus amniocentesis for prenatal diagnosis (Cochrane Review). In: *The Cochrane library*, issue 2. Oxford: Update Software. Meta-analysis of studies including more than 9000 women. Pregnancy loss was more common after first-trimester chorion villus sampling (CVS) than after second trimester amniocentesis (AC) (OR 1.33, 95% CI 1.17–1.52). If early diagnosis is required then transabdominal CVS is preferable to transcervical CVS. Pregnancy loss in transabdominal CVS versus AC (OR 0.9, 95% CI 0.65–1.24) and pregnancy loss in transcervical CVS versus AC (OR 1.32, 95% CI 1.12–1.55). **Ia A**

6 Wong SF, Ho LC (1998) Labour outcome of low-risk multiparas of 40 years and older. A case-control study. *Aust N Z J Obstet Gynecol* **38**, 388–390. Case-control study of 76 multiparous women of 40 years and older and 152 multiparous controls between 25 and 30 years. Incidence of intrapartum fetal distress and cesarean section rate were significantly higher among older multiparas (6.6% vs 1.3%, $p < 0.05$ and 5.3% vs 0.7%, $p < 0.05$ respectively). **III B**

4.3 Pregnancy in women at the extremes of parity

Jeroen van de Riet

Management option		Quality of evidence	Strength of recommendations	References
Prepregnancy	Discussion of the risks with emphasis on the effects of parity alone and nulliparity/ 'grand multiparity'	III	B	1,2
Prenatal	Encourage regular attendance for care in those of high parity	III	B	2
	Vigilance for pregnancy-induced hypertension in those of nulliparity	III	B	2
	Vigilance for abnormal presentation from 36 weeks in those of high parity	III	B	3,4
	Plan for care of existing children for labor/delivery	–	✔	–
Labor/delivery	Nothing specific on the grounds of parity alone	III	B	1,2
	Higher chance of post-partum hemorrhage with increasing parity	III	B	1
Postnatal	Discussion of long-term contraception	–	✔	–

References

1 Babinszki A, Kerenyi T, Torok O *et al.* (1999) Perinatal outcome in grand and great-grand multiparity: effects of parity on obstetric risk factors. *Am J Obstet Gynecol* **181**, 669–674. Observational study involving 133 great-grand multiparous, 314 grand multiparous and 2195 multiparous women (all ≥35 years). The incidence of postpartum hemorrhage increased significantly between multiparous and grand multiparous women (0.3% and 1.9% respectively, $p = 0.001$). The rate of cesarean section decreased with higher parity; 20.6%, 15.6% and 11.3% in multiparous, grand multiparous and great-grand multiparous women respectively ($p < 0.05$ and p = NS respectively). There was no significant difference in maternal diabetes, peripartum infections and neonatal mortality between these three groups. **III B**

2 Juntunen K, Kirkinen P, Kauppila A (1997) The clinical outcome in pregnancies of grand grand multiparous women. *Acta Obstet Gynecol Scand* **76**, 755–759. Longitudinal observational study of 1200 pregnancies in 96 grand-grand multiparous women. 13.5% developed preeclampsia in their first pregnancy in contrast to 2–3% in their following pregnancies. Hypertension occurred more often in grand-grand multiparous women than in other pregnancies. Antepartum anemia was found in 3–4% of all pregnancies but postpartum anemia was twice as high (6%) after delivery in the group of grand-grand multiparous women. The cesarean section rate increased with parity, mostly because of hypertensive complications (2.3% vs 7.1% in grand multiparous and grand-grand multiparous pregnancies respectively). **III B**

3 Dildy GA, Jackson GM, Fowers GK *et al.* (1996) Very advanced maternal age: pregnancy after age 45. *Am J Obstet Gynecol* **75**, 668–674. Retrospective analysis of 79 births in women over 45 years (0.63/1000 births). Obstetric complications occurred in 46.8%; most common were gestational diabetes (12.7%) and preeclampsia (10.1%). Eight cases had chromosomal disorders. The most frequent indications for cesarean section (total 31.7%) were abnormal lie ($n = 9$), fetal distress ($n = 5$), and previous cesarean section ($n = 5$). **III B**

4 Ozumba BC, Igwegbe AO (1992) The challenge of grandmultiparity in Nigerian obstetric practice. *Int J Gynaecol Obstet* **37**, 259–264. Retrospective analysis of 733 grandmultiparas. Anemia, hypertensive diseases, abruptio placentae, breech presentation and abnormal lie were the most common complications found. **III B**

4.4 Pregnancy in women with poor socioeconomic background

Jeroen van de Riet

Management option		Quality of evidence	Strength of recommendations	References
Prepregnancy	Health education measures especially directed at antismoking and family planning	Ib	A	1
Prenatal	Extra specific and directed social support	Ia	A	2
	Plan for care for existing children for labor/delivery	–	✓	–
	Vigilance for clinical evidence of poor fetal growth	Ia IIa	A B	2 3
Labor/delivery	No additional measures on the basis of adverse socioeconomic factors alone	III	B	4
Postnatal	Encourage breastfeeding	III	B	5
	Extra specific and directed social support	Ib	A	2,6
	Discussion of contraception	–	✓	–

References

1. Ershoff DH, Quinn VP, Mullen PD (1990) Pregnancy and medical cost outcomes of a self-help prenatal smoking cessation program in a HMO. *Pub Health Rep* **105**, 340–347. Randomized clinical trial of 242 pregnant women who smoked cigarettes. Those who stopped smoking were 45% less likely to deliver an infant with a low birthweight. **Ib A**
2. Hodnett ED (2000) Support during pregnancy for women at increased risk of low birthweight babies (Cochrane Review). In: *The Cochrane library*, issue 4. Oxford: Update Software. Meta-analysis of randomized trials involving over 11 000 pregnant women at risk of preterm delivery or giving birth to a low-birthweight baby. Programs offering social support to these women showed no improvements in medical outcomes for the index pregnancy. **Ia A**
3. Nieto A, Matorras R, Serra M *et al.* (1994) Multivariate analysis of determinants of fetal growth retardation. *Eur J Obstet Gynecol Reprod Biol* **53**, 107–113. Case-control study on 185 women with intrauterine growth retardation and 185 controls. Of the 25 factors taken into account, the following were five were found to be independent risk factors in a multiple logistic regression analysis: tobacco (OR 23.50, 95% CI 3.01–183.18), low prepregnancy weight (OR 4.01, 95% CI 2.14–7.51), low socioeconomic status (OR 2.91, 95% CI 1.72–4.90), little gestational weight gain (OR 2.52, 95% CI 1.21–5.22) and urinary infection (OR 3.83, 95% CI 1.49–9.87). **IIa B**
4. Leon DA (1991) Influence of birth weight on differences in infant mortality by social class and legitimacy. *Br Med J* **303**, 964–967. Cohort study on the influence of social class on neonatal morbidity and mortality. The relative risk of neonatal mortality increased with lower social class. (RR 1.11, 95% CI 0.88–1.4; and RR 1.36, 95% CI 1.04–1.79 in the highest and lowest social class respectively). Postneonatal mortality showed a similar correlation (RR 1.21, 95% CI 0.91–1.6; and RR 2.15, 95% CI 1.57–2.96 for the highest and lowest social class respectively). **III B**
5. Donath S, Amir L (2000) Rates of breastfeeding in Australia by state and socio-economic status: evidence from the 1995 National Health Survey. *J Paediatr Child Health* **36**, 164–168. Retrospective analysis of data from the 1995 Australian National Health Survey. It was found that the rates of breastfeeding varied according to the socioeconomic status of the geographical area, with a strong inverse relationship between rates of breastfeeding and socioeconomic status. **III B**
6. Langer A, Campero L, Garcia C *et al.* (1998) Effects of psychosocial support during labour and childbirth on breastfeeding, medical interventions, and mothers' wellbeing in a Mexican public hospital: a randomised clinical trial. *Br J Obstet Gynaecol* **105**, 1056–1063. Randomized clinical trial of 724 women receiving either routine care or psychosocial support during delivery and postpartum. The frequency of breastfeeding 4 weeks postpartum was higher in the social-supported group (RR 1.64, 95% CI 1.01–2.64). **Ib A**

4.5 Pregnancy in women from different ethnic backgrounds

Jeroen van de Riet

Management option		Quality of evidence	Strength of recommendations	References
Prepregnancy	Education, screening and counseling for communities at specific risk	III	B	1
Prenatal	Overcoming language and cultural barriers	–	✔	–
	Screening and counseling where specific risk	III IIa	B B	1,2 3
	Offering prenatal diagnosis if appropriate	III	B	1
	Maternal surveillance appropriate to any specific risk	IIa	B	3
	Fetal surveillance appropriate to any specific risk	IIa	B	4
Labor/delivery	Interpreter who can be present for the whole labor and delivery	–	✔	–
	Consideration of cultural norms in provision of care	–	✔	–
Postnatal	Encourage breastfeeding	–	✔	–
	Contraceptive advice taking account of individual sociocultural norms and values	–	✔	–

References

1 Cao A, Rosatelli MC, Galanello R (1996) Control of beta-thalassaemia by carrier screening, genetic counselling and prenatal diagnosis: the Sardinian experience. *Ciba Found Symp* **197**, 137–151; discussion 151–155. Report on the Sardinian education, genetic counseling and screening program of prospective parents and pregnant women for the prevention of homozygous beta-thalassemia over the previous 20 years in an at-risk population (Sardinians). Following counseling, the large majority of parents accepted prenatal diagnosis. The program resulted in a reduction of the birth rate of babies with thalassemia major from 1:250 live births to 1:4000. **III B**

2 Kadkhodaei Elyaderani M, Cinkotai KI, Hyde K *et al.* (1998) Ethnicity study and non-selective screening for haemoglobinopathies in the antenatal population of central Manchester. *Clin Lab Haematol* **20**, 207–211. Retrospective epidemiological study of 6718 patients to evaluate the effect of an hemoglobinopathy service. 62.3% were white, 13.2% Asian, 7.9% black, 3.8% Chinese or 'other' and 12.7% gave no information about their ethnicity. 1144 patients were screened for hemoglobinopathies. The incidence of hemoglobinopathies within the screened population was 2.62% and comprised beta-thalassemia trait (0.69%), sickle-cell trait (1.22%), hemoglobin-C trait (0.43%) and hemoglobin-D trait (0.26%). The total incidence of hemoglobinopathies was highest within the black population (18.2%), followed by the no-information group (5.6%), Asian (3.35%) and white (0.26%). **III B**

3 Rey, E (1997) Preeclampsia and neonatal outcomes in chronic hypertension: comparison between white and black women. *Ethnicity Dis* **7**, 5–11. Case-control study of 208 white and 74 pregnant black women with mild chronic hypertension compared to 17677 white and 2400 black normotensive controls. Superimposed preeclampsia (32.4% vs 14.9%; $p<0.01$), perinatal mortality (9.5% vs 2.9%; $p<0.05$) and prematurity (32.4% vs 19.7%; $p<0.05$) were more frequent in black women with chronic hypertension. **IIa B**

4 James SA (1993) Racial and ethnic differences in infant mortality and low birth weight. A psychosocial critique. *Ann Epidemiol* **3**, 130–136. Review on ethnic differences in infant mortality involving over 6 million pregnancies. Infant mortality was significantly higher among black pregnant women than among white pregnant women, 18 per 1000 live births versus 8 per 1000 live births respectively (RR 2.1, $p<0.05$). **III B**

Chapter 5

Maternal weight and weight gain

5.1 Pregnancy in underweight women

Tim Overton

Management option		Quality of evidence	Strength of recommendations	References
Prepregnancy	Improve calorie intake	III	B	1,2
	Multidisciplinary approach for eating disorders	III	B	1
Prenatal	Check for fetal growth restriction	IIa	B	3
	Multidisciplinary treatment for women with eating disorders not yet in remission	III	B	4
Labor and delivery	Continuous electronic fetal heart rate monitoring if fetus is small	III IIa	B B	5 6
Postnatal	Encourage breastfeeding	III	B	7

References

1 Stewart DE, Raskin J, Garfinkel PE *et al.* (1987) Anorexia nervosa, bulimia, and pregnancy. *Am J Obstet Gynecol* **157**, 1194–1198. Retrospective study of 74 women treated for anorexia nervosa and bulimia in whom 15 had conceived a total of 23 pregnancies. Women in remission gained more weight in pregnancy, had heavier babies and had higher 5 min Apgar scores. On the basis of this the authors recommended delaying pregnancy until the eating disorder was in remission. **III B**

2 Clark PM, Atton C, Law CM *et al.* (1998) Weight gain in pregnancy, triceps skinfold thickness, and blood pressure in offspring. *Am J Obstet Gynecol* **91**, 103–107. Study correlating blood pressure in 296 11-year-old children of mothers who had taken part in a study of nutrition in pregnancy and had been weighed at 18 and 28 weeks gestation and had had their triceps skinfold thickness measured at 18 weeks. There was a weak non-significant inverse relation between triceps skinfold thickness and weight gain between 18 and 28 weeks with the child's blood pressure. However, the offspring of those women with a skinfold thickness below the median value at 18 weeks who also exhibited reduced pregnancy weight gain had significantly higher blood pressures. They concluded that, in women who were poorly nourished in early pregnancy, reduced weight gain is associated with higher blood pressure in offspring. Although only 60% of offspring were followed up and were felt to be representative of the group as a whole, the women enrolled in the original study were not typical of all women attending antenatal clinics. The authors recognize the need for caution in interpreting their results. This was an observational study that could not establish causation but the authors suggested that the results could be the consequence of fetal adaptation to poor maternal nutrition and highlighted the need for interventional studies. **III B**

3 Van der Spuy ZM, Steer PJ, McCusker M *et al.* (1988) Outcome of pregnancy in underweight women after spontaneous and induced ovulation. *Br Med J* **296**, 962–965. Study comparing 41 women who achieved pregnancy following ovulation induction with 1212 in whom ovulation was spontaneous. Women of normal weight who ovulated spontaneously and showed a normal weight gain in pregnancy had the lowest incidence of small-for-gestational-age (SGA) babies (6%). Underweight women who ovulated spontaneously had a threefold increase in delivering SGA babies (18%). Overall, the women who had ovulation induced had a 25% incidence of SGA babies and those who were underweight had the highest incidence, 54%. **IIa B**

4 Franko DL, Blais MA, Becker AE *et al.* (2001) Pregnancy complications and neonatal outcomes in women with eating disorders. *Am J Psychiatry* **158**, 1461–1466. Prospective descriptive study on pregnancy complications and neonatal outcomes in 49 live births in 246 women with eating disorders over a period of 12 years. Most women had normal pregnancies and normal babies. The mean birth weight was 7.6 lb (3.45 kg). 13 (26.5%) had a cesarean section and postpartum depression occurred in 17 (34.7%) cases. Symptomatic women more often had a cesarean section and postpartum depression. It was concluded that pregnant women with a history of eating disorders should be considered to be high-risk. **III B**

5 Strauss A, Kirz D, Modanlou HD *et al.* (1985) Perinatal events and intraventricular/subependymal hemorrhage in the very low-birth weight infant. *Am J Obstet Gynecol* **151**, 1022–1027. Prospective study on 119 very-low-birthweight infants to assess the relationship between intrapartum fetal distress with or without acidosis and the development of intraventricular and subependymal hemorrhage. Intraventricular/subependymal hemorrhage occurred in 24% (27/112); 4.4% (5/112) had severe hemorrhage (grade 3/4). Ominous fetal heart rate patterns occurred in 50% of infants with severe intraventricular/subependymal hemorrhage compared to 8% of matched controls ($p < 0.01$). Normal fetal heart rate patterns occurred more often in infants without intraventricular/subependymal hemorrhage ($p < 0.05$). Antepartum and intrapartum complications, fetal presentation, cesarean section, duration of labor, hyaline membrane disease and volume expansion appeared to play no role in the incidence of intraventricular/subependymal hemorrhage. This study suggests that intrapartum fetal distress and acidosis may predict which very-low-birthweight infants will develop intraventricular/subependymal hemorrhage. The condition of the infant at birth may be predictive of the extent of intraventricular/subependymal hemorrhage. **III B**

6 Lin CC, Mowawad AH, River P *et al.* (1980) Acid–base characteristics of fetuses with intrauterine growth retardation during labor and delivery. *Am J Obstet Gynecol* **137**, 553–559. Prospective study on the maternal and fetal cord blood in 37 growth-retarded neonates (IUGR) and 108 normally grown controls (AGA) comparing lactate, pH and blood gas measurements during labor and delivery. With normal fetal heart rate tracings, there was no difference between the outcome measures between both groups. However, in cases with abnormal tracings, IUGR fetuses demonstrated a significantly higher lactate level than AGA fetuses. It was concluded that IUGR fetuses tolerate labor less well than AGA fetuses, urging for a lower threshold for intervention. **IIa B**

7 Atalah E, Lagos I, Grez M *et al.* (1983) Effect of lactation on the weight and body composition of wet nurses. *Arch Latinoam Nutr* **33**, 649–663. Cohort study on 134 women (95 breastfeeding and 39 bottlefeeding) to assess the impact of lactation on the nutritional status and body composition of mothers. It was found that dietary intake was deficient in calories, protein, calcium, iron and vitamin A when compared to the FAO/WHO standards. Given the excellent growth curves of the children as well as the minimal changes observed in maternal nutrition and body composition, it was concluded that the current recommended dietary allowances (FAO/WHO) are overestimated for a population of the type studied. **III B**

5.2 Pregnancy in overweight women

Tim Overton

Management option		Quality of evidence	Strength of recommendations	References
Prepregnancy	Weight reduction with diet and exercise regime	III	B	1, 2
	Explain risks of hypertension, diabetes, urinary infections, large fetal size and postpartum hemorrhage	III	B	3, 4
Prenatal	Avoid attempts to manipulate diet during pregnancy	III Ib	B A	2 5
	Screen for hypertension, diabetes and bacteriuria	III	B	3
	Monitor for fetal growth using ultrasound	III	B	1, 4
Labor and delivery	Vigilance for cephalopelvic disproportion and shoulder dystocia	III	B	1
	Cesarean section: ❑ Regional rather than general anesthesia ❑ Prophylactic methods ❑ Prophylactic low-dose subcutaneous heparin ❑ No agreement over which incision is best ❑ Value of wound drains is debated	 IIa IIa IV – IIa	 B B C ✔ B	 6 7, 8, 9 – 10

➡

Management option		Quality of evidence	Strength of recommendations	References
Postnatal	Subcutaneous heparin until fully ambulatory	IV	C	11
	Early mobilization	–	✔	–
	Continue with measures to lose weight	–	✔	–

References

1 Garbaciak JA, Richter M, Miller S *et al.* (1985) Maternal weight and pregnancy complications. *Am J Obstet Gynecol* **152**, 238–245. Well conducted, retrospective study assessing the effect of obesity alone (by dividing the study population into those with antenatal and those without antenatal complications, thus eliminating many confounding variables that have affected the accuracy of other studies) on perinatal mortality, primary cesarean section and infant birth weight. In the group with antenatal complications there was a significant increase in all three in the obese (120–150% of ideal body weight) and morbidly obese (>150%). In the group without antenatal complications there was a significant increase in only the primary cesarean rate and infant birthweight. **III B**

2 Campbell DM (1982) Dietary restriction in obesity and its effects on neonatal outcome. In: *Nutrition in pregnancy. Proceedings of the Tenth Study Group of the Royal College of Obstetricians and Gynaecologists.* London: Royal College of Obstetricians and Gynaecologists, 243–254. This small study failed to show that dietary restriction in obese women (1) decreased the production of fat babies without causing growth restriction, (2) prevented the onset of preeclampsia or (3) resulted in any changes in metabolism or in body fat in the mother and baby. **III B**

3 Richards DS, Miller DK, Goodman GN (1987) Pregnancy after gastric bypass for morbid obesity. *J Reprod Med* **32**, 172–176. Small retrospective study comparing the pregnancy outcome in 57 obese women following gastric bypass surgery with a similar number of controls from a preoperative group. There was a significant reduction in hypertension and large-for-gestational-age babies in the postoperative group. Unfortunately, the study relied on patient-completed questionnaires rather than careful review of the medical records. **III B**

4 Scott A, Moar V, Ounstead M *et al.* (1982) The relative contribution of different maternal factors in large-for-gestational-age pregnancies. *Eur J Obstet Gynecol Reprod Biol* **13**, 269–277. Prospective study of women delivering in one institution between 1966 and 1977 attempting to identify risk factors that predict the delivery of large-for-dates infants. In multiparous women the most important predictor was of having given birth to a large-for-dates (LGA) infant in the past. Other factors included nonsmoking, increased height and weight, and multiparity. Significant obesity was noted to have a relative risk for LGA of 9. An attempt was made to produce a scoring system to predict the chances of a LGA pregnancy. This was noted to be of limited value and in any case has now been superseded by modern-day ultrasound. **III B**

5 Kramer MS (2000) Energy/protein restriction for height-for-weight or weight gain during pregnancy (Cochrane Review). In: *The Cochrane library*, issue 4. Oxford: Update Software. Meta-analysis assessing the effect of prescribing a low-energy diet in pregnancy to women who were either overweight or exhibited high weight gain early in pregnancy on subsequent weight gain, preeclampsia and the outcome of pregnancy. Only three studies involving a total of 266 patients were studied. Energy/protein restriction led to a significant reduction in weekly maternal weight gain and in birthweight. There was no effect on pregnancy-induced hypertension or preeclampsia but certain outcomes, including fetal/infant mortality and measures of maternal morbidity, were not discussed. It was concluded that protein/energy restriction is unlikely to be beneficial and may be harmful to the developing fetus. **Ia A**

6 Hood DD, Dewan DM (1993) Anesthetic and obstetric outcome in morbidly obese parturients. *Anesthesiology* **79**, 1210–1218. Prospective case-control study on the anesthetic and obstetric outcome in 117 morbidly obese parturients (>300 lb (136.4 kg)). 62% versus 24% had a cesarean section ($p < 0.05$) (48% vs 9%, $p < 0.05$, were intrapartum). Initial epidural anesthesia failure was significantly more likely in the study group, warranting resiting, difficult tracheal intubation occurred in 6/17, compared with 0/8 of the controls. Morbidly obese women had increased incidences of antepartum medical disease, prolonged cesarean section operation times, serious postoperative complications and increased hospital stays. **IIa B**

7 Smaill F, Hofmeyr GJ (2000) Antibiotic prophylaxis for caesarean section. In: *Cochrane pregnancy and childbirth database. Cochrane library*, issue 4. Oxford: Update Software. This meta-analysis was updated in 1998. This conclusively shows that routine administration of prophylactic antibiotics at the time of both elective and nonelective cesarean section reduces the chance of postpartum infection, particularly endometritis (by between two thirds and three quarters). **Ia A**

8 Perlow JH, Morgan MA (1994) Massive maternal obesity and perioperative cesarean morbidity. *Am J Obstet Gynecol* **170**, 560–565. Retrospective case-control study on the impact of weight on perioperative morbidity in 43 massively obese pregnant women (<300 lb) undergoing cesarean section and 43 controls. The study group was found

to have a significantly increased risk for emergency cesarean section (32.6% vs 9.3%, $p = 0.02$), prolonged delivery interval (25.6% vs 4.6%, $p = 0.01$), and total operative time (48.8% vs 9.3%, $p < 0.0001$), blood loss of more than 1000 ml (34.9% vs 9.3%, $p = 0.009$), multiple epidural placement failures (14.0% vs 0%), postoperative endometritis (32.6% vs 4.9%, $p = 0.002$) and prolonged hospitalization (34.9% vs 2.3%, $p = 0.0003$). **IIa B**

9 Greer IA (1997) Epidemiology, risk factors and prophylaxis of venous thrombo-embolism in obstetrics and gynaecology. *Baillière's Clin Obstet Gynaecol* **11**, 403–430. Review of specific thromboprophylactic measures in patients considered to have significant risk for developing venous thromboembolism. It discusses the pros and cons of the various options. **IV C**

10 Allaire AD, Fisch J, McMahon MJ, *et al.* (2000) Subcutaneous drain vs. suture in obese women undergoing cesarean delivery. A prospective, randomized trial. *J Reprod Med* **45**, 327–331. Prospective randomized study on the skin-closure technique at cesarean section in 76 obese women comparing closure of the subcutaneous tissue with placement of a subcutaneous closed suction drain with a group without suture closure or drainage. It was concluded that the use of closed suction drainage in the subcutaneous space may reduce the incidence of postoperative cesarean section wound complications in obese women who have at least 2 cm of subcutaneous fat. **IIa B**

11 Kakkar VV, De Lorenzo F (1998) Prevention of venous thromboembolism in general surgery. *Baillière's Clin Haematol* **11**, 605–619. Review of venous thromboembolism and low-molecular-weight heparin preparations in hospitalized patients undergoing major elective surgery. It is stated that low-molecular-weight heparin is highly effective in preventing postoperative venous thromboembolism. Further, it is underlined that prophylaxis is started preoperatively and the usual duration for the postoperative period is 7 days, or until the patient is discharged from the hospital. **IV C**

5.3 Abnormal weight gain in pregnancy

Tim Overton

Management option		Quality of evidence	Strength of recommendations	References
Prenatal	Check for abnormal fetal growth	III	B	1
	Consider physical or psychological pathology	IIb	B	2
	Advice on improving diet	Ia III	A B	1 3, 4
	Advice on reducing weight is not useful	IIb	B	2
	Other prenatal measures			
	For poor weight gain: as for women who are underweight	III	B	3, 4
	For excessive weight gain: as for women who are overweight	III	B	5
Labor and delivery	For poor weight gain: as for women who are underweight	-	✔	-

References

1 Scott A, Moar V, Ounstead M *et al.* (1982) The relative contribution of different maternal factors in large-for-gestational-age pregnancies. *Eur J Obstet Gynecol Reprod Biol* **13**, 269–277. Prospective study of women delivering in one institution between 1966 and 1977 attempting to identify risk factors that predict the delivery of large-for-dates infants. In multiparous women the most important predictor was of having given birth to a large-for-dates (LGA) infant in the past. Other factors included nonsmoking, increased height and weight, and multiparity. Significant obesity was noted to have a relative risk for LGA of 9. An attempt was made to produce a scoring system to predict the chances of a LGA pregnancy. This was noted to be of limited value and in any case has now been superseded by modern-day ultrasound. **III B**

2 Theron GB, Thompson ML (1998) The usefulness of a weight gain spurt to identify women who will develop preeclampsia. *Eur J Obstet Gynecol Reprod Biol* **78**, 47–51. Case-control study on 99 women and 675 controls to assess sudden weight gain as a predictor of developing preeclampsia in early pregnancy. It was concluded that sudden weight gain spurts are not reliable signs of impending preeclampsia and that routine weighing of pregnant women for this purpose is not useful. **IIa B**

3 Clark PM, Atton C, Law CM *et al.* (1998) Weight gain in pregnancy, triceps skinfold thickness, and blood pressure in offspring. *Am J Obstet Gynecol* **91**, 103–107. Study correlating blood pressure in 296 11-year-old children of mothers who had taken part in a study of nutrition in pregnancy and had been weighed at 18 and 28 weeks gestation and had had their triceps skinfold thickness measured at 18 weeks. There was a weak non-significant inverse relation between triceps skinfold thickness and weight gain between 18 and 28 weeks with the child's blood pressure. However, the offspring of those women with a skinfold thickness below the median value at 18 weeks who also exhibited reduced pregnancy weight gain had significantly higher blood pressures. They concluded that, in women who were poorly nourished in early pregnancy, reduced weight gain is associated with higher blood pressure in offspring. Although only 60% of offspring were followed up and were felt to be representative of the group as a whole, the women enrolled in the original study were not typical of all women attending antenatal clinics. The authors recognize the need for caution in interpreting their results. This was an observational study that could not establish causation but the authors suggested that the results could be the consequence of fetal adaptation to poor maternal nutrition and highlighted the need for interventional studies. **III B**

4 Shiell AW, Campbell DM, Hall MH *et al.* (2000) Diet in late pregnancy and glucose–insulin metabolism of the offspring 40 years later. *Br J Obstet Gynaecol* **107**, 890–895. Small retrospective study examining how the diets of women in pregnancy influenced the glucose–insulin metabolism of their offspring in adult life some 40 years later. In all a total of 168 women were studied. The authors found that low birthweight and low maternal body mass index in early and late pregnancy were associated with insulin resistance in adult life. In addition, the offspring of women who had high intakes of fat and protein in late pregnancy had lower 30 min plasma insulin concentrations and higher 30 min glucose concentrations and thus lower insulin increments. While concluding that high intakes of protein and fat during pregnancy may impair development of fetal pancreatic beta cells, the authors acknowledged that only tentative conclusions could be reached. **III B**

5 Lawrence M, McKillop FM, Durnin JV *et al.* (1991) Women who gain more fat during pregnancy may not have bigger babies: implications for recommended weight gain during pregnancy. *Br J Obstet Gynaecol* **98**, 254–259. Prospective study correlating the infant birthweight in multiparous women with uncomplicated pregnancies with fat gained during pregnancy. There was very little correlation suggesting that women who gained more fat in pregnancy gave birth to heavier babies. The authors concluded that attempts to increase birthweight by encouraging greater weight gain may be unsuccessful. However, the sample size was small (n = 115) and the power of the study would not have been sufficient to detect small effects. In addition, the study did not look at the effect of gain in weight in undernourished individuals embarking on pregnancy. **III B**

EARLY PREGNANCY

Chapter 6

Bleeding in early pregnancy

6.1 Bleeding in early pregnancy

Christianne Lok

Initial/general management

Management option	Quality of evidence	Strength of recommendation	References
Identify cause by combination of history, examination, hCG assay and ultrasound	–	✔	–
Assess amount and rate of blood loss	–	✔	–
Regular recordings of pulse and blood pressure	–	✔	–
Intravenous access if actual or risk of hemodynamic instability	–	✔	–
FBC for all; clotting screening if coagulopathy suspected or excess blood loss; cross-match blood if excess blood loss	–	✔	–
Anti-D administration <28 w	III	B	1–3
Anti-D administration >28 w	Ia	A	4,5

References

1 Gjode P, Rasmussen TB, Jorgensen J *et al.* (1982) Low dose rhesus immunoprophylaxis after early induced abortions. *Acta Obstet Gynecol Scand* **61**, 105–106. Clinical trial in 463 patients with induced abortion. A dose of 50µg anti-D immunoglobulin was administered as rhesus immunoprophylaxis following suction curettage before the 13th week of pregnancy. After 6 months, a follow-up of 381 patients (82%) showed that none of these patients was rhesus-immunized. Conclusion: a low dose of anti-D is recommended for rhesus immunoprophylaxis after first trimester abortion. **III B**

2 Stewart FH, Burnhill MS, Bozorgi N *et al.* (1978) Reduced dose of Rh immunoglobulin following first trimester pregnancy termination. *Obstet Gynecol* **51**, 318–322. Clinical trial in 1027 women undergoing vacuum abortion to test the efficacy and safety of a 50µg dose of anti-D. Follow-up after 6 months in 755 (73.5%) patients showed no serological evidence of rhesus sensitization. No serious adverse reactions to the drug were observed. Conclusion: anti-D can prevent sensitization after first trimester abortion. **III B**

3 Keith L, Bozorgi N (1977) Small-dose anti-Rh therapy after first trimester abortion. *Int J Gynaecol Obstet* **15**, 235–237. Pilot study of 315 patients given 50µg or 300µg anti-Rh immunoglobulin after first trimester abortion. At 6 months no patient had developed atypical blood group antibodies. Conclusion: 50µg of the used product is also protective after first trimester abortion. **III B**

4 Crowther C, Middleton P (2000) Anti-D administration after childbirth for preventing Rhesus alloimmunisation (Cochrane Review). In: *The Cochrane library*, Issue 2. Oxford: Update Software. Review of 6 RCTs comparing anti-D prophylaxis with no treatment or placebo. Anti-D given within 72 hours of birth, lowered the incidence of RhD alloimmunization 6 months after birth (RR 0.04) and in subsequent pregnancy (RR 0.12). Higher doses were more effective. Conclusion: anti-D reduces risk of alloimmunization, evidence on optimal dose is limited. **Ia A**

5 Crowther CA, Keirse MJ (2000) Anti-D administration in pregnancy for preventing Rhesus alloimmunisation (Cochrane Review). In: *The Cochrane library*, Issue 2. Oxford: Update Software. Review of 2 RCTs comparing anti-D after 28 weeks of pregnancy with no treatment or placebo. Administration of 500IU at 28 and 34 weeks gestation in the first pregnancy can reduce the risk of alloimmunization from 1.5% to 0.2% without adverse effects. With lower dose (250IU) no significant benefit was detected. Conclusion: anti-D (500IU) can reduce alloimmunization. **Ia A**

Miscarriage/spontaneous abortion

Management option		Quality of evidence	Strength of recommendations	References
First trimester	Expectant management	Ia	A	1,2
	Medical evacuation	Ib	A	1–7
	Surgical evacuation	Ia	A	1,3
	Expectant management as first choice	Ia	A	1,2
	Medical management before recourse to surgical management	Ib	A	3,7
Second trimester	Prostaglandins	Ib	A	8–10
	Prostaglandins management of first choice	III	B	8
	Vaginal prostaglandins management of first choice	Ib	A	9
	Cervical suture to prolong pregnancy			
	❑ Elective	Ib	A	11
	❑ Emergency	III	B	12–14
	Indomethacin as tocolytic to prolong pregnancy	Ib	A	15–17

See also Preterm labour, Section 46.1.

References

1 Geyman JP, Oliver LM, Sullivan SD *et al.* (1999) Expectant, medical, or surgical treatment of spontaneous abortion in first trimester of pregnancy? A pooled quantitative literature evaluation. *J Am Board Fam Pract* **12**, 55–64. Meta-analysis of RCTs or observational studies about treatment for spontaneous abortion in the first trimester. Of 31 studies, 18 met the inclusion criteria. There were 545 pooled patients for expectant management, 198 for medical treatment and 1408 for surgical therapy. In the first group, 92% had a complete abortion within 2 weeks without complications, in the surgical group 93.6% and in the medical group 51.5%. Conclusion: expectant management is safe and effective. There is insufficient evidence to support medical therapy and more research is needed to clarify the more limited role of surgical treatment. **Ia A**

2 Nielsen S, Hahlin M, Platz-Christensen J (1999) Randomised trial comparing expectant with medical management for first trimester miscarriages. *Br J Obstet Gynaecol* **106**, 804–807. RCT in 122 women with first-trimester miscarriages. Randomization to mifepristone 400 mg orally, repeated 48 hours later, or expectant management. Evaluation 5 days later showed 82% in the treatment group versus 76% in expectant group had an empty uterine cavity. Conclusion: no significant difference between expectant and medical management. **Ib A**

3 Chung TK, Lee DT, Cheung LP *et al.* (1999) Spontaneous abortion: a randomized, controlled trial comparing surgical evacuation with conservative management using misoprostol. *Fertil Steril* **71**, 1054–1059. RCT in 635 women with spontaneous abortion. Randomization to routine surgical evacuation or medical evacuation with misoprostol. Significantly lower incidence of immediate and short-term complications in misoprostol group. 50% of the misoprostol group subsequently needed surgical evacuation. Conclusion: misoprostol can reduce demand for surgical intervention and has fewer complications. **Ib A**

4 Creinin MD, Moyer R, Guido R *et al.* (1997) Misoprostol for medical evacuation of early pregnancy failure. *Obstet Gynecol* **89**, 768–772. RCT of 20 women with early pregnancy failure with closed cervical os and minimal vaginal bleeding. They either had 400 μg orally or 800 μg vaginally, repeated once if necessary. Complete evacuation occurred in 25% in the first group and 88% in the second group. Conclusion: vaginal misoprostol 800 μg is more effective than 400 μg orally. **Ib A**

5 Autry A, Jacobson G, Sandhu R *et al.* (1999) Medical management of non-viable early first trimester pregnancy. *Int J Gynaecol Obstet* **67**, 9–13. RCT in 21 women with non-viable pregnancy up to 49 days gestation. They received either methotrexate intramuscularly and misoprostol or misoprostol alone. Complete abortion occurred in 100% in the first group and 89% in the second group. Conclusion: both treatments are alternatives to surgery or expectant management. **Ib A**

6 Nielsen S, Hahlin M, Platz-Christensen JJ *et al.* (1997) Unsuccessful treatment of missed abortion with a combination of an antiprogesterone and a prostaglandin E_1 analogue. *Br J Obstet Gynaecol* **104**, 1094–1096.

Prospective clinical trial in which 31 women with missed abortion were included and received 400mg mifepristone and 400μg misoprostol orally. 52% had an empty uterine cavity 6 days later, 35% needed surgery. Conclusion: mifepristone and misoprostol does not resolve miscarriage quickly. **III B**

7 Herabutya, Y, Prasersawat P (1997) Misoprostol in the management of missed abortion. *Int J Gynaecol Obstet* **56**, 263–266. RCT in 84 women with missed abortion. They were randomized to 200μg vaginal misoprostol or placebo the day before dilatation and aspiration. In the misoprostol group 83.3% aborted spontaneously and in the placebo group 17.1%. Conclusion: misoprostol reduces the need for surgical treatment. **Ib A**

8 Hill NC, MacKenzie IZ (1989) 2308 second trimester terminations using extra-amniotic prostaglandin E_2: an analysis of efficacy and complications. *Br J Obstet Gynaecol* **96**, 1424–1431. 2308 mid-trimester terminations using prostaglandin E_2 extra-amniotically or intra-amniotically were compared for efficacy and morbidity. Morbidity rates and induction-to-abortion interval were similar and morbidity rate was not higher than with surgical therapy. **III B**

9 Cameron IT, Michie AF, Baird DT (1984) The use of 16,16-dimethyl-trans delta 2 prostaglandin E_1 methyl ester (gemeprost) vaginal pessaries for the termination of pregnancy in the early second trimester. *Br J Obstet Gynaecol* **91**, 1136–1140. RCT in which patients were randomized to gemeprost pessaries or extra-amniotic infusion of prostaglandin E_2 for termination of pregnancies between 12 and 16 weeks. In the first group, 77% had a successful termination and in the second group 79%. There were no differences in induction–delivery interval. Women in the pessary group needed less analgesia. Conclusion: gemeprost is an effective alternative to extra-amniotic infusion of prostaglandin E_2. **Ib A**

10 Wong KS, Ngai CS, Chan KS *et al.* (1996) Termination of second trimester pregnancy with gemeprost and misoprostol: a randomized double-blind placebo-controlled trial. *Contraception* **54**, 23–25. RCT in 70 women with termination of second trimester pregnancy. They received either misoprostol 400μg orally or placebo before the administration of gemeprost vaginally. There was no difference in induction–abortion interval. Conclusion: oral misoprostol is not useful as pretreatment before gemeprost. **Ib A**

11 Anonymous (1993) Final report of the Medical Research Council/Royal College of Obstetricians and Gynaecologists multicentre randomised trial of cervical cerclage. MRC/RCOG Working Party on Cervical Cerclage. *Br J Obstet Gynaecol* **100**, 516–523. Multicenter RCT in 1292 women who would possibly benefit from cerclage. Randomization to cerclage or expectant policy. There were 13% deliveries before 33 weeks in the cerclage group and 17% in the expectant group ($p = 0.03$). Conclusion: there is a beneficial effect in 1 in 25 cases of suspected cervical incompetence. There is increased risk of medical intervention and puerperal pyrexia. **Ib A**

12 Kurup M, Goldkrand JW (1999) Cervical incompetence: elective, emergent, or urgent cerclage. *Am J Obstet Gynecol* **181**, 240–246. Retrospective analysis of all cerclages placed between 1993 and 1997. Emergency cerclages had a prolongation of 8.3 ± 0.9 weeks, urgent cerclage 12.2 ± 0.9 weeks and elective cerclage 20.2 ± 0.9 weeks. Conclusions: emergency cerclage confers some benefit in cervical incompetence. **III B**

13 Yip SK, Fung HY, Fung TY (1998) Emergency cervical cerclage: a study between duration of cerclage in situ with gestation at cerclage, herniation of forewater, and cervical dilatation at presentation. *Eur J Obstet Gynecol* **78**, 63–67. Retrospective review of 19 patients who had emergency cerclage for cervical incompetence. Mean gestation at delivery was 30.5 ± 6.6 weeks. Duration of cerclage *in situ* was longer when placed before 20 weeks and when no herniation of forewaters was present. Conclusion: gestation and herniation of forewaters influence duration of cerclage *in situ*. **III B**

14 Olatunbosun OL, al-Nuaim L, Turnell RW (1995) Emergency cerclage compared with bed rest for advanced cervical dilatation in pregnancy. *Int Surg* **80**, 170–174. Prospective study of 43 women with cervical dilatation more than 4cm between 20 and 27 weeks gestation. 22 underwent emergency cerclage and 15 elected for bed rest. Cerclage resulted in a longer gestational age at delivery, shorter stay in hospital and less need for tocolysis and fewer premature rupture of membranes. Conclusion: cerclage is superior to bed rest. **III B**

15 Besinger RE, Niebyl JR, Keyes WG *et al.* (1991) Randomized comparative trial of indomethacin and ritodrine for the long-term treatment of preterm labor. *Am J Obstet Gynecol* **164**, 981–986. RCT comparing ritodrine and indomethacin in 40 patients. They were equally successful in delaying delivery. Conclusion: both ritodrine and indomethacin can be used for long-term treatment for preterm labor. **Ib A**

16 Niebyl JR, Blake DA, White RD *et al.* (1980) The inhibition of premature labor with indomethacin. *Am J Obstet Gynecol* **5**, 136. RCT with indomethacin and placebo for the treatment of preterm labor in 30 patients. Indomethacin was significantly more effective than placebo during a 24h course of therapy. No difference in gestational age at delivery, birthweight and neonatal morbidity. Conclusion: indomethacin is effective in inhibition of labor but is still experimental. **Ib A**

17 Panter KR, Hannah ME, Aman Kwah KS *et al.* (1999) The effect of indomethacin tocolysis in preterm labour on perinatal outcome: a randomised placebo-controlled trial. *Br J Obstet Gynecol* **106**, 467–473. RCT in 34 women with preterm labor between 23 and 30 weeks. In the indomethacin group 81% had a delay in delivery of more than 48h versus 56% in the placebo group. Perinatal mortality and morbidity was the same. Conclusion: no evidence that indomethacin tocolysis is beneficial. **Ib A**

Ectopic pregnancy

Management option		Quality of evidence	Strength of recommendations	References
Expectant		Ib	A	1–3
Medical	Methotrexate local	Ib	A	1
	Methotrexate systemic	Ib	A	1,4
	Hyperosmolar glucose	Ib	A	1,3–6
	Prostaglandins and methotrexate	Ib	A	1,6–8
Laparoscopy	Salpingostomy/salpingectomy	Ib	A	1,9–11
Laparotomy	Salpingostomy/salpingectomy	Ib	A	1,9–11
Laparoscopy management of first choice	Salpingostomy	Ib	A	1,9–11

References

1 Hajenius PJ, Mol BW, Bossuyt PM *et al.* (2000) Interventions for tubal ectopic pregnancy (Cochrane Review). In: *The Cochrane library*, issue 2. Oxford: Update Software. A review of 39 RCTs comparing treatments in women with ectopic pregnancy. Laparoscopic conservative surgery is significantly less successful than the open surgical approach because of a higher persistent trophoblast rate. Subsequent intrauterine pregnancy and ectopic pregnancy rates are comparable. Local methotrexate is not a treatment option compared to laparoscopic salpingostomy. Systemic single-dose methotrexate is not effective enough. Systemic intramuscular methotrexate in multiple doses is as effective but is more expensive and causes greater impairment of health-related quality of life. Conclusion: laparoscopic surgery is the first-choice treatment; intramuscular multiple-dose methotrexate is a good alternative. **Ib A**

2 Korhonen J, Stenman UH, Ylostalo P. (1996) Low-dose oral methotrexate with expectant management of ectopic pregnancy. *Obstet Gynecol* **88**, 775–778. RCT in 60 women with ectopic pregnancy. They received either 5 days 2.5 mg oral methotrexate or placebo. In both groups, 77% recovered without the need for laparoscopy and no difference in recovery time. Conclusion: Oral methotrexate is not more effective than placebo in women with ectopic pregnancy eligible for expectant management. **Ib A**

3 Lang PF, Makinen JI, Irjala KM *et al.* (1997) Laparoscopic instillation of hyperosmolar glucose vs. expectant management of tubal pregnancies with serum hCG < or = 2500 mIU/mL. *Acta Obstet Gynecol Scand* **76**, 797–800. Prospective non-randomized comparative trial in 128 patients with laparoscopically confirmed tubal pregnancy and serum human chorionic gonadotropin ≤2500. They were treated with laparoscopic instillation of glucose solution or were followed expectantly. In the first group, 92% of the ectopic pregnancies resolved and in the second group 75%. Conclusion: glucose instillation is superior to expectant management. **IIb B**

4 Laatkainen, Tuomivaara L, Kaar K (1993) Comparison of a local injection of hyperosmolar glucose solution with salpingotomy for the conservative treatment of tubal pregnancy. *Fertil Steril* **60**, 80–84. RCT in 40 women with unruptured tubal pregnancy. They either underwent local injection of hyperosmolar glucose or laparoscopic salpingostomy. Persistent ectopic pregnancy rates were 20% in the first group and 10% in the second group. Conclusion: local injection of hyperosmolar glucose does not offer advantages over salpingotomy but can be used in selected cases. **Ib A**

5 Gjelland K, Hordnes K, Tjugum J *et al.* (1995) Treatment of ectopic pregnancy by local injection of hypertonic glucose: a randomized trial comparing administration guided by transvaginal ultrasound or laparoscopy. *Acta Obstet Gynecol Scand* **74**, 629–634. RCT in 80 women with ectopic pregnancy. They underwent either sonography-guided injection transvaginally or laparoscopy-guided glucose injection. In the first group 74.4% were successfully treated and in the second group 51.2%. Conclusion: local injection of hyperosmolar glucose guided by transvaginal ultrasound is an effective treatment for ectopic pregnancy. **Ib A**

6 Lang PF, Weiss PA, Mayer HO *et al.* (1990) Conservative treatment of ectopic pregnancy with local injection of hyperosmolar glucose solution or prostaglandin-F2 alpha: a prospective randomised study. *Lancet* **336**, 78–81. RCT in 31 patients with unruptured tubal pregnancy. They were treated with either local and systemic prostaglandins or local instillation of glucose solution. The first treatment was successful in 86.7% and the second in 100%. Conclusion: hyperosmolar glucose is an option in the laparoscopic management of tubal pregnancy. **Ib A**

7 Gazvani MR, Christmas S, Quenby S *et al.* (1998) Mifepristone in combination with methotrexate for the medical treatment of tubal pregnancy: a randomized, controlled trial. *Hum Reprod* **13**, 1987–1990. RCT in 50 patients with unruptured tubal pregnancy that was laparoscopically confirmed. They received a combination of 600 mg oral mifepristone and methotrexate 50 mg/m^2 intramuscularly or methotrexate only. A second injection was

necessary in 4% and 16% respectively. A complete resolution was achieved in 23/25 and 22/25 respectively. Conclusion: unruptured ectopic pregnancy resolves faster with a combination of methotrexate and mifepristone. **Ib A**

8 Paulsson G, Kuint S, Labecker BM *et al.* (1995) Laparoscopic prostaglandin injection in ectopic pregnancy: success rates according to endocrine activity. *Fertil Steril* **63**, 473–477. Prospective study in 108 patients with 127 tubal pregnancies. Prostaglandin $F_{2\alpha}$ was injected in the surrounding tubal wall and the corpus-luteum-bearing ovary. In 7.5%, laparotomies were subsequently necessary. Conclusion: prostaglandin injection can be a simple and financially attractive alternative for treating ectopic pregnancy. **III B**

9 Murphy AA, Nager CW, Wujek JJ *et al.* (1992) Operative laparoscopy versus laparotomy for the management of ectopic pregnancy: a prospective trial. *Fertil Steril* **57**, 1180–1185. Controlled clinical trial in 63 patients with suspected ectopic pregnancy. Operative times did not differ significantly. Laparoscopic treated patients had less intraoperative blood loss, hospital stay, narcotic requirement and costs. No difference in subsequent intrauterine pregnancy or ectopic pregnancy rates. Conclusion: laparoscopy is a safe alternative for the management of selected patients with ectopic pregnancy. **IIa B**

10 Vermesh M, Silva PD, Rosen GF *et al.* (1989) Management of unruptured ectopic gestation by linear salpingostomy: a prospective, randomized clinical trial of laparoscopy versus laparotomy. *Obstet Gynecol* **73**, 400–404. RCT in 60 women with laparoscopy-confirmed ectopic pregnancy. They underwent linear salpingostomy laparoscopically or by laparotomy. Blood loss was less in the laparoscopy group; one patient in each group had persistent trophoblastic activity. Human chorionic gonadotropin decline rates were similar. Hospital stay was shorter in the laparoscopic group. Subsequent patency of the involved tube was 80% in the laparoscopic group and 89% in the laparotomy group. Subsequent pregnancy rates were 56% and 58% respectively. Conclusion: laparoscopy is a good alternative to laparotomy. **Ib A**

11 Lundorff P (1997) Laparoscopic surgery in ectopic pregnancy. *Acta Obstet Gynecol Scand Suppl* **164**, 81–84. RCT comparing laparotomy and laparoscopy in 105 women with tubal pregnancy. The laparoscopy group had shorter operation times, hospital stays and convalescence periods. Human chorionic gonadotropin elimination rates were similar. Conclusion: Laparoscopy has the same success rate as open surgery but results in a shorter stay in hospital and convalescence period. **Ib A**

Gestational trophoblastic disease

Management option		Quality of evidence	Strength of recommendations	References
Surgical	Evacuation	III	B	1
Medical	Methotrexate	III	B	2
	Actinomycin-D	III	B	2
	Combination therapy	III	B	3,4

References

1 Horn LC, Bilek K (1997) Clinicopathologic analysis of gestational trophoblastic disease, report of 158 cases. *Gen Diagn Pathol* **143**, 173–178. Descriptive study of 158 cases of gestational trophoblastic disease. 63.9% had spontaneous regression after curettage, 36.1% had persistent or metastatic disease. **III B**

2 Matsui H, Iitsuka Y, Seji K *et al.* (1998) Comparison of chemotherapies with methotrexate, VP-16 and actinomycin-D in low risk gestational trophoblastic disease. Remission rates and drug toxicities. *Gynecol Obstet Invest* **46**, 5–8. Retrospective study to compare efficiency and toxicity of four chemotherapeutic regimens – (a) 5 days MTX intramuscularly; (b) 5 days VP-16 intravenously; (c) 5 days Act-D intravenously; or (d) 8 days MTX and folic acid – in 247 patients. The primary remission rates were 73.6%, 90.1%, 84.0% and 60.0% respectively. Conclusion: Higher remission rates with lower toxicity occur with VP-16 and Act-D. **III B**

3 Newlands ES, Bower M, Holden L et al. (1998) Management of resistant gestational trophoblastic tumors. J Reprod Med 43, 111–118. Analysis of 272 patients with high-risk gestational trophoblastic disease. They were all treated with etoposide, methotrexate and actinomycin-D (EMA)/cyclophosphamide, vincristine (CO). The 5-year survival rate was 86.2%; 78% achieved complete remission. In patients resistant to EMA/CO (17%), EP (etoposide, cisplatin)/EMA with or without surgery produced 70% survival rates. The early death rate (within 1 year) was 4%. **III B**

4 Dobson LS, Lorigan PC, Coleman RE *et al.* (2000) Persistent gestational trophoblastic disease: results of MEA (methotrexate, etoposide and dactinomycin) as first-line chemotherapy in high risk disease and EA (etoposide and dactinomycin) as second-line therapy for low risk disease. *Br J Cancer* **82**, 1547–1552. Retrospective analysis in 73 patients with gestational trophoblastic disease. 38 had high-risk disease and were treated with MEA and 35 had low-risk disease and were treated with EA as second-line treatment. Overall the complete response rate was 85% (75% and 97% respectively). Conclusion: MEA and EA have high success rates and are well tolerated. **III B**

Chapter 7

Recurrent miscarriage

7.1 Recurrent miscarriage *Katinka Overmars*

'Prepregnancy' (at the time of the third miscarriage)

Management option		Quality of evidence	Strength of recommendation	References
Additional information that may be helpful in caring for the next pregnancy	Carefully document any suspected uterine abnormality at surgical evacuation	III	B	1, 2
	Send products of conception for histology or autopsy and karyotype	–	✔	–
	Offer follow-up assessment and counseling	IV	C	3
	General approach is important (e.g. see couple together, sympathy, etc.)	–	✔	–
History and examination for causative and associated factors	Obstetric history to confirm true diagnosis of 'recurrent miscarriage' (gestations of former losses, previous confirmation of pregnancy: biochemical, ultrasonographic and/or histological)	–	✔	–
	General medical history	–	✔	–
	Family history (polycystic ovaries, hereditary thrombophilia)	–	✔	–
	Physical examination: identifying signs of endocrine disease, opportunistic screening (blood pressure, cervical cytology, breast palpation), rubella antibodies, checking special risk factors raised by history	–	✔	–
Routine investigations	Karyotype both partners	III	B	4
	Hysterosalpingography, transvaginal ultrasonography, hysteroscopy	III	B	1, 5
	Anticardiolipin antibodies (IgG and IgM)	IIb	B	6
	Venereal Diseases Research Laboratory test, activated partial thromboplastin time, dilute Russell viper venom time	IIa	B	7, 8
	Antinuclear factor	IIb	B	6
	Mid-follicular LH, FSH, testosterone	IIa	B	8
	Thrombophilia screening: antithrombin III, factor XII, protein C, protein S, activated protein C resistance	IIb IIa	B B	9–11 12,13
	Others determined by positive features in history	III	B	14

➡

Management option		Quality of evidence	Strength of recommendation	References
Counseling with the following key principles/ guidelines	The true rate of recurrent miscarriage is affected by a reproductive compensation effect	IV	C	3
	After three consecutive losses, intensive investigation will identify a probable cause in about 50% of couples	III	B	15
	The remaining 50% probably result from repeated but sporadic chromosome abnormalities occurring consecutively by chance	IIa	B	16
	Anatomical defects of the uterine fundus and cervix, parental chromosomal rearrangements,gene mutations, phospholipid antibodies and hypersecretion of luteinizing hormone also play a role	III	B	1–3,5,17
	Progesterone deficiency, infective agents and immune rejection are very uncommon causes	IV	C	3,18
	Subclinical thyroid disorders or diabetes mellitus are rare	IV	C	3
	Psychological stress is probably not relevant	IV	C	3
	Even after three consecutive losses, the chance of success without treatment exceeds 55% apart from women with antiphospholipid antibodies, where it is lower	III	B	1,19

References

1 Van Iddekinge B, Hofmeyr GJ (1991) Recurrent spontaneous abortion: aetiological factors and subsequent reproductive performance in 76 couples. *South Afr Med J* **80**, 223–226. Retrospective study where possible etiological factor of recurrent miscarriage (three or more consecutive abortions) was found in 32 of 76 couples (42%). The abnormalities most commonly observed were endocervical infections (18%), cervical incompetence (11%) and uterine abnormality (9%). Hypothyroidism was present in 3 women and chromosomal abnormality in 2. None were positive for lupus anticoagulant. **III B**

2 Heinonen PK (1997) Reproductive performance of women with uterine anomalies after abdominal or hysteroscopic metroplasty or no surgical treatment. *J Am Assoc Gynecol Laparosc* **4**, 311–317. Retrospective evaluation of reproductive outcome in 405 women with a uterine anomaly treated by hysteroscopic or abdominal metroplasty, or by no surgical treatment. Fetal survival improved from 13% to 91% after hysteroscopic and from 3% to 86% after abdominal metroplasty. A live child was born in 67% of 264 pregnancies in 116 women with a septate uterus without surgical treatment. Conclusion: hysteroscopic metroplasty is better than abdominal metroplasty in the treatment of septate uterus in women with repeated miscarriage. **III B**

3 Stirrat GM (1990) Recurrent miscarriage. II: Clinical associations, causes and management. *Lancet* **336**, 728–733. Review on the causes of recurrent miscarriage. Commonest direct cause is repeated sporadic chromosome abnormalities. Congenital and acquired anatomical anomalies of the uterus and cervix, parental chromosomal rearrangements, gene mutations, antibodies to cardiolipin, and luteal phase defects each make a small contribution. Reassurance and clear statements about prognosis are important and psychological support must be offered throughout investigation and subsequent pregnancy. **IV C**

4 Sachs ES, Jahoda MG, Van Hemel JO *et al.* (1985) Chromosome studies of 500 couples with two or more abortions. *Obstet Gynecol* **65**, 375–378. Retrospective study on the chromosomal analysis of 500 couples with recurrent (two or more) spontaneous abortions. Abnormal karyotypes – translocations (44%), mosaicisms (48%), and deletions or inversions (8%) – were found in 50 partners (10%). There was no relation with the absolute number of abortions. Conclusion: couples should have chromosome studies after two spontaneous abortions. **III B**

5 Jurkovic D, Geipel A, Gruboeck K *et al.* (1995) Three-dimensional ultrasound for the assessment of uterine anatomy and detection of congenital anomalies: a comparison with hysterosalpingography and two-dimensional sonography. *Ultrasound Obstet Gynecol* **5**, 233–237. Prospective study of three-dimensional

ultrasound in 61 patients with a history of recurrent miscarriage or infertility previously investigated by hysterosalpingography (HSG). Comparison between HSG and ultrasound showed that five false-positive diagnoses of arcuate uterus and three of major uterine anomalies were made on two-dimensional scans. Three-dimensional ultrasound agreed with hysterosalpingography in all cases of arcuate uterus and major congenital anomalies. **III B**

6 Reznikoff-Etievant MF, Cayol V, Zou GM *et al.* (1999) Habitual abortions in 678 healthy patients: investigation and prevention. *Hum Reprod* **14**, 2106–2109. Prospective study on 678 healthy patients with a history of habitual abortion and the presence of antiphospholipid antibodies, antinuclear and antithyroid antibodies (total 33.9% positive) who were given either prednisone and aspirin or aspirin alone during the first trimester. Prednisone and aspirin seemed to be as efficient as aspirin in autoantibody-positive women but better than aspirin alone in autoantibody-negative women. **IIb B**

7 Ogasawara M, Aoki K, Katano K *et al.* (1998) Activated partial thromboplastin time is a predictive parameter for further miscarriages in cases of recurrent fetal loss. *Fertil Steril* **70**, 1081–1084. Prospective cohort study of coagulation status in 261 nonpregnant patients with a history of two consecutive first-trimester abortions (without antiphospholipid antibodies or other autoimmune diseases or anatomical anomalies). Only a shortened activated partial thromboplastin time before conception was found to be significantly associated with further miscarriages. **IIb B**

8 Bussen S, Sutterlin M, Steck T *et al.* (1999) Endocrine abnormalities during the follicular phase in women with recurrent spontaneous abortion. *Hum Reprod* **14**, 18–20. Case-control study of endocrine status of 42 consecutive nonpregnant women with recurrent spontaneous abortion with no parental chromosome rearrangement or uterine abnormality and 42 controls. Mean concentrations of prolactin and androstenedione and body mass index were significantly higher in the study group. Conclusion: reduction of body weight and correction of hyperprolactinemia and of hyperandrogenism may reduce the rate of miscarriage in a subsequent pregnancy in these women. **IIa B**

9 Younis JS, Brenner B, Ohel G *et al.* (2000) Activated protein C resistance and factor V Leiden mutation can be associated with first- as well as second-trimester recurrent pregnancy loss. *Am J Reprod Immunol* **43**, 31–35. Prospective study on the prevalence of activated protein C resistance (aPCR) and the factor V Leiden in 78 consecutive nonpregnant women with two or more unexplained miscarriages and 139 nonpregnant women with at least one successful pregnancy and no abortions. aPCR and factor V Leiden mutations were significantly more prevalent in all recurrent-pregnancy-loss patients than in controls: 38% and 19% compared to 8% and 6% respectively. **IIb B**

10 Coumans AB, Huijgens PC, Jakobs C *et al.* (1999) Haemostatic and metabolic abnormalities in women with unexplained recurrent abortion. *Hum Reprod* **14**, 211–214. Prospective study on 52 patients with a history of unexplained habitual abortion who were tested for protein S, protein C and antithrombin III deficiency, activated protein C resistance, hyperhomocystinemia and anticardiolipin antibodies (ACA). The control group consisted of 67 healthy women with only uncomplicated pregnancies. Parous women with a history of unexplained recurrent abortion had an increased incidence of hyperhomocysteinemia and a trend towards an increased incidence of ACA. **IIb B**

11 Rai R, Regan L, Hadley E *et al.* (1996) Second-trimester pregnancy loss is associated with activated C resistance. *Br J Haematol* **92**, 489–490. Prospective study on the prevalence of activated protein C resistance (aPCR) in second trimester miscarriage. The prevalence of aPCR was found to be significantly higher in 50 women with a history of second-trimester miscarriage (20%) than in 70 women with a history of first-trimester miscarriages only (5.7%) or a control group of 70 parous women with no previous history of pregnancy losses (4.3%) ($p < 0.02$). **IIb B**

12 Gris JC, Ripart-Neveu S, Maugard C *et al.* (1997) Respective evaluation of the prevalence of haemostasis abnormalities in unexplained primary early recurrent miscarriages. The Nimes Obstetricians and Haematologists (NOHA) Study. *Thromb Haemost* **77**, 1096–1103. Prospective study on the prevalence of hemostasis abnormalities in 500 consecutive women with unexplained recurrent miscarriages and two control groups of 100 healthy parous and 50 nulliparous women with no history of miscarriage. In the study group 9.4% had an isolated factor XII deficiency and 7.4% had antiphospholipid antibodies. Von Willebrand disease, fibrinogen deficiency, antithrombin, protein C or protein S deficiencies were not more frequent in recurrent aborters than control groups. **IIa B**

13 Sarig G, Younis JS, Hoffman R *et al.* (2002) Thrombophilia is common in women with idiopathic pregnancy loss and is associated with late pregnancy wastage. *Fertil Steril* **77**, 342–347. Prospective observational study of the thrombophilia status (activated protein C (APC) resistance, protein C, protein S and antithrombin III, antiphospholipid antibodies, factor V Leiden, factor II G20210A and MTHFR C677T mutations) of 145 patients with repeated pregnancy loss and 145 matched controls. At least one thrombophilic defect was found in 66% of the study group compared with 28% in the control group. Combined thrombophilic defects were documented in 21% and 5.5% of study and control patients respectively. Late pregnancy wastage occurred more frequently in women with thrombophilia compared with women without thrombophilia (37% vs 24% respectively). **IIa B**

14 Mavragani CP, Ioannidis JP, Tzioufas AG *et al.* (1999) Recurrent pregnancy loss and autoantibody profile in autoimmune diseases. *Rheumatology* **38**, 1228–1233. A retrospective cohort study on 70 unselected anti-Ro/SSA-positive women. 40 anti-Ro/SSA-positive women were age matched to an equal number of women with autoimmune disorders who were anti-Ro/SSA-negative. In women with autoimmune disorders, a history of recurrent pregnancy loss was independently associated with reactivity against each of three antigen specificities and also with the presence of antithyroglobulin antibodies, suggesting that cumulative autoimmune responses against these antigens correlate with the risk of stillbirth and spontaneous abortion. **III B**

15 Stray-Pedersen B, Stray-Pederson S (1984) Etiologic factors and subsequent reproductive performance in 195 couples with a prior history of habitual abortion. *Am J Obstet Gynecol* **148**, 140–146. A diagnostic screening program was applied to 195 couples with a prior history of habitual abortion (three or more consecutive abortions). Abnormalities were identified in 110 (56%) of the couples (anomalies of the uterine body, endometrial infections and cervical incompetence, hormonal dysfunctions and, rarely, chromosomal anomalies. Women with abnormalities were offered surgical or medical treatment. Among women with no abnormalities, specific antenatal counseling and psychological support was given. In this group, the pregnancy success rate was 86% compared to 33% observed in women who were given no specific antenatal care ($p < 0.001$). **III B**

16 Stern JJ, Dorfmann AD, Gutierrez-Najar AJ *et al.* (1996) Frequency of abnormal karyotypes among abortuses from women with and without a history of recurrent spontaneous abortion. *Fertil Steril* **65**, 250–253. Prospective study on the products of conception in 94 women with a history of recurrent abortion and a control group of 130 women without such a history. No differences in frequency of abnormal karyotype were observed in products of conception from women with recurrent spontaneous abortion compared with women without recurrent spontaneous abortion. **IIa B**

17 Guzman ER, Mellon R, Vintzileos AM *et al.* (1998) Relationship between endocervical canal length between 15–24 weeks gestation and obstetric history. *J Matern Fetal Med* **7**, 269–272. Retrospective cohort study of 155 multigravidas (singleton pregnancies) with normal and abnormal obstetric histories on the correlation between the obstetric history and the ultrasonographically determined cervical canal length between 15 and 24 weeks gestation. There was a significant correlation between the measurements between 15 and 20 weeks and 21–24 weeks in the studied pregnancy and the earliest gestational age at delivery of prior pregnancies. There was also a significant relationship between the ultrasound diagnosis of cervical incompetence (canal length < 2 cm) and the obstetric history category. Conclusion: women with a prior delivery before 30 weeks gestation should be followed with second-trimester serial cervical sonography. **III B**

18 Hensleigh PA, Fainstat T (1979) Corpus luteum dysfunction: serum progesterone levels in diagnosis and assessment of therapy for recurrent and threatened abortion. *Fertil Steril* **32**, 396–400. Clinical experience of serum progesterone (P) measurements in the diagnosis and treatment of patients with recurrent and threatened abortion. Patients were treated with clomiphene, gonadotropins and/or progesterone in order to correct serum P levels. When treatment of patients with subnormal P levels resulted in normalization of serum P, successful pregnancies occurred. **IV C**

19 Knudsen UB, Hansen V, Juul S *et al.* (1991) Prognosis of a new pregnancy following previous spontaneous abortions. *Eur J Obstet Gynaecol Reprod Biol* **39**, 31–36. Retrospective cohort study to determine the risk of a miscarriage following 0–4 consecutive spontaneous abortions (total of about 300 500 pregnancies in Denmark). The overall risk of a spontaneous abortion was 11%, 16%, 25%, 45% and 54% after 0–4 consecutive spontaneous abortions respectively. For women over 35 years the risk of a spontaneous abortion was significantly increased, but the virtually identical abortion rates after repeated abortions in both young and old women indicate a risk factor that is not age-related. **III B**

Prepregnancy treatment options

Management option		Quality of evidence	Strength of recommendation	References
Do not advocate 'unproven' treatments		–	✔	–
Parental translocations	Genetic counseling of couple and relatives	IV	C	1
	Gamete donation	III	B	2,3
Uterine abnormalities	Hysteroscopic resection/division	III	B	4,5
	Temporary intrauterine device	III	B	6,7
Cervical incompetence	Serial cervical ultrasonography	III	B	8
	Primary cervical cerclage	Ib	A	9
	Emergency cerclage	III	B	10
Hormonal treatments	Human chorionic gonadotropin	Ib	A	11
	In-vitro fertilization: desensitization with buserelin in women with polycystic ovaries	III	B	12
	Gonadotropin-releasing hormone-α with HMG for anovulatory women with polycystic ovaries	III	B	13

Management option		Quality of evidence	Strength of recommendation	References
Diabetes mellitus	Good metabolic control	IIb	B	14, 15
Antiphospholipid syndrome	Low-dose aspirin (in combination with heparin) better than aspirin plus prednisone	Ib	A	16, 17
	Heparin with low-dose aspirin is superior to low-dose aspirin alone	Ib	A	18, 19
Thrombophilia	Low-dose aspirin and/or low-dose heparin	IIb	B	20
Immunological therapy	No evidence of benefit	Ia	A	21

References

1. De Braekeleer M, Dao TN (1990) Cytogenetic studies in couples experiencing repeated pregnancy losses. *Hum Reprod* **5**, 519–528. Retrospective analysis of a computerized database generated from the literature that consisted of cytogenetic data from 22 199 couples (44 398 individuals). Overall, 4.7% of the couples with two or more spontaneous abortions included one carrier of a chromosomal abnormality. Only translocations and inversions were associated with a higher risk of pregnancy wastage. To these couples genetic counseling should be offered and investigations performed on their extended families. **IV C**
2. Sachs ES, Jahoda MG, Van Hemel JO *et al.* (1985) Chromosome studies of 500 couples with two or more abortions. *Obstet Gynecol* **65**, 375–378. Retrospective study on the chromosomal analysis of 500 couples with recurrent (two or more) spontaneous abortions. Abnormal karyotypes – translocations (44%), mosaicisms (48%) and deletions or inversions (8%) – were found in 50 partners (10%). There was no relation with the absolute number of abortions. Conclusion: couples should have chromosome studies after two spontaneous abortions. **III B**
3. Remohi J, Gallardo E, Levy M *et al.* (1996) Oocyte donation in women with recurrent pregnancy loss. *Hum Reprod* **11**, 2048–2051. Case study on 12 oocyte donations in eight couples in whom the woman was a low responder to gonadotropin stimulation with a history of recurrent abortion. Pregnancy and delivery rates per cycle were 75% and 67% respectively. The results of ovum donation compared favorably with low responders without a history of recurrent abortion undergoing this treatment during the study period. These results strongly suggest that the oocyte may be the origin of infertility in women with idiopathic recurrent miscarriages. **III B**
4. Heinonen PK (1997) Reproductive performance of women with uterine anomalies after abdominal or hysteroscopic metroplasty or no surgical treatment. *J Am Assoc Gynecol Laparosc* **4**, 311–317. Retrospective evaluation of reproductive outcome in 405 women with a uterine anomaly treated by hysteroscopic or abdominal metroplasty, or by no surgical treatment. Fetal survival improved from 13% to 91% after hysteroscopic and from 3% to 86% after abdominal metroplasty. A live child was born in 67% of 264 pregnancies in 116 women with a septate uterus without surgical treatment. Conclusion: hysteroscopic metroplasty is better than abdominal metroplasty in the treatment of septate uterus in women with repeated miscarriage. **III B**
5. Porcu G, Cravello L, D'Ercole C *et al.* (2000) Hysteroscopic metroplasty for septate uterus and repetitive abortions: reproductive outcome. *Eur J Obstet Gynecol Reprod Biol* **88**, 81–84. Retrospective study to assess reproductive outcome and obstetrical prognosis of 63 patients undergoing hysteroscopic resection of uterine septa for women with a history of recurrent abortion or abnormal fetal presentation. There were 45 pregnancies in 54 cases with 28 children born alive of which 26 at term. Treatment improved the obstetrical prognosis significantly ($p = 0.001$). **III B**
6. Sanfilippo JS, Fitzgerald MR, Badawy SZ *et al.* (1982) Asherman's syndrome. A comparison of therapeutic methods. *Reprod Med* **27**, 328–330. Retrospective study on Asherman's syndrome in which 35 patients were treated with dilatation and curettage, followed by conjugated estrogens and progestins. 26 patients also had hysteroscopic evaluation of the procedure, an intrauterine contraceptive device inserted and prophylactic antibiotics. The pregnancy rate was higher in the second group. **III B**
7. Ismajovich B, Lidor A, Confino E *et al.* (1985) Treatment of minimal and moderate intrauterine adhesions (Asherman's syndrome). *J Reprod Med* **30**, 769–772. Case reports on 51 women with intrauterine adhesions who underwent lysis of adhesions and insertion of an intrauterine contraceptive device (IUD). A pregnancy rate of 90% is reported. In 85% of these a viable infant was delivered, and 15% had a miscarriage. It was concluded that, in mild to moderate Asherman's syndrome, IUD insertion after adhesiolysis without estrogen administration yields satisfactory results. **III B**
8. Guzman ER, Mellon R, Vintzileos AM *et al.* (1998) Relationship between endocervical canal length between 15–24 weeks gestation and obstetric history. *J Matern Fetal Med* **7**, 269–272. Retrospective cohort study of 155

multigravidas (singleton pregnancies) with normal and abnormal obstetric histories on the correlation between the obstetric history and the ultrasonographically determined cervical canal length between 15 and 24 weeks gestation. There was a significant correlation between the measurements between 15 and 20 weeks and 21–24 weeks in the studied pregnancy and the earliest gestational age at delivery of prior pregnancies. There was also a significant relationship between the ultrasound diagnosis of cervical incompetence (canal length < 2 cm) and the obstetric history category. Conclusion: women with a prior delivery before 30 weeks gestation should be followed with second-trimester serial cervical sonography. **III B**

9 Medical Research Council/Royal College of Obstetricians and Gynaecologists (1988) Multicentre Randomized Trial of Cervical Cerclage. Interim Report. *Br J Obstet Gynaecol* **95**, 437–445. Randomized controlled trial in 905 women with a history of early delivery or cervical surgery who were randomly allocated to cerclage or no surgery. The group with cervical cerclage had fewer deliveries before 33 weeks (13% vs 18%, $p = 0.03$), fewer miscarriages and stillbirths or neonatal death (8% vs 12%, $p = 0.06$). Conclusion: primary cervical cerclage may be beneficial to pregnancy outcome but the interpretation of the results is to be taken with care because of marginal statistical significances. **Ib A**

10 MacDougall J, Siddle N (1991) Emergency cervical cerclage. *Br J Obstet Gynaecol* **98**, 1234–1238. Case reports on 19 women who underwent emergency cerclage between 16 and 28 weeks with cervical dilatation between 3 cm and 10 cm. Outcome: prolongation of gestation from between 1 and 19 weeks. 15 live babies (survival rate 63%). Infection responsible for 8 intrauterine or neonatal deaths. **III B**

11 Quenby S, Farquharson RG (1994) Human chorionic gonadotrophin supplementation in recurring pregnancy loss: a controlled trial. *Fertil Steril* **62**, 708–710. Randomized controlled trial to investigate the efficacy of human chorionic gonadotropin (hCG) in the management of early recurrent miscarriage. 81 women with idiopathic recurrent pregnancy loss were randomized to receive supplementation of hCG or placebo during early pregnancy. In women with regular menstrual cycles, no beneficial effect of hCG was seen but there was an improvement of pregnancy success rate in women with oligomenorrhea (from 40% in the placebo group to 86% in the hCG-supplemented grou **Ib A**

12 Balen AH, Tan SL, MacDougall J *et al.* (1994) Miscarriage rates following in vitro fertilisation are increased in women with polycystic ovaries and reduced by pituitary desensitization with buserelin. *Hum Reprod* **8**, 959–964. Retrospective study of 1060 pregnancies from 7623 cycles of *in-vitro* fertilization (IVF) to assess the risk of miscarriage after IVF in relation to different variables. A total of 26.6% spontaneous abortions. Women who miscarried were significantly older (32.2 vs 33.2 years, $p = 0.008$), had more often polycystic ovaries (miscarriage rate 23.6% vs 35.8%; $p = 0.0038$, 95% CI 4.68–23.1%). Reduction of the miscarriage rate was seen in women with polycystic ovaries when treated with the long buserelin protocol compared with clomiphene citrate (20.3% vs 47.2%, $p = 0.0003$, 95% CI 13.82–40.09%) **III B**

13 Homburg R, Levy T, Berkovitz D *et al.* (1993) Gonadotrophin-releasing hormone agonist reduces the miscarriage rate for pregnancies achieved in women with polycystic ovarian syndrome. *Fertil Steril* **59**, 527–531. Retrospective study on the effect of gonadotropin-releasing hormone agonist (GnRH-a) decapeptyl and human menopausal gonadotropins (hMG) compared to gonadotropins only on the miscarriage rate in 239 women with anovulatory polycystic ovarian syndrome (PCOS). The miscarriage rate after ovulation induction was 16.7% with and 39.4% without GnRH-α. Cumulative live birth rate after four cycles for GnRH-α was 64% compared to 26% for gonadotropins only. It was concluded that co-treatment with GnRH-α/hMG of anovulatory women with PCOS reduces the miscarriage rate and improves the live birth rate compared to treatment with gonadotropins alone. **III B**

14 Mills JL, Simpson JL, Driscoll SG *et al.* (1988) (National Institute of Child Health and Human Development/ Diabetes in Early Pregnancy Study.) Incidence of spontaneous abortion among normal women and insulin-dependent diabetic women whose pregnancies were identified within 21 days of conception. *N Engl J Med* **319**, 1617–1623. Prospective case-control study on the risk of miscarriage in pregnant women with insulin-dependent diabetes and nondiabetic women as controls. Diabetic women with good metabolic control are not more likely than nondiabetic women to lose a pregnancy. Diabetic women with elevated blood glucose and glycosylated hemoglobin levels in the first trimester were found to have an increased risk of spontaneous abortion. **IIa A**

15 Rosenn B, Miodovnik M, Combs CA *et al.* (1991) Pre-conception management of insulin-dependent diabetes: improvement of pregnancy outcome. *Obstet Gynecol* **77**, 846–849. Prospective study on pregnancy outcome in 99 pregnant insulin-dependent diabetic women, of which 28 attended a preconception clinic to optimize early glycemic control (study group). The 71 women in the control group were enrolled after conception but before 9 weeks gestation. Early glycemic control was significantly better in the study group (significantly lower Hb1Ac in the 9th and 14th week). The rate of spontaneous abortion was significantly lower in the study group (7%) than in the controls (24%). **IIb A**

16 Cowchock FS, Reece EA, Balaban D *et al.* (1992) Repeated fetal losses associated with antiphospholipid antibodies: a collaborative randomized trial comparing prednisone with low-dose heparin treatment. *Am J Obstet Gynecol* **166**, 1318–1323. Randomized trial on 20 patients with antiphospholipid antibody and recurrent fetal loss comparing low-dose heparin with 40 mg prednisone (both with low-dose aspirin). Live birth rates were the same (75%) but maternal morbidity and preterm delivery occurred more often in women using prednisone ($p = 0.02$ vs $p = 0.006$). It was concluded that in this group of patients low-dose heparin is to be preferred to prednisone. **Ib A**

17 Silver RK, MacGregor SN, Farrell EE *et al.* (1993) Comparative trial of prednisone plus aspirin versus aspirin alone in the treatment of anti-cardiolipin antibody-positive obstetric patients. *Am J Obstet Gynecol* **169**,

1411–1417. Randomized trial in pregnant women with antiphospholipid antibodies and a poor obstetric history comparing 81 mg aspirin daily (n = 22) with low-dose aspirin (81 mg) in combination with prednisone (started with 20 mg/day and adjusted according to changes in antibody levels; n = 12). Preterm delivery occurred more often in patients receiving prednisone plus aspirin (8/12 vs 3/22 respectively; p = 0.003. Prednisone exposure appeared to be an independent risk factor for preterm birth. **Ib A**

18 Kutteh WH (1996) Antiphospholipid antibody-associated recurrent pregnancy loss: treatment with heparin and low-dose aspirin is superior to low-dose aspirin alone. *Am J Obstet Gynecol* **174**, 1584–1589. Randomized trial with alternate allocation of treatment on pregnant women with antiphospholipid syndrome and three or more miscarriages comparing low-dose aspirin only with low-dose aspirin with heparin. The live birth rate was 44% versus 80% respectively (p< 0.05). No significant differences were seen in gestational age at delivery, number of cesarean sections or complications. It was concluded that in this group of patients heparin plus low-dose aspirin provides a significantly better pregnancy outcome than low-dose aspirin alone. **Ib A**

19 Rai R, Cohen H, Dave M *et al.* (1997) Randomised controlled trial of aspirin and aspirin plus heparin in pregnant women with recurrent miscarriage associated with phospholipid antibodies (or antiphospholipid antibodies). *Br Med J* **314**, 253–257. Randomized controlled trial of aspirin (75 mg daily) and aspirin (75 mg daily) plus heparin (5000 U 12-hourly) in 90 women with recurrent miscarriage and phospholipid antibody syndrome. Treatment was stopped at 34 weeks or at the time of miscarriage. The rate of live births with aspirin plus heparin was 71% (32/45 pregnancies) and 42% (19/45 pregnancies) with aspirin only (OR 3.37 with 95% CI 1.40–8.10). There was no difference in outcome between the two treatments in pregnancies that advanced beyond 13 weeks gestation. **Ib A**

20 Brenner B, Hoffman R, Blumenfeld Z *et al.* (2000) Gestational outcome in thrombophilic women with recurrent pregnancy loss treated by enoxaparin. *Thromb Haemost* **83**, 693–697. Retrospective study on enoxaparin in 50 women with recurrent pregnancy and thrombophilia. 61 pregnancies were treated with enoxaparin throughout gestation until 4 weeks after delivery. Aspirin was given in addition to women with antiphospholipid syndrome. 75% (46/61) pregnancies treated with enoxaparin resulted in live births, compared to 20% (38/193) prior to the diagnosis of thrombophilia (p < 0.00001). **IIb B**

21 Scott JR (2000) Immunotherapy for recurrent miscarriage. *Cochrane Database Syst Rev* **2**, CD000112. Meta-analysis of 18 randomized trials of immunotherapy in women with three or more miscarriages, no more than one live birth, all nonimmunological causes ruled out and no simultaneous treatment intervention. The various forms of immunotherapy did not show significant differences between treatment and control groups. It was concluded that paternal cell immunization, third-party donor leukocytes, trophoblast membranes and intravenous immunoglobulin provide no significant beneficial effect over placebo in preventing further miscarriages. **Ia A**

Management during subsequent pregnancy, delivery and puerperium

Management option		Quality of evidence	Strength of recommendation	References
Psychological support, reassurance, etc.		III	B	1,2
First trimester	Transvaginal ultrasound scan to confirm fetal viability	–	✔	–
	Serial scans for reassurance	–	✔	–
	Progesterone measurement to detect uncommon cases of deficiency	IV	C	3
Second trimester	Serial transvaginal ultrasound scan to monitor suspected cervical incompetence	III	B	4
	Serial vaginal swabs for pathogens	–	✔	–
	Consider prophylactic dexamethasone and formal glucose tolerance test at 27 weeks in selected cases	–	✔	–
Third trimester	Serial ultrasound scans for fetal growth	III	B	2,5
	Anticipate increased risk of preeclampsia in some cases	III	B	5
	Consider elective lower-segment section/ induction of labor at term in some cases	III	B	5
Specific options for specific conditions		–	✔	–

References

1 Liddell HS, Pattison NS, Zanderigo A (1991) Recurrent miscarriage – outcome after supportive care in early pregnancy. *Aust N Z J Obstet Gynaecol* **31**, 320–322. Case-control study on couples with a history of unexplained recurrent miscarriage treated with formal emotional support and close supervision ($n = 44$) or regular controls without formal support ($n = 9$) during their pregnancy after an initial investigation. In the group receiving emotional support, 86% (38/44) had a good pregnancy outcome compared to 33% (3/9) in the group getting no formal emotional support ($p = 0.005$). **III B**

2 Reginald PW, Beard RW, Chapple J *et al.* (1987) Outcome of pregnancies progressing beyond 28 weeks gestation in women with a history of recurrent miscarriage. *Br J Obstet Gynaecol* **94**, 643–648. Retrospective study on the outcome of ongoing pregnancies beyond 28 weeks in 97 women who had had three or more miscarriages. 30% were small-for-gestational age, 28% were born preterm and the perinatal mortality, excluding babies of less than 28 weeks gestation, was 16.1%. It was concluded that pregnancies in women with a history of recurrent miscarriage are at high risk for these complications. **III B**

3 Hensleigh PA, Fainstat T (1979) Corpus luteum dysfunction: serum progesterone levels in diagnosis and assessment of therapy for recurrent and threatened abortion. *Fertil Steril* **32**, 396–400. Clinical experience of serum progesterone (P) measurements in the diagnosis and treatment of patients with recurrent and threatened abortion. Patients were treated with clomiphene, gonadotropins and/or progesterone in order to correct serum P levels. When treatment of patients with subnormal P levels resulted in normalization of serum P, successful pregnancies occurred. **IV C**

4 Guzman ER, Mellon R, Vintzileos AM *et al.* (1998) Relationship between endocervical canal length between 15–24 weeks gestation and obstetric history. *J Matern Fetal Med* **7**, 269–272. Retrospective cohort study of 155 multigravidas (singleton pregnancies) with normal and abnormal obstetric histories on the correlation between the obstetric history and the ultrasonographically determined cervical canal length between 15 and 24 weeks gestation. There was a significant correlation between the measurements between 15 and 20 weeks and 21–24 weeks in the studied pregnancy and the earliest gestational age at delivery of prior pregnancies. There was also a significant relationship between the ultrasound diagnosis of cervical incompetence (canal length < 2 cm) and the obstetric history category. Conclusion: women with a prior delivery before 30 weeks gestation should be followed with second-trimester serial cervical sonography. **III B**

5 Lima F, Khamashta MA, Buchanan NM *et al.* (1996) A study of sixty pregnancies in patients with the antiphospholipid syndrome. *Clin Exp Rheumatol* **14**, 131–136. Retrospective study on maternal and fetal outcome in 47 women with antiphospholipid syndrome and recurrent miscarriage treated with low-dose aspirin (75 mg) daily or subcutaneous unfractionated or low-molecular-weight heparin and low-dose aspirin (75 mg) daily in case of a history of thrombotic events. The live birth rate increased from 19% of their previous nontreated pregnancies to 70% despite a high incidence of obstetric and fetal complications: preeclampsia (18%), prematurity (43%), fetal distress (50%) and intrauterine growth restriction (31%). Two predictors of fetal outcome were observed: the previous obstetric history and the presence of thrombocytopenia. **III B**

Chapter 8

Screening for fetal abnormality

8.1 Serum alpha-fetoprotein screening for neural tube defects *Mike Wyldes and Sharon Hodgkiss*

Management option	Quality of evidence	Strength of recommendation	References
Maternal serum alpha-fetoprotein (MSAFP) estimation for neural tube defects (NTD) screening in isolation from routine midpregnancy ultrasound scanning is cost-effective	IV	C	1
The optimal timing for MSAFP screening for NTD is 16–18 weeks	III	B	2
The diagnosis of neural tube defects is made using ultrasound (not amniocentesis) but relies upon the quality of the machine, the skill of the operator and patient characteristics. Diagnostic images can be achieved in almost all circumstances at 18–20 weeks	III III	B B	3 4
MSAFP adds little or nothing to the sensitivity of the prenatal diagnosis of NTD when routine mid-pregnancy fetal anomaly ultrasound scanning is used. MSAFP is therefore only a cost-effective method for screening for NTD if routine mid-pregnancy ultrasound is not being undertaken	III	B	5
Pre-test counseling: The population being screened should be fully informed about the purpose of the serum screening, the conditions being screened for and the diagnostic process that would follow a high-risk result	III III IV	B B C	6 7 8
The laboratory undertaking the screening should adhere to national standards, with a named individual responsible	IV	C	9,10
A positive screening result should lead rapidly to a diagnostic ultrasound scan. That should be conducted where there are facilities to both establish the diagnosis and to deal with all possible outcomes	IV	C	10
The diagnostic ultrasound scan should be comprehensive. Unsuspected twins, structural malformations, abnormal measurements, evidence of bleeding, abnormal blood flow studies in both maternal and fetal placental circulations and oligohydramnios are potential sonographic abnormalities or conditions associated with an abnormal MSAFP	III	B	11,12
Repeating high MSAFP levels is not recommended. It tends to reduce the sensitivity by introducing a regression to the mean for borderline values	–	✔	–
Facilities should be available for dealing with other outcomes from a raised MSAFP – including other structural anomalies, fetal death, intrauterine growth restriction and preeclampsia	IIa III	A B	13 11,14

Management option		Quality of evidence	Strength of recommendation	References
Counseling by a fetal medicine specialist and midwife/nurse should include a disclosure interview, explanation of the findings and implications. Consultation with pediatric specialists is also helpful		IV	C	15
Clear documentation		IV	C	8
Written and other illustrative information should be available to women following the diagnostic ultrasound scan		IV	C	8
Genetic counseling should include a discussion of neonatal treatment, and prognosis. A non-directive approach should be used in providing the family with their options, including termination		IV	C	9
Style	Professionals must show sensitivity and flexibility with a clear focus on the individual pregnant woman. Repeat ultrasound scans, review with other people and second-opinion confirmation will all be required at certain times	IV	C	8
Prognosis	Anencephaly is universally lethal, often during pregnancy. Open spina bifida and encephalocele frequently lead to significant mental and physical handicap but the prediction of the precise degree and nature of disability are difficult to predict from the serum AFP levels or ultrasound appearances	–	✔	–
Prevention	Recurrence of neural tube defect can be reduced by folate supplementation in the 12 weeks before conception and the first 12 weeks of pregnancy	Ib	A	16
	Women themselves and their primary care team should be informed of the requirement to take folate 5 mg daily for at least 3 months before trying to conceive in future	IV	C	17
See also Section 18.1.				

References

1 Shackley P (1996) Economic evaluation of prenatal diagnosis: a methodological review. *Prenat Diagn* **16**, 389–395. A review of the role of economic evaluation in prenatal diagnosis. As the availability of new and improved techniques of prenatal diagnosis increases, so does the relevance of economic evaluation. The various methods of economic evaluation are discussed in the context of amniocentesis and chorionic villus sampling. It is argued that, in view of the potentially wide range of benefits from prenatal diagnosis, more sophisticated measures of benefit should be incorporated into economic evaluations. Further development of utility-based measures and monetary valuation is suggested. **IV C**

2 Greenberg F, James LM, Oakley GP Jr *et al.* (1983) Estimates of birth prevalence rates of spina bifida in the United States from computer generated maps. *Am J Obstet Gynecol* **145**, 570–573. A computer-generated mapping procedure was developed to estimate geographical and race-specific birth prevalence rates of open spina bifida. The estimates are based on birth certificate data adjusted for under ascertainment. Separate maps were produced for white births and black births. For both races there is a general decreasing rate of spina bifida from east to west. The highest rate is 8/10000 total births for whites in southern Appalachia and the lowest rate is less than 1/10000 for blacks in the Rocky Mountain states and the Pacific northwest. Until more exact data are available, these maps represent the best current available data on racial and geographical birth prevalence rates in the USA. They are useful for program planning and as an aid in interpreting maternal serum alpha-fetoprotein levels to detect neural tube defects. **III B**

3 Sepulveda W, Donaldson A, Johnson RD *et al.* (1995) Are routine alpha-fetoprotein and acetylcholinesterase determinations still necessary at second-trimester amniocentesis? Impact of high-resolution ultrasonography. *Obstet Gynecol* **85**, 107–112. Retrospective study of 1737 amniotic fluid (AF) samples obtained at second-trimester amniocentesis. High-resolution ultrasonography was performed prior to amniocentesis. Details of pregnancy outcome of all cases with AF alpha-fetoprotein (AFP) levels greater than 2.0 multiples of the median and a positive or faint acetylcholinesterase band were obtained. There were 31 abnormal results. Ultrasonography identified all fetuses with anomalies associated with abnormal biochemical markers, including neural tube defects. The conclusion was that high-resolution ultrasonography was more accurate than AF biochemistry in the detection of congenital anomalies associated with elevated AFP levels and acetylcholinesterase in the AF. Routine measurement of these biochemical markers appears to have a very low yield and would therefore not be cost-effective in practices where high-resolution ultrasonography is performed before amniocentesis. **III B**

4 Kyle PM et al. (1994) Life without amniocentesis: elevated maternal serum alpha-fetoprotein in the Manitoba program 1986–91. *Ultrasound Obstet Gynecol* **4**, 199–204. Retrospective study of the years 1986–91 inclusive. Women demonstrating a raised maternal serum alpha-fetoprotein (MSAFP) level were referred at 17–24 weeks gestation for an ultrasound examination. 49982 women were screened. 1671 (3.3%) were shown to have a raised MSAFP level. Of the latter group, 1325 (79%) went on to have a detailed fetal assessment. Of this group, 4.8% were shown to have incorrect dates and 26.3% had a pregnancy abnormality. Multiple pregnancy accounted for 50% of these abnormalities. There were 70 fetal structural anomalies – 42 were neural tube defects (NTDs). 18 amniocenteses were performed specifically because of poor visualization of the fetus or accentuated maternal risk. Maternal obesity was one limiting factor. No NTDs were missed by ultrasound examination. The authors concluded that high-resolution ultrasound by skilled and experienced personnel allows fetal anatomy to be examined thoroughly to make, or exclude, a diagnosis of spina bifida. The authors therefore recommended a policy of 'restricted' amniocentesis for an elevated MSAFP value. **III B**

5 Jorgensen FS (1999) MULTISCAN – a Scandinavian multi-centre second trimester obstetric ultrasound and serum screening study. *Acta Obstet Gynecol Scand* **78**, 501–510. Multicenter cohort study of 27844 low-risk pregnancies in which routine ultrasound scanning was undertaken between 17 and 19 weeks gestation. Maternal serum alpha-fetoprotein (MSAFP) was taken at the same time in 10264 cases and the resulting prenatal diagnosis rates were compared. The study was undertaken in 1989–1991, in women booking for pregnancy care in maternity units in Scandinavia. The sensitivity for ultrasound detection of neural tube defects was 80% and, although the detection rate was increased in those women having both investigations, the additional sensitivity from MSAFP was small. The improving image quality of prenatal ultrasound can only make the additional sensitivity from MSAFP compared to routine ultrasound scanning alone diminish over time. **III B**

6 Drugan A, Dvorin E, Koppitch FC III *et al.* (1989) Counseling for low maternal serum alpha-fetoprotein should emphasize all chromosome anomalies, not just Down syndrome. *Obstet Gynecol* **73**, 271–274. This study performed diagnostic amniocentesis on 1154 patients who had age-adjusted low maternal serum alpha-fetoprotein (AFP). 13 chromosomally abnormal conceptions were found, with half the cases diagnosed as autosomal trisomies. Additional abnormalities included numbers of sex-chromosome aberrations, deletions or triploidy consistent with numbers seen in an advanced-maternal-age population. The authors' recommendation was that all patients with low serum AFP should be counseled that not just Down syndrome but other aneuploidies might be diagnosed. The risk quoted should be that of all chromosomal abnormalities, which is about twice the risk calculated for Down syndrome. **III B**

7 Gekas J, Gondry J, Mazur S *et al.* (1999) Informed consent to serum screening for Down syndrome: are women given adequate information? *Prenat Diagn* **19**, 1–7. A survey conducted to assess the information given to women during a maternal serum screening (MSS) program. A questionnaire was given to 504 pregnant women attending for amniocentesis after a screen-positive result. The survey was based on 200 useable questionnaires (39.7% of the study sample). Issues pertinent to the amount and quality of information given and informed consent were included. The results revealed the need for a routine consultation with an antenatal care professional before testing to enable pregnant women to give their informed consent to MSS. **III B**

8 Anon (1997) *Fetal abnormalities: guidelines for screening, diagnosis and management.* London: Royal College of Obstetricians and Gynaecologists/Royal College of Paediatrics and Child Health. Report of the joint Working Party of the RCOG and RCPCH. Guidelines based on a critical review of the available evidence, in addition to expert-based recommendations to ensure parents receive the best information and support to make appropriate decisions. **IV C**

9 Accreditation Standards. Presently there is no professional or government requirement for a laboratory to be monitored concerning its own standard of working or publication of results. There is an accreditation system, the Clinical Pathology Accreditation (CPA). Specific test standards are assessed by the UK External Quality Assurance Scheme (UKEQAS). **IV C**

10 Maternal Serum Screening (1996) *ACOG Educ Bull 228*, **September**. This bulletin summarized recognized methods and techniques of clinical practices relative to maternal serum screening. **IV C**

11 Milunsky A, Jick SS, Bruell CL *et al.* (1989) Predictive values, relative risks, and overall benefits of high and low maternal serum α-fetoprotein screening in singleton pregnancies: New epidemiologic data. Am J Obstet Gynecol 161, 291–297. Prospective study of maternal serum alpha-fetoprotein (MSAFP) screening for both high and low values. 13486 women with singleton pregnancies were included in the study – 3.9% had an elevated MSAFP. A high maternal serum alpha-fetoprotein was associated with the following adverse outcomes: neural tube defects (RR = 224), other major congenital defects (RR = 4.7), fetal death (RR = 8.1), neonatal death (RR = 4.7), low birth weight (RR = 4.0), newborn complications (RR = 3.6), oligohydramnios (RR = 3.4), abruptio placentae (RR = 3.0) and preeclampsia (RR = 2.3). **III B**

12 Kelly RB, Nyberg DA, Mack LA *et al.* (1989) Sonography of placental abnormalities and oligohydramnios in women with elevated alpha-fetoprotein levels: comparison with control subjects. *AJR* **153**, 815–819. Observational study: the ultrasound examination that was performed between 18 and 24 weeks gestation in 76 women with an elevated maternal serum alpha-fetoprotein (MSAFP) level was compared with a control group. Patients with fetal malformations, incorrect dates, twins or lack of follow-up were excluded. 27 (36%) of 76 patients with elevated MSAFP levels had placental or amniotic fluid abnormalities compared with only 3 (3%) of 87 control subjects. **III B**

13 Waller DK, Lustig LS, Cunningham GC *et al.* (1991) Second-trimester maternal serum alpha-fetoprotein levels and the risk of subsequent fetal death. *N Engl J Med* **325**, 6–10. Case-control study of 612 women whose pregnancies ended in a fetal death and 2501 women who gave birth to live infants. All of the women had singleton pregnancies and an alpha-fetoprotein (AFP) screening in the second trimester. The authors found that the women with an elevated level of serum AFP in the second trimester of pregnancy had an increased risk of fetal death and the risk was increased until term. Women with an AFP of 3 or more had an odds ratio of 10.4 (95% CI 4.9–22.0) as compared with women who had normal levels of AFP. **IIa B**

14 Yaron Y, Cherry M, Kramer RL *et al.* (1999) Second-trimester maternal serum marker screening: maternal serum α-fetoprotein, β-human chorionic gonadotropin, estriol, and their various combinations as predictors of pregnancy outcome. *Am J Obstet Gynecol* **181**, 968–974. The authors reviewed 60040 patients who underwent maternal serum screening. They found that an increased maternal serum alpha-fetoprotein (>2.5 multiples of the median) was associated with pregnancy-induced hypertension, an increased miscarriage rate, preterm delivery, intrauterine growth restriction, intrauterine fetal death, oligohydramnios and abruptio placentae. **III B**

15 The UK National Screening Committee (NSC) Antenatal Subgroup is formulating standards and guidelines with the recommendation that a regional and local infrastructure is established in England. The introduction of Specialist Coordinators in each maternity unit to manage clinical, educational and audit programs is advocated by 2004. For further information see http://www.nsc.nhs.uk www.nelh.nhs.uk. **IV C**

16 Wald N, Hackshaw AD, Stone R *et al.* (1996) Blood folic acid and vitamin B_{12} in relation to neural tube defects. *Br J Obstet Gynaecol* **103**, 319–324. RCT performed to determine the relation between blood folic acid and serum vitamin B_{12} in neural tube defect pregnancies. Stored blood samples were retrieved from affected pregnancies (27 cases) and unaffected pregnancies (108 matched controls). Samples were collected at entry to the trial, immediately before the woman became pregnant and at around 12 weeks of pregnancy. Results were combined with those from other studies to obtain an overall assessment. Results revealed serum and red-cell folic acid and serum vitamin B_{12} levels were lower in the cases at all three sample collections. This was consistent with other evidence that folic acid and vitamin B_{12} levels are lower in women with neural tube defect pregnancies and consistent with evidence that folic acid is protective. **Ib A**

17 Department of Health (2000) *Folic acid and the prevention of disease. Report of the Committee on Medical Aspects of Food and Nutrition Policy.* London: Department of Health. The Committee on Medical Aspects of Food and Nutrition Policy (COMA), a committee of independent experts, reviewed the role of folic acid in the prevention of disease. Guidelines were issued to women planning a pregnancy to take folate supplements and consume more folate-rich foods. **IV C**

8.2 Serum screening for fetal chromosomal abnormality

Mike Wyldes and Sharon Hodgkiss

Management option	Quality of evidence	Strength of recommendation	References
Serum screening has been focused on Down syndrome, although it has the potential to detect other chromosomal anomalies (e.g. trisomy 18)	III	B	1
Cost–benefit analysis for screening for Down syndrome relies on the premise that many women will chose to terminate an affected pregnancy	III	B	2
Triple analysis screening – human chorionic gonadotropin (hCG), maternal serum alpha-fetoprotein (MSAFP) and estriol (E3) – at 16–20 weeks is cost-effective	III	B	3

➡

Management option	Quality of evidence	Strength of recommendation	References
Quadruple-analyte screening (hCG, E3, inhibin A and MSAFP) at 16–20 weeks has similar characteristics to triple-analyte screening, with a higher detection rate for Down syndrome	III	B	4
Different centers have adopted different approaches to reporting the risk for trisomy 21: ❑ An arbitrary cut-off point and values above that are 'screen-positive' and those below are 'screen-negative' ❑ Report the actual calculated risk and allow the patient to decide whether that is an acceptable risk, perhaps in comparison with her age-related risk ❑ Combination of the above with women below a certain cut-off being told they are 'low risk', while those who are high risk are given their individual risk, during counseling	–	✓	–
Nuchal translucency measurement at 11–14 weeks is at least as effective as second-trimester serum screening	III	B	5
First-trimester serum screening using free βhCG and pregnancy associated plasma protein (PAPP)-A is as effective as second trimester screening with hCG, MSAFP and E3	III	B	5
Nuchal translucency, first-trimester hCG and PAPP-A and second-trimester hCG MSAFP and E3 seem to be independent, may therefore work together synergistically to further enhance efficiency, and may be the most cost-effective method of screening for Down syndrome	III	B	5
All screening programs for fetal chromosomal abnormality should include			
❑ Written agreed protocols for screening, diagnosis and management of elevated risk	IV	C	6
❑ Appropriate and adequate training for all staff involved (pre- and post-test)	III	B	7
❑ Adequate time for presenting and discussing different options and results in a non-directive manner	IV	C	6,8
❑ Adequate documentation and communication	III	B	9
❑ An adequately regulated laboratory and ultrasound department	IV	C	10
❑ Confirmation of abnormality after termination/ delivery by postmortem/neonatal examination	IV	C	6
❑ Ongoing follow-up and support of parents whether choice is to terminate or continue with pregnancy	IV	C	11

References

1 Drugan A, Dvorin E, Koppitch FC III *et al.* (1989) Counseling for low maternal serum alpha-fetoprotein should emphasize all chromosome anomalies, not just Down syndrome. *Obstet Gynecol* **73**, 271–274. This study performed diagnostic amniocentesis on 1154 patients who had age-adjusted low MSAFP. 13 chromosomally abnormal conceptions were found, with half the cases diagnosed as autosomal trisomies. Additional abnormalities included numbers of sex-chromosome aberrations, deletions or triploidy consistent with numbers seen in an advanced maternal-age population. The authors' recommendation was that all patients with low serum AFP should be counseled that not just Down syndrome but other aneuploidies might be diagnosed. The risk quoted should be that of all chromosomal abnormalities, which is about twice the risk calculated for Down syndrome. **III B**

2 Waitzman NJ, Romano PS, Scheffler RM (1994) Estimates of the economic costs of birth defects. *Inquiry* **31**, 188–205. This analysis produces an economic model for a variety of congenital anomalies and addresses the question of cost-effectiveness, assuming sensitivity for identification and estimating the rate of termination following prenatal diagnosis. Using an incidence approach, a comprehensive estimate of 18 of the most clinically significant birth defects in the USA was undertaken, providing the basis for assessing competing strategies for research and prevention. There is no consideration of the negative effects of pregnancies lost through invasive testing, nor the anxiety caused by a

prenatal screening program with high false-positive rates, but there is evidence of cost-effectiveness, especially for non-lethal neural tube defects that carry a high burden of handicap. **III B**

3 Gilbert RE, Augood C, Gupta R et al. (2001) Screening for Down's syndrome: effects, safety and cost effectiveness of first and second trimester strategies. *Br Med J* **323**, 423–425. The study consisted of a comparative analysis of incremental cost-effectiveness of antenatal screening strategies for Down syndrome. Outcome measures, such as the number of liveborn babies with Down syndrome, miscarriages due to diagnostic procedures and health-care costs of a screening program were considered. The study concluded that the choice of screening strategy should be between the integrated test, first-trimester combined test and the quadruple test, or nuchal translucency measurement depending on the service provider's budget and values on safety. Screening based on maternal age, the second-trimester double test and the first-trimester serum test were less effective and more costly than the other four options. **III B**

4 Wenstrom KD, Owen J, Chu D *et al.* (1999) Prospective evaluation of free β-subunit of human chorionic gonadotropin and dimeric inhibin A for aneuploidy detection. *Am J Obstet Gynecol* **181**, 887–892. The study group consisted of women who had a second-trimester multiple-marker screening test (alpha-fetoprotein, unconjugated estriol, human chorionic gonadotropin) and genetic amniocentesis from August 1996 to August 1998. The serum was analyzed for inhibin and the free β-subunit of human chorionic gonadotropin. The authors evaluated 1256 patients, including 23 with aneuploidy. The multiple-marker screening test plus inhibin detected 85% of Down syndrome cases, in comparison with 69% with the multiple-marker screening test alone. The multiple-marker screening test plus inhibin also detected 60% of the other aneuploidies. **III B**

5 SURRUS: The Serum, Urine and Ultrasound Study (expected publication date early 2002). A national 5-year study that looks at the effectiveness of the range of antenatal screening methods available throughout the UK. A comprehensive study that it is envisaged will influence future recommendations for service provision and practice through the National Screening Committee and the National Institute for Clinical Effectiveness. **III B**

6 Anon (1997) *Fetal abnormalities: guidelines for screening, diagnosis and management.* London: Royal College of Obstetricians and Gynaecologists/Royal College of Paediatrics and Child Health. Report of the joint Working Party of the RCOG and RCPCH. Guidelines based on a critical review of the available evidence, in addition to expert-based recommendations to ensure parents receive the best information and support to make appropriate decisions. **IV C**

7 Fairgrieve S, Magnay D, White I *et al.* (1997) Maternal serum screening for Down's syndrome: a survey of midwives' views. *Publ Health* **111**, 383–385. This study was designed to ascertain midwives' views about maternal serum screening and assess whether the introduction of screening coordinators had affected the widespread variation in practice relating to antenatal screening. 133 midwives were surveyed and 90 (67.7%) responded. 51.2% reported that the introduction of a coordinator had improved staff education but 76.6% requested further input. The study recommended the ongoing training provision. **III B**

8 Lawrence S (1999) Counselling for Down's syndrome screening. *Br J Midwifery* **7**, 368–370. This article reviews several studies relating to psychotherapy and non-directive counseling for Down's syndrome screening. Recommendations are made, based on the review by eminent counselors and geneticists, for future practice. It emphasized the importance of effective, evidence-based training to enable health professionals to facilitate parents in the decision-making process. **IV C**

9 Murray J, Cuckle H, Sehmi I *et al.* (2001) Quality of written information in Down syndrome screening. *Prenat Diagn* **21**, 138–142. A qualitative assessment was performed on 81 leaflets used in maternal serum screening from the National Health Service obstetric units and private screening services. Quality was assessed and scored using different variables. 14% included all eight factual items as recommended by the Royal College of Obstetricians and Gynaecologists, 7% were well presented and 12% easy to interpret. The overall quality score of 40% or less was allocated to 19% of leaflets. Generally the standard was poor and recommendations were made for a national peer-reviewed leaflet that can be modified to suit local policy. **III B**

10 Standards for laboratory and ultrasound. Currently, biochemical laboratories have no recognized national standards. However, they can become a member of an external quality assurance scheme such as the UK External Quality Assurance Scheme (UKEQAS), and accreditation with the Clinical Pathology Accreditation (CPA) for biochemistry. Ultrasound departments also have no national requirements at present but adhere to guidelines from the Royal Colleges and can achieve quality assurance from the Fetal Medicine Foundation on nuchal translucency measurements. **IV C**

11 There are many voluntary agencies relevant to specific abnormalities, which offer support through the full experience for parents and their families. ARC (Antenatal Results and Choices), previously known as SAFTA (Support Around Termination for Abnormality), offers a comprehensive, unbiased support structure through a national and local network. **IV C**

8.3 The routine obstetric ultrasound scan

Ellen Knox and Mike Wyldes

Management option		Quality of evidence	Strength of recommendation	References
General	**Prerequisites**			
	❑ Details of history, examination, and routine investigations for pregnancy completed and known relevant risk factors identified	–	✔	–
	❑ Relevant serology and genetic concerns specified	–	✔	–
	❑ Prescan interview, discussions and counseling	–	✔	–
	Preparation			
	❑ High resolution real-time gray-scale ultrasound machine	IV	C	1
	❑ Experienced sonographer	III	B	2
	❑ Semirecumbent comfortable mother	–	✔	–
	❑ Screen visible to mother and sonographer	IIb	B	3
	❑ Documentation (varies)	III	B	4
	❑ Written report	–	✔	–
	❑ Hard copy/video/image capture system to preserve image	–	✔	–
	❑ Appropriate follow-up of problems	Ib	A	5
	It is considered to be safe in both short and long term	Ib IV	A C	6 7
	Benefits			
	❑ Diagnosis of certain abnormalities (but not all)	Ib	A	8
	❑ Earlier diagnosis of multiple pregnancy	Ib	A	9
	❑ Location of placental site enhanced	IIb	B	10
	❑ Maternal bonding and psychological wellbeing enhanced	IIb	B	11
	❑ Accurate dating of pregnancy	III	B	12
First-trimester scan	**Comment**			
	❑ Currently complementary to mid-trimester scan (and serum screening, if offered) for detection of fetal anomalies	IIb	B	13
	Content			
	❑ Nuchal translucency thickness	IIb	B	14
	❑ Establish dating (CRL)	III	B	15
	❑ Number of fetuses, and chorionicity if multiple	IIb	B	16
	❑ Establish viability	IIb	B	17
	❑ Evaluate gross fetal anatomy	IIb	B	13
	❑ Examine uterus and adnexal structures	IV	C	18
18–20 week scan	**Comment**			
	❑ If offered, serum screening result should be known before this scan	IIb	B	19
	❑ Benefit of bonding	III	B	20
	❑ Importance of documentation	III	B	4
	Content			
	❑ Confirm viability	–	✔	–
	❑ Check dating/gestational age	IIb	B	21
	❑ Confirm fetal number	IIa	B	22

➡

Management option		Quality of evidence	Strength of recommendation	References
18–20 week scan (cont'd)	**Content (cont'd)**			
	❑ Examine anatomy	Ib	A	23
	❑ Apply the local policy for soft markers	Ia	A	24
	❑ Specific examinations with indications,			
	e.g. fetal echocardiography	IV	C	25
	maternal cervical length	IIb	B	26
Third-trimester scan	**Comment**			
	❑ Generally these are targeted scans; no evidence of benefit from 'routine' scans	Ib	A	27
	Content depends on indication			
	❑ Anatomy	IIb	B	28
	❑ Growth	IIb	B	29
	❑ Doppler: no evidence of benefit in 'routine' use	Ia	A	30
	but evidence of benefit in 'high risk'	Ia	A	31
	❑ Biophysical profile score (no evidence of benefit but small trial numbers)	Ia	A	32
	❑ Amniotic fluid (trials show no evidence of benefit and increased intervention rates)	Ib	A	33
	❑ Presentation	IIa	B	34
	❑ Placenta	IIb	B	10
	❑ Uterus and adnexa	IIb	B	35

References

1 Morgan CL, Trought WS, Haney A *et al.* (1979) Applications of real-time ultrasound in obstetrics: the linear and dynamically focused phased arrays. *J Clin Ultrasound* **7**, 108–114. The authors' experience of real-time ultrasound compared with linear arrays is discussed and it is concluded that the former provide greater resolution and an improved gray scale. The advantages of this system are discussed. **IV C**

2 Bernaschek G, Steumpflen I, Deutinger J (1996) The influence of the experience of the investigator on the rate of sonographic diagnosis of fetal malformations in Vienna. *Prenat Diagn* **16**, 807–811. Evaluation of all 323 cases of fetal malformations registered by the obstetric departments of Vienna or registered by the Vienna perinatal mortality statistics of 1990–91. The medical charts or patient hand-held antenatal records were used for analysis. Obstetricians in private hospitals detected 22% of abnormalities, hospital examiners 40% and the examiner in the center for prenatal diagnosis and therapy 90%. The detection rate before the 24th week of gestation was significantly different. **III B**

3 Hyde B (1986) An interview study of pregnant women's attitudes to ultrasound scanning. *Soc Sci Med* **22**, 587–592. Interview study of 404 women in the antenatal clinics of two hospitals – one with a routine ultrasound policy, the other with a selective policy. Most who had been scanned were positive about the procedure but the inability to see the screen and receive feedback was an important source of dissatisfaction. **IIb B**

4 Smulian JC, Vintzileos AM, Rodis JF *et al.* (1996) Community-based obstetrical ultrasound reports: documentation of compliance with suggested minimum standards. *J Clin Ultrasound* **24**, 123–127. The minimum standards were those published by the American College of Obstetricians and Gynecologists and the American Institute of Ultrasound in Medicine. First-trimester reports from both obstetric offices and radiological facilities showed poor compliance with either standard. None of the second- or third-trimester reports had completed compliance with either set of standards. The importance of clear documentation is highlighted. **III B**

5 Saari-Kemppainen A (1995) Use of antenatal care services in a controlled ultrasound screening trial. *Acta Obstet Gynecol Scand* **74**, 12–14. 9310 women were randomized to an ultrasound screening or a control group. The screening group had an ultrasound scan at 16–20 weeks gestation but otherwise antenatal care was identical. Ultrasound screening reduced the need for antenatal outpatient services but increased the use of maternal health centers, emphasizing the need for adequate follow up. **Ib A**

6 Kieler H, Ahlsten G, Haglund B et al. (1998) Routine ultrasound screening in pregnancy and the children's subsequent neurologic development. *Obstet Gynecol* **91**, 750–756. Follow-up study of 3265 children aged 8–9 whose mothers participated in a randomized controlled trial of ultrasound screening during pregnancy. There was no significant difference in the frequency of impaired neurological development in either exposed or nonexposed groups. **Ib A**

7 Barnett SB, Rott HD, ter Haar GR *et al.* (1997) The sensitivity of biological tissue to ultrasound. *Ultrasound Med Biol* **23**, 805–812. The known effects of ultrasound on pre- and postnatal tissues are evaluated. There is a biologically significant increase in temperature at or near the bone of the fetus if the beam is held stationary for more than 30s. However, a consequent deleterious effect has not been demonstrated. **IV C**

8 Saari-Kemppainen A, Karjalainen O, Ylostalo P et al. (1994) Fetal anomalies in a controlled one-stage ultrasound screening trial. A report from the Helsinki Ultrasound Trial. J Perinat Med 22, 279–289. RCT of 4691 screened and 4619 control groups of women in Helsinki 1986–87. The screened group underwent one ultrasound examination between 16 and 20 weeks of pregnancy including a systematic search for fetal anomalies. This resulted in an increased detection rate for fetal anomalies and a reduction in the perinatal mortality rate because of an increase in terminations. Most central nervous system and genitourinary system abnormalities were detected but far fewer anomalies of the heart and gastrointestinal tract were visualized. **Ib A**

9 Neilson JP (2001) Ultrasound for fetal assessment in early pregnancy (Cochrane Review). In: *The Cochrane library*, issue 4. Oxford: Update Software. Review of nine trials of women scanned routinely in early pregnancy (usually before 20 weeks) compared to those with scans for specific indications. Those scanned routinely had better detection of gestational age, earlier detection of clinically unsuspected fetal malformations and earlier detection of multiple pregnancy. The odds ratio of undiagnosed twins in the routinely scanned group at 26 weeks was 0.08 (95% CI 0.04–0.16). **Ia A**

10 Tan NH, Abu M, Woo JL *et al.* (1995) The role of transvaginal sonography in the diagnosis of placenta praevia. *Aust N Z J Obstet Gynecol* **35**, 42–45. Transvaginal ultrasonography was performed on 70 patients diagnosed to have placenta previa on transabdominal ultrasound. The diagnosis was confirmed either by digital examination in theater at term or by operative findings at delivery. The diagnostic accuracy of transabdominal ultrasound was 75.5% and transvaginal ultrasound was 92.8%. There were no complications or exacerbations of bleeding. **IIb B**

11 Reading AE, Platt LD (1985) Impact of fetal testing on maternal anxiety. *J Reprod Med* **30**, 907–910. The maternal impact of high-feedback ultrasonography, low-feedback ultrasonography, fetal heart rate monitoring and video of an ultrasound were compared. There was a significant reduction in maternal anxiety before and after testing, the most pronounced of which was in those women undergoing high-feedback ultrasonography. **IIb B**

12 Chervenak FA, Skupski DW, Romero R *et al.* (1998) How accurate is fetal biometry in the assessment of fetal age? *Am J Obstet Gynecol* **178**, 678–687. Retrospective study of 152 singleton, 67 twin and 19 triplet gestations resulting from *in-vitro* fertilization, comparing gestational age as defined by fetal biometry at 14–22 weeks and a gestation age prediction equation. Fetal biometry proved accurate and head circumference was the most accurate parameter. **III B**

13 Whitlow BJ, Chatzipapas IK, Lazanakis ML *et al.* (1999) The value of sonography in early pregnancy for the detection of fetal abnormalities in an unselected population. *Br J Obstet Gynaecol* **106**, 923–936. Prospective cross sectional study of 6634 sequential unselected women. All underwent transabdominal sonography and, if the anatomy scan was considered incomplete, they also underwent a transvaginal examination. Nuchal translucency was also performed. The overall detection rate for structurally abnormal fetuses was 59% in early pregnancy (11–14 weeks) and 81% in combination with a second trimester scan. **IIb B**

14 Snijders RJ, Noble P, Sebire N *et al.* (1998) UK multicentre project on the assessment of risk of trisomy 21 by maternal age and fetal nuchal translucency thickness at 10–14 weeks of gestation. *Lancet* **352**, 343–346. Multicentre study of 96127 women, investigated for their risk of trisomy 21 by a combination of maternal age and nuchal translucency thickness at 10–14 weeks gestation. Risk was calculated by maternal age, gestational-age-related prevalence and multiplied by a likelihood ratio derived from the deviation from normal of the nuchal translucency measurement. The sensitivity of a cut-off risk of 1/300 was investigated. Phenotype was derived from fetal karyotype or clinical examination of liveborn infants. The estimated trisomy 21 risk was more than 1/300 for 8.3% of normal pregnancies, 82.2% of those with trisomy 21 and 77.9% of those with other chromosomal defects. 80% of affected pregnancies were identified using the above screening method to determine those offered invasive testing. **IIb B**

15 Evans J (1991) Fetal crown–rump length values in the first trimester based upon ovulation timing using the luteinizing hormone surge. *Br J Obstet Gynaecol* **98**, 48–51. Fetal crown–rump length (CRL) was measured weekly in 33 singleton pregnancies conceived after *in-vitro* fertilization, gamete intrafallopian transfer or natural intercourse in monitored infertility treatment cycles. There was no difference in the CRL between different infertility groups. However the CRL was found to be smaller than the CRL measurement from pregnancies where the gestational age was based on the last menstrual period. **III B**

16 Sepulveda W, Sebire NJ, Hughes K *et al.* (1996) The lambda sign at 10–14 weeks of gestation as a predictor of chorionicity in twin pregnancies. *Ultrasound Obstet Gynecol* **7**, 421–423. Prospective determination of chorionicity in 369 twin pregnancies at 10–14 weeks using absence of the lambda sign within a single placental mass to demonstrate monochorionicity. Dichorionicity was defined as presence of the lambda sign or nonadjacent placentas. Pregnancy outcome was available in 279 cases and all 63 pregnancies classified as monochorionic resulted in the delivery of single-sex twins. There were 100 different sex pairs that were correctly classified as dichorionic. **IIb B**

17 Pandya PP, Snijders RJ, Psara N *et al.* (1996) The prevalence of non-viable pregnancy at 10–13 weeks of gestation. *Ultrasound Obstet Gynecol* **7**, 170–173. Cross-sectional ultrasound study of 17870 women at 10–13 weeks gestation. Early pregnancy failure was found in 2.8%. **IIb B**

18 Fleischer AC, Shah DM, Entman SS (1990) Sonographic evaluation of maternal disorders during pregnancy. *Radiol Clin North Am* **28**, 51–58. Review of the role of ultrasonography in pregnancy, concluding that there is a role in detecting and monitoring pelvic masses that appear in pregnancy. **IV C**

19 Jorgensen FS, Valentin L, Salvesen KA *et al.* (1999) MULTISCAN – a Scandinavian multicentre second trimester obstetric ultrasound and serum screening study. *Acta Obstet Gynecol Scand* **78**, 501–510. Prospective multicenter study of 27844 low-risk women, undertaken between 1989 and 1991, to determine detection rates for neural tube defects (NTD), abdominal wall defects (AWD) and Down syndrome using ultrasound and serum screening. All had ultrasound in the second trimester and a subgroup (10264) had both ultrasound and serum screening. Ultrasound produced a low detection for Down syndrome (6.3%) and an acceptable rate for NTD (79.4%) and AWD (85.7%). However, in the group that had both tests, serum screening performed better than ultrasound, especially regarding Down syndrome. **IIb B**

20 Cox DN, Wittmann BK, Hess M *et al.* (1987) The psychological impact of diagnostic ultrasound. *Obstet Gynecol* **70**, 673–676. The psychological impact of scanning in pregnancy was examined in both high- and low-risk pregnancies. Both had either high feedback in the form of extensive visual and verbal interaction or low feedback in which they were denied access to the monitor. Those in the former group had more positive emotional experiences and less anxiety as assessed by the State Anxiety Inventory and the Subjective Stress scale. **III B**

21 Campbell S, Warsof SL, Little D *et al.* (1985) Routine ultrasound screening for the prediction of gestational age. *Obstet Gynecol* **65**, 613–620. The consecutive pregnancies of 4527 women were scanned and the gestational age was determined by both menstrual age and crown–rump length or biparietal diameter. The estimated delivery dates based on menstrual history and ultrasound measurements were compared. Crown–rump length measurements were as predictive as optimal menstrual history but biparietal diameter measurements between 12 and 18 weeks gestation were significantly more accurate. **IIb B**

22 Hughey MJ, Olive DL (1985) Routine ultrasound scanning for the detection and management of twin pregnancies. *J Reprod Med* **30**, 427–430. Routine scanning of 1551 private patients to detect twins, compared with 5950 private patients who acted as controls and underwent scanning only when indicated. There was a significant increase in the early detection of twins in the study group. In addition there was a significant improvement in outcome in the study group due to a reduction in the incidence of low birth weight, smallness for gestational age, prematurity, depressed Apgar scores and stillbirths. **IIa B**

23 Saari-Kemppainen A, Karjalainen O, Ylostalo P *et al.* (1994) Fetal anomalies in a controlled one-stage ultrasound screening trial. A report from the Helsinki Ultrasound Trial. *J Perinat Med* **22**, 279–289. RCT of women at 16–20 weeks gestation randomized to either ultrasound scan (4691) or not (4619). Otherwise their care was identical. Screening included a search for fetal anomalies. In the screening group 40% of abnormalities were detected, most of the anomalies of the central nervous system and genitourinary system but far fewer of the heart and gastrointestinal tract. In this study detection of major fetal abnormalities in the screening group caused a reduction in perinatal mortality. **Ib A**

24 Smith-Bindman R, Hosmer W, Feldstein VA *et al.* (2001) Second trimester ultrasound to detect fetuses with Down Syndrome – a meta analysis. *JAMA* **285**, 1044–1055. Meta-analysis of the accuracy of the soft markers: nuchal fold, echogenic bowel, echogenic foci in the fetal heart, renal pyelectasis, choroid plexus cyst and humeral and femoral shortening, in the detection of Down syndrome. Using any soft marker in isolation as an indication for karyotyping results in more fetal losses than cases of Down syndrome detected. The likelihood of Down syndrome does not decrease substantially after normal ultrasound findings. **Ia A**

25 Copel JA, Pilu G, Kleinman CS (1986) Congenital heart disease and extra cardiac anomalies: associations and indications for fetal echocardiography. *Am J Obstet Gynecol* **154**, 1121–1132. Review of the associations and indications for fetal echocardiography. They provided an outline of the specific congenital anomalies with a higher association of cardiac abnormalities. Maternal diabetes and phenylketonuria, as well as exposure to specific medications were also discussed as possible indications for fetal echocardiography. Because of the 5% risk of a chromosome abnormality in fetuses with congenital heart disease, the authors recommended genetic amniocentesis for all patients when a fetal congenital heart defect is diagnosed. **IV C**

26 Heath VC, Daskalakis G, Zagaliki A *et al.* (2000) Cervicovaginal fibronectin and cervical length at 23 weeks of gestation: relative risk of early preterm delivery. *Br J Obstet Gynecol* **107**, 1276–1281. Prospective observational study of 5146 singleton pregnancies assessed at 23 weeks by transvaginal ultrasound to measure cervical length. Of those with a cervical length less than 15 mm managed conservatively the risk of premature delivery (< 33 weeks) was highly significant (odds ratio 46.2, CI 18.8–113.6). **IIb B**

27 Bricker L, Neilson JP (2001) Routine ultrasound in late pregnancy (after 24 weeks gestation) (Cochrane review). In: *The Cochrane library*, issue 4. Oxford: Update Software. Review of seven studies of 25036 women. There was no difference in obstetric, antenatal or neonatal interventions between those women undergoing routine Doppler ultrasound compared with those who did not. Likewise there was no difference in outcome measures and long-term safety was not assessed. **Ia A**

28 Economou G, Egginton JA, Brookfield DS *et al.* (1994) The importance of late pregnancy scans for renal tract abnormalities. *Prenat Diagn* **14**, 177–180. A 12-month prospective population study of 6497 pregnant women to assess ultrasound scanning in late pregnancy for the detection of nonlethal renal anomalies. All women underwent 18–20- and 28–32-week ultrasound scans. 40 fetuses had abnormal antenatal scans and of those 29 had renal abnormalities confirmed postnatally. Only 6 were detected at the earlier scan, suggesting that a late scan is needed to detect nonlethal renal abnormalities. **Ib B**

29 Harding K, Evans S, Newnham J (1995) Screening for the small fetus: a study of the relative efficiency of ultrasound biometry and symphysiofundal height. *Aust N Z Obstet Gynaecol* **35**, 160–164. 1135 women were screened for birthweight below the 10th centile using three different methods, alone and in combination: symphysiofundal height measurement, amniotic fluid index and ultrasound imaging, at 18, 24, 28, 34 and 38 weeks. The best test was fetal abdominal circumference measurement by ultrasound. Selecting at-risk pregnancies by symphysiofundal height measurement first prior to ultrasound reduces the false-positive rate at the expense of sensitivity. **IIb B**

30 Bricker L, Neilson JP (2001) Routine Doppler ultrasound in pregnancy (Cochrane Review). In: *The Cochrane library*, issue 4. Oxford: Update Software. Review of five randomized trials of 14 338 women. Three trials were involved in a meta-analysis of perinatal mortality. There was no difference in antenatal, obstetric or neonatal intervention and no differences in short-term outcomes such as perinatal mortality. Long-term neurodevelopmental outcomes and maternal psychological outcomes were not addressed. **Ia A**

31 Neilson JP, Alfirevic Z (2001) Doppler ultrasound for fetal assessment in high risk pregnancies (Cochrane review). In: *The Cochrane library*, issue 4. Oxford: Update Software. Review of 11 randomized studies involving nearly 7000 women. Doppler ultrasound compared with no Doppler ultrasound in high-risk pregnancy was associated with a trend in reduction in perinatal deaths. There was also a reduction in induction of labour and admissions to hospital. There was no difference in fetal distress in labour or cesarean section rate between the two groups. **Ia A**

32 Alfirevic Z, Neilson JP (2001) Biophysical profile for fetal assessment in high risk pregnancies (Cochrane review). In: *The Cochrane library*, issue 4. Oxford: Update Software. Meta-analysis of four trials including 2839 women showed no benefit or harm of the use of the biophysical profile on outcome measures in high-risk pregnancy. However the sample size was too small to show any difference in serious outcome measures such as perinatal death or low Apgar score. One small trial showed an increase in the number of inductions of labor in the biophysical profile group. **Ia A**

33 Alfirevic Z, Luckas SM, Walkinshaw SA *et al.* (1997) A randomised comparison between amniotic fluid index and maximum pool depth in the monitoring of post term pregnancy. *Br J Obstet Gynaecol* **104**, 207–211. RCT of 500 singleton uncomplicated pregnancies at term + 10, showing that amniotic fluid index was more likely to label the pregnancy as abnormal and lead to subsequent intervention. **Ib A**

34 Tadmor OP, Rabinowitz R, Alon L *et al.* (1994) Can breech presentation at birth be predicted from ultrasound examinations during the second or third trimesters? *Int J Gynaecol Obstet* **46**, 11–14. Retrospective longitudinal investigation of ultrasound examination in the second and third trimester of 157 breech deliveries and 1325 controls (vertex deliveries). At the 15–19-week ultrasound, 63.2% of the breech delivery group and 55.2% of the vertex group were presenting as breech. However, after 25 weeks there was a statistically significant difference between those in the breech delivery group (70.6%) and those in the vertex delivery group (28.9%) presenting as breech on ultrasound scan. Therefore patients found to be breech on ultrasound at 25 weeks or later are at high risk for malpresentation at delivery. **IIa B**

35 Hill LM, Martin JG, Deutsch K *et al.* (1996) Sonographic visualization of the ovaries throughout pregnancy. *Obstet Gynecol* **88**, 830–832. Cross-sectional study of 5617 pregnant women at 5.0–39.9 weeks gestation. The visualization rate for one or both normal ovaries, as well as their position above or below the umbilicus, was recorded for one examination in each patient. As gestational age advanced there was a significant decrease in the visualization of the ovaries and an increase in the percentage seen above the ovaries. **IIb B**

Chapter 9

Invasive fetal procedures

9.1 Chorion villus sampling and placental biopsy

Simon Grant

Chorion villus sampling in comparison with amniocentesis

Management option	Quality of evidence	Strength of recommendation	References
Inconsistent evidence over comparative safety:			
❑ Overall loss rate similar at equivalent gestation	Ib	A	1
	III	B	2
❑ Loss rate higher with chorion villus sampling (OR: 1.33)	Ia	A	3
Higher loss rate with multiple attempts	III	B	4
Operator experience affects loss rate with:			
❑ Chorion villus sampling	IIb	B	2
❑ Amniocentesis	III	B	5

References

1 Canadian Collaborative CVS–Amniocentesis Clinical Trial Group (1989) Multicentre randomised clinical trial of chorion villus sampling and amniocentesis. *Lancet* **1**, 1–6. Multicentre RCT including 2787 women over 35 years at expected date of delivery, randomized to transcervical chorion villus sampling (CVS) at 9–12/40 or amniocentesis at 15–17 weeks, with 396 excluded after randomization, leaving comparable groups, demographically and numerically. More women allocated to amniocentesis did not have the procedure (13% vs. 9%) but overall loss rates were similar (7.6% CVS vs. 7.0% amniocentesis, spontaneous/induced), with maximum possible difference in loss rates of 2.4%, based on 95% CI. There was a nonsignificant trend towards later loss in the CVS group, with a higher rate of late pregnancy loss (higher crude perinatal mortality rate and rate of stillbirth after 28/40) for no obvious reason. **Ib A.**

2 Young SR, Shipley CF, Wade RV *et al.* (1991) Single center comparison of 1000 prenatal diagnoses with chorionic villus sampling and 1000 diagnoses with amniocentesis. *Am J Obstet Gynecol* **165**, 255–263. Comparative study of 1000 each chorion villus sampling (CVS) and amniocentesis. Indicates CVS to be safe and accurate alternative to amniocentesis. **IIb B.**

3 Alfirevic Z, Gosden CM, Neilson JP *et al.* (2000) Chorion villus sampling versus amniocentesis for prenatal diagnosis. In: *Cochrane database of systematic reviews*, issue 3. Oxford: Update Software. Systematic review of randomized trials comparing first-trimester chorion villus sampling (CVS) and second-trimester sampling and technical failures, more false-positive and false-negative results. Pregnancy loss was also more common after CVS (OR 1.33, 95% CI 1.17–1.52). Concluded that benefits of earlier diagnosis with CVS must be set against increased chance of pregnancy loss. **Ia A**

4 Rhoads GG, Jackson LG, Schlesselman SE *et al.* (1989) The safety and efficacy of chorionic villus sampling for early prenatal diagnosis of cytogenetic abnormalities. *N Engl J Med* **320**, 609–617. Multicenter observational study of 2278 women undergoing transcervical chorion villus sampling (CVS) and 671 undergoing amniocentesis. Cytogenetic diagnosis made in 97.8% of those who had CVS and 99.4% who had amniocentesis, ($p < 0.05$), with respectively aneuploidy in 1.8% and 1.4% of diagnoses made. 0.8% of women who had CVS subsequently had amniocentesis because of diagnostic ambiguity. Two diagnoses of aneuploidy were false positives (one of tetraploidy and one of T22). No errors in identification of major trisomies (13, 18, 21). Combined loss rate for all reasons of 7.2% in CVS group, compared with 5.7% in amniocentesis group, adjusted to an excess of only 0.8% allowing for differences in maternal age and gestation (80% CI 0.6–2.2). There was a higher rate of loss of normal fetuses if three or four CVS attempts were made, compared to those with only one (10.8% vs 2.9%, $p < 0.01$). No serious maternal infections. **III B** – underpowered according to Firth 1997.

5 Wiener JJ, Farrow A, Farrow SC *et al.* (1990) Audit of amniocentesis from a district general hospital: is it worth it? *Br Med J* **300**, 1243–1245. Retrospective audit of 469 procedures. Showed higher rate of failure to obtain amniotic fluid among several obstetricians carrying out just over 12% of the procedures, compared to the remaining 87%+ performed by one individual. Draws conclusions about audit of individuals' practice that are questionable as they rely on outdated information systems. **III B**

Chorion villus sampling alone

Management option	Quality of evidence	Strength of recommendation	References
Conflicting evidence over risk of limb deficiencies			
❑ Not procedure-related	III	B	1
❑ Limb deficiencies increase if procedure before 9 weeks gestation	Ia	A	2
Transcervical versus transabdominal: no difference in outcome	Ib	A	3
Transabdominal chorion villus sampling safer than early amniocentesis	Ia	A	4

References

1 Schloo R, Miny P, Holzgreve W *et al.* (1992) Distal limb deficiency following chorionic villus sampling? *Am J Med Genet* **42**, 404–413. Descriptive study of 2537 women undergoing transcervical and 763 transabdominal chorion villus sampling (CVS) in the first trimester and 548 transabdominal placental biopsies in the second. 85 transabdominal and 551 transcervical procedures were done at 66 days or earlier. Outcome data available on 2836 pregnancies after first trimester CVS, with 137 spontaneous abortions before 28 weeks. 16 anatomical defects were found: 5 heart defects, 4 isolated cleft lip/palate, 4 limb defects, one each of hypospadias, gastroschisis and multiple malformation. Two cases of limb defects had a family history of limb defects. Concluded that it was doubtful that defects were all due to CVS and suggested other possible mechanisms for abnormalities noted in previously reported literature. **III B**

2 Firth H (1997) Chorion villus sampling and limb deficiency – cause or coincidence? *Prenat Diagn* **17**, 1313–1330. Review of recent data on true incidence of abnormalities, previous trials, cohort studies, meta-analyses of cohort and case-controlled studies and international voluntary registry of chorion villus sampling (CVS). Also reviewed data relating to temporal association between CVS and limb defects and information relating to possible mechanisms of injury. Points out limits of sensitivity of clinical trials in identifying rare outcomes and importance of gestational age in assessing safety of procedures. Suggests diminishing risk for transverse limb defects with advancing gestation. The risk extends through the period of limb morphogenesis and slightly beyond, with a 10–20× risk at 9 weeks and below and levels approaching or only a few-fold above background at 11 weeks. **Ia A**

3 Brambati B, Terzian E, Tognoni G (1991) Randomized clinical trial of transabdominal versus transcervical chorionic villus sampling methods. *Prenat Diagn* **11**, 285–293. RCT of transcervical and transabdominal chorion villus sampling, including 1194 women and producing demographically and numerically similar groups. Randomized at 7–12 weeks at time of sampling. Overall fetal loss rate after randomization 16.5% transabdominal (TA) and 15.5% transcervical (TC), with procedures equally effective, with no failures or diagnostic errors. Fewer insertions with TA, more material with TC. Comment that numbers limit the interpretation of the data and that results in some ways inconclusive, with choice between procedures dependent on operator choice. **Ib A**

4 Alfirevic Z (2000) Early amniocentesis versus transabdominal chorion villus sampling for prenatal diagnosis. In: *Cochrane database of systematic reviews*, issue 3. Oxford: Update Software. Systematic review of randomized trials comparing early amniocentesis with transabdominal chorion villus sampling (CVS), again identifying three studies. No difference in laboratory failures, or women with chromosomal abnormalities. Total pregnancy loss (6.2% versus 5%, RR 1.24, 95% CI 0.85–1.81), spontaneous miscarriage (4.4% versus 2.3%, RR 1.92, 95% CI 1.14–3.23) and talipes were all more common in the amniocentesis group. Sampling failure was more common in the CVS group, in which more women therefore required repeat procedures, as were hemangiomas. Concludes that CVS is safer but associated with more technical failures. **Ia A**

9.2 Amniocentesis

Simon Grant

Management option	Quality of evidence	Strength of recommendation	References
Higher rate of miscarriage than in control group	Ib	A	1
Early amniocentesis (11–12 weeks): higher loss rate than amniocentesis in second trimester	Ib	A	2
Ultrasound guidance increases the success rate	III	B	3
Transplacental versus nontransplacental: no difference in the miscarriage rate	III	B	4
Transplacental amniocentesis increases the feto–maternal hemorrhage rate	III	B	3
Experience increases the success rate	III	B	5

References

1 Tabor A, Philip J, Madsen M et al. (1986) Randomised controlled trial of genetic amniocentesis in 4606 low-risk women. *Lancet* **1**, 1287–1293. RCT of 4606 women at no known increased risk of genetic disease, assessing procedure related risk of miscarriage and the hypothesis that amniocentesis predisposes to postural deformities and neonatal respiratory disorders. Population-based study excluding high-risk groups, those with complicating factors and those declining, randomizing to either ultrasound-guided amniocentesis or ultrasound alone, with a small number (66) excluded after randomization. Amniocentesis between less than 14 and over 20 weeks. Higher rate of miscarriage in study group, after 16th week associated with raised serum alpha-fetoprotein, placental puncture, 'miscolored' amniotic fluid and also higher rate of pregnancy complications (pain, amniotic fluid leakage) and of respiratory distress syndrome, pneumonia, intubation and treatment with antibiotics **Ib A**

2 The Canadian Early and Midtrimester Amniocentesis Trial (CEMAT) Group (1998) Randomised trial to assess safety and fetal outcome of early and midtrimester amniocentesis. *Lancet* **351**, 242–247. Randomized study allocating women to amniocentesis between 11 + 0 and 12 + 0 weeks or between 15 + 0 and 16 + 0 weeks gestation. Same criteria for amniocentesis at both times. Showed early amniocentesis to be associated with increased risks of fetal loss and talipes. **Ib A**

3 Crandon AJ, Peel KR (1979) Amniocentesis with and without ultrasound guidance. *Br J Obstet Gynaecol* **86**, 1–3. Comparative study of amniocentesis under ultrasound guidance (284) and without ultrasound guidance (140). Ultrasound guidance increased the success rate from 80% to 99.6%, decreased the incidence of feto–maternal hemorrhage from 8.5% to 2.8% and decreased bloodstaining of amniotic fluid from 43.5% to 17.6%. **III B**

4 Giorlandino C, Mobili L, Bilancioni E *et al.* (1994) Transplacental amniocentesis: is it really a higher-risk procedure? *Prenat Diagn* **14**, 803–806. Prospective descriptive study of transplacental and nontransplacental amniocentesis and associated complications. Showed no difference in miscarriage rate but higher rate of amniotic fluid leakage in nontransplacental amniocentesis. Raises concern over risk of feto–maternal hemorrhage in transplacental procedure, although making no comment on the rate of transplacental hemorrhage. **III B**

5 Wiener JJ, Farrow A, Farrow SC *et al.* (1990) Audit of amniocentesis from a district general hospital: is it worth it? *Br Med J* **300**, 1243–1245. Retrospective audit of 469 procedures. Showed higher rate of failure to obtain amniotic fluid among several obstetricians carrying out just over 12% of the procedures, compared to the remaining 87%+ performed by one individual. Draws conclusions about audit of individuals' practice that are questionable as they rely on outdated information systems. **III B**

9.3 Fetal blood sampling before labor

Simon Grant

Advances in molecular genetics, cytogenetic techniques and Doppler imaging have greatly reduced the list of indications for fetal blood sampling. It continues to play a pivotal role in the management of isoimmunized pregnancies (see **Section 15.1**).

Management option	Quality of evidence	Strength of recommendation	References
Procedure-related pregnancy loss rate, 1.4–4.3%,	III	B	1,2,3
❑ Is related to:			
- gestational age	III	B	2,3
- procedure duration, i.e. operator experience	III	B	2,3
- number of needle insertions	III	B	2
- umbilical artery puncture rather than intrahepatic	III	B	4
- indication for procedure – increased for intrauterine growth restriction and karyotypically abnormal fetuses	III	B	3,4,5
❑ Is increased if free loop rather than placental cord insertion is sampled	III	B	6

References

1 Orlandi F, Damiani G, Jakil C *et al.* (1990) The risks of early cordocentesis (12–21 weeks): analysis of 500 cases. *Prenat Diagn* **10**, 425–428. Descriptive study of 500 cases of cordocentesis between 12 and 21 weeks and the associated risks. Safety data related to 370 continuing pregnancies, for which follow-up data could be obtained. There were 16 (4.3%) fetal losses, 22 (5.9%) premature deliveries and no other reported complications. Identified four adverse prognostic factors and found fall in fetal loss rate (to 2.5%) after 19–21 weeks. **III B**

2 Levi-Setti PE, Buscaglia M, Ferrazzi E *et al.* (1989) Evaluation of the fetal risk after echo-guided blood sampling from the umbilical cord in the second trimester of pregnancy. *Ann Obstet Ginecol Med Perinat* **110**, 89–97. Descriptive study of 222 pregnancies with normal fetuses that had undergone cordocentesis in the second trimester, because of suspicion of disease. Fetal loss rate was 4.1%. Fetal risk related to gestational age, duration of procedure and number of needle insertions to the abdomen. **III B**

3 Ghidini A, Sepulveda W, Lockwood CJ *et al.* (1993) Complications of fetal blood sampling. *Am J Obstet Gynecol* **168**, 1339–1344. Review of literature on complications of fetal blood sampling. Three main indicators of risk: gestational age, operator's experience and the indication for procedure. Loss rate estimated for low-risk population (after excluding fetuses with pathology) from pooled data from series with more than 100 cases. Loss rate with experienced operator carries about a 1.4% risk of fetal loss before 28 weeks and 1.4% risk of perinatal death after 28 weeks. **III B**

4 Weiner CP, Okamura K (1996) Diagnostic fetal blood sampling – technique related losses. *Fetal Diagn Ther* **11**, 169–175. Observational study of cordocentesis using fixed needle guide (25 operators in two centers). 1260 procedures, 12 losses (0.9%). No relationship between losses and number of prior procedures performed by operator. Losses associated with umbilical artery puncture. For diagnoses excluding chromosome abnormality or severe fatal intrauterine growth restriction, loss rate was 0.2%. Compared with loss rates of 1–7% for freehand technique, suggest technique is a variable in loss rates. **III B**

5 Maxwell DJ, Johnson P, Hurley P *et al.* (1991) Fetal blood sampling and pregnancy loss in relation to indication. *Br J Obstet Gynaecol* **98**, 892–897. Descriptive report of relation between indication for procedure and procedure-related loss. Four groups, freehand technique: normal ultrasound, structural abnormality, fetal assessment, nonimmune hydrops. 253 samples, 268 procedures and 51 pregnancy terminations. 51/202 pregnancy losses, 19 (9%) within 2 weeks of procedure, with rates of 1%, 7%, 14% and 25% in the four groups respectively. Risk of procedure increased in abnormal pregnancies, reflecting underlying pathology. **III B**

6 Weiner CP, Wenstrom KD, Sipes SL *et al.* (1991) Risk factors for cordocentesis and fetal intravascular transfusion. *Am J Obstet Gynecol* **165**, 1020–1025. Descriptive study (retrospective review) of 594 cordocenteses and 156 intravascular transfusions over 6 years, using needle guide. Number of needle punctures not related to procedure success but lower if placental cord origin used rather than free loop. Bleeding not significant, although longer if artery punctured and after transfusion rather than cordocentesis. Amnionitis complicated 0.5% of procedures, preterm premature rupture of membranes in 0.4%. Fetal bradycardia in 6.6%. Five perinatal losses, all associated with bradycardia, uncorrected rate 0.8%, but all in unsalvageable fetuses. Two independent risk factors for bradycardia, arterial puncture and intrauterine growth restriction. Pancuronium reduced incidence of bradycardia. **III B**

9.4 Fetal tissue biopsy

Simon Grant

There are, to date, no comparative or randomized trials assessing the safety or efficacy of fetal tissue biopsy. This technique has an extremely limited application and is generally restricted to perinatal referral centers.

9.5 Selective reduction of pregnancy

Shantala Vadeyar

Multifetal reduction

Management option		Quality of evidence	Strength of recommendation	References
Careful prior discussion and counseling		–	✔	–
Ideally at 10–12 weeks, although one report of late multifetal pregnancy reduction (MFPR) at 20 weeks		III	B	1
Choice of fetus to be reduced ❑ Technical grounds (avoid fetuses lying over the cervix) ❑ Prenatal cytogenetic diagnosis prior to MFPR		III	B	2
Reduce to two fetuses		–	✔	–
Technique	Transcervical potassium chloride	III	B	3
	Transcervical suction	III	B	3
	Transabdominal potassium chloride	III	B	4
Outcome	MFPR for quadruplets and higher-order multiple pregnancies has an improved perinatal outcome	III	B	5
	MFPR (triplets to twins) has similar perinatal mortality, gestational age at delivery and 'take home' infant rates as expectantly managed triplets	III	B	6
	MFPR (triplets to twins) has better perinatal morbidity than expectantly managed triplet pregnancies (prematurity, low birthweight)	IIa III	B B	7 8–11
	Twin pregnancies following MFPR have similar perinatal outcome to nonreduced twin pregnancies	III	B	11,12
	Twin pregnancies following MFPR have a poorer outcome (fetal and maternal) than spontaneous twin pregnancies	IIa	B	13,14

References

1 Hartoov J, Geva E, Wolman I *et al.* (1998) A 3-year, prospectively designed study of late selective multifetal pregnancy reduction. *Hum Reprod* **13**, 1996–1998. Prospective observational study of 28 patients who underwent multifetal pregnancy reduction (MFPR) at a mean gestational age of 20.2 weeks. The mean gestation at delivery was 36.6 weeks. The authors concluded that late MFPR may facilitate the detection of structural and chromosomal anomalies prior to MFPR and thus selective reduction of the affected fetus, without being associated with an unfavorable perinatal outcome. **III B**

2 DeCatte L, Camus M, Bonduelle M *et al.* (1998) Prenatal diagnosis by chorionic villus sampling in multiple pregnancies prior to fetal reduction. *Am J Perinatol* **15**, 339–343. Descriptive study reporting the results of prenatal diagnosis by chorionic villous sampling (CVS) in 32 pregnancies prior to multifetal pregnancy reduction (MFPR). CVS was carried out at 10.5 weeks followed by MFPR 1 week later. The authors concluded that prenatal cytogenetic diagnosis prior to MFPR is feasible, accurate and safe. Abnormal chromosomal results can indicate the fetus to be reduced but some parents may opt to continue the multifetal pregnancy with the knowledge that the chromosomes are normal. **III B**

3 Mansour RT, Aboulghar MA, Serour GI *et al.* (1999) Multifetal pregnancy reduction: modification of the technique and analysis of outcome. *Fertil Steril* **71**, 380–384. Study describing modified techniques for multifetal pregnancy reduction (MFPR) using transvaginal ultrasonically directed intracardiac KCl (30 cases) and transvaginal ultrasound-guided aspiration of embryonic parts without prior use of KCl (45 cases). The outcome (miscarriage rate, gestational age at delivery, birthweight and pregnancy complications) of these 75 pregnancies was then compared to that of 40 nonreduced twins and 22 higher-order multiple pregnancies. All outcome measures were significantly better in the MFPR group than in the nonreduced high-order multiple pregnancy group and were similar to the outcomes of the nonreduced twin group. **III B**

4 Evans MI, May M, Drugan A *et al.* (1990) Selective termination: clinical experience and residual risks. *Am J Obstet Gynecol* **16**, 1568–1575. Descriptive paper of 22 multifetal pregnancy reductions done by the transabdominal (intracardiac KCl) route. One octuplet, 5 quintuplets, 12 quadruplets and 4 triplets were reduced. There were one early and 4 late pregnancy losses. **III B**

5 Collins MS, Bleyl JA (1990) 71 quadruplet pregnancies: management and outcome. *Am J Obstet Gynecol* **162**, 1384–1392. Observational study of the epidemiology, management and outcome of 71 quadruplet pregnancies from 1980–89. Interventions included bed rest from 16 weeks, cervical cerclage (14%) and tocolytics from 24 weeks (83%). The mean gestational age at delivery was 31.4 weeks and the mean birthweight was 1482 g. The neonatal mortality was 37/1000 and the perinatal mortality was 67/1000 births. **III B**

6 Leonidires MP, Ernst SD, Miller BT *et al.* (2000) Triplets: outcomes of expectant management versus multifetal reduction for 127 pregnancies. *Am J Obstet Gynecol* **183**, 454–459. Comparative multicenter study of triplets conceived via assisted reproductive technology. Outcomes for 81 patients in the expectant group compared with 46 patients in the reduced group showed no significant differences in perinatal mortality, gestation age at delivery or 'take home' infant rates. However, mean birthweights for babies delivered after 24 weeks were significantly lower in the expectant group as compared to the reduced group. **III B**

7 Lipitz S, Reichman B, Uval J *et al.* (1994) A prospective comparison of the outcome of triplet pregnancies managed expectantly or by multifetal reduction to twins. *Am J Obstet Gynecol* **170**, 874–879. Prospective controlled study comparing the outcome of 106 triplet pregnancies managed expectantly versus 34 multifetal pregnancy reduction (MFPR) twin pregnancies. The fetal loss rate before 25 weeks was significantly lower in the MFPR group as were other outcomes such as: prematurity, low birthweight, pregnancy complications, neonatal mortality and morbidity. The authors conclude that MFPR of triplet pregnancies resulted in an improved pregnancy outcome without a concomitant increase in the loss of the entire pregnancy. **IIa B**

8 Boulot P, Vignal J, Vergnes C *et al.* (2000) Multifetal reduction of triplets to twins: a prospective comparison of pregnancy outcome. *Hum Reprod* **15**, 1619–1623. Comparative monocentric study of triplets – 83 with expectant management and 65 undergoing multifetal pregnancy reduction. No statistical difference was noted between the loss rate prior to 24 weeks in the two groups, and the neonatal and perinatal mortality. However, reducing triplets was associated with a significantly lowered incidence of the following: prematurity before 28, 32 and 34 weeks, infant weights under 3rd centile and/or less than 1000, 1500 and 2000 g. The authors concluded that reduction from triplets to twins is effective in improving preterm birth and fetal growth. **III B**

9 Haning RV Jr, Seifer DB, Wheeler CA *et al.* (1996) Effects of fetal number and multifetal reduction on length of in vitro fertilization pregnancies. *Obstet Gynecol* **87**, 964–968. Observational study comparing gestational age at delivery between 162 singletons, 64 twins, 25 twins resulting from multifetal pregnancy reduction (MFPR) from triplets and 9 triplet pregnancies, all resulting from *in-vitro* fertilization in a single center. Triplets delivered 4.9 weeks earlier than nonreduced twins and 3.7 weeks earlier than twins resulting from MFPR. Only 14% of triplet pregnancies underwent spontaneous reduction. The authors concluded that MFPR from triplets was beneficial and increased the duration of gestation. **III B**

10 Macones GA, Schemmer G, Pritts E *et al.* (1993) Multifetal reduction of triplets to twins improves perinatal outcome. *Am J Obstet Gynecol* **169**, 982–986. Comparative study of 63 nonreduced twins, 14 nonreduced triplets and 47 reduced twins (from triplets). The mean gestational age was significantly higher and the perinatal mortality was significantly lower in the reduced group. The authors concluded that multifetal pregnancy reduction from triplets to twins yields an improved outcome. **III B**

11 Yaron Y, Bryant-Greenwood PK, Dave N *et al.* (1999) Multifetal pregnancy reduction of triplets to twins: comparison with nonreduced triplets and twins. *Am J Obstet Gynecol* **180**, 1268–1271. Observational study comparing outcomes of 143 triplet pregnancies reduced to twins, 12 nonreduced triplet pregnancies and 812 nonreduced twin pregnancies over a 10-year period. The mean gestational age at delivery was significantly shorter and the mean birthweights were significantly lower for expectantly managed triplet pregnancies as compared to the multifetal pregnancy reduction (MFPR) group. Pregnancy loss rates, mean length of gestation and mean birthweight did not vary significantly between the MFPR twins and nonreduced twins. **III B**

12 Lipitz S, Uval J, Achiron R et al. (1996) Outcome of twin pregnancies reduced from triplets compared with nonreduced twin gestations. Obstet Gynecol 87, 511–514. Comparative study between 43 multifetal pregnancy reduction (MFPR; triplet to twins) pregnancies that reached 24 weeks, and 134 dichorionic twin pregnancies. Maternal complications such as premature contractions and pregnancy-induced hypertension were the same in both groups. A higher incidence of preterm premature rupture of membranes was noted in the MFPR group, which was of borderline significance. The mean gestational age, low birthweight prevalence and respiratory disorders were not significantly different in the two groups. **III B**

13 Groutz A, Yovel I, Amit A *et al.* (1996) Pregnancy outcome after multifetal pregnancy reduction to twins compared with spontaneously conceived twins. *Hum Reprod* **11**, 1334–1336. Prospective case-control study comparing pregnancy outcomes in three groups – 10 quadruplet pregnancies reduced to twins, 30 triplet pregnancies

reduced to twins and 30 consecutive spontaneously conceived twins (chorionicity?) matched by maternal age and parity. The initial number of fetuses was found to be inversely correlated with gestational age at delivery and birth weight, and positively correlated with pregnancy complications such as premature contractions and pregnancy-induced hypertension. Twin pregnancies following multifetal pregnancy reduction have a higher incidence of pregnancy complications, lower mean gestational age at delivery and lower birth weights than spontaneously conceived twins. **IIa B**

14 Silver RK, Helfand BT, Russell TL *et al.* (1997) Multifetal reduction increases the risk of preterm delivery and fetal growth restriction in twins: a case-control study. *Fertil Steril* **67**, 177–178. Case-control study comparing outcomes in twin gestations resulting from multifetal pregnancy reduction (MFPR) to 'primary' twin gestations. Significant differences were noted for outcomes in the above groups. The authors concluded that twin gestations resulting from MFPR are at increased risk for preterm birth, fetal growth restriction and discordancy compared with nonreduced twins. **IIa B**

Selective termination of abnormal twin (or as an option in severe twin-to-twin transfusion syndrome)

Management option	Quality of evidence	Strength of recommendation	References
Careful prior discussion and counseling	–	✔	–
Second trimester, although first-trimester termination following chorionic villous sampling at 11 weeks is possible	III	B	1
Safe in dichorionic twins	IV	C	2
Monoamniotic twins are a contraindication, few reports of umbilical cord banding/ transection	IV	C	3–5
Technique ❑ Intracardiac KCl ❑ Umbilical cord ligation/banding	IV	C	3–5
If other twin survives: ❑ Monitor fetal growth and health	–	✔	–

References

1 DeCatte L, Camus M, Bonduelle M *et al.* (1998) Prenatal diagnosis by chorionic villus sampling in multiple pregnancies prior to fetal reduction. *Am J Perinatol* **15**, 339–343. Descriptive study reporting the results of prenatal diagnosis by chorionic villous sampling (CVS) in 32 pregnancies prior to multifetal pregnancy reduction (MFPR). CVS was carried out at 10.5 weeks followed by MFPR 1 week later. The authors concluded that prenatal cytogenetic diagnosis prior to MFPR is feasible, accurate and safe. Abnormal chromosomal results can indicate the fetus to be reduced but some parents may opt to continue the multifetal pregnancy with the knowledge that the chromosomes are normal. **III B**

2 Lipitz S, Peltz R, Achiron R *et al.* (1997) Selective second-trimester termination of an abnormal fetus in twin pregnancies. *J Perinatol* **17**, 301–304. Observational paper describing the outcome of 14 dichorionic twins where selective feticide was performed for structural (10) and chromosomal (4) abnormalities. No major problems were seen in terms of preterm premature rupture of membranes. The mean gestational age at delivery was 34 weeks. The authors concluded that selective termination for dichorionic twins was a safe and effective procedure. **III B**

3 Lopoo JB, Paek BW, Maichin GA *et al.* (2000) Cord ultrasonic transection procedure for selective termination of a monochorionic twin. *Fetal Diagn Ther* **15**, 177–179. Two case reports of monochorionic twins discordant for abnormality in which the cords were transected using a harmonic scalpel under ultrasonic guidance. This procedure may also prove to be useful in monoamniotic twins to prevent entanglement of the dead fetus around the cord of the normal twin. **IV C**

4 Quintero RA, Romero R, Reich H *et al.* (1996) In utero percutaneous umbilical cord ligation in the management of complicated monochorionic gestations. *Ultrasound Obstet Gynecol* **8**, 16–22. A report of 13 cases of monochorionic twins discordant for abnormality (11) or severe twin-to-twin transfusion syndrome (2). Percutaneous umbilical cord ligation was performed under combined endoscopic and sonographic guidance. The procedure was accomplished in 84% of cases, 64% of which had living children, but preterm rupture of membranes was seen in 30% of cases. **IV C**

5 Deprest JA, Van Ballaer PP, Evrard VA *et al.* (1998) Experience with fetoscopic cord ligation. *Eur J Obstet Gynecol Reprod Biol* **81**, 157–164. A review article on the efficacy of fetoscopic cord ligation in salvaging the co-twin in a monochorionic twin pregnancy with one non-viable or abnormal fetus. 23 reported cases were analyzed, with a survival rate of 71% and a high risk for preterm premature rupture of membranes (40%). **IV C**

FETAL PROBLEMS

Chapter 10

Fetal health

10.1 Assessing fetal health

Jim Dornan

Management option		Quality of evidence	Strength of recommendation	References
Indications	**Low-risk patients** – implement surveillance program to identify when the risk ceases to be 'low'; this might include:			
	❑ Ultrasound in first half of pregnancy (insufficient evidence to show the value of routine US screening pregnancy)	Ia	A	1,2
	❑ Serum alpha-fetoprotein	III	B	3
	❑ Fetal movement counting (evidence suggests that this identifies fetuses at risk rather than improving outcome)	Ib	A	4
	❑ Fundal height measurement (insufficient evidence of value in improving outcome)	Ib	A	5
	High-risk patients – where there is a risk of chronic hypoxemia:	IV	C	6
	❑ *Mother*: cyanotic heart disease, diabetes, autoimmune disease, renal disease, hypertension, inadequate nutrition, smoking (often synergistic with other factors), alcohol and other drug abuse			
	❑ *Placenta*: 'idiopathic' growth restriction; recurrent abruption; pre-eclampsia			
	❑ *Fetus*: congenital anomalies (monitoring not likely for these); acquired (infection, anemia, hydrops, metabolic)			
Principles	Integrated comprehensive evaluation of maternal and fetal conditions	III IV	B C	7 8
	Multiple repeated fetal assessment methods more likely to be informative than single test	III IV	B C	7 8
	Select test appropriate for pathology/problem if possible/known	–	✔	–
Methods – mother	Clinical, e.g. evaluation of hypertension, cardiac disease	–	✔	–
	Laboratory, e.g. diabetes, Kleihauer, renal and liver function	–	✔	–
Methods – fetus	Biophysical profile score (gives best prediction of both acute and chronic fetal compromise) (insufficient Grade A evidence to support use)	III Ia	B A	9–11 12,13
	Umbilical artery Doppler velocimetry (only test shown in randomized trials to reduce perinatal mortality)	Ia	A	14
	Growth/size (see Chapter 11)	–	✔	–
	Normality			
	❑ Ultrasound	Ia	A	1
	❑ Invasive procedure (for, e.g., karyotype)	–	✔	–

References

1. Bucher H, Schmidt JG (1993) Does routine ultrasound scanning improve outcome of pregnancy? Meta-analysis of various outcome measures. *Br Med J* 307, 13–17. Meta-analysis of four randomized controlled trials that included 15935 pregnancies (7992 had routine scanning and 7943 controls were selectively scanned). Differences in perinatal morbidity were not significant between the two groups. Perinatal mortality was significantly lower in the routinely scanned group (OR 0.64) as a result of the termination of fetuses with lethal congenital anomalies. The live birth rate between the two groups was unaffected. The subgroup analyses indicated that the correction of inaccurate dating, early detection of twins and improved diagnosis of small-for-gestational-age fetuses did not equate to improved outcome. The failure to find an effect from routine ultrasound may have been due to: (1) the studies having insufficient subgroup power to appropriately test this hypothesis and (2) the lack of a cohesive management plan once a diagnosis was made. **Ia A**
2. Bricker L, Neilson JP (2001) Routine Doppler ultrasound in pregnancy. In: *The Cochrane library*, issue 2. Oxford: Update Software. Review of five trials including 14338 women. Based on their review of these studies, the authors concluded that routine Doppler ultrasound in low-risk or unselected populations does not confer benefit to either the mother or fetus. **Ia A**
3. Aickin DR, Duff GB, Evans JJ *et al.* (1983) Antenatal biochemical screening to predict low birthweight Infants. *Br J Obstet Gynaecol* 90, 129–133. Urine and plasma estriol, plasma progesterone, human placental lactogen, β_1-glycoprotein and serum cystyl aminopeptidase were measured at intervals during 608 pregnancies. The predictive accuracy of low values for identification of pregnancies with low-birthweight outcomes was assessed for each test at various gestations. No test was superior to the others at all centiles and gestations. Biochemical screening of pregnant populations to identify high-risk groups for intensive fetal monitoring has limited potential. Combining any pair of tests with values below the 10th centile did not reduce false-positive and false-negative predictions any more than could be achieved by movement of centiles up or down for a single test. **III B**
4. Grant A, Elbourne D, Valentin L *et al.* (1989) Routine formal fetal movement counting and risk of antepartum late death in normally formed singletons. *Lancet* **2**, 345–349. Multicenter RCT: 68000 women were randomly allocated within 33 pairs of clusters either to a policy of routine counting or to standard care, which might involve selective use of formal counting or informal noting of movements. Antepartum death rates for normally formed singletons were similar in the two groups, regardless of cause of prior risk status. Despite the counting policy, most of these fetuses were dead by the time the mothers received medical attention. The study does not rule out a beneficial effect but, at best, the policy would have to be used by about 1250 women to prevent one unexplained antepartum late fetal death, and an adverse effect is just as likely. In addition, formal routine counting would use considerable extra resources. **Ib A**
5. Neilson JP (2001) Symphysis–fundal height measurement in pregnancy. In: *Cochrane database of systematic reviews*, issue 3. Oxford: Update Software. One trial involving 1639 women was included. No differences were detected in any of the outcomes measured. There is not enough evidence to evaluate the use of symphysis–fundal height measurements during antenatal care. **Ib A**
6. Bernstein PS, Divon MY (1997) Etiologies of fetal growth restriction. *Clin Obstet Gynecol* **40**, 723–729. Review of conditions associated with an increased incidence of fetal growth restriction. **IV C**
7. James DK, Parker MJ, Smoleniec JS (1992) Comprehensive fetal assessment with three ultrasonographic characteristics. *Am J Obstet Gynecol* **166**, 1486–1495. Observational study of 103 fetuses (100 mothers) referred to a tertiary center for fetal assessment because of suspected chronic fetal asphyxia, performed with three ultrasonographic characteristics, umbilical artery Doppler recording, measurement of abdominal circumference and documenting the biophysical profile score. The order of deterioration (which had a very variable time-scale) was umbilical artery Doppler recording, followed by abdominal circumference and finally biophysical profile score. Normal characteristics or an abnormal umbilical artery Doppler recording alone or an abnormal abdominal circumference alone was associated with an excellent prognosis. The worst outcome was found in the 28 fetuses with abnormality of all three ultrasonographic features before delivery. The main suggested implications for management are avoidance of preterm delivery with normal ultrasonographic characteristics, an abnormal umbilical artery Doppler recording alone, or an abnormal abdominal circumference alone; delivery of fetuses at 34 weeks or more with abnormal umbilical artery Doppler recording and abdominal circumference before the biophysical profile score becomes abnormal; and implementation of specific measures to prevent necrotizing enterocolitis in newborns when all three characteristics are abnormal. **III B**
8. Harrington KF (2000) Making best and appropriate use of fetal biophysical and Doppler ultrasound data in the management of the growth restricted fetus. *Ultrasound Obstet Gynecol* **16**, 399–401. Review examining largely observational studies that suggest that monitoring the 'at-risk' fetus is best undertaken using a comprehensive approach with multiple rather than single tests. **IV C**
9. Manning FA, Morrison I, Harman CR *et al.* (1987) Fetal assessment based on fetal biophysical profile scoring: experience in 19221 referred high-risk pregnancies. *Am J Obstet Gynecol* **157**, 880–884. 19221 referred high-risk patients who were followed with biophysical profile scores were retrospectively studied. The corrected false-negative fetal death rate after a last normal biophysical profile score within 1 week was 0.7/1000. The authors concluded that a normal biophysical profile score confers a high probability of perinatal survival. **III B**

10 Manning FA, Snijders R, Harman CR *et al.* (1993) Fetal biophysical profile score VI. Correlation with antepartum umbilical venous fetal pH. *Am J Obstet Gynecol* **169**, 755–763. This was a prospective observational study. A total of 493 paired observations of biophysical profile score and pH were made; 104 observations were of fetuses with intrauterine growth restriction and 389 of fetuses with alloimmune anemia. The pH was always greater than 7.20 when the biophysical profile score was 10 of 10. The fetal biophysical profile score accurately predicts antepartum umbilical venous pH. **III B**

11 Manning FA, Bondaji N, Harman CR *et al.* (1998) Fetal assessment based on fetal biophysical profile scoring VIII. The incidence of cerebral palsy in tested and untested perinates. *Am J Obstet Gynecol* **178**, 696–706. This was a comparative clinical study. The incidence of cerebral palsy among the 84947 live births was 3.68/1000 live births. The rate of cerebral palsy in the 26290 referred high-risk tested patients was 1.33/000 compared with a rate of 4.74/1000 live births in the 48657 untested mixed low-risk/high-risk patients. These differences were highly significant. The authors concluded that the antepartum assessment by fetal biophysical profile scoring is associated with a significant reduction in the incidence of cerebral palsy compared with untested patients. **IIb B**

12 Alfirevic Z, Neilson JP (2000) Biophysical profile for fetal assessment in high-risk pregnancies. In: *The Cochrane library*, issue 4. Oxford: Update Software. Four studies with a total population of 2849 patients. The randomized controlled trials do not support the use of the biophysical profile score as a test of fetal wellbeing in high-risk pregnancies. However, these studies combined have insufficient power to prove that the biophysical profile score is without value. **Ia A**

13 Pattison N, McCowan, L (2000) Cardiotocography for antepartum fetal assessment. In: *The Cochrane library*, issue 4. Oxford: Update Software. Four studies, 1588 patients, studies performed on patients at risk. The use of cardiotocography had no significant effect on perinatal morbidity or mortality. However, the number of patients studied was insufficient to determine the presence or absence of a significant affect of testing on perinatal outcome. Furthermore, all the studies were from the 1980s and may not be appropriate for current practice. **Ia A**

14 Alfirevic Z, Neilson JP (1995) Doppler ultrasonography in high-risk pregnancies: systematic review with meta-analysis. *Am J Obstet Gynecol* **172**, 1379–1387. A total of 20 randomized control trials of Doppler ultrasonography were reviewed. The authors found that the clinical action guided by Doppler ultrasonography reduced the odds of perinatal death by 38%. **Ia A**

Chapter 11

Fetal growth

11.1 Fetal growth restriction

Jim Dornan

Management option		Quality of evidence	Strength of recommendation	References
Screening	**Biochemical:** alpha-fetoprotein clinically most useful (if raised and no fetal abnormality, risk of intrauterine growth restriction increased five- to 10-fold)	III	B	1
	Clinical:			
	❑ Fundal–symphysial height (relatively poor sensitivity and specificity, also insufficient data to assess value at improving outcome)	Ib	A	2
	❑ Increased surveillance in at-risk groups	IV	C	3
	Ultrasound biometry: insufficient evidence to show value of routine biometric screening on outcome; furthermore there is controversy as to whether two ultrasound measurements in late pregnancy are better than clinical methods. Problem of studies being of insufficient power and largely looking at one ultrasound scan in late pregnancy	Ia	A	4
	Ultrasound Doppler recordings:			
	❑ Uterine artery (conflicting data over value in screening)	III	B	5
	❑ Umbilical artery (insufficient data to show value; but studies of insufficient power and largely looking at only one Doppler measurement in late pregnancy)	Ia	A	6
Diagnosis and evaluation	Diagnosis is by ultrasound	–	✔	–
	Exclude abnormality by: ❑ Ultrasound ❑ Karyotype (especially if in early pregnancy and/or with hydramnios)	–	✔	–
	Doppler velocimetry … umbilical artery, middle cerebral artery	Ia	A	7
	and ductus venosus …helps differentiate causes and can identify the hypoxic fetus with cardiac decompensation	III	B	8
Management – prenatal	**In those at risk:**			
	❑ Serial ultrasound scans for growth and	–	✔	–
	umbilical artery Doppler recordings	Ia	A	7
	❑ Encourage cessation of smoking	Ia	A	9
	❑ Low-dose aspirin in women with history of preeclampsia	Ia	A	10

➡

Management option		Quality of evidence	Strength of recommendation	References
Management – prenatal (cont'd)	**Early onset:**			
	❑ Detailed scan to exclude fetal anomaly	–	✔	–
	❑ Progressive serial Doppler evaluation	Ia	A	7
	❑ Consider fetal karyotype especially if ultrasound markers and/or hydramnios	–	✔	–
	❑ Serial biophysical assessment – non-stress tests (NST), amniotic fluid volume (AFV), biophysical profile score (BPS) – if normal fetus	III	B	11–13
	(insufficient Grade A data to support use)	Ia	A	14,15
	❑ Steroids to aid pulmonary maturation if needed	Ia	A	16
	❑ Hospitalization, bedrest, stop smoking, etc.	–	✔	–
	❑ Value of fetal blood sampling for blood gases and viral infection is unclear	–	✔	–
	❑ Maternal oxygenation and hyper-alimentation are experimental	–	✔	–
	Late onset:			
	❑ Serial ultrasound growth scans for growth and Doppler flow	Ia	A	7
	❑ Serial biophysical assessment – NST,	III	B	11,12
	AFV, BPS	IIb	B	13
	(insufficient Grade A data to support use)	Ia	A	14,15
	❑ Steroids to aid pulmonary maturation if needed	Ia	A	16
Management – labor and/or delivery	Timing when risks from prematurity are low	III	B	17
	or when acute fetal 'distress' is present	IV	C	18
	Method determined by gestation, fetal wellbeing and severity of pathology	–	✔	–

References

1 Aickin DR, Duff GB, Evans JJ *et al.* (1983) Antenatal biochemical screening to predict low birthweight Infants. *Br J Obstet Gynaecol* **90**, 129–133. Urine and plasma estriol, plasma progesterone, human placental lactogen, β_1-glycoprotein and serum cystyl aminopeptidase were measured at intervals during 608 pregnancies. The predictive accuracy of low values for identification of pregnancies with low-birthweight outcomes was assessed for each test at various gestations. No test was superior to the others at all centiles and gestations. Biochemical screening of pregnant populations to identify high-risk groups for intensive fetal monitoring has limited potential. Combining any pair of tests with values below the 10th centile did not reduce false-positive and false-negative predictions any more than could be achieved by movement of centiles up or down for a single test. **III B**

2 Neilson JP (2001) Symphysis–fundal height measurement in pregnancy. In: *Cochrane database of systematic reviews*, issue 3. Oxford: Update Software. One trial involving 1639 women was included. No differences were detected in any of the outcomes measured. There is not enough evidence to evaluate the use of symphysis–fundal height measurements during antenatal care. **Ib A**

3 Bernstein PS, Divon MY (1997) Etiologies of fetal growth restriction. *Clin Obstet Gynecol* **40**, 723–729. Review of conditions associated with an increased incidence of fetal growth restriction. **IV C**

4 Bucher H, Schmidt JG (1993) Does routine ultrasound scanning improve outcome of pregnancy? Meta-analysis of various outcome measures. *Br Med J* **307**, 13–17. Meta-analysis of four randomized controlled trials that included 15 935 pregnancies (7992 had routine scanning and 7943 controls were selectively scanned). Differences in perinatal morbidity were not significant between the two groups. Perinatal mortality was significantly lower in the routinely scanned group (OR 0.64) as a result of the termination of fetuses with lethal congenital anomalies. The live birth rate between the two groups was unaffected. The subgroup analyses indicated that the correction of inaccurate dating, early detection of twins and improved diagnosis of small-for-gestational-age fetuses did not equate to improved outcome. The failure to find an effect from routine ultrasound may have been due to: (1) the studies having insufficient subgroup power to appropriately test this hypothesis and (2) the lack of a cohesive management plan once a diagnosis was made. **Ia A**

5 Coleman MA, McCowan LM, North RA (2000) Mid-trimester uterine artery Doppler screening as a predictor of adverse pregnancy outcome in high-risk women. *Ultrasound Obstet Gynecol* **15**, 7–12. A total of 116 pregnancies in 114 women at high risk of preeclampsia and/or small-for-gestational-age (SGA) babies had uterine artery Doppler screening performed as part of clinical practice between 22 and 24 weeks gestation. 32 (27.5%) women developed preeclampsia, 31 (26.7%) had SGA babies, 23 (20%) were delivered before 34 weeks because of pregnancy complications and there were three (2.6%) placental abruptions and three (2.6%) perinatal deaths. The sensitivity of any RI of more than 0.58 for preeclampsia, SGA, 'all' outcomes and 'severe' outcome was 91%, 84%, 83% and 90% respectively. The specificity of any RI of more than 0.58 for these outcomes was 42%, 39%, 47% and 38% respectively. The positive predictive value of any RI of more than 0.58 for the same outcomes was 37%, 33%, 58% and 24% respectively. Among women with both RI values 0.7 or more, 58%, 67%, 85% and 58% developed preeclampsia, SGA, 'all' and 'severe' outcomes respectively. In women with bilateral notches, 47%, 53%, 76% and 65% developed the respective outcomes. Women with both RI values 0.7 or more and women with bilateral notches had relative risks of 11.1 (95% CI 2.6–46.4) and 12.7 (95% CI 4.0–40.4) for developing severe outcome respectively. Only 5% of women with both RI values below 0.58 developed a severe outcome. **III B**

6 Bricker L, Neilson JP (2001) Routine Doppler ultrasound in pregnancy. In: *The Cochrane library*, issue 2. Oxford: Update Software. Review of five trials including 14 338 women. Based on their review of these studies, the authors concluded that routine Doppler ultrasound in low-risk or unselected populations does not confer benefit to either the mother or fetus. **Ia A**

7 Alfirevic Z, Neilson JP (1995) Doppler ultrasonography in high-risk pregnancies: systematic review with meta-analysis. *Am J Obstet Gynecol* **172**, 1379–1387. A total of 20 randomized control trials of Doppler ultrasonography were reviewed. The authors found that the clinical action guided by Doppler ultrasonography reduced the odds of perinatal death by 38%. **Ia A**

8 Baschat AA, Gembruch U, Reiss I *et al.* (2000) Relationship between arterial and venous Doppler and perinatal outcome in fetal growth restriction. *Ultrasound Obstet Gynecol* **16**, 407–413. Observational study in 121 fetuses with intrauterine growth restriction (IUGR). Doppler velocimetry of the umbilical artery (UA), middle cerebral artery (MCA), inferior vena cava (IVC), ductus venosus (DV) and free umbilical vein was performed. All 121 IUGR fetuses had an UA pulsatility index (PI) more than 2 SD above the gestational age mean and subsequent birth weight below the 10th centile for gestational age. Three groups were identified based on the last Doppler examination: (1) abnormal UA-PI only ($n = 42$, 34.7%); (2) MCA-PI more than 2 SD below the gestational age mean (= 'brain sparing'), in addition to abnormal UA-PI ($n = 29$, 24.0%); (3) DV or IVC peak velocity index more than 2 SD above the gestational age mean and/or pulsatile UV flow ($n = 50$, 41.3%). Z-scores (delta indices) were calculated for Doppler indices. Perinatal mortality, respiratory distress, bronchopulmonary dysplasia, intraventricular hemorrhage, necrotizing enterocolitis, circulatory failure and umbilical artery blood gases were recorded. Absence or reversal of umbilical artery end-diastolic flow was observed in 4 (9.5%) fetuses in group 1, 10 (34.5%) fetuses in group 2 and 41 (82%) fetuses in group 3. A low middle cerebral artery pulsatility index was found in 39 (78%) fetuses in group 3. Multiple regression analysis with gestational age at delivery, delta indices and cord artery blood gas as independent parameters and individual perinatal outcomes as dependent variables was performed. In this analysis the association was strongest with gestational age for each complication. There were no significant differences in Apgar scores between groups. At delivery, 'brain sparing' was associated with hypoxemia and abnormal venous flows with acidemia. Perinatal mortality was highest in group 3 and stillbirth was only observed when venous flow was abnormal. All postpartum complications were more frequent in fetuses with abnormal venous flows. The only statistically significant relation between Doppler indices and outcome was the association between abnormal DV flow and fetal death ($r^2 = 0.24$, $p < 0.05$). The authors conclude that: (1) Growth-restricted fetuses with abnormal venous flow have worse perinatal outcome than those where flow abnormality is confined to the UA or MCA; (2) in fetuses with low MCA pulsatility, venous Doppler allows detection of further deterioration; (3) while abnormal venous flows can be significantly associated with fetal demise, gestational age at delivery significantly impacts on all short-term outcomes. **III B**

9 Lumley J, Oliver S, Waters E (2000) Interventions for promoting smoking cessation during pregnancy. In: *The Cochrane library*, issue 4. Oxford: Update Software. Systematic review of 34 randomized trials. There was a significant reduction in smoking in the intervention group (OR 0.53). The subset of trials with information on fetal outcome revealed a reduction in low-birthweight (OR 0.80) and preterm birth (OR 0.83). **Ia A**

10 Duley L, Henderson-Smart D, Knight M *et al.* (2001) Antiplatelet drugs for prevention of pre-eclampsia and its consequences: systematic review. *Br Med J* **222**, 329–333. Meta-analysis of 39 trials (30 563 women). Use of antiplatelet drugs was associated with a 15% reduction in the risk of preeclampsia (32 trials, 29 331 women; relative risk 0.85, 95% CI 0.78–0.92; number needed to treat 100, 59–167). There was also an 8% reduction in the risk of preterm birth (23 trials, 28 268 women; 0.92, 0.88–0.97; 72, 44–200), and a 14% reduction in the risk of fetal or neonatal death (30 trials, 30 093 women; 0.86, 0.75–0.98; 250, 125 to > 10 000) for women allocated antiplatelet drugs. Small-for-gestational-age babies were reported in 25 trials (20 349 women), with no overall difference between the groups (relative risk 0.92, 0.84–1.01). There were no significant differences in other measures of outcome. It is concluded that antiplatelet drugs, largely low-dose aspirin, have small to moderate benefits when used for prevention of preeclampsia. **Ia A**

11 Manning FA, Morrison I, Harman CR *et al.* (1987) Fetal assessment based on fetal biophysical profile scoring: experience in 19 221 referred high-risk pregnancies. *Am J Obstet Gynecol* **157**, 880–884. 19 221 referred high-risk patients who were followed with biophysical profile scores were retrospectively studied. The corrected false-negative fetal death rate after a last normal biophysical profile score within 1 week was 0.7/1000. The authors concluded that a normal biophysical profile score confers a high probability of perinatal survival. **III B**

12 Manning FA, Snijders R, Harman CR *et al.* (1993) Fetal biophysical profile score VI. Correlation with antepartum umbilical venous fetal pH. *Am J Obstet Gynecol* **169**, 755–763. This was a prospective observational study. A total of 493 paired observations of biophysical profile score and pH were made; 104 observations were of fetuses with intrauterine growth restriction and 389 of fetuses with alloimmune anemia. The pH was always greater than 7.20 when the biophysical profile score was 10 of 10. The fetal biophysical profile score accurately predicts antepartum umbilical venous pH. **III B**

13 Manning FA, Bondaji N, Harman CR *et al.* (1998) Fetal assessment based on fetal biophysical profile scoring VIII. The incidence of cerebral palsy in tested and untested perinates. *Am J Obstet Gynecol* **178**, 696–706. This was a comparative clinical study. The incidence of cerebral palsy among the 84 947 live births was 3.68/1000 live births. The rate of cerebral palsy in the 26 290 referred high-risk tested patients was 1.33/1000 compared with a rate of 4.74/1000 live births in the 48 657 untested mixed low-risk/high-risk patients. These differences were highly significant. The authors concluded that the antepartum assessment by fetal biophysical profile scoring is associated with a significant reduction in the incidence of cerebral palsy compared with untested patients. **IIb B**

14 Alfirevic Z, Neilson JP (2000) Biophysical profile for fetal assessment in high-risk pregnancies. In: *The Cochrane library*, issue 4. Oxford: Update Software. Four studies with a total population of 2849 patients. The randomized controlled trials do not support the use of the biophysical profile score as a test of fetal wellbeing in high-risk pregnancies. However, these studies combined have insufficient power to prove that the biophysical profile score is without value. **Ia A**

15 Pattison N, McCowan L (2000) Cardiotocography for antepartum fetal assessment. In: *The Cochrane library*, issue 4. Oxford: Update Software. Four studies, 1588 patients, studies performed on patients at risk. The use of cardiotocography had no significant effect on perinatal morbidity or mortality. However, the number of patients studied was insufficient to determine the presence or absence of a significant effect of testing on perinatal outcome. Furthermore, all the studies were from the 1980s and may not be appropriate for current practice. **Ia A**

16 Crowley P (2001) Prophylactic corticosteroids for preterm birth (Cochrane Review). In: *The Cochrane library*, Issue 2. Oxford: Update Software. Systematic review (of 18 trials including more than 3700 babies) of the effects of corticosteroids administered to pregnant women to accelerate fetal lung maturity prior to preterm delivery. Antenatal administration of 24 mg betamethasone, 24 mg dexamethasone, or 2 g hydrocortisone to women expected to give birth preterm was associated with a significant reduction in mortality (OR 0.60, 95% CI 0.48–0.75), respiratory distress syndrome (OR 0.53, 95% CI 0.44–0.63) and intraventricular hemorrhage in preterm infants. No adverse consequences of prophylactic corticosteroids for preterm birth were identified. **Ia A**

17 James DK, Parker MJ, Smoleniec JS (1992) Comprehensive fetal assessment with three ultrasonographic characteristics. *Am J Obstet Gynecol* **166**, 1486–1495. Observational study of 103 fetuses (100 mothers) referred to a tertiary center for fetal assessment because of suspected chronic fetal asphyxia, performed with three ultrasonographic characteristics, umbilical artery Doppler recording, measurement of abdominal circumference and documenting the biophysical profile score. The order of deterioration (which had a very variable time-scale) was umbilical artery Doppler recording, followed by abdominal circumference and finally biophysical profile score. Normal characteristics or an abnormal umbilical artery Doppler recording alone or an abnormal abdominal circumference alone was associated with an excellent prognosis. The worst outcome was found in the 28 fetuses with abnormality of all three ultrasonographic features before delivery. The main suggested implications for management are avoidance of preterm delivery with normal ultrasonographic characteristics, an abnormal umbilical artery Doppler recording alone, or an abnormal abdominal circumference alone; delivery of fetuses at 34 weeks or more with abnormal umbilical artery Doppler recording and abdominal circumference before the biophysical profile score becomes abnormal; and implementation of specific measures to prevent necrotizing enterocolitis in newborns when all three characteristics are abnormal. **III B**

18 The GRIT Study Group (1996) When do obstetricians recommend delivery for a high-risk preterm growth-retarded fetus? Growth Restriction Intervention Trial. *Eur J Obstet Gynecol Reprod Biol* **67**, 121–126. A total of 49 obstetricians from three European countries were asked when they would advise delivery for a preterm fetus failing to thrive *in utero*, given various gestational ages and a range of either umbilical artery Doppler flow velocity waveforms or CTG variability measures. Their responses indicated a wide area of disagreement about the correct timing of delivery and a willingness to randomize patients to clinical trials of management. The area of uncertainty corresponded to the gestational age and Doppler bands at which participants have been entered to the pilot phase of a randomized trial of timed delivery, the Growth Restriction Intervention Trial (GRIT). **IV C**

Chapter 12

Abnormalities of amniotic fluid

12.1 Abnormalities of amniotic fluid

David James

Hydramnios

Management option		Quality of evidence	Strength of recommendation	References
Identify the cause (if possible)	History taking with emphasis on maternal symptoms, diabetes mellitus, red blood cell alloimmunization and diabetes insipidus	–	✔	–
	Ultrasound to assess: ❑ The degree of hydramnios (amniotic fluid index) ❑ Presence of multiple gestation, growth deficiency or macrosomia ❑ Fetal thorax ❑ Fetal central nervous system ❑ Fetal gastrointestinal system ❑ Fetal bladder dynamics ❑ Chorionicity in multiple pregnancy	–	✔	–
	Fetal specimens for karyotyping and viral infection	–	✔	–
Relieve maternal symptoms and prolong gestation	Indomethacin (50–200 mg daily)	III Ib	B A	1 2,3
	Sulindac (200 mg 12-hourly)	Ib	A	2,3
	Therapeutic amniocentesis (to maintain an acceptable/normal amniotic fluid volume; see also relevant chapters for management of specific causes of hydramnios, e.g. twin–twin transfusion syndrome, fetal intestinal obstruction)	III	B	4

References

1 Mamopoulos M, Assimakopoulos E, Reece EA *et al.* (1990) Maternal indomethacin therapy in the treatment of polyhydramnios. *Am J Obstet Gynecol* **68**, 1225–1229. Uncontrolled study in 15 patients with hydramnios. Gestational age at commencement of treatment was 27–33 weeks. Dose was 2.0–2.2 mg/kg. Reduction in fluid volume was noted. All fetuses were delivered at term and were healthy. **III B**

2 Carlan SJ, O'Brien WF, O'Leary TD *et al.* (1992) Randomised comparative trial of indomethacin and sulindac for the treatment of refractory preterm labor. *Obstet Gynecol* **79**, 223–228. Randomized trial of 36 women refractory to magnesium sulfate subsequently treated with indomethacin or sulindac. Sulindac had comparable efficacy in preventing preterm delivery with fewer fetal/neonatal side effects. **Ia A**

3 Rasanen J, Jouppila P (1995) Fetal cardiac function and ductus arteriosus during indomethacin and sulindac therapy for threatened preterm labor: a randomized study. *Am J Obstet Gynecol* **173**, 20–25. Randomized clinical trial in 20 patients (28–32 weeks) with threatened preterm labour. Sulindac cases had less severe disturbances of cardiac function and ductus arteriosus constriction than indomethacin. All effects were reversed with cessation of the drugs. **Ia A**

4 Elliott JP, Sawyer AT, Radin TG *et al.* (1994) Large-volume therapeutic amniocentesis in the treatment of hydramnios. *Obstet Gynecol* **84**, 1025–1027. Observational study of 94 patients with hydramnios having 200

therapeutic amniocenteses in one center over 6 years. Therapeutic amniocentesis was defined as an attempt to remove enough amniotic fluid (AF) in pregnancies complicated by symptomatic hydramnios to leave a normal volume of AF (AF index less than 25 cm). The most common condition treated with therapeutic amniocentesis was twin–twin transfusion syndrome (36 patients). The mean volume of fluid removed was 1666 ± 1245 ml (mean ± SD). The median volume of fluid removed was 1500 ml (range 350–10 000). The fluid was removed at a mean rate of 54 ± 22 ml/min. Complications were limited to one patient with ruptured membranes one day after therapeutic amniocentesis, one patient who developed chorioamnionitis and one patient with an anencephalic fetus who had an abruption following removal of 10 200 ml of fluid. The authors concluded that large-volume therapeutic amniocentesis could be used to treat hydramnios, with a 1.5% complication rate. **III B**

Oligohydramnios

Management option		Quality of evidence	Strength of recommendation	References
Identify the cause (if possible)	History-taking with emphasis on maternal symptoms of hypertension, membrane rupture and congenital infection	–	✔	–
	Ultrasonography (transvaginal may be helpful) to assess: ❑ Degree of oligohydramnios (amniotic fluid index) ❑ Presence of growth deficiency ❑ Presence and appearance of the kidneys ❑ Genitourinary and other malformations	III	B	1
	Color Doppler ultrasonography to: ❑ Visualize fetal renal arteries ❑ Determine the severity of oligohydramnios by excluding loops of cord	III	B	2
	Fetal intraperitoneal infusion to outline renal beds if necessary	III	B	3
	Amnioinfusion, if necessary, to improve ultrasonographic resolution	III	B	4,5
	Fetal specimens for karyotyping and viral infection	–	✔	–
Management depends on etiology	Premature preterm rupture of the membranes (see Section 46.2)	–	✔	–
	Growth deficiency (see Section 11.1)			
	Prolonged pregnancy (see Section 47.3)			
	Fetal renal anomalies (see Section 19.1)			
	Treatments tried in mid-trimester oligohydramnios to maintain amniotic fluid volume and promote lung development:			
	❑ Infusion of fluid via a transcervical catheter	III	B	5
	❑ Serial transabdominal therapeutic amnioinfusions	III	B	4
	– Prenatal (insufficient evidence to advocate)	Ib	A	6
	– Intrapartum (good evidence to advocate)	Ia	A	7,8
	❑ Vesicoamniotic shunting in obstructive uropathies	III	B	9,10
	❑ Cervical canal occlusion with fibrin gel	III	B	11
	❑ Maternal hydration	Ib	A	12,13

References

1 Benacerraf BR (1990) Examination of the second-trimester fetus with severe oligohydramnios using transvaginal scanning. *Obstet Gynecol* **75**, 491–493. Two cases are reported of second-trimester oligohydramnios in which the fetal abnormalities were visible only with the vaginal probe. The vaginal scan permitted a definitive diagnosis of Potter syndrome not possible with the poorer resolution of the transabdominal approach. **III B**

2 Sepulveda W, Stagiannis KD, Flack NJ *et al.* (1995) Accuracy of prenatal diagnosis of renal agenesis with color flow imaging in severe second-trimester oligohydramnios. *Am J Obstet Gynecol* **173**, 1788–1792. Prospective study of 33 consecutive second-trimester pregnancies referred with severe oligohydramnios using high-resolution color Doppler ultrasonography to establish the presence or absence of renal arteries. Prenatal findings were correlated with the presence or absence of fetal kidneys at postmortem or postnatal examination. Neither renal artery was visualized in 8 fetuses; postmortem examination confirmed bilateral renal agenesis in 7 and unilateral renal agenesis with a contralateral atrophic multicystic kidney in the other. Only one renal artery was seen in 3; postmortem examination demonstrated unilateral renal agenesis in 2 fetuses and bilateral multicystic dysplastic kidneys in the other. Postmortem or postnatal evaluation confirmed the presence of both kidneys in all 22 fetuses in which both renal arteries were identified prenatally. Color Doppler ultrasonography is useful in the prenatal evaluation of fetuses with severe second-trimester oligohydramnios to demonstrate the presence or absence of renal arteries. **III B**

3 Nicolini U, Santolaya J, Hubinont C *et al.* (1989) Visualization of fetal intraabdominal organs in second trimester severe oligohydramnios by intraperitoneal infusion. *Prenat Diagn* **9**, 191–194. Fetal intraperitoneal infusion of saline was performed in two patients with severe oligohydramnios at 24 and 25 weeks gestation in order to enhance visualization of intra-abdominal organs. Renal agenesis was easily diagnosed. The technique can be considered as an alternative to artificial instillation of amniotic fluid in the differential diagnosis of conditions associated with severe oligohydramnios. **III B**

4 Fisk NM, Ronderos-Dumit D, Soliani A *et al.* (1991) Diagnostic and therapeutic transabdominal amnioinfusion in oligohydramnios. *Obstet Gynecol* **78**, 270–278. Report of 92 antenatal amnioinfusion procedures. In order to facilitate ultrasound visualization, a diagnostic infusion was attempted at a median of 22 weeks (range 16–36) in 61 pregnancies with oligohydramnios in the absence of ruptured membranes on clinical examination. The procedure was successful in 58 (95%). Infusion (mean volume 181 ml, range 40–64) significantly increased ($p < 0.001$) the deepest pool of amniotic fluid to a mean of 3.2 cm. Suspected fetal anomalies were then confirmed in 27/30 cases, whereas kidneys were clearly demonstrated in 3 fetuses suspected of renal agenesis. In addition, previously unsuspected anomalies were identified in 5. Vaginal leakage indicating ruptured membranes occurred in 16 women. Leakage occurred in 0/24 patients with, compared to 16/35 without, fetal urinary disorders ($p < 0.001$), which does not support the recent suggestion that amnioinfusion causes rather than unmasks rupture of the membranes. Membranous detachment was observed by ultrasound in 13 patients, 11 of whom leaked vaginally. Information obtained at amnioinfusion led to a change of etiological diagnosis in 8 (13% of subjects). 40 serial infusions were performed in 9 women as a pilot study to prevent oligohydramnios sequelae. There were no skeletal deformities; 3 neonates survived, and 5 of the 6 perinatal deaths had normal lung–bodyweight ratios. Overall, only 2/89 infusions (2.2%) were complicated by clinical amnionitis. The findings support a role for amnioinfusion in oligohydramnios. **III B**

5 Imanaka M, Ogita S, Sugawa T (1989) Saline solution amnioinfusion for oligohydramnios after premature rupture of the membranes. *Am J Obstet Gynecol* **161**,102–106. Observational study of amnioinfusion to prevent adverse fetal effects of prolonged oligohydramnios. Physiological saline solution was infused continuously into the amniotic cavity at a flow rate of 10–20 ml/h with a new cervical indwelling catheter (PROM-fence). As a result the average pocket size of the amniotic cavity was 2.7 cm before amnioinfusion, 5.9 cm 1 day after, 5.8 cm 5 days after and 5.0 cm 10 days after amnioinfusion. The saline solution amnioinfusion made it possible to keep the amniotic cavity fluid level adequate. Variable decelerations disappeared in one case. No side effects such as uterine contractions were observed. **III B**

6 Hofmeyr GJ (2001) Amnioinfusion for preterm rupture of membranes. In: *Cochrane database of systematic reviews*, issue 2. Oxford: Update Software. Systematic review that included only one trial of 66 women. No significant differences between amnioinfusion and no amnioinfusion were detected for cesarean section (RR 0.32, 95% CI 0.07–1.40); low Apgar scores (RR 0.28, 95% CI 0.03–2.33) or neonatal death (RR 0.55, 95% CI 0.05–5.77). In the amnioinfusion group, the number of severe fetal heart rate decelerations per hour during the first stage of labour were reduced (weighted mean difference –1.20, 95% CI –1.83 to –0.57). It is concluded that there is not enough evidence concerning the use of amnioinfusion for preterm rupture of membranes. **Ib A**

7 Hofmeyr GJ (2001) Amnioinfusion for umbilical cord compression in labour. In: *Cochrane database of systematic reviews*, issue 2. Oxford: Update Software. Systematic review of 12 studies. Transcervical amnioinfusion for potential or suspected umbilical cord compression was associated with the following reductions: fetal heart rate decelerations (RR 0.54, 95% CI 0.43–0.68); cesarean section for suspected fetal distress (RR 0.35, 95% CI 0.24–0.52); neonatal hospital stay greater than 3 days (RR 0.40, 95% CI 0.26–0.62); maternal hospital stay greater than 3 days (RR 0.46, 95% CI 0.29–0.74). Transabdominal amnioinfusion showed similar results. Transcervical amnioinfusion to prevent infection in women with membranes ruptured for more than 6 hours was associated with a reduction in puerperal infection (RR 0.50, 95% CI 0.26–0.97). While it is concluded that amnioinfusion appears to reduce the occurrence of variable heart rate decelerations and lower the use of cesarean section, the studies were done in settings where fetal distress was not confirmed by fetal blood sampling. The results may therefore only be relevant where

cesarean sections are commonly done for abnormal fetal heart rate alone. The trials reviewed are too small to address the possibility of rare but serious maternal adverse effects of amnioinfusion. **Ia A**

8 Hofmeyr GJ (2001) Prophylactic versus therapeutic amnioinfusion for oligohydramnios in labour. In: *Cochrane database of systematic reviews*, issue 2. Oxford: Update Software. Two studies of 285 women were included in this systematic review. No differences were found in the rate of cesarean section (RR 0.98, 95% CI 0.58–1.66) or forceps delivery. There were no difference in Apgar scores, cord arterial pH, oxytocin augmentation, meconium aspiration, neonatal pneumonia or postpartum endometritis. Prophylactic amnioinfusion was associated with increased intrapartum fever (RR 3.48, 95% CI 1.21–10.05). It is concluded that there appears to be no advantage of prophylactic amnioinfusion over therapeutic amnioinfusion carried out only when fetal heart rate decelerations or thick meconium-staining of the liquor occur. **Ia A**

9 Johnson MP, Bukowski TP, Reitleman C *et al.* (1994) In utero surgical treatment of fetal obstructive uropathy: A new comprehensive approach to identify appropriate candidates for vesicoamniotic shunt therapy. *Am J Obstet Gynecol* **170**, 1770–1779. Retrospective review of 34 fetuses with megacystis and hydronephrosis between 14 and 24 weeks evaluated using ultrasound, rapid karyotyping and a minimum of three bladder taps at 48–72 h intervals to assess urinary biochemical values in addition to observing the rate of bladder refilling after vesicocentesis. If there was a sequential fall in biochemical values these were considered to have a good prognosis, with a rise suggesting progressive dysplasia. The authors showed that the third or fourth bladder tap was the best predictor. Using an integrated approach of the above they achieved a 100% rate in predicting the presence of significant underlying renal pathology. In spite of this, 4 such cases underwent shunting, a fact not consistent with the proposed algorithm. Of interest, of the initial 34 assessed, after termination (11) and other perinatal losses (12) only 11 survived, 2 of whom were on dialysis awaiting renal transplant, illustrating that, in spite of the above approach, morbidity and mortality is very high with this condition. **III B**

10 Freedman AL, Johnson MP, Smith CA *et al.* (1999) Long-term outcome in children after antenatal intervention for obstructive uropathies. *Lancet* **354**, 374–377. Observational study, from the same group as in reference 9, reviewing the long-term follow-up for 34 patients who underwent vesicoamniotic shunt placement between 1987 and 1996. 13 died and 21 survived, of whom 14 were more than 2 years old. Height was below 25th centile in 86% with 50% below the 5th centile. 36% had renal failure requiring transplantation, with 43% having normal renal function. 50% are acceptably continent with 14% incontinent. 3 of 4 children with valves needed bladder augmentation surgery. Although the numbers are relatively small the results are somewhat disappointing but should enable more informed parental counseling before intervention. **III B**

11 Baumgarten K, Moser S (1986) The technique of fibrin adhesion for premature rupture of the membranes during pregnancy. *J Perinat Med* **14**, 43–49. Report of a new technique of fibrin adhesion for premature rupture of the membranes in pregnancy in 28 patients. Unless cerclage had been carried out earlier, it was necessary to suture the cervical canal immediately after rupture of the membranes in order to be able to insert a fibrin clot. The author's modified cerclage technique (reverse McDonald procedure) was described. The perceived advantages were minimal trauma to the lower uterine segment and a more 'physiological' fixation of the synthetic suture material. The technique was claimed to carry no risk to mother or child. No cases of amniotic infection syndrome had been observed. **III B**

12 Kilpatrick SJ, Safford KL (1991) Maternal hydration increases amniotic fluid index. *Obstet Gynecol* **78**, 1098–1102. Randomized blinded trial examining whether maternal hydration would increase the amniotic fluid index (AFI) in women with low AFIs. Women seen in the authors' testing centers were randomized into control or hydration groups. The control group was instructed to drink their normal amount of fluid; the hydration group was instructed to drink 2 liters of water, in addition to their usual amount of fluid, 2–4 h before the posttreatment AFI. The women returned for the posttreatment AFI the same or following day. The mean posttreatment AFI was significantly greater in the hydration group (6.3 versus 5.1; $p < 0.01$), as was the mean change in AFI (posttreatment AFI–pretreatment AFI: 1.5 versus 0.31; $p < 0.01$). These findings suggest that maternal oral hydration increases amniotic fluid volume in women with decreased fluid levels. **Ib A**

13 Flack NJ, Sepulveda W, Weiner E *et al.* (1995) Acute maternal hydration in third-trimester oligohydramnios: effects on amniotic fluid volume, uteroplacental perfusion, and fetal blood flow and urine output. *Am J Obstet Gynecol* **173**, 1186–1191. Prospective RCT of acute maternal hydration in pregnancies with third-trimester oligohydramnios. 10 women with third-trimester oligohydramnios (amniotic fluid index ≤5 cm) and 10 controls with normal amniotic fluid volume (amniotic fluid index >7 cm) were prospectively recruited for this study. There was a significant reduction in maternal plasma ($p < 0.05$) and urine osmolality ($p < 0.0001$) in both groups after short-term oral hydration. Hydration increased amniotic fluid volume in women with oligohydramnios (mean change in amniotic fluid index 3.2 cm, 95% CI 1.1–5.3; $p < 0.02$) but not in those with normal amniotic fluid volume (mean change in amniotic fluid index –2.0, 95% CI –4.1 to +0.2). The hourly fetal urine production rate, however, did not increase in either group. Hydration was also associated with a significant increase in uterine artery mean velocity in the oligohydramnios group but not in controls. There was no change in pulsatility index or in velocity in any of the fetal vessels studied in either group. The mechanism for this effect remains unclear: it could not be accounted for by fetal urination in this study but instead was associated with improved uteroplacental perfusion. **Ib A**

Chapter 13

Fetal death

13.1 Fetal death

David Penman

Management option		Quality of evidence	Strength of recommendation	References
Risk factors	Increasing maternal age	III	B	1
	Smoking	III	B	1
	Intrauterine growth restriction	III	B	1,2
	Prior induced abortion	III	B	1
	Prematurity	III	B	1
	Insulin-dependent diabetes mellitus	III	B	2
Etiology	Placental factors/cord complications	III	B	2
	Congenital anomalies	III	B	2,3
	Chromosome abnormalities	III	B	3
	Syndromes	III	B	3
	Mendelian (single-gene defect)	III	B	3
	Infection	III	B	2
	Conditions associated with multiple births	III	B	3
	Etiology not determined in 12–60%	III	B	1,4
Maternal investigation	Kleihauer–Betke	IV	C	5
	Anticardiolipins, lupus anticoagulant	III	B	1
Fetal investigation	Amniotic fluid culture	IV	C	5
	Karyotype	III	B	1
	Postmortem and placental examination	III	B	1,3
Delivery	< 13 weeks			
	❑ Vacuum evacuation/curettage	–	✔	–
	❑ Oral mifepristone followed by oral or vaginal prostaglandin 48 h later	Ib	A	6
	13–22 weeks			
	❑ Ripen cervix with laminaria and:	–	✔	–
	– dilatation and evacuation (not formally compared to contemporary medical methods but safer in comparison to older methods)	III	B	7
	or			
	– high-dose oxytocin induction	III	B	8

Management option		Quality of evidence	Strength of recommendation	References
Delivery (cont'd)	13–22 weeks (cont'd)			
	❑ Prostaglandin E_2 vaginal pessaries	III	B	8
	❑ Oral mifepristone followed by oral or vaginal prostaglandin 48h later. This regimen may need to be supplemented by oxytocin infusion	Ib	A	6
	❑ Vaginal misoprostol is very effective, followed by gemeprost or oral misoprostol	Ib	A	6,9
	22–28 weeks			
	❑ Ripen cervix with laminaria and:	–	✔	–
	– oxytocin induction	III	B	8
	❑ Prostaglandin E_2 vaginal pessaries with oxytocin augmentation	III	B	10,11
	❑ Oral mifepristone followed by oral or vaginal prostaglandin 48h later; this regimen may need to be supplemented by oxytocin infusion	Ib	A	6
	❑ Vaginal misoprostol is very effective, followed by gemeprost or oral misoprostol	Ib	A	6,9
	>28 weeks	IV	C	12
	❑ Cervix favorable: – oxytocin induction			
	❑ Cervix unfavorable: – ripen cervix with low-dose prostaglandin E_2 vaginal suppositories without concurrent oxytocin			
	❑ Overall, vaginal prostaglandin E_2 is superior to oxytocin at inducing labor	Ia	A	13,14
Screen for coagulopathy	Particularly if death before 4 weeks	III	B	15
Perinatal grief		III	B	16
	❑ Discongruent grieving between spouses			
	❑ May be a long-term process without a predictable end-point			

References

1 Ogunyemi D, Jackson U, Buyske S *et al.* (1998) Clinical and pathologic correlates of stillbirths in a single institution. *Acta Obstet Gynecol Scand* **77**, 722–728. Retrospective analysis of stillbirths at 25 weeks gestation or earlier. 115 stillbirths and 193 controls were analyzed. The authors found that maternal age, nulliparity, tobacco use, prior induced abortions, anticardiolipin antibodies, elevated maternal alpha-fetoprotein, twins and amniocentesis were significantly associated with stillbirth. Primary pathological diagnoses were placental factors (37%), cord complications (28%) and fetal causes (15%). **III B**

2 Fretts RC, Boyd ME, Usher RH *et al.* (1992) The changing pattern of fetal death, 1961–1988. *Obstet Gynecol* **79**, 35–39. Study of 709 stillbirths occurring among 88651 births in a tertiary care unit. The authors noted a significant decline in unexplained antepartum fetal deaths and in those caused by intrauterine growth restriction. The incidence of fetal death from infection and placental abruption did not change over the time interval of the study. **III B**

3 Pauli RM, Reiser CA (1994) Wisconsin stillbirth service program II. Analysis of diagnosis and diagnostic categories in the first 1,000 referrals. *Am J Med Genet* **50**, 135–153. Study evaluating the first 1000 referrals in the Wisconsin stillbirth service program. Among all those referred, 24.5% were found to have an identifiable intrinsic fetal cause of death. **III B**

4 Ahlenius I, Floberg J, Thomassen P (1995) Sixty-six cases of intrauterine fetal death. *Acta Obstet Gynecol Scand* **74**,109–117. Prospective study performed to elucidate the etiology of intrauterine fetal death and to evaluate diagnostic procedures. The authors evaluated 66 stillbirths. The cause of death was certain in 57%, probable in 20% and possible in 11% of the cases. In only 12% did the cause of death remain entirely unexplained. The principal causes

of intrauterine fetal death were infection, including premature rupture of the membranes (15%), anomalies (11%), preeclampsia-associated conditions (9%) and intrauterine growth restriction of unknown etiology (8%). **III B**

5 Pitkin RM (1987) Fetal death: diagnosis and management. *Am J Obstet Gynecol* **157**, 583–589. Review article that discusses both diagnosis and management of an intrauterine fetal death. The author discusses dilatation and curettage, intrauterine oxytocin and intravaginal prostaglandins as potential means for delivery. The author suggests that, in any case of intrauterine fetal death, a fetal karyotype, a Kleihauer–Betke test for fetal maternal hemorrhage and lupus anticoagulant be obtained. **IV C**

6 Rodger MW, Baird DT (1990) Pretreatment with mifepristone (RU 486) reduces interval between prostaglandin administration and expulsion in second trimester abortion. *Br J Obstet Gynaecol* **97**, 41–45. The effect of pretreatment with mifepristone on prostaglandin-induced abortion was investigated in a double-blind randomized trial involving 100 women in the second trimester of pregnancy. The women were randomly allocated to receive either 600mg oral mifepristone or placebo tablets 36h before the administration of gemeprost pessaries. The median interval between administration of prostaglandin and abortion was significantly shorter in the mifepristone group (6.8h) compared with the placebo group (15.8h). The women pretreated with mifepristone required significantly fewer gemeprost pessaries to induce abortion and experienced significantly less pain than the women who had received placebo. **Ib A**

7 Peterson WF, Berry FN, Grace MR *et al.* (1983) Second-trimester abortion by dilatation and evacuation: an analysis of 11,747 cases. *Obstet Gynecol* **62**, 185–190. The dilatation and evacuation procedure was explored in 1971 as an alternative method of second-trimester abortion. The results in 11747 cases from 1972–81 are presented. Although complications did occur – most notably hemorrhage, cervical laceration, fever and perforation – the overall complication rate was lower than that reported for saline or prostaglandin in other large series. Further study and refinement of technique may help bring this shorter, safer and more convenient procedure within the reach of larger numbers of women seeking second-trimester abortion. **III B**

8 Winkler CL, Gray SE, Hauth JC (1991) Mid-second trimester labor induction: concentrated oxytocin compared with prostaglandin E_2 vaginal suppositories. *Obstet Gynecol* **77**, 297–300. Retrospective review of labor induction between 17 and 24 weeks gestation with either prostaglandin E_2 vaginal suppositories or a concentrated intravenous oxytocin infusion. The authors concluded that a concentrated oxytocin infusion was a reasonable alternative to prostaglandin E_2 vaginal suppositories for induction of labor in the mid-second trimester. **III B**

9 Frydman R, Fernandez H, Pons JC *et al.* (1988) Mifepristone (RU486) and therapeutic late pregnancy termination: a double-blind study of two different doses. *Hum Reprod* **3**, 803–806. An antiprogesterone, mifepristone (RU486), was administered to 35 patients undergoing a therapeutic interruption of pregnancy during the second and third trimester for maternal or fetal indications. A randomized double-blind study test was performed using 150 and 450mg of mifepristone as pretreatment prior to prostaglandins. No toxicity or maternal morbidity were recorded. In three patients the onset of labor occurred spontaneously before prostaglandin administration. Mifepristone produced a modification in the consistency of the cervix with a statistical improvement in cervical calibration in the two groups, but the cervical effect was independent of the dose. **Ib A**

10 Lauersen NH, Cederqvist LL, Wilson KH (1980) Management of intrauterine fetal death with prostaglandin E_2 vaginal suppositories. *Am J Obstet Gynecol* **137**, 753–757. The study reviewed 78 intrauterine fetal deaths at between 13 and 14 weeks gestation that were treated with prostaglandin E_2 vaginal suppositories. A concomitant oxytocin infusion was utilized in 38 patients. In gestations of less than 24 weeks, the oxytocin was administered via intravenous drip at a rate of 10U/h. However, in cases of intrauterine fetal death and a gestation of 24 weeks or more, oxytocin was administered via a constant-rate infusion pump, a targeted dose of 1mU/min and careful titration of the dose to uterine activity. **III B**

11 Scher J, Jeng DY, Moshirpur J *et al.* (1980) Comparison between vaginal prostaglandin E_2 suppositories and intrauterine extra-amniotic prostaglandins in the management of fetal death. *Am J Obstet Gynecol* **137**, 769–772. Retrospective study that compared the efficacy and side effects and complications of prostaglandin E_2 (PGE_2) given as a vaginal suppository with those of PGE_2 administered by the intrauterine extra-amniotic route to induce labor after fetal death. 23 patients who were treated with vaginal suppositories had a mean gestational age at induction of 26.1 weeks. Oxytocin was used in 30.4% of this group for augmentation purposes. Most of the augmentation was performed after the fetus had been expelled and while the placenta was still retained. The side effects of vomiting, diarrhea and fever as well as complications (incomplete abortion, uterine rupture, oxytocin augmentation) occurred more frequently with the use of PGE_2 vaginal suppositories. **III B**

12 Kochenour NK (1987) Management of fetal demise. *Clin Obstet Gynecol* **30**, 322–330. Review article outlining the management of fetal demise. The pros and cons of prostaglandins for induction are specifically addressed. **IV C**

13 Tan BP, Hannah ME (2001) Prostaglandins versus oxytocin for prelabour rupture of membranes at term. In: *Cochrane database of systematic reviews*, issue 3. Oxford: Update Software. Systematic review of eight RCTs. On the basis of three trials, prostaglandins compared to oxytocin were associated with increased chorioamnionitis (OR 1.51, 95% CI 1.07–2.12) and neonatal infections (OR 1.63, 95% CI 1.00–2.66). From the results of four trials, prostaglandins were associated with a decrease in epidural analgesia (OR 0.86, 95% CI 0.73–1.00) and internal fetal heart rate monitoring (based on one trial). Cesarean section, endometritis and perinatal mortality were not significantly different between the groups. **Ia A**

14 Tan BP, Hannah ME (2001) Prostaglandins for prelabour rupture of membranes at or near term. In: *Cochrane database of systematic reviews*, issue 3. Oxford: Update Software. Review of 15 trials of moderate to good quality. Induction of labor by prostaglandins was associated with a decreased risk of chorioamnionitis (OR 0.77, 95% CI 0.61–0.97) based on eight trials and admission to neonatal intensive care (OR 0.79, 95% CI 0. 66–0.94) based on seven trials. No difference was detected for rate of cesarean section, although induction by prostaglandins was associated with a more frequent maternal diarrhea and use of anesthesia and/or analgesia. Based on one trial, women were more likely to view their care positively if labor was induced with prostaglandins. **Ia A**

15 Maslow AD, Breen TW, Sarna MC *et al.* (1996) Prevalence of coagulation abnormalities associated with intrauterine fetal death. *Can J Anaesth* **43**, 1237–1243. Study reviewing 238 patients diagnosed with an intrauterine fetal death over a 10-year period. In most pregnancies, the fetus and placenta delivered within 1 week of fetal demise. The previously reported severe coagulation disturbances are usually eliminated by early delivery. Placental abruption and uterine perforation were found to significantly increase the likelihood of a coagulopathy. **III B**

16 Schapp AHP, Wolf H, Bruinse HW *et al.* (1997) Long-term impact of perinatal bereavement. Comparison of grief reactions after intrauterine versus neonatal death. *Eur J Obstet Gynecol Reprod Biol* **75**, 161–167. Retrospective matched study. There were 10 in the intrauterine death group and 9 in the neonatal death group. The authors found that discongruent grieving between partners was more pronounced in the intrauterine death group. **III B**

Chapter 14

Fetal hydrops

14.1 Fetal hydrops

Stephen Carroll

See also Chapter 15, Fetal hemolytic disease.

Management option		Quality of evidence	Strength of recommendation	References
Etiology	Many causes but a diagnosis can be established in 90% of cases; chromosomal abnormalities are commoner with decreased gestational age	III	B	1–6
Prognosis	Determined by underlying etiology	III	B	4
	The earlier it is detected, the worse the prognosis	III	B	2,7
	Presence of a congenital anomaly worsens the prognosis	III	B	8
	Bilateral pleural effusions are a poor prognostic sign	III	B	9–11
	Mortality varies between 50% and 95%	III	B	10,12
	Generally a good prognosis for psychomotor development in survivors	III	B	11,13
	Prevention of prematurity improves long-term outcome	III	B	11
Evaluation	Maternal history (ethnic origin, previous fetal hydrops, baby with jaundice) and investigations (CBC, group, antibody titer, electrophoresis, G-6-PD and pyruvate kinase carrier status, alpha-fetoprotein, serological test for syphilis, parvovirus B19, toxoplasmosis, cytomegalovirus, herpes simplex virus, Coxsackie virus, urate, urea and electrolytes, liver function including albumin, Kleihauer, lupus anticoagulant and anti-Ro if fetal bradycardia)	III	B	12
	Fetal ultrasound (sites and severity of hydrops, fetal/placental/cord abnormality, Doppler studies including middle cerebral with anemia, amniotic fluid volume, biophysical assessment) and fetal blood (CBC, electrophoresis, group, Coombs, acute-phase serology for infection, EM for rapid parvovirus B19, blood gas and pH estimation, karyotype, white cell enzymes)	III	B	12,14
Management	Preconceptual and prenatal screening for thalassemia	–	✔	–

Management option		Quality of evidence	Strength of recommendation	References
Management (cont'd)	Counseling about prognosis before and after investigations; multidisciplinary approach may be necessary	-	✔	-
	In-utero therapy can be effective in selected cases (about one third): ❑ Intrauterine transfusions for fetal anemia (hemolytic disease – see Section15.1, fetal bleed, parvovirus) ❑ Antiarrhythmic medication ❑ Specific treatments for twin–twin transfusion syndrome (see Section 45.2) ❑ Pleuroamniotic shunts for primary hydrothorax, cystic adenomatous malformation ❑ Open surgery for chest lesions should be regarded as experimental	III	B	2,4,8,9,15–19
	Consider termination in those with severe hydrops at a previable gestation, with a condition with no effective treatment	-	✔	-

References

1 Holzgreve W, Miny P (1989) Nonimmune hydrops fetalis: diagnosis and management. *Semin Perinatol* **9**, 52–67. Data on causes of 103 cases of nonimmune hydrops are given. The data show that prenatal investigations and postpartum evaluation can lead to a diagnosis in 85% of cases of nonimmune hydrops. The authors discuss the associated maternal complication of preeclampsia. Successful treatment of prenatal fetal tachyarrhythmias is discussed. **III B**

2 Hansmann M, Gembruch U, Bald R *et al.* (1989) New therapeutic aspects in nonimmune hydrops fetalis based on 402 prenatally diagnosed cases. *Fetal Ther* **4**, 29–36. Report of 402 cases of prenatally diagnosed hydrops fetalis: cardiovascular disorders were present in 18%, chromosomal defects in 11% and hematological disorders in 10%. Important treatments such as intravascular blood transfusion, thoracoamniotic shunting and antiarrhythmic agents can improve outcome. The survival rate was 19.4% before 24 weeks and 28.5% after this gestation. The majority of survivors were in the tachyarrhythmic, hematological and hydrothorax groups (53 of 78 survivors, 68%). **III B**

3 Boyd PA, Keeling JW (1992) Fetal hydrops. *J Med Genet* **29**, 91–97. A total of 72 fetuses or neonates with nonimmune hydrops were reviewed. The most common association was chromosomal abnormality; 11 fetuses had a 45,X karyotype and 11 autosomal trisomy. In five twin pairs, hydrops was the result of twin–twin transfusion syndrome. **III B**

4 Anandakumar C, Biswas A, Wong YC *et al.* (1996) Management of non-immune hydrops: 8 years' experience. *Ultrasound Obstet Gynecol* **8**, 196–200. During a period of 8 years, 100 fetuses with nonimmune hydrops were evaluated using a set protocol including Doppler ultrasound examination of the fetal vessels and cordocentesis. Cardiovascular anomalies (23%) and alpha-thalassemia (22%) were the most common causes in the south-east Asian population. 26 fetuses were suitable for *in-utero* therapy, which included intrauterine blood transfusions for anemia, direct fetal drug therapy with digoxin for tachyarrhythmias, and thoracoamniotic shunting for pleural effusions. 18 of the 26 fetuses (69%) survived and were well 1 month after delivery. The authors conclude that fetal therapy in appropriate cases can lead to increased survival. **III B**

5 Lallemand AV, Doco-Fenzy M, Gaillard DA *et al.* (1999) Investigation of non-immune hydrops fetalis: multidisciplinary studies are necessary for diagnosis – review of 94 cases. *Pediatr Develop Pathol* **2**, 432–439. Review of 94 cases of nonimmune fetal hydrops over a 10-year period. The most common causes of nonimmune hydrops were chromosome abnormalities (38%), infections (16%) and cardiac pathology (13.8%). The authors were able to establish a diagnosis in 90.4% of the cases based on a systematic examination of both fetus and placenta. **III B**

6 Iskaros J, Jauniaux E, Rodeck C (1997) Outcome of non-immune hydrops fetalis diagnosed during the first half of pregnancy. *Obstet Gynecol* **90**, 321–325. Review of 45 cases of nonimmune fetal hydrops presenting between 11 and 17 weeks gestation. They found that nonimmune fetal hydrops diagnosed before 18 weeks gestation is associated with a higher incidence of aneuploidy than hydrops diagnosed during the second half of pregnancy. **III B**

7 McCoy MC, Katz VL, Gould N *et al.* (1995) Non-immune hydrops after 20 weeks' gestation: review of 10 years' experience with suggestions for management. *Obstet Gynecol* **85**, 578–582. A total of 82 cases of nonimmune hydrops presenting after 20 weeks gestation were reviewed. Overall perinatal mortality was 86.6%. The survival rates before and after 24 weeks were 5% and 20% respectively. The cause of hydrops was identified in 51% of cases before autopsy. Before 24 weeks, 32% were found to have chromosomal abnormalities. The cause was more likely to be cardiovascular after 24 weeks. **III B**

8 Machin GA (1989) Hydrops revisited: literature review of 1,414 cases published in the 1980s. *Am J Med Genet* **34**, 366–390. Review of 610 cases of hydrops fetalis providing guidelines for prenatal diagnosis and management. Prenatal treatment is successful in anemia, tachyarrhythmias and chylothorax and consideration should be given to cordocentesis in addition to detailed ultrasound for diagnosis. **III B**

9 Smoleniec J, James D (1995) Predictive value of pleural effusions in fetal hydrops. *Fetal Diagn Ther* **10**, 95–100. Fetal therapy was confined to three conditions – fetal anemia, fetal tachyarrhythmias and chylothorax. 28 cases of hydrops are reported and fetal therapy was undertaken in 12 (43%). The overall fetal survival was 36.8%. When normal fetuses presenting after 20 weeks were considered the overall survival was 64%. Fetal ascites was the most common ultrasound sign in anemia-related hydrops. Pleural effusions predicted death with a sensitivity of 67% and specificity of 53%. **III B**

10 Castillo RA, Devoe LD, Hadi HA *et al.* (1986) Non-immune hydrops fetalis: clinical experience and factors related to a poor outcome. *Am J Obstet Gynecol* **55**, 812–816. Review of 21 cases of nonimmune fetal hydrops. Two factors were associated with a poor perinatal outcome – the presence of a congenital malformation and the presence of persistent pleural effusions. **III B**

11 Nakayama H, Kukita J, Hikino S *et al.* (1999) Long-term outcome of 51 liveborn neonates with non-immune hydrops fetalis. *Acta Paediatr* **88**, 24–28. Clinical outcome of 51 newborns with nonimmune hydrops fetalis was retrospectively assessed in a single center. The survival rate of the patients with pleural effusions was significantly lower than those without it. 13 of 19 (68.4%) of patients who survived beyond 1 year of age showed normal development, 2 mild developmental delay at 1 year of age and one mental retardation at 8 years of age, while 3 (15.8%) had severe psychomotor retardation. However, 2 of the last 3 patients were born as very-low-birthweight infants. The authors concluded that the prevention of premature birth could improve the long-term outcome of fetuses with nonimmune hydrops fetalis. **III B**

12 Carlton DP, McGillivray BC, Schreiber MD (1989) Nonimmune hydrops fetalis: a multidisciplinary approach. *Clin Perinatol* **16**, 839–851. Review article in which issues in antenatal and delivery room management of nonimmune hydrops are discussed. The causes are listed and include chromosomal abnormalities, abnormalities of cardiac structure and rhythm, pulmonary defects such as diaphragmatic hernia and cystic adenomatoid malformation, intrauterine infection such as parvovirus and cytomegalovirus, alpha-thalassemia and twin–twin transfusion syndrome. Antenatal assessment includes ultrasound evaluation, maternal blood specimens and fetal blood sampling. Mortality is discussed, giving figures of 50–98% depending on etiology. Delivery-room management includes tracheal intubation, paracentesis and thoracocentesis. **IV C**

13 Haverkamp F, Noeker M, Gerresheim G *et al.* (2000) Good prognosis for psychomotor development in survivors with non-immune hydrops fetalis. *Br J Obstet Gynaecol* **107**, 282–284. Observational study of the psychomotor development of 33 of 61 surviving children from a series of 107 consecutive liveborn cases with nonimmune hydrops fetalis. The majority had a normal outcome. **III B**

14 Mari G (2000) Non-invasive diagnosis by Doppler ultrasonography of fetal anemia due to maternal red-cell alloimmunization. *N Engl J Med* **342**, 9–14. Multi-institutional study that measured the hemoglobin concentration in blood obtained by cordocentesis as well as the peak systolic velocity in the middle cerebral artery in the 111 fetuses at risk for anemia due to maternal red-cell alloimmunization. The authors found that the sensitivity of an increased peak systolic velocity in the middle cerebral artery for the prediction of moderate or severe anemia was 100% either in the presence of or in the absence of hydrops, with a false positive rate of 12%. **III B**

15 Fairley CK, Smoleniec JS, Caul OE *et al.* (1995) Observational study of effect of intrauterine transfusions on outcome of fetal hydrops after parvovirus B19 infection. *Lancet* **346**, 1335–1337. Study claiming that intrauterine transfusion will benefit fetuses with hydrops due to parvovirus B19 infection. The study population consisted of 66 cases reported to the Communicable Diseases Surveillance Centre. 12 of 38 cases alive at the first abnormal ultrasound scan received intrauterine transfusions and 9 survived. In 26 cases intrauterine transfusions were not performed and 13 died. The odds of death among those who received an intrauterine transfusion was significantly less than among those who did not. **III B**

16 Bullard KM, Harrison MR (1995) Before the horse is out of the barn: fetal surgery for hydrops. *Semin Perinatol* **19**, 462–473. Review of the pathophysiology and surgical management of hydrops secondary to thoracic lesions and sacrococcygeal teratoma. Thoracoamniotic shunting may improve outcome in cases of large unilocular cystic adenomatoid malformation (CAM) lung lesions; however in only one of four cases was long-term decompression obtained. *In-utero* fetal surgical resection was performed in six cases of CAM with four survivors. The authors refer to the literature and describe thoracoamniotic shunting in eight cases with fetal pleural effusion where six survived. Two cases of *in-utero* surgery for sacrococcygeal teratoma are described and neonatal death occurred in both. The major risk of *in-utero* surgery appears to be preterm labor. **III B**

17 Rodeck CH, Fisk NM, Fraser DI *et al.* (1988) Long-term in utero drainage of fetal hydrothorax. *N Engl J Med* **319**, 1135–1138. Observational study of thoracoamniotic shunting in eight fetuses with hydrothorax. Five of the cases presented with hydrops and resolution of the hydrops occurred in three and these infants survived. The other three cases without hydrops survived. Polyhydramnios resolved in six of the eight fetuses following treatment. To prevent pulmonary hypoplasia long-term drainage is necessary, particularly if the hydrothorax occurs in the second trimester, which is the critical time for lung development. One of the other benefits of thoracoamniotic shunting appears to be facilitation of neonatal resuscitation. **III B**

18 Frohn-Mulder IM, Stewart PA, Witsenburg M *et al.* (1995) The efficacy of flecainide versus digoxin in the management of fetal supraventricular tachycardia. *Prenat Diagn* **15**, 1297–1302. Retrospective analysis of fetal supraventricular tachycardia treated transplacentally was carried out. Of 35 cases, 22 presented without hydrops and 13 with hydrops. Restoration of normal sinus rhythm occurred in 73% of the nonhydropic cases compared with 30% with hydrops ($p < 0.001$) and the mortality was 0% in the nonhydropic fetuses compared with 46% in the hydropic ones ($p < 0.001$). Digoxin was effective in restoring sinus rhythm in 55% of the nonhydropic fetuses but in only 8% of the cases with hydrops. Flecainide caused conversion to sinus rhythm in all nonhydropic fetuses where digoxin treatment failed, and in 43% of hydropic fetuses. Postnatal antiarrhythmic treatment was necessary in 23 infants. Treatment could be withdrawn within 1 year in 22 of the 23 cases. **III B**

19 Van Engelen AD, Weijtens O, Brenner JI *et al.* (1994) Management outcome and follow-up of fetal tachycardia. *J Am Coll Cardiol* **24**, 1371–1375. Study involving 51 fetuses with a tachyarrhythmia where 33 had supraventricular tachycardia (SVT), 15 atrial flutter, one with both SVT and atrial flutter and two with ventricular tachycardia, showed that either digoxin or flecainide as the first administered drug established rhythm control in 84% of cases without hydrops and in 80% with hydrops. Of the 22 fetuses with hydrops, three died. Postnatal drug therapy was needed in 78% by 1 month of age and in 14% by 3 years. The authors concluded that fetal tachycardia can be adequately treated in the majority of cases, even in the presence of hydrops, and that emergency delivery may not be indicated. **III B**

Chapter 15

Fetal hemolytic disease

15.1 Fetal hemolytic disease

Peter McParland

Management option		Quality of evidence	Strength of recommendation	References
Prevention of rhesus hemolytic disease	Antenatal prophylaxis at delivery	III IIb	B	1 2
	Antenatal prophylaxis at 28–34 weeks and at delivery	IIb	B	3
	Prophylaxis after amniocentesis etc.	III	B	4
Prediction of disease severity	Prenatal determination of fetal RhD	III	B	5
	Maternal serum anti-D antibody concentration	III	B	6
	Sonographic prediction of severity of disease – poor without evidence of frank hydrops	III	B	7
	Middle cerebral Doppler appears to be reliable noninvasive technique to determine severity of anemia	III	B	8
	Amniocentesis bilirubin from 27–41 weeks – three zones helpful in managing patients (true level of anemia not known)	III	B	9
	Liley curves of amniotic fluid bilirubin between 18 and 25 weeks detected only 32% of fetuses with a Hb of less than 6 g/dl (appropriate management and survival may not be directly correlated with Hb less than 6 g/dl)	III	B	10
	An extrapolated Liley curve from 20–27 weeks can be used to appropriately manage patients	III	B	11
Treatment	Intravascular transfusion is associated with more than 90% survival	III IIa	B B	12 13
	Intraperitoneal transfusion is a second-line procedure	IIa	B	13
	Fetal transfusion via intrahepatic vein has similar success rates to intravascular sites; possibly less morbidity	III	B	14
	Decline in donor red cells is approximately 2%/day	III	B	15
	The efficacy of intravenous immunoglobulin as a treatment for severe fetal hemolytic disease has not been established	IIb	B	16

Management option		Quality of evidence	Strength of recommendation	References
Treatment (cont'd)	Long-term neurodevelopmental outcome after intravascular transfusion is normal in most cases	III	B	17
	Kell sensitization does not behave like rhesus disease	IV	C	18
	Kell sensitization is due to inhibition of erythroid progenitor cells by anti-Kell antibodies	III	B	19

References

1 Clarke CA (1966) Prevention of Rh haemolytic disease. *Vox Sang* **11**, 641–655. Series of 256 postpartum women unaffected for ABO blood group and parity but containing 206 Rh-negative mothers. Fetal bleeding was assessed by the recently described Keilhauer–Betke test. Of the 85 RhD-negative mothers who had Rh-positive infants, 10 had fetal cells in their blood and 3 of these had formed Anti-D. None of the 75 mothers without evidence of fetal cells in the maternal circulation were sensitized. Clarke concluded that 'transplacental hemorrhage at delivery was the most important factor in sensitizing Rh-negative women'. **III B**

2 Bowman JM, Chown B, Lewis M *et al.* (1978) Rh immunization during pregnancy: antenatal prevention. *Can Med Assoc J* **118**, 623–629. Largest study demonstrating that antenatal prophylaxis is effective in preventing rhesus isoimmunization. Nearly 10000 Rh-negative women delivering RhD-positive fetuses had been given either 300mg of anti-D intramuscularly or 240–300mg intravenously at 28 weeks gestation. Less than 0.1% of women developed anti-D at delivery. These were compared with historical controls given only postnatal anti-D who had an isoimmunization rate of 1.8% (62/3533). **IIb B**

3 Tovey LA, Townley A, Stevenson BJ *et al.* (1983) The Yorkshire antenatal anti-D immunoglobulin trial in primigravidae. *Lancet* **2**, 244–246. Prospective study of over 2000 rhesus-negative women (of whom 1238 were subsequently shown to be carrying a rhesus-positive fetus) in their first pregnancy received 100μg doses of anti-D immunoglobulin at 28 and 34 weeks gestation and a further dose at delivery if the infant was positive in 1980–81. This group was compared with a historical control group of 2000 primigravidae who only received the standard postdelivery dose in 1978–79. There was a nine-fold increase (18 vs 2, $p < 0.01$) in the number of those who did not receive anti-D in the antenatal period who became immunized during the first pregnancy. This is one of several studies supporting the use of routine antenatal anti-D in rhesus-negative mothers. **IIb B**

4 Bowman JM, Pollock JM (1985) Transplacental fetal haemorrhage after amniocentesis. *Obstet Gynecol* **66**, 749–754. Retrospective survey of over 2000 women undergoing amniocentesis and immediate Kleihauer testing between 1981 and 1984 at varying gestations, which showed that 2.3–2.6% of all cases had a fetal–maternal transplacental hemorrhage greater than or equal to 0.1ml of fetal red cells. In 1.8% of cases the fetal maternal hemorrhage was greater than 1ml. Even with placental localization prior to amniocentesis there was an appreciable risk. The authors recommended that 300μg of Rh immune globulin should be administered to all nonimmunized rhesus-negative women after amniocentesis. **III B**

5 Bennett PR, Le Van Kim C, Colin Y *et al.* (1993) Prenatal determination of fetal RhD type by DNA amplification. *N Engl J Med* **329**, 607–610. Prospective study that determined the RhD type in 15 fetuses using polymerase chain reaction in amniotic cells and serological methods in fetal blood collected simultaneously and in a further 15 cases utilizing chorionic villus sampling. With the prior knowledge that RhD is absent on both chromosomes of RhD-negative subjects they were able to identify the Rh D typing correctly in all 30 cases. They suggested that amniocentesis for fetal Rh typing be carried out in the first, or early in the second, trimester when the putative partner is heterozygous. **III B**

6 Nicolaides KH, Rodeck CH (1992) Maternal serum anti-D antibody concentration and assessment of Rhesus isoimmunisation. *Br Med J* **304**, 1155–1156. Observational study in which fetal blood was obtained by fetoscopy or cordocentesis from 237 untreated pregnancies in which rhesus isoimmunization had occurred at 17–38 weeks gestation. In all 42 pregnancies with a maternal anti-D concentration below 15IU/ml the fetuses were at most mildly anemic (as assessed by a hemoglobin deficit below 30g/l). On this basis they suggested that, with anti-D antibody concentrations of less than 15IU/ml, invasive testing was not warranted. In contrast, with a concentration of more than 15IU/ml the fetus could be severely anemic and cordocentesis should be considered. **III B**

7 Nicolaides KH, Fontanarosa M, Gabbe SG *et al.* (1988) Failure of ultrasonographic parameters to predict the severity of fetal anemia in rhesus isoimmunization. *Am J Obstet Gynecol* **158**, 920–926. Observational study measuring placental thickness, extrahepatic and intrahepatic umbilical vein diameters, abdominal circumference, head

circumference, head/abdominal circumference ratio and intraperitoneal volume in 50 rhesus-isoimmunized pregnancies at 18–26 weeks with the severity of fetal anemia being assessed by fetal blood sampling at the same time as the ultrasound assessment. In the absence of fetal hydrops none of the above parameters could reliably distinguish mild from severe fetal hemolytic disease. **III B**

8 Mari G (2000) Noninvasive diagnosis by Doppler ultrasonography of fetal anemia due to maternal red-cell alloimmunization. *N Engl J Med* **342**, 9–14. Observational study correlating middle cerebral artery velocities just before fetal blood sampling in 111 fetuses at risk for anemia due to red-cell immunization in a multicenter prospective trial to determine the predictive value of these measurements. Fetuses with values below 1.5 multiples of the median did not have anemia or had only mild anemia. By using this as a cut-off level the test had 100% sensitivity and 88% specificity for the prediction of moderate to severe anemia. This 12% false-positive rate seems to be lower than amniocentesis and Liley charts. **III B**

9 Liley AW (1961) Liquor amnii analysis in the management of the pregnancy complicated by rhesus sensitization. *Am J Obstet Gynecol* **82**, 1359–1368. Observational study describing the spectrophotometric findings in amniotic fluid from 101 sensitized pregnancies between 27 and 41 weeks. Liley demonstrated, by reported tests, that the 450 mU peak usually diminishes gradually as pregnancy advances. By plotting the measured peaks semi-logarithmically against maturity, he was able to establish three clinically helpful prediction zones separated by lines sloping in accordance with the usual fall in the peak. The size and trend of the 450 mU peak provided an indication of the severity of the anemia and prognosis for the fetus. A limitation of this seminal work was that, because fetal blood sampling was not yet available, the actual degree of fetal disease at the time of amniocentesis was not assessed. **III B**

10 Nicolaides KH, Rodeck CH, Mibashan R (1986) Have Liley charts outlived their usefulness? *Am J Obstet Gynecol* **155**, 90–94. Observational study challenging the assumption that the Liley charts could be simply extrapolated back into the second trimester. Fetal blood and amniotic fluid were obtained fetoscopically from 59 sensitized pregnancies at 18–25 weeks. The sensitivity and specificity of using the extrapolated Liley charts for diagnosing fetal anemia was shown to be 44% and 82% respectively. Of 31 severely anemic fetuses (Hb < 6 g/dl) only 10 (32%) would have received intrauterine transfusion using the extrapolated Liley criteria. **III B**

11 Spinnato JA, Clark AL, Ralston KK *et al.* (1998) Hemolytic disease of the fetus: a comparison of the Queenan and extended Liley methods. *Obstet Gynecol* **92**, 441–445. Amniotic fluid bilirubin was evaluated spectrophotometrically in 73 women sensitized to red-cell antigens. Values in the four Queenan zones were compared with the four zones of the Liley graph (middle zone subdivided). Overestimation of risk occurred with greater frequency when using the Queenan method. In 13% of cases, the Queenan graph and method would have prompted unnecessary or premature fetal blood sampling, with its attendant risks. **III B**

12 Weiner CP, Williamson RA, Wenstrom KD *et al.* (1991) Management of fetal hemolytic disease by cordocentesis. II. Outcome of treatment. *Am J Obstet Gynecol* **165**, 1302–1307. A group of 48 fetuses received a total of 142 intravascular transfusions (range 1–7) for treatment of severe anemia (hematocrit of < 30%). 13 (27%) fetuses had hydrops when therapy was initiated. The overall survival rate was 96%. They demonstrated that, after the second transfusion, on average less than 1% of circulating red blood cells were fetal and also showed suppression of fetal erythropoiesis with a mean reticulocyte count of less than 1% within 3 weeks of the second transfusion. Two hydropic fetuses died shortly after the first transfusion. **III B**

13 Harman CR, Bowman JM, Manning FA *et al.* (1980) Intrauterine transfusion – intraperitoneal versus intravascular approach: a case-control comparison. *Am J Obstet Gynecol* **162**, 1053–1059. Well-matched case-control study (44 pairs) comparing intraperitoneal (IPT) and intravascular transfusion (IVT) in the management of severe rhesus disease. The intravascular approach was better with regard to all objective endpoints, including greater maturity at survival, improved neonatal constitution, fewer transfusions as neonates, less time on ventilators and in intensive care units. Overall survival was 91% with IVT compared with 66% with IPT. The authors concluded that intraperitoneal transfusion was a second-line procedure to be used in very limited circumstances. **IIa B**

14 Nicolini U, Nicolaidis P, Fisk NM *et al.* (1990) Fetal blood sampling from the intrahepatic vein: analysis of safety and clinical experience with 214 procedures. *Obstet Gynecol* **76**, 47–53. Retrospective report described the usefulness of intrahepatic vein transfusion on 214 occasions in 177 fetuses. The success rate of obtaining blood was 91% and the overall survival was 86%. The authors felt that this approach reduced the risk of fetal blood loss, fetomaternal hemorrhage, arterial vasospasm and cord tamponade as well as acting as an alternate site when difficulties arise with the placental cord insertion. **III B**

15 Egberts J, van Kamp IL, Kanhai HH *et al.* (1997) The disappearance of fetal and donor red blood cells in alloimmunised pregnancies: a reappraisal. *Br J Obstet Gynaecol* **104**, 818–824. Retrospective study of 302 transfusions in 101 fetuses to determine the rate of fall of both fetal and donor red blood cells after intrauterine intravascular transfusions. The interval between the first and second transfusion (15.5 days) was shorter than between subsequent transfusions (21.4–21.9 days). This rate of fall in numbers of donor red cells equated to about 2% per day. The authors suggest using the above criteria for timing transfusions as a rule of thumb but did acknowledge exceptions necessitating close fetal surveillance in between transfusions. **III B**

16 Voto LS, Mathet ER, Zapaterio JL *et al.* (1997) High-dose gammaglobulin (IVIG) followed by intrauterine transfusions (IUT): a new alternative for the treatment of severe fetal hemolytic disease. *J Perinat Med* **25**, 85–88. Largest case-controlled study assessing the value of high-dose intravenous immunoglobin (IVIG) as adjunct treatment to intravascular transfusion in very severely isoimmunized fetuses. 30 cases were treated with IVIG before 21 weeks but still needed IUTs after 20–21 weeks; they were compared with 39 patients receiving similar IUT treatment without IVIG. The percentage of severely anemic fetuses was higher in the IUT-alone group and fetal mortality was 36% lower than in the IVIG and IUT group. The authors concluded that RCTs were necessary to confirm these results. **IIb B**

17 Hudon L, Moise KJ Jr, Hegemier SE *et al.* (1998) Long-term neurodevelopmental outcome after intrauterine transfusion for the treatment of fetal hemolytic disease. *Am J Obstet Gynecol* **179**, 858–863. Prospective observational study using well-established methods of neurodevelopmental assessment in 40 neonatal survivors of severe hemolytic disease treated with intrauterine transfusion (IUT), up to 62 months of age (median number of IUTs was four, with first IUT at 26 weeks). Although there was one case of severe bilateral deafness and one case of right spastic hemiplegia, all other neurodevelopmental assessments were reassuring, suggesting normal developmental outcome in children treated for severe disease. A limitation of this study is lack of follow-up for all children. **III B**

18 Berkowitz RL, Beyth Y, Sadovsky E (1982) Death in utero due to Kell sensitization without excessive elevation of the delta od450 value in amniotic fluid. *Obstet Gynecol* **60**, 746–749. First case report to suggest that Kell sensitization might not behave in the same fashion as rhesus sensitization. Three amniocenteses were carried out between 21 and 24 weeks, demonstrating a downward trend in zone II. An intrauterine death with evidence of gross hydrops was diagnosed around the time of the third amniocentesis. **IV C**

19 Vaughan JI, Manning M, Warwick RM *et al.* (1998) Inhibition of erythroid progenitor cells by anti-Kell antibodies in fetal alloimmune anemia. *N Engl J Med* **338**, 789–803. Observational study comparing the growth *in vitro* of Kell-positive and Kell-negative hematopoietic progenitor cells from cord blood in the presence of anti-Kell antibodies and anti-D antibodies and serum from 22 women with anti-Kell antibodies. The growth of Kell-positive erythroid progenitor cells from cord blood was markedly inhibited by monoclonal IgG and IgM anti-Kell antibodies but in a dose-dependent fashion, while anti-D antibodies had no effect. This finding supported a hypothesis put forward by the same group previously that anti-Kell antibodies cause fetal anemia mainly by suppressing erythropoiesis at the progenitor-cell level. **III B**

Chapter 16

Fetal thrombocytopenia

16.1 Fetal thrombocytopenia

Jane Rutherford

Autoimmune thrombocytopenia

Management option		Quality of evidence	Strength of recommendation	References
Prenatal	Laboratory investigations: ❑ Monitor maternal platelet counts ❑ Exclude other causes	–	✔	–
	Treatment: ❑ Corticosteroids when the maternal platelet count falls below 50 ❑ Consider splenectomy with severe immune thrombocytopenic purpura (ITP) in early pregnancy with no response to steroids ❑ Immunoglobulin is best reserved for administration between 36 and 37 weeks	–	✔	–
Labor and delivery	Cordocentesis at 38–39 weeks and fetal scalp blood sampling have been proposed to assess fetal risk of thrombocytopenia. However, there are no reports of fetal intracerebral hemorrhage in women with ITP and no convincing evidence that cesarean delivery is protective, although one review suggests a higher incidence of postnatal intracranial hemorrhage (ICH) with *vaginal* delivery (2% vs 0.5% respectively)	–	✔	–
	Cesarean section is performed entirely for obstetric indications	III	B	1–3
	Avoidance of assisted vaginal delivery, especially by vacuum extraction	–	✔	–
	Episiotomy should be avoided if possible with low maternal platelet counts	–	✔	–
	Maternal platelet transfusion to cover delivery if the platelet count is below 50	–	✔	–
	Epidural analgesia is reasonable if the platelet count is above 70	III	B	4
Postnatal	Neonatal platelet count; transfusion of platelets low and clinically indicated	–	✔	–

References

1 Song TS, Lee JY, Kim YH *et al.* (1999) Low neonatal risk of thrombocytopenia in pregnancy associated with immune thrombocytopenic purpura. *Fetal Diagn Ther* **14**, 216–219. Retrospective survey of 32 pregnancies complicated by immune thrombocytopenic purpura. Cordocentesis was performed in 16. No neonates had severe thrombocytopenia. **III B**

2 Burrows RF, Kelton JG (1993) Fetal thrombocytopenia and its relation to maternal thrombocytopenia. *N Engl J Med* **329**, 1463–1466. Cross-sectional prospective study of 1027 mothers with thrombocytopenia due to various causes (immune thrombocytopenic purpura, ITP, hypertensive disorders of pregnancy, gestational thrombocytopenia). Only 19 infants had severe thrombocytopenia (9 due to alloimmune thrombocytopenia, 5 with hypertensive disorders, 4 due to ITP and one due to incidental thrombocytopenia). None of the infants born to women with ITP had intracranial hemorrhage. **III B**

3 Payne SD, Resnik R, Moore TR *et al.* (1997) Maternal characteristics and risk of severe neonatal thrombocytopenia and intracranial hemorrhage in pregnancies complicated by autoimmune thrombocytopenia. *Am J Obstet Gynecol* **177**, 149–155. Retrospective observational study in 41 women with immune thrombocytopenic purpura (ITP). There was an increased incidence of neonatal thrombocytopenia in women with a previous splenectomy. A review of literature with regard to mode of delivery includes 601 neonates born to women with ITP; 12% had severe thrombocytopenia. 51% of the total delivered vaginally; 6 cases had intracranial hemorrhage (2 were delivered by caesarean section, 4 vaginally). **III B**

4 Beilin Y, Zahn J, Comerford M (1997) Safe epidural analgesia in thirty parturients with platelet counts between 69,000 and 98,000 mm^{-3}. *Anesth Analg* **85**, 385–388. Retrospective case note review of 80 women with platelet counts below100 000/mm^3. 30 of these had an epidural catheter sited. Platelet count ranged from 69 000 to 98 000/mm^3. No neurological complications were noted. **III B**

Alloimmune thrombocytopenia

Management option		Quality of evidence	Strength of recommendation	References
Prepregnancy	Once alloimmunization is suspected (usually after the birth of an affected child), type parents' platelets, screen mother for antibodies against the paternal platelets	–	✔	–
	Establish human leukocyte antigen (HLA) status of the mother	–	✔	–
	The maternal antibody level may help predict the severity in future pregnancies	III	B	1
	Careful counseling of parents	–	✔	–
	In addition to the parents, members of the mother's family should be typed to establish whether her sisters are at similar risk during their pregnancies	–	✔	–
Prenatal	Early contact with a specialist is essential once conception is confirmed	–	✔	–
	Cordocentesis for fetal platelet typing is no longer necessary	–	✔	–
	If the partner is heterozygous for the human platelet antigen (HPA) in question, the fetal genotype can be determined by DNA analysis using polymerase chain reaction technology on amniocytes	–	✔	–
	No further action is necessary if the fetus types as HPA-negative (accuracy 95–99%)	–	✔	–
	At-risk pregnancies should be managed in a specialist center	–	✔	–
	The two main treatment regimens are			
	❑ Maternal administration of immunoglobulin ± oral corticosteroids	IIb	B	2
	❑ Repeated fetal platelet sampling and intravascular transfusion of fresh platelets	IIa	B	3
	❑ Various combinations of these two regimens have also been used	III	B	4–6

➡

Management option		Quality of evidence	Strength of recommendation	References
Labor and delivery	Mode of delivery depends on the fetal platelet count. A trial of labor is reasonable if the count exceeds 50. A transfusion of platelets just before delivery may be considered even if a cesarean section is contemplated; abdominal delivery is not always atraumatic	–	✔	–
Postnatal	Neonatal platelet count; transfusion of platelets low and clinically indicated	–	✔	–

References

1 Williamson LM, Hackett G, Rennie J *et al.* (1998) The natural history of fetomaternal alloimmunisation to the platelet specific antigen HPA-1α (P1A1, Zwa) as determined by antenatal screening. *Blood* **92**, 2280–2287. Prospective observational study of 385 HPA-1-negative women. Anti HP-1α was detected in 46 of 387 pregnancies. There was one *in-utero* fetal death. 26 HPA-1α-positive babies were born of which 9 were severely thrombocytopenic. Severe thrombocytopenia was significantly associated with third trimester anti-HPA-1α titers of 1:32 or more. **III B**

2 Bussel JB, Berkowitz RL, Lynch L *et al.* (1996) Antenatal management of alloimmune thrombocytopenia with intravenous gamma-globulin: a randomized trial of the addition of low-dose steroid to intravenous gamma-globulin. *Am J Obstet Gynecol* **174**, 1414–1423. Prospective randomized multicenter study in alloimmune thrombocytopenia of giving intravenous immunoglobulin to all, with or without dexamethasone. No difference with dexamethasone. Increased platelet counts were found with any treatment. There were no cases of intracranial hemorrhage. **IIb B**

3 Paidas MJ, Berkowitz RL, Lynch L *et al.* (1995) Alloimmune thrombocytopenia: fetal and neonatal losses related to cordocentesis. *Am J Obstet Gynecol* **172**, 475–479. Retrospective case control (44 controls). Increased fetal death following cordocentesis if platelets less than 20 (5 cases). Authors recommended prophylactic platelet transfusion. **IIa B**

4 Giers G, Hoch J, Bauer H *et al.* (1996) Therapy with intravenous immunoglobulin G during pregnancy for fetal alloimmune thrombocytopenic purpura. *Prenat Diagn* **16**, 495–502. Observational study in seven patients. Fetal blood sampling regularly from 20 weeks. Platelet transfusions were given to prevent hemorrhage. Intravenous immunoglobulin was also given. The platelet count remained unchanged in three, fell in two and rose in two. **III B**

5 Wenstrom KD, Weiner CP, Williamson RA (1992) Antenatal treatment of fetal alloimmune thrombocytopenia. *Obstet Gynecol* **80**, 433–435. Retrospective review of six pregnancies. All had a previous pregnancy with a history suggestive of alloimmune thrombocytopenia. Serial fetal platelet counts were performed. Maternal treatment with intravenous immunoglobulin (IVIG) was performed in three women and using IVIG + dexamethasone in three women. Five had counts adequate for vaginal delivery (97–257). **III B**

6 Murphy MF, Waters AH, Doughty HA *et al.* (1994) Antenatal management of fetomaternal alloimmune thrombocytopenia – report of 15 affected pregnancies. *Transfusion Med* **4**, 281–292. Observational study of 15 pregnancies in 11 women. Fetal platelet transfusions and steroids and/or intravenous immunoglobulin (IVIG) were used. One case had an intracerebral hemorrhage before 32 weeks; five were severely affected requiring serial platelet transfusions and five were mildly affected (four were maintained with IVIG and steroids but one also required platelets). Four pregnancies were unsuccessful. **III B**

Chapter 17

Fetal cardiac problems

17.1 Fetal arrhythmias

Helena Gardiner

Bradycardias

Management option		Quality of evidence	Strength of recommendation	References
Prepregnancy	Counseling of women with risk factors for complete atrioventricular block (CAVB)			
	❑ Previous child with CAVB	III	B	1,2
	❑ Maternal anti-SSA (Ro) or anti-SSB (La) antibodies	III IV	B C	3 4,5
	❑ Maternal heart block	–	✔	–
	❑ Previous child with left atrial isomerism	–	✔	–
Prenatal – diagnosis	Detailed and serial fetal echocardiography of antibody-positive mothers and those with a positive family history	–	✔	–
	Fetal echocardiography for persistent fetal heart rate below 100	–	✔	–
	Serial echocardiography for emerging block (second or third degree heart block)	–	✔	–
	Irregular rhythms			
	❑ If occasional, clinical follow-up	–	✔	–
	❑ If persistent, fetal echocardiography and intensify follow-up	–	✔	–
	Evaluation of asymptomatic mothers for autoimmune disease (rheumatoid arthritis, Sjögren syndrome, systemic lupus erythematosus or undifferentiated autoimmune syndrome)	III	B	1
Prenatal – treatment	Controversial: early steroids and/or plasmapheresis?	IV	C	4,5
	Inotropic/chronotropic support of limited benefit	III	B	6
	Fetal pacing has been attempted	IV	B	7
	Consider early delivery in tertiary center if hydrops is evident but generally try to avoid preterm delivery	–	✔	–
	Mode of delivery: intrapartum monitoring of fetal distress may be difficult in CAVB	III	B	8
Postnatal	Temporary pacing may be needed	IV	C	9
	Permanent pacemaker for rate below 60, symptoms or structural disease	III	B	10

References

1 Waltuck J, Buyon JP (1994) Autoantibody-associated congenital heart block: outcome in mothers and children. *Ann Intern Med* **120**, 544–551. Longitudinal review of 55 children with complete atrioventricular block to ascertain the development of maternal illness. 11 (48%) of the 23 initially asymptomatic mothers developed symptoms of a rheumatic disease (6 (26%) developed an undifferentiated autoimmune syndrome, 2 (9%) developed Sjögren syndrome and 3 (13%) developed systemic lupus erythematosus). Of 25 subsequent pregnancies in 22 women, 4 (16%) were complicated by heart block. 17 affected children died, 12 within 1 month of birth. Pacemakers were implanted in 37 (67%) of the 55 children, 27 within 3 months after birth. **III B**

2 Julkunen H, Kaaja R, Siren MK *et al.* (1998) Immune-mediated congenital heart block (CAVB): identifying and counseling patients at risk for having children with CAVB. *Semin Arthritis Rheum* **28**, 97–106. Retrospective study of 46 women with a complete atrioventricular block (CAVB) child, comparing the strength and specificity of the immune response to SSA/Ro and SSB/La, in 44 affected women with 85 women with systemic lupus erythematosus and 32 women with primary Sjögren syndrome with healthy children. High levels of anti-SSA/Ro and anti-SSB/La were associated with a significantly increased risk of having a CAVB child. The relative risk for a female child compared with a male child to have CAVB was 1.9 (1.2–2.9, $p = 0.009$), and the risk of the mother having another child with CAVB was 12% (4 of 34). **III B**

3 Buyon JP, Waltuck J, Kleinman C *et al.* (1995) In utero identification and therapy of congenital heart block. *Lupus* **4**, 116–121. A retrospective postal questionnaire study of 72 affected pregnancies to identify the gestational age at detection and outcome. More than half of the cases were detected between 16 and 24 weeks. Progression of block was documented, as was improvement in 3 of 19 fetuses whose mothers were given steroids to prevent CAVB. In 8 of the others, effusions resolved, perhaps reflecting an improvement in active myocarditis. **III B**

4 Buyon JP, Roubey R, Swersky S *et al.* (1988) Complete congenital heart block: risk of occurrence and therapeutic approach to prevention. *J Rheumatol* **15**, 1104–1108. Case report of a fetus whose previous sibling had complete atrioventricular block. Recurrence was not seen in this pregnancy and the authors propose that maternal plasmapheresis and steroid therapy prevented harmful transplacental transfer of antibodies. **IV C**

5 Reichlin M (1998) Systemic lupus erythematosus and pregnancy. *J Reprod Med* **43**, 355–360. Review of disease activity at the time of conception and its effect on pregnancy. **IV C**

6 Groves ANM, Allan LD, Rosenthal E (1995) Therapeutic trial of sympathomimetics in three cases of complete heart block in the fetus. *Circulation* **92**, 3394–3396. A nonrandomized therapeutic study of three fetuses with complete atrioventricular block given isoprenaline and salbutamol (albuterol). No changes in fetal heart rate were observed with isoprenaline but maternal salbutamol increased the heart rate and shortening fraction in all three and reversed fetal hydrops in one case. **III B**

7 Walkinshaw SA, Welch CR, McCormack J *et al.* (1994) In utero pacing for fetal congenital heart block. *Fetal Diagn Ther* **9**, 183–185. Case report of attempted fetal pacing demonstrating its feasibility and the technical improvements necessary to permit long-term success. **IV B**

8 Kleinman CS, Copel JA, Hobbins JC (1987) Combined echocardiographic and Doppler assessment of fetal congenital atrioventricular block. *Br J Obstet Gynaecol* **94**, 967–974. Echocardiographic assessment of atrial reactivity during labour in five fetuses with second- or third-degree heart block, demonstrating that echocardiography, combined with external atrial monitoring, is suitable for monitoring fetal wellbeing during vaginal delivery if performed by an appropriately trained operator. **III B**

9 Weindling SN, Saul P, Triedman JK *et al.* (1994) Staged pacing therapy for congenital complete heart block in premature infants. *Am J Cardiol* **74**, 412–413. Two case reports of preterm delivery of fetuses with complete heart block. Ventricular pacing took place on days 1 and 2 respectively. Both infants survived. **IV C**

10 Villain E, Martelli H, Bonnet D *et al.* (2000) Characteristics and results of epicardial pacing in neonates and infants. *Pacing Clin Electrophysiol* **12**, 2052–2056. The results of epicardial pacing in 34 children with complete atrioventricular block in a single center are reported, concluding that this is a safe and effective method of pacing small children with few complications. **III B**

Tachycardias

Management option		Quality of evidence	Strength of recommendation	References
Prepregnancy	Counseling of those with history of:			
	❑ Wolff–Parkinson–White syndrome (WPW)	IV	C	1
	❑ Familial long QT syndrome	IV	C	2
Prenatal – diagnosis	Fetal echocardiography for sustained fetal heart rate above 180	–	✔	–

➡

Management option		Quality of evidence	Strength of recommendation	References
Prenatal – diagnosis (cont'd)	Evaluate cardiac structure, function, presence of hydrops and mechanism (1:1 conduction vs evidence of block)	III IV	B C	3 4,5
Prenatal – treatment	Nonsustained tachycardia requires monitoring but no treatment unless hydrops is present	–	✔	–
	Medical (transplacental) control of sustained tachycardia	IV	C	5,6
	❑ Digoxin given orally to the mother is usually effective, occasionally it may not be and some prefer the maternal intravenous route	III	B	7,8
	❑ If no response in 48 hours, flecainide or verapamil may be helpful (some use flecainide as first choice)	III IV	B C	9,10 11
	❑ Therapy delivered directly to the fetus has been effective, particularly in the setting of hydrops	IV	C	12
	❑ Long-term effects of fetal drug administration should be sought	III	B	13
Postnatal	12-lead electrocardiogram to confirm WPW or long QT syndrome	–	✔	–
	Take local advice re prophylactic treatment for tachycardia – some will not use this routinely. Some centers will treat asymptomatic neonates for 6–12 months and review	–	✔	–
	Treat recurrent tachycardia in infancy	III	B	14

References

1. Gollob MH, Green MS, Tang AS *et al.* (2001) Identification of a gene responsible for familial Wolff–Parkinson–White syndrome. *N Engl J Med* **344**, 1823–1831. Study permitting the identification of a candidate gene on chromosome 7 in two families. This may permit further investigation of the mechanisms involved and further identification of cases. **IV C**
2. Yamada M, Nakazawa M, Momma K (1998) Fetal ventricular tachycardia in long QT syndrome. *Cardiol Young* **8**, 119–122. Case report of a fetus with intermittent ventricular tachycardia during mid-gestation. The mother had long QT syndrome. The arrhythmia disappeared spontaneously, and the electrocardiogram of the baby after birth showed prolonged QTc. **IV C**
3. Naheed ZJ, Strasburger JF, Deal BJ (1996) Fetal tachycardia: mechanisms and predictors of hydrops fetalis. *J Am Coll Cardiol* **27**, 1736–1740. Single-center observational study of 30 patients to elucidate the electrophysiological mechanisms of fetal tachycardia, the predictors of hydrops and the outcome. 22 fetuses showed 1:1 conduction and 8 an atrial tachycardia with atrioventricular block. Electrophysiological studies showed AVRT in 25/27 in whom tachycardia was inducible postnatally using transesophageal pacing with an intra-atrial tachycardia in 2. They confirmed that AVRT is the predominant mechanism of supraventricular tachycardia in the fetus despite the presence of block. Hydrops was more common with sustained tachycardia but the mechanism of tachycardia and the heart rate were not shown to be important and the outcome (1–7 years) excellent regardless of the severity of illness at presentation. **III B**
4. Kleinman CS, Copel JA, Weinstein EM *et al.* (1985) Treatment of fetal supraventricular tachyarrhythmias. *J Clin Ultrasound* **13**, 265–273. This review documents noninvasive methods of diagnosis and treatment strategies for fetal supraventricular tachycardia. **IV C**
5. Meijboom EJ, van Engelen AD, van de Beek EW *et al.* (1994) Fetal arrhythmias. *Curr Opin Cardiol* **9**, 97–102. This review describes the methods of diagnosis and treatment options of fetuses in arrhythmias. **IV C**
6. Ward RM (1989) Maternal–placental–fetal unit: unique problems of pharmacologic study. *Pediatr Clin North Am* **36**, 1075–1088. Review article of changes in pharmacokinetics during pregnancy and the implications of transplacental treatment of the fetus. **IV C**

7 Van Engelen AD, Weijtens O, Brenner JL *et al.* (1994) Management outcome and follow-up of fetal tachycardia. *J Am Coll Cardiol* **24**, 1371–1375. Retrospective multicenter study of treatment and outcome of 51 fetuses with tachycardia confirming successful control in 82% even in the presence of hydrops. Although 50% had tachycardia after delivery, only 14% were on treatment at 3 years. **III B**

8 Azancot-Benisty A, Jacqz-Aigrain E, Guirgis NM *et al.* (1992) Clinical and pharmacologic study of fetal supraventricular tachyarrhythmias. *J Pediatr* **121**, 608–613. Small single-center observational study of different therapeutic regimens to control fetal tachycardia. The authors found little success with oral digoxin therapy and recommend routine intravenous use (this is not in line with most other centers and may suggest noncompliance), while flecainide was thought useful in flutter. **III B**

9 Allan LD, Chita SK, Sharland GK *et al.* (1991) Flecainide in the treatment of fetal tachycardias. *Br Heart J* **65**, 46–48. Single-center series of 14 mothers treated with flecainide for fetal atrial tachycardias associated with intrauterine cardiac failure. 12/14 fetuses responded with one subsequently dying in utero. The 2 failures were successfully treated with digoxin. The authors caution the use of flecainide, limiting it to patients with severe fetal hydrops and supraventricular tachycardias, particularly in atrial flutter. **III B**

10 Frohn-Mulder IME, Stewart PA, Witsenburg M *et al.* (1995) The efficacy of flecainide versus digoxin in the management of fetal supraventricular tachycardia. *Prenat Diagn* **15**, 1297–1302. Retrospective analysis of 49/51 fetuses with supraventricular tachycardia. 14 were not treated but 9 needed postnatal treatment. Transplacental treatment was reported in 35 fetuses (22 without and 13 with hydrops). Those with hydrops had a high mortality (0% vs 46%; $p < 0.001$). Digoxin restored sinus rhythm in 55% of the nonhydropic fetuses but in only 8% of the hydropic fetuses. Flecainide was effective in restoring sinus rhythm in all nonhydropic fetuses where digoxin treatment failed and in 43% of hydropic fetuses. Administration of flecainide resulted in a significantly reduced mortality ($p < 0.001$) compared with digoxin treatment. No adverse effects were seen. Postnatal antiarrhythmic treatment was necessary in 23 infants. Treatment could be withdrawn within one year in all cases but one. **III B**

11 Fish FA, Gillette PC, Benson Jr DW (1991) Proarrhythmia, cardiac arrest, and death in young patients receiving encainide and flecainide. *J Am Coll Cardiol* **18**, 356–365. Multicenter audit of class 1C sodium-channel blockers in children, highlighting the proarrhythmic effects. Children with structural heart defects and poor function were more likely to suffer a proarrhythmic event or cardiac arrest. **IV C**

12 Kohl T, Tercanli S, Kececioglu D *et al.* (1995) Direct fetal administration of adenosine for the termination of incessant supraventricular tachycardia. *Obstet Gynecol* **85**, 873–874. Single case report of direct intravenous administration of adenosine via the fetal hepatic vein to temporarily stop fetal tachycardia with control achieved by digoxin and flecainide. This approach is used diagnostically and therapeutically postnatally for AVRT, which is the commonest mechanism of fetal supraventricular tachycardia, and is a possible alternative to gain rapid control of tachycardia in a hydropic fetus. **IV C**

13 Magee LA, Downar E, Sermer M *et al.* (1995) Pregnancy outcome after gestational exposure to amiodarone in Canada. *Am J Obstet Gynecol* **172**, 1307–1311. Retrospective study of 12 children who had received fetal amiodarone, showing that first-trimester exposure might be associated with thyroid dysfunction and neurological abnormalities. Four of the cases had received beta-blockers, which might explain their additional smallness. **III B**

14 O'Sullivan JJ, Derrick G, Foxall RJ *et al.* (1995) Digoxin or flecainide for prophylaxis of supraventricular tachycardia in infants? *J Am Coll Cardiol* **26**, 991–994. Study comparing the safety and efficacy of digoxin and flecainide in the prophylaxis of supraventricular tachycardia (SVT) in 39 infants with SVT due to atrioventricular reentry. Patients treated with oral digoxin showed breakthrough tachycardia that responded to flecainide, while the converse was not seen. The authors conclude that comparison with previous natural history studies suggests that digoxin is ineffective in the prophylaxis of SVT while oral flecainide was effective with no adverse effects and may now be preferred as the primary prophylactic agent in infancy. **III B**

17.2 Cardiac malformations

Helena Gardiner

Management option		Quality of evidence	Strength of recommendation	References
Prepregnancy	All women should be counseled that there is about 1% risk of congenital heart defects (CHD) in pregnancy and that most babies with CHD are born to mothers perceived to be low risk. Multifetal pregnancies are at increased risk of CHD (3%). All women considering pregnancy should take periconceptual folic acid	Ib IIa	A B	1 2

Management option		Quality of evidence	Strength of recommendation	References
	High-risk groups: ❑ Maternal/paternal CHD; sibling or relatives with CHD ❑ Maternal insulin-dependent diabetes mellitus ❑ Maternal illness (phenylketonuria; epilepsy; autoimmune antibodies, e.g. systemic lupus erythematosus; drugs, e.g. lithium) ❑ Possibility of multifetal pregnancy (assisted conception)	 III III	 B B	 3 4
Prenatal – diagnosis	Nuchal translucency screening will generate a new 'high-risk' group with normal karyotype who will require a cardiac scan in second trimester	III	B	5
	Routine level 2 anomaly scanning should include assessment of situs, four-chamber view, crossover of great arteries and 'three-vessel' view of transverse aorta, ductus arteriosus and superior vena cava	III	B	6
	Refer all high-risk groups for fetal echocardiography	–	✔	–
Prenatal – management	Morphological diagnosis and severity of circulatory compromise (joint evaluation by obstetrician and cardiologist)	–	✔	–
	Search for extracardiac anomalies	IV III	C B	7 8
	Offer fetal karyotyping, including 22q deletion	IV III III	C B B	7 8 9
	Multidisciplinary counseling, including the cardiac surgeon and psychological support for parents	–	✔	–
	Monitoring of defect may document progression of disease (worsening)	–	✔	–
	Monitor fetal growth (usually normal in the absence of karyotypic abnormalities) and wellbeing by nonstress test, biophysical profile and Doppler of peripheral vessels	–	✔	–
Labor and delivery	Delivery in center with appropriate obstetric, pediatric and cardiology facilities	III	B	10
	Vaginal delivery usually appropriate for isolated cardiac defects	–	✔	–
	Fetal monitoring advised but may not be useful, e.g. in fetal complete heart block	–	✔	–
	Elective delivery at 38 weeks may be appropriate for fetuses with complex defects such as hypoplastic left heart syndrome	III	B	11,12

➡

Management option		Quality of evidence	Strength of recommendation	References
Postnatal	After termination of pregnancy or perinatal death obtain autopsy whenever possible and arrange for bereavement counseling and to discuss the full diagnosis and implications for future pregnancies	–	✔	–
	Stabilize the neonate, confirm the diagnosis by detailed echocardiography, adjust management plan according to any new findings	–	✔	–

References

1 Czeizel AE (1996) Reduction of urinary tract and cardiovascular defects by periconceptional multivitamin supplementation. *Am J Med Genet* **62**, 179–183. Randomized double-blind controlled trial to study the preventive effect of periconceptional multivitamin supplementation on neural-tube defects and other congenital abnormalities. The authors documented a marked reduction in the total rate of major congenital abnormalities when multivitamins (including 0.8 mg of folic acid) were given compared with trace element supplementation alone (20.6/1000 vs 40.6/1000). Following exclusion of the neural-tube defects in the trace element group, the difference in urinary tract defects and congenital heart disease, mostly septal defects, was highly significant ($p = 0.0003$, relative risk 0.54, 95% CI 0.39–0.76). **Ib A**

2 Botto LD, Mulinare J, Erickson JD (2000) Occurrence of congenital heart defects in relation to maternal multivitamin use. *Am J Epidemiol* **151**, 878–884. Population-based case-control study to examine the effect of preconceptual vitamin use and cardiac defects in the offspring born to mothers in Atlanta, Georgia from 1968–80. Periconceptual vitamin use (regular use for at least 3 months before pregnancy and during the first trimester) was associated with a reduced odds ratio for nonsyndromic cardiac defects in the offspring (0.76; 95% CI 0.60–0.97). This was greatest for conotruncal defects and ventricular septal defects. No risk reduction was evident if vitamins were started during pregnancy. The authors postulate that one in four cardiac defects could be prevented by preconceptual vitamin use. **IIa B**

3 Burn J, Brennan P, Little J *et al.* (1998) Recurrence risks in offspring of adults with major heart defects: results from first cohort of British collaborative study. *Lancet* **351**, 311–316. Prospective study assessing the recurrence risks of congenital heart disease in offspring of survivors of major congenital heart disease in a collaborative British study. There were 393 live offspring from a participating cohort of 727 of 1094 individuals identified as surviving surgery for major cardiac defects before 1970. The recurrence risk for heart defects overall was 4.1%, which was twice that of sibling risk (2.1%) and heart defects were twice as common following maternal as paternal heart disease. There was an excess of miscarriages in affected women (20%) with an overall rate of 15.3% (71/469 pregnancies). **III B**

4 Gladman G, McCrindle BW, Boutin C *et al.* (1997) Fetal echocardiographic screening of diabetic pregnancies for congenital heart disease. *Am J Perinatol* **14**, 59–62. Prospective observational study in one center investigating the relationship between the hemoglobin A1c levels of diabetic women and cardiac malformations between 1988 and 1995. Cardiac defects were detected in 7/328 pregnancies (incidence 2.1% 95% CI 0.6–3.6%). A wide range of HbA1c levels was associated with fetal cardiac abnormality but no significant difference between those with and without cardiac defects. The authors conclude that the incidence of cardiac defects in diabetic mothers is low and did not appear to be associated with diabetic control in this study. **III B**

5 Hyett J, Perdu M, Shareland G *et al.* (1999) Using fetal nuchal translucency to screen for major congenital cardiac defects at 10–14 weeks of gestation: population based cohort study. *Br Med J* **318**, 81–85. Population-based cohort study of 29154 singleton pregnancies with chromosomally normal fetuses at 10–14 weeks gestation. The relationship of increased nuchal translucency and the presence of congenital heart disease (CHD) was reported. 56% (95% CI 42–70%) had nuchal translucency measurements above the 95th centile. The authors propose this as a useful early screening for CHD. **III B**

6 Stumpflen I, Stumpflen A, Wimmer M *et al.* (1996) Effect of detailed fetal echocardiography as part of routine prenatal ultrasonographic screening on detection of congenital heart disease. *Lancet* **348**, 854–857. Unselected consecutive detailed fetal echocardiography was performed in a single institution over a 21-month period in 3085 pregnant women, 2181 with no known risk factors for congenital heart disease (CHD). 364 of the fetuses had abnormalities detected sonographically. 46 cases of CHD were detected, 28 in the group with sonographic abnormality and 15 in those with no risk factors. The authors conclude that the incidence of CHD in those with no risk factors is 6.9 per 1000 and is not significantly altered by maternal disease or a family history of CHD (5.6 per

1000). The detection of a sonographic abnormality was significantly more likely to be associated with CHD (79.9 per 1000) and underscores the need for detailed cardiac scanning in all pregnancies. **III B**

7 Copel JA, Pilu G, Kleinman CS *et al.* (1986) Congenital heart disease and extra cardiac anomalies: associations and indications for fetal echocardiography. *Am J Obstet Gynecol* **154**, 1121–1132. Review of the prevalence of congenital heart disease with specific extracardiac anomalies. The bottom line: whenever an extracardiac anomaly is found, fetal echocardiography is recommended. The most common sonographic diagnoses that should prompt fetal echocardiography include: ventriculomegaly, microcephaly, agenesis of the corpus callosum, esophageal atresia, duodenal atresia, omphalocele, diaphragmatic hernia and dysplastic kidneys. **IV C**

8 Allan LD, Sharland GK, Chita SK *et al.* (1991) Chromosomal anomalies in fetal congenital heart disease. *Ultrasound Obstet Gynecol* **1**, 8–11. Series of 467 cases of congenital heart disease (CHD) detected prenatally – 77 (16.5%) had a chromosomal anomaly. The authors therefore concluded that all continuing pregnancies with CHD should be karyotyped. **III B**

9 Ryan AK, Goodship JA, Wilson DI *et al.* (1997) Spectrum of clinical features associated with interstitial chromosome 22q11 deletions: a European collaborative study. *J Med Genet* **34**, 798–804. Multicenter study detailing the clinical features associated with 22q11 deletion in 558 patients. It emphasizes the variety of phenotypic expression and its lack of association with specific size deletions. **III B**

10 Bonnet D, Cottri A, Butera G F *et al.* (1999) Detection of transposition of the great arteries reduces morbidity and mortality in newborn infants. *Circulation* **99**, 916–918. This prospective series compares the morbidity and mortality of transposition of the great arteries (TGA) over 10 years in two groups of patients with (68) and without (250) an antenatal diagnosis. Those with a postnatal diagnosis had increased morbidity (metabolic acidosis, multiorgan failure) and, despite identical risk factors for surgery, a longer hospital stay and increased mortality (20/235 vs 0/68). The authors conclude that training to detect TGA sonographically before birth is essential and that delivery of such infants in or near a cardiac unit is desirable and influences outcome. **III B**

11 Brackley KJ, Kilby MD, Wright JG *et al.* (2000) Outcome after prenatal diagnosis of hypoplastic left-heart syndrome: a case series. *Lancet* **356**, 1143–1147. The authors highlight the poor early outcome of a relatively large series of antenatally diagnosed fetuses with hypoplastic left heart syndrome (HLHS). It is a retrospective study of 87 fetuses with HLHS diagnosed in a single center between 1994 and 1999. 61% of the parents chose karyotyping which was abnormal in 12%, and 21% of the cohort (18/87) had associated structural malformations. 38/87 parents chose termination of pregnancy and a further 11 babies (23%) were not considered for surgery because of parental choice after birth and died. 12/36 babies undergoing stage 1 Norwood survived. They stress the importance of using survival figures from prenatal rather than postnatal series when counseling pregnant women whose fetuses have been found to have HLHS. **III B**

12 Tworetzky W, McElhinney DB, Reddy VM *et al.* (2001) Improved surgical outcome after fetal diagnosis of hypoplastic left heart syndrome. *Circulation* **103**, 1269–1273. Retrospective review of three outcome variables (preoperative clinical status; outcome of surgery following Stage 1 Norwood and parental choices) in a cohort of 88 fetuses and newborn infants with a diagnosis of hypoplastic left heart syndrome (HLHS) evaluated in one institution between 1992 and 1999. 33 had had an antenatal diagnosis, with 14 of the 22 liveborn infants surviving stage 1 Norwood compared with 25 of the 38 whose diagnosis was made after birth. Parents opted for termination of pregnancy in one-third of antenatally diagnosed cases and one-third chose no surgery after the birth of their child. Of those with a postnatal diagnosis, similar proportions (one-third) did not undergo surgery after birth because of either parental wishes or significant multiorgan failure. All fetally diagnosed cases that were offered surgery survived to discharge (14) while only 66% (25/38) of those diagnosed after birth survived. Postnatal diagnosis, preoperative acidosis and poor ventricular function were significantly associated with poor survival. The authors conclude that a prenatal diagnosis is associated with improved preoperative clinical status and survival after stage 1 Norwood but the eventual numbers are small and there is insufficient information on parental decision-making versus clinical indication to refuse surgery in the cohort who had a postnatal diagnosis. **III B**

Chapter 18

Craniospinal and facial abnormalities

18.1 Open neural tube defects: anencephaly, cephalocele and spina bifida

Jane Rutherford

Management option		Quality of evidence	Strength of recommendation	References
Prenatal	Search for skull defect in cephalocele and associated anomalies in all cases of open neural tube defects (especially hydrocephalus)	–	✔	–
	Prognosis for cephalocele dependent on amount of herniated brain tissue; prognosis for spina bifida difficult to predict early on, dependent on level and extent of lesion	–	✔	–
	Karyotype	–	✔	–
	Watch for development of hydrocephalus	–	✔	–
	Interdisciplinary approach	–	✔	–
	Termination may be chosen	–	✔	–
Labor and delivery	Vaginal route for anencephaly and cephalocele; cephalocentesis for encephaloceles if parents wish	–	✔	–
	Optimal route of delivery unknown for spina bifida	III	B	1,2
	Care with delivery of the back regardless of delivery route	–	✔	–
Postnatal	Necropsy for abortuses/stillbirths	–	✔	–
	Karyotype if not already done	–	✔	–
	Assess for diabetes, teratogens (anticonvulsants, vitamin A)	–	✔	–
	Counseling	–	✔	–
	Periconceptual high-dose folate	Ia	A	3

References

1 Merrill DC, Goodwin P, Burson JM *et al.* (1998) The optimal route of delivery for fetal myelomeningocele. *Am J Obstet Gynecol* **179**, 235–240. Retrospective case note review of 60 consecutive cases of myelomeningocele. Multiple abnormalities and abnormal karyotypes were excluded. 36 cases were available for long-term follow-up. Overall, 21 delivered vaginally, 15 by cesarean section. No obvious differences detected in the maternal or neonatal characteristics between the two groups. No obvious differences detected in the long-term neurological outcome between the two groups. **III B**

2 Bensen JT, Dillard RG, Burton BK (1988) Open spina bifida: does cesarean section improve prognosis? *Obstet Gynecol* **71**, 532–534. Retrospective case note review. 72 infants with isolated open spina-bifida lesions were followed

up to age 1 year. Comparison was made between 40 infants born vaginally and 32 by cesarean section. Distribution and size of lesion similar in the two groups although mode of delivery not randomly assigned. No differences in outcome in cesarean section group when subdivided into those exposed to labour and those not exposed to labour. No significant difference in the neurological and developmental findings between the vaginal delivery group and the cesarean section group. **III B**

3 Lumley J, Watson L, Watson M *et al.* (2000) Periconceptional supplementation with folate and/or multivitamins for preventing neural tube defects. In: *Cochrane database of systematic reviews*, issue 1. Oxford: Update Software. A systematic review of four RCTs were included with a total of 6425 women. Comparisons of multivitamins with placebo, folate with placebo, different doses of the above or dietary advice with standard care. Women were included whether or not they had a previous affected fetus. Folate supplementation resulted in a significant reduction in neural tube defects whether or not the mother had had a previously affected fetus. Doses used varied significantly, from 0.36 mg/day to 4 mg/day. **Ia A**

18.2 Hydrocephalus

Jane Rutherford

Management option		Quality of evidence	Strength of recommendation	References
Prenatal	Search for other anomalies including karyotype, full work-up for congenital infection	–	✔	–
	Cautious counseling regarding prognosis if isolated finding	III	B	1–5
	Termination remains an option	–	✔	–
	In continuing pregnancy: ❑ Serial scans to identify progressive dilatation ❑ Deliver fetus when risk of prematurity low ❑ Interdisciplinary care ❑ No evidence to support fetal shunt placement	–	✔	–
Labor and delivery	No evidence for cesarean delivery *a priori*	–	✔	–
	Cephalocentesis is potentially destructive but a medically acceptable option in severest cases	–	✔	–
Postnatal	Establish cause and type	–	✔	–
	Counseling	–	✔	–
	Pediatric neurosurgical management	–	✔	–

References

1 Beke A, Csabay L, Rigo J Jr *et al.* (1999) Follow-up studies of newborn babies with congenital ventriculomegaly. *J Perinat Med* **27**, 495–505. Prospective cohort study of 30 cases of prenatally diagnosed ventriculomegaly. Divided into groups according to the etiology and complications of the ventriculomegaly. A 4-year follow-up of neurological condition, motor and sensory development was undertaken. 13 patients were symptomless, 10 moderately handicapped and 7 severely handicapped. The group with isolated moderate ventriculomegaly had the best prognosis. **III B**

2 Jamjoom AB, Khalaf NF, Mohammed AA *et al.* (1998) Factors affecting the outcome of fetal hydrocephaly. *Acta Neurochir* **140**, 1121–1125. Retrospective observational study of factors affecting prognosis in 26 fetuses with hydrocephalus. Hydrocephalus was in association with myelomeningocele in 35%. Mean follow-up period was 2 years. The authors reported better prognosis when hydrocephalus does not progress *in utero*, delivery is not preterm, the neonate is not small for gestational age, head circumference is less than 95th centile and there is a cortical mantle of greater than 2 cm on computed tomography scanning. **III B**

3 Rosseau GL, McCullough DC, Joseph AL (1992) Current prognosis in fetal ventriculomegaly. *J Neurosurg* **77**, 551–555. Retrospective case review of 37 cases of antenatally diagnosed ventriculomegaly in which the pregnancy was continued and follow-up information was available. 10 cases had incorrect antenatal diagnosis when reviewed after birth. 26 had associated abnormalities. 26 were treated with ventriculoperitoneal shunts. There were no cases of progressive ventriculomegaly. The overall survival was 28 out of 37. Of 26 shunted patients, 10 had satisfactory cognitive development. 6 of 11 patients who did not have shunt placement had satisfactory cognitive development; 3 of these had resolution of ventriculomegaly *in utero*. **III B**

4 Oi S, Matsumoto S, Katauama K *et al.* (1990) Pathophysiology and postnatal outcome of hydrocephalus. *Childs Nerv Syst* **6**, 338–345. Retrospective observational case series of 24 cases of fetal hydrocephalus of varying etiology. Overall the mortality was 25%. 16 underwent postnatal shunting procedures. Follow-up varied from 4 months to 6 years. Mean IQ or developmental quotient was 45.2. **III B**

5 Drugan A, Krause B, Canady A *et al.* (1989) The natural history of prenatally diagnosed cerebral ventriculomegaly. *JAMA* **261**, 1785–1788. Retrospective observational case series carried out from 1984–87 of 43 cases of antenatally diagnosed ventriculomegaly. 26 pregnancies were continued and the neonates were divided into four groups for the purpose of analysis. 5 cases had borderline isolated ventriculomegaly and all were neurologically normal at follow-up. 6 cases with isolated ventriculomegaly had ventriculoperitoneal shunts inserted; of 5 available for follow-up, 3 were neurologically normal and 2 had moderate developmental delay. 8 neonates had associated anomalies: 3 had severe neurological impairment, 5 had mild developmental delay. 7 neonates were severely affected at birth. **III B**

18.3 The holoprosencephaly sequence

Jane Rutherford

Management option		Quality of evidence	Strength of recommendation	References
Prenatal	Karyotype	–	✔	–
	Offer pregnancy termination (prognosis poor), induction of labor	–	✔	–
Labor and delivery	Vaginal delivery; cephalocentesis ethically justified in cases of severe macrocephaly to avoid cesarean section	–	✔	–
Postnatal	Necropsy	–	✔	–
	Karyotype if not already done	–	✔	–
	Family history	–	✔	–
	Screen for diabetes	–	✔	–
	Counseling	–	✔	–

18.4 Facial clefts

Jane Rutherford

Management option		Quality of evidence	Strength of recommendation	References
Prenatal	Careful search for other anomalies	–	✔	–
	Karyotype	–	✔	–
	Prognosis depends on cause (good if isolated)	–	✔	–
Postnatal	Counseling	–	✔	–
	Special measures for infant feeding	–	✔	–
	Pediatric surgery	–	✔	–

18.5 Dandy–Walker malformation

Jane Rutherford

Management option		Quality of evidence	Strength of recommendation	References
Prenatal	Cautious counseling, prognosis difficult to predict	III	B	1–3
	Pregnancy termination remains an option	–	✔	–

References

1 Kalidasan V, Carroll T, Allcutt D *et al.* (1995) The Dandy–Walker syndrome – a 10 year experience of its management and outcome. *Eur J Pediatr Surg* **5**(Suppl 1), 16–18. Retrospective case review series of 12 children with Dandy–Walker syndrome over 10 years. 35% had reasonable outcome; 65% had mental retardation. There were 2 deaths. 9 patients had ventriculoperitoneal shunting and 2 had cystoperitoneal shunting in addition. **III B**

2 Osenbach RK, Menezes AH (1992) Diagnosis and management of the Dandy Walker malformation: 30 years of experience. *Pediatr Neurosurg* **18**, 179–189. Retrospective observational case review series of 37 cases with Dandy–Walker malformation treated between 1959 and 1989. 70% presented in the first year of life, 80% in first 3 years of life. Hydrocephalus present in 91% at diagnosis. 30% showed developmental delay and 48% had associated congenital abnormalities. 8 patients had posterior fossa craniectomy with membrane excision, 13 had lateral ventricle shunting, 4 had cyst shunt insertion and 12 had combined shunting. Combined shunting had the best outcome. Overall, the mortality was 28% with the majority being before 1970. 27 of the 28 survivors were shunt-dependent. **III B**

3 Pascual-Castroviejo I, Velvez A, Pascual-Pascual SI *et al.* (1991) Dandy Walker malformation: analysis of 38 cases. *Childs Nerv Syst* **7**, 88–97. Review of 38 cases of Dandy–Walker malformation. 32 cases were diagnosed in the first year of life, 17 at birth. Macrocephaly present in 31 cases. Associated abnormalities were common. The mortality was 44.7%. Mental retardation was reported in 58% of survivors. Only 2 patients showed normal intellectual development. **III B**

18.6 Aneurysm of the vein of Galen

Jane Rutherford

Management option		Quality of evidence	Strength of recommendation	References
Prenatal	Color flow Doppler used to differentiate from hydrocephalus and porencephalic cyst	–	✔	–
	Careful search for hydrops, hydrocephalus or other abnormalities	–	✔	–
	Prognosis difficult to predict	–	✔	–

18.7 Hydranencephaly

Jane Rutherford

Management option		Quality of evidence	Strength of recommendation	References
Prenatal	Karyotype	–	✔	–
	Offer termination or induction of labor	–	✔	–

18.8 Microcephaly

Jane Rutherford

Management option		Quality of evidence	Strength of recommendation	References
Prenatal	Careful search for other anomalies	–	✔	–
	Karyotype and full work up for congenital infection	–	✔	–
	Look for history of teratogens, alcohol, family history, infection	–	✔	–
	Caution with counseling	–	✔	–
Labor and delivery	Aim for vaginal delivery	–	✔	–
	Beware shoulder dystocia	–	✔	–
Postnatal	Establish cause if not already done (teratogens, alcohol, family history, karyotype, infection serology, necropsy)	–	✔	–
	Counseling depending on cause	–	✔	–

18.9 Agenesis of the corpus callosum

Jane Rutherford

Management option		Quality of evidence	Strength of recommendation	References
Prenatal	Careful search for other anomalies	–	✔	–
	Counseling depends on other lesions; prognosis for isolated condition difficult to predict	–	✔	–
	Pregnancy termination remains an option	–	✔	–

18.10 Intracranial hemorrhage and porencephaly

Jane Rutherford

Management option		Quality of evidence	Strength of recommendation	References
Prenatal	May be associated with severe maternal illness	–	✔	–
	In absence of identifiable cause, work-up for alloimmune thrombocytopenia and congenital infection	–	✔	–
	Prognosis related to location and degree of tissue loss; usually poor with larger lesions	–	✔	–

18.11 Choroid plexus cyst

Jane Rutherford

Management option		Quality of evidence	Strength of recommendation	References
Prenatal	Careful search for other structural abnormalities	III	B	1–3
	Karyotype if other anomalies found	III	B	1–3
	Careful counseling; ?50% increased risk of aneuploidy; benign if isolated with normal chromosomes	III	B	1–5

References

1 Sohn C, Gast AS, Krapfl E (1997) Isolated fetal choroid plexus cysts: not an indication for genetic diagnosis? *Fetal Diagn Ther* **12**, 255–259. Prospective case series of 41 fetuses with choroid plexus cysts diagnosed by ultrasound in the second trimester from a total of 4326 pregnancies scanned in one center between January 1994 and August 1995. 34 had bilateral and 7 unilateral cysts. 38 of 41 had karyotyping procedures performed. Only one fetus had associated abnormalities on ultrasound, was confirmed to have trisomy 18 and termination of pregnancy was carried out. No other chromosomal abnormalities were detected. In all 40 surviving fetuses, the cysts had disappeared by 30 weeks. In an additional 19 cases of trisomy18 diagnosed between 1990 and 1996 and analyzed retrospectively, there were no cases of isolated choroid plexus cysts. **III B**

2 Reinsch RC (1997) Choroid plexus cysts – association with trisomy: prospective review of 16,059 patients. *Am J Obstet Gynecol* **176**, 1381–1383. Prospective case series in which 301 cases of choroid plexus cysts (CPC) from a total of 16059 patients who had screening ultrasound scans performed (1.9%). Cysts were unilateral in 55%. 263 had isolated choroid plexus cysts, 38 had CPC plus one or more risk factor (advanced maternal age, additional ultrasound abnormality, family history, past obstetric history) and all of these opted to have amniocentesis. There were 3 with abnormal karyotype (one trisomy 21, 2 trisomy 18). 92 patients with isolated CPC had amniocentesis performed and all were normal. All 163 fetuses with isolated CPCs followed up until delivery were normal (8 patients with isolated CPCs were lost to follow-up). **III B**

3 Nadel AS, Bromley BS, Frigoletto FD Jr *et al.* (1992) Isolated choroid plexus cysts in the second trimester fetus: is amniocentesis really indicated? *Radiology* **185**, 545–548. Prospective cohort study of 242 fetuses at one center scanned between February 1988 and February 1992 shown to have choroid plexus cysts. 8 were lost to follow-up, making a study group of 234 fetuses. 220 had no other ultrasound detected fetal anomalies and none of these had aneuploidy at amniocentesis or an anomaly at birth. 14 had other major anomalies: 11 had trisomy 18, one had triploidy and 2 had major structural abnormalities but normal karyotype. The size and bilaterality of the cysts were not statistically different between normal and abnormal karyotypes. **III B**

4 Bakos O, Moen KS, Hansson S (1998) Prenatal karyotyping of choroid plexus cysts. *Eur J Ultrasound* **8**, 79–83. Retrospective descriptive study of 50 cases of choroid plexus cysts diagnosed on ultrasound scanning. All were offered karyotyping and 46 accepted. In 10 cases there were additional abnormalities including one trisomy 13 and one trisomy 18. There was no relationship between abnormalities and the diameter, complexity or bilaterality of the cysts. **III B**

5 Bromley B, Lieberman R, Banacerraf BR (1996) Choroid plexus cysts: not associated with Down syndrome. *Ultrasound Obstet Gynecol* **8**, 232–235. Prospective cohort study over 7 years of 473 fetuses with choroid plexus cysts (CPCs) identified from 32053 mid-trimester ultrasound scans (1.38% incidence excluding trisomy 18). 16 were lost to follow-up, 3 had structural defects and normal karyotypes, 21 had abnormal karyotypes, 2 of which were trisomy 21. The remaining 433 either had normal karyotype or were normal neonates. Over the same time period, scans and reports of all fetuses with trisomy 21 were reviewed. During the study period 143 fetuses with trisomy 21 were karyotyped and 2 had CPCs (1.4%). No significant difference was detected in the prevalence of CPCs in those fetuses with and without trisomy 21. **III B**

18.12 Cystic hygroma

Jane Rutherford

Management option		Quality of evidence	Strength of recommendation	References
Prenatal	Careful search for evidence of fetal hydrops, other anomalies	–	✔	–
	Investigate as for non-immune hydrops, including karyotype (see Section 14.1)	–	✔	–
	Prognosis and management dependent on cause	–	✔	–
	Pregnancy termination an option	–	✔	–
Labor and delivery	If pregnancy continues and cyst massive, transabdominal aspiration of cyst fluid may allow vaginal delivery; cesarean section is alternative	–	✔	–
Postnatal	Establish cause	–	✔	–
	Counseling	–	✔	–
	'Cosmetic' surgery	–	✔	–

18.13 Caudal regression syndrome

Jane Rutherford

Management option		Quality of evidence	Strength of recommendation	References
Prenatal	Determine degree of malformation	–	✔	–
	Offer termination	–	✔	–
	Screen for diabetes	–	✔	–
Postnatal	Screen for diabetes	–	✔	–
	Counseling	–	✔	–

Chapter 19

Genitourinary malformations

19.1 Genitourinary malformations

Peter McParland

Management option		Quality of evidence	Strength of recommendation	References
Make diagnosis	Checklist of questions: ❑ Oligohydramnios? ❑ Dilatation of the urinary tract (or urinoma or urinary ascites)? ❑ Renal cysts? ❑ Size, shape and echogenicity of kidneys? ❑ Bladder present?	III	B	1–3
	❑ Associated abnormalities (including karyotype)?	III	B	4,5
	Establish whether family history of renal disease	III	B	6
Management options	Counseling	–	✔	–
	If isolated pyelectasis consider using cut-off of >8 mm in the second trimester and >10 mm during the third trimester as a basis for follow-up	III	B	7–13
	If anteroposterior >20 mm possible need for surgery or long-term follow-up	III	B	14
	Consideration of invasive procedure if bladder outlet obstruction:			
	❑ To clarify diagnosis	III	B	15,16
	❑ For possible therapeutic benefit	III	B	17
	Consideration of termination if appropriate	–	✔	–
	Plan place, timing and method of delivery	–	✔	–
	Pediatric involvement			
	❑ Prenatally for counseling	–	✔	–
	❑ After birth for further evaluation, confirmation of diagnosis and planning subsequent management	Ib	A	18
	Post-mortem examination if lethal abnormality	–	✔	–

References

1 Levi S, Schaaps JP, De Havay P *et al.* (1995) End-result of routine ultrasound screening for congenital anomalies: the Belgian Multicentre Study 1984–92. *Ultrasound Obstet Gynecol* **5**, 366–371. Ultrasound identifies most renal abnormalities and this study demonstrated excellent ability with sensitivities of 86–90% for identification of obstructive uropathy, unilateral and bilateral agenesis and cystic and polycystic disease. Less frequently encountered genitourinary anomalies such as duplication, ectopia, horse-shoe kidney, ovarian and penile cysts, intersex, gonad and duct duplication were less well identified with a sensitivity of 40%. **III B**

2 Isaksen CV, Eik-Nes SH, Blaas HG *et al.* (2000) Fetuses and infants with congenital urinary system anomalies: correlation between prenatal ultrasound and postmortem findings. *Ultrasound Obstet Gynecol* **15**, 177–185.

Urinary tract anomalies were found in 112 (27%) of 408 fetuses with congenital anomalies who subsequently underwent post-mortem examination. In 97 (87%) of the 112 cases there was full agreement between the ultrasound observations and the autopsy findings, illustrating the accuracy with which ultrasound can discriminate between various types of genitourinary anomaly. **III B**

3 Podevin G, Mandelbrot L, Vuillard E *et al.* (1996) Outcome of urological abnormalities prenatally diagnosed by ultrasound. *Fetal Diagn Ther* **11**, 181–190. Retrospective evaluation of the usefulness of antenatal diagnosis and subsequent management of 142 cases of genitourinary malformations. There were 107 children born alive, with 35 intrauterine deaths. The latter group comprised 27 fetuses with multiple defects and, of the 8 cases with urological defects, only 7 had urethral anomalies. The overall positive predictive value (PPV) for urinary tract anomaly was 83%, with a PPV of 94% for cystic kidney disease and a PPV of 100% for urethral anomalies. They were, however, unable to distinguish between posterior urethral valves, urethral atresia or stenosis. **III B**

4 Snidjers R, Sebire NJ, Faria M *et al.* (1995) Fetal mild hydronephrosis and chromosomal defects: relation to maternal age and gestation. *Fetal Diagn Ther* **10**, 349–355. Report of a series of 1177 fetuses with mild hydronephrosis at 16–26 weeks gestation. The fetal karyotype was abnormal in 7.3% of cases. In the 805 fetuses with apparently isolated hydronephrosis there were only 5 (0.62%) cases of trisomy 21. On the basis of the maternal age and gestational age distribution of the population, the expected frequency of trisomy 21 was 0.4%. This was not significantly different from the observed frequency of 0.62%, suggesting no association between isolated antenatal hydronephrosis and trisomy 21. **III B**

5 Thompson MO, Thilaganathan B (1998) Effect of routine screening for Down's syndrome on the significance of isolated fetal hydronephrosis. *Br J Obstet Gynaecol* **105**, 860–864. Isolated fetal hydronephrosis (anteroposterior diameter ≥4 mm) was diagnosed in 423 (3.9%) pregnancies of 10 971 scanned at 18–23 weeks. None of these pregnancies were affected by Down syndrome, suggesting that isolated fetal hydronephrosis does not increase the risk for Down syndrome. **III B**

6 Degani S, Leibovitz Z, Shapiro I *et al.* (1997) Fetal pyelectasis in consecutive pregnancies: a possible genetic predisposition. *Ultrasound Obstet Gynecol* **10**, 19–21. The recurrence rate of mild fetal pyelectasis was assessed in 420 women who otherwise had uncomplicated pregnancies. Pyelectasis was defined as a fetal pelvis of 4 mm or more. Of 64 pregnancies with fetal pyelectasis, 43 (67%) had a recurrence of this finding in the next pregnancy. Compared with normal fetuses, those with pyelectasis had a relative risk of 6.1 to have a recurrence (95% CI 4.3–7.5, $p < 0.001$). The authors suggested a genetic and/or environmental risk. **III B**

7 Persutte WH, Koyle M, Lenke RR (1997) Mild pyelectasis ascertained with prenatal ultrasonography is pediatrically significant. *Ultrasound Obstet Gynecol* **10**, 12–18. A total of 306 fetuses with mild pyelectasis defined as a pelvicalyceal fluid-filled space with the smallest of two transverse perpendicular measurements 4 mm or greater but less than10 mm were studied. 27% of these cases progressed to 'frank hydronephrosis' (>10 mm) and in only 5% did the measurement diminish to less than 4 mm. The overall incidence of mild pyelectasis was a high 5.5%, possibly reflecting a selected referred population. On postnatal follow-up only 84 underwent voiding videocystourethrography with an abnormal finding in 19% (16/84) and surgery being necessary in only 4 cases. The authors argued for all cases of mild pyelectasis in utero (≥4 mm) to have postnatal ultrasound, videocystourethrography and possible prophylactic antibiotics. **III B**

8 Sairam S, Al-Habib A, Sasson S *et al.* (2001) Natural history of fetal hydronephrosis diagnosed on mid-trimester ultrasound. *Ultrasound Obstet Gynecol* **17**, 191–196. Prospective study of 11 465 unselected women undergoing an anomaly scan at 18–23 weeks. Hydronephrosis was identified in 2.3%, being mild (≥4 and < 7 mm) in 81% and moderate/severe (≥7 mm) in 19%. Hydronephrosis resolved in the antenatal or early neonatal period in 88% of fetuses, with only 5/39 (13%) who had hydronephrosis at delivery needing prophylactic antibiotics. None of the fetuses with mild hydronephrosis and approximately 15% with persistent hydronephrosis required postnatal surgery with, overall, 1/1000 total births requiring postnatal urological surgery. The outcome in the group with mild hydronephrosis was excellent, 96% of pregnancies demonstrating spontaneous resolution either antenatally or postnatally. **III B**

9 Langer B, Simeoni U, Montoya Y *et al.* (1996) Antenatal diagnosis of upper urinary tract dilatation by ultrasonography. *Fetal Diagn Ther* **11**, 191–198. A total of 95 fetuses with pyelectasis, defined as a mean renal pelvic dimension of more than 5 mm before 28 weeks or more than 10 mm after 28 weeks, were included in this prospective study. In 13 (13.7%) cases an obstructive urinary tract abnormality, a severe vesicoureteral reflux or a megaureter was diagnosed postnatally. On the basis that nearly all cases that are below 10 mm before 28 weeks result in normal neonatal findings, the authors suggest that all cases between 5 and 10 mm during the second trimester should be confirmed in the third. Postnatal complementary investigations could then be limited to cases with persistent pyelectasis above 10 mm. **III B**

10 Aviram R, Pomeron A, Sharoney R *et al.* (2000) The increase of renal pelvis dilatation in the fetus and its significance. *Ultrasound Obstet Gynecol* **16**, 60–62. A total of 56 fetuses with fetal renal anteroposterior (AP) diameters of 4 mm or more in the second trimester that persisted to 7 mm or more in the third trimester were evaluated postnatally. In 39 babies, urinary tract pathology was confirmed. The authors demonstrated that when the renal pelvis maintains a stable diameter through pregnancy there is no significant pathology. Fetuses with pelvis diameters of 10 mm or more in the second trimester are likely to have postnatal renal tract pathology, even if there is no further pelvic dilatation in the third trimester. **III B**

Comment: there are at least 20 papers in the literature addressing the prevalence of fetal pyelectasis and its clinical significance. The definition of pyelectasis varies from an AP diameter of 3–10 mm at differing gestations in selected, routine and mixed populations. The prevalence, not surprisingly, varies from 0.37% to 18%. Considerable controversy exists as to what cut-offs should be used, with the above papers illustrating the gap in opinions. The interested reader is referred to an editorial 'Is fetal hydronephrosis overdiagnosed?' by Shearer (2000) in Ultrasound Obstet Gynecol 16, 601–606. In reviewing the current available evidence, he suggests that using a cut-off of an anteroposterior diameter of 8 mm or more in the second trimester and more than 10 mm during the third trimester would reduce the high false-positive rate, limit parental anxiety and reduce costs, with no significant reduction in identifying those with significant postnatal renal pathology.

11 Persutte WH, Hussey M, Chyu J *et al.* (2000) Striking findings concerning the variability in the measurement of the fetal renal collecting system. *Ultrasound Obstet Gynecol* **15**, 186–190. Some of the apparent confusion, outlined above, that exists in the relationship between prenatal pyelectasis and progression to frank hydronephrosis, postnatal vesicoureteric reflux and postnatal surgery is explained in this study. 20 second- and third-trimester patients with varying degrees of fetal pyelectasis were studied every 15 min for a 2 h period. The mean variation over time in the anteroposterior diameter was 3.8 mm. 70% of cases (14/20) had both normal (<4 mm) and abnormal values (≥ 4 mm) during the 2 h study period. The authors suggest that maternal hydration may explain the variable findings. **III B**

12 Robinson JN, Tice K, Kolm P *et al.* (1998) Effect of maternal hydration on fetal renal pyelectasis. *Obstet Gynecol* **92**, 137–141. The wide variability reported between antenatal hydronephrosis and postnatal renal outcome may be partly explained by this study of 13 pregnant women with fetal pyelectasis and 13 matched controls. Ultrasound was performed before and after maternal oral hydration. After hydration the amniotic fluid index increased and the fetal renal pelvis diameter increased significantly in both groups, and this increase was independent of the state of the fetal bladder; thus simple hydration could convert an individual with normal renal characteristics to one with pyelectasis. Interestingly the mean anteroposterior diameter after maternal hydration was 7 mm, highlighting the fact that this effect in this study was seen in those with mild hydronephrosis. A similar incremental change in those with anteroposterior diameters of more than 10 mm would not have the same effect, supporting the view that a cutoff of more than 7 mm should be used to define abnormality. **III B**

13 Jaswon MS, Dibble L, Puri S *et al.* (1999) Prospective study of outcome in antenatally diagnosed renal pelvis dilatation. *Arch Dis Child Neonat Ed* **80**, 135–138. The relationship between antenatal hydronephrosis and postnatal vesicoureteric reflux is unclear. This prospective study had a clear follow-up protocol involving a micturating cystogram at 2–3 months in all babies who had antenatal pyelectasis (anteroposterior diameter >5 mm). Vesicoureteric reflux (VUR) was the most common clinical significant pathology (22%, 23/104). There was no correlation between the degree of either antenatal or postnatal renal pelvic dilatation and the severity of VUR. Of interest, a diagnosis of VUR was made in 14 babies who had a normal postnatal ultrasound scan. **III B**

14 Gotoh H, Masuzaki H, Fukuda H *et al.* (1998) Detection and assessment of pyelectasis in the fetus: relationship to postnatal renal function. *Obstet Gynecol* **92**, 226–231. This study prospectively evaluated the relationship between the severity of pyelectasis in 36 fetuses at 30–40 weeks gestation and postnatal renal function. Renal pelvic diameters were at least 20, 25 and 26 mm respectively, during late fetal life in those neonates who needed corrective surgery. The mean anteroposterior diameter in those fetuses who did not require surgery was significantly less (11 ± 6 mm) than in those requiring surgery (33 ± 14 mm, $p < 0.01$). In this study, surgery was not necessary when the diameter was less than 20 mm. **III B**

15 Nicolaides KH, Cheng HH, Snijders RJ *et al.* (1992) Fetal urine biochemistry in the assessment of obstructive uropathy. *Am J Obstet Gynecol* **166**, 932–937. This was one of the first studies to evaluate the role of sampling fetal urine in cases with obstructive uropathy. 60 fetuses were retrospectively assigned to two groups according to whether the outcome was good or poor. None of the fetuses underwent shunting as this would have influenced the natural history of the disease. Reference ranges for sodium, total calcium, urea and creatinine were calculated from fetuses with obstructive uropathy who either survived with normal postnatal renal function or who died with no histological evidence of renal dysplasia. The best prediction of outcome was the combination of either high calcium or high sodium with a positive predictive value of 91%. **III B**

16 Johnson MP, Bukowski TP, Reitleman C *et al.* (1994) In utero surgical treatment of fetal obstructive uropathy: a new comprehensive approach to identify appropriate candidates for vesicoamniotic shunt therapy. *Am J Obstet Gynecol* **170**, 1770–1779. In this retrospective review, 34 fetuses with megacystis and hydronephrosis between 14 and 24 weeks were evaluated using ultrasound, rapid karyotyping and a minimum of three bladder taps at 48–72 h intervals to assess urinary biochemical values in addition to observing the rate of bladder refilling after vesicocentesis. If there was a sequential fall in biochemical values these were considered to have a good prognosis, with a rise suggesting progressive dysplasia. The authors showed that the third or fourth bladder tap was the best predictor. Using an integrated approach of the above they achieved a 100% rate in predicting the presence of significant underlying renal pathology. In spite of this, 4 such cases underwent shunting, a fact not consistent with the proposed algorithm. Of interest, of the initial 34 assessed, after termination (11) and other perinatal losses (12) only 11 survived, 2 of whom were on dialysis awaiting renal transplant, illustrating that, in spite of the above approach, morbidity and mortality are very high with this condition. **III B**

17 Freedman AL, Johnson MP, Smith CA *et al.* (1999) Long-term outcome in children after antenatal intervention for obstructive uropathies. *Lancet* **354**, 374–377. This study, from the same group in reference 16, reviewed the long-term follow-up for 34 patients who underwent vesicoamniotic shunt placement between 1987 and 1996. 13 died and 21 survived, of whom 14 were more than 2 years old. Height was below the 25% centile in 86% with 50% below the 5th centile. 36% had renal failure requiring transplantation and 43% had normal renal function. 50% were acceptably continent with 14% incontinent. 3 of 4 children with valves needed bladder augmentation surgery. Although the numbers were relatively small the results were somewhat disappointing but should enable more informed parental counseling before intervention. **III B**

18 Smellie JM, Barratt TM, Chantler C *et al.* (2001) Medical versus surgical treatment in children with severe bilateral vesicoureteric reflux and bilateral nephropathy: a randomised trial. *Lancet* **357**, 1329–1333. Of interest to all obstetricians involved in counseling parents is this randomized study comparing a medical versus a surgical approach in 52 children with severe bilateral vesicoureteric reflux (grades III–IV) and bilateral nephropathy. Medical treatment consisted of antibiotic prophylaxis while surgery was left to the preference of the individual surgeon, with most adopting a Cohen ureteric advancement. The change in the glomerular filtration rate at 4-year follow-up did not differ between the groups, suggesting that surgery for vesicoureteric reflux does not improve the outcome for renal function. The authors suggest most damage in these cases may have occurred at a very early stage and that severely damaged or dysplastic kidneys will either remain stable or progress to end-stage renal failure despite all efforts to cure the reflux. **Ib A**

Chapter 20

Gastrointestinal abnormalities

20.1 Omphalocele

Bryan Beattie

Management option		Quality of evidence	Strength of recommendation	References
Prenatal	Offer karyotyping	III	B	1–3
	Chromosomal abnormalities more likely with bowel rather than liver containing omphalocele	III	B	4
	Ultrasound examination for other structural defects	III	B	1–3
	Vigilance for risk of prematurity	III	B	2
Delivery	Mode of delivery does not affect outcome	III	B	5–7
	Rupture of covering membrane with exposed liver increases mortality	III	B	8
	Respiratory insufficiency at birth significant clinical predictor of mortality	III	B	9
Neonatal care	Necrotizing enterocolitis associated with increased mortality	III	B	7

References

1 Calzolari E, Bianchi F, Dolk H *et al.* and the Eurocat Working Group (1995) Omphalocele and gastroschisis in Europe: a survey of 3 million births 1980–1990. *Am J Med Genet* **58**, 187–194. A total of 732 cases of omphalocele and 274 cases of gastroschisis were registered in 21 regional registers in Europe during the period 1980–90. Omphalocele was an isolated malformation in 46% of cases; gastroschisis was isolated in 79% of cases. The average birthweight and gestational age of both isolated and multiply malformed cases of both omphalocele and gastroschisis were low. Isolated gastroschisis is associated with a significantly younger age than isolated omphalocele. Omphalocele is associated with a high association of other malformations and chromosomal abnormalities (21.0% vs 7.3% for gastroschisis cases). **III B**

2 Mayer T, Black R, Matlak ME *et al.* (1980) Gastroschisis and omphalocele. An eight-year review. *Ann Surg* **192**, 783–787. This was an 8-year review of 75 fetuses with gastroschisis and omphalocele. The authors found that gastroschisis occurred approximately twice as often as omphalocele and was increasing in frequency. Prematurity occurred in 65% of the fetuses with gastroschisis. Although the incidence of malformations associated with gastroschisis was 23%, the vast majority of these were due to jejunoileal or colonic atresias. The mortality rate for fetuses with gastroschisis was 12.7%. Omphalocele was associated with a 23% prematurity rate and an associated anomaly rate of 66%. Major cardiac malformations and chromosomal defects were quite common in fetuses with omphalocele. The mortality rate with omphalocele (34%) was primarily due to major cardiac malformations or chromosomal anomalies. The survival rate in fetuses with omphalocele who did not have either a cardiac malformation or a chromosomal defect was 94%. **III B**

3 Moore TC, Nur K (1986) An international survey of gastroschisis and omphalocele (490 cases). I. Nature and distribution of additional malformations. *Pediatr Surg Int* **1**, 46–50. This is an international survey of 16 pediatric surgery centers on four continents. In 203 cases of gastroschisis, additional malformations were infrequent and were primarily restricted to bowel atresias or stenosis. In 287 cases of omphalocele 14% were classified as syndromes. Additional malformations were found in approximately 74% of fetuses; approximately 5% of the fetuses had a karyotypic abnormality. **III B**

4 Hughes MD, Nyberg DA, Mack LA *et al.* (1989) Fetal omphalocele: prenatal US detection of concurrent anomalies and other predictors of outcome. *Radiology* **173**, 371–376. This study evaluated 46 consecutive cases of omphalocele. In 43 of the fetuses with adequate follow-up, 67% had additional malformations. Fetal mortality was strongly associated with the presence of concurrent malformations and an abnormal amniotic fluid volume. Chromosome abnormalities correlated with the absence of liver in the omphalocele sac ($p < 0.001$). **III B**

5 Kirk EP, Wah RM (1983) Obstetric management of the fetus with omphalocele or gastroschisis. A review of one-hundred and twelve cases. *Am J Obstet Gynecol* **146**, 512–518. Review of 112 cases with anterior abdominal wall defects admitted to a neonatal surgical unit prior to 1983. No cesarean sections were performed because of the antenatal diagnosis of an anterior abdominal wall defect (only made in four cases). The overall cesarean section rate was 16%. Decisions about delivery were made in the absence of the existence of the condition in 118 (97%) cases and there were no adverse effects on outcome from vaginal delivery. **III B**

6 Moretti M, Khoury A, Rodriquez J *et al.* (1990) The effect of mode of delivery on the perinatal outcome in fetuses with abdominal wall defects. *Am J Obstet Gynecol* **163**, 833–838. Review of 56 cases with gastroschisis and 69 cases of omphalocele. There were no significant differences between the groups in terms of cesarean section rate (26% vs 22%) and prematurity rate (30% vs 26%). There was a lower incidence of infant deaths (7% vs 22%), associated congenital abnormalities (5% vs 29%) and long-term infant morbidity (8.9% vs 14.5%). In either group there was no difference in infant mortality, acute or long-term infant outcome or frequency of associated major abnormalities between those delivered vaginally and those delivered by cesarean section. **III B**

7 Snyder CL (1999) Outcome analysis for gastroschisis. *J Pediatr Surg* **34**, 1253–1256. Retrospective study of 185 infants with gastroschisis who were treated at a single institution between 1969 and 1999. The mean birthweight was 2501 grams and the mean gestational age was 36.6 weeks. The overall survival rate was 91%. The survival rate improved over the last two decades. Neonatal sepsis, bowel obstruction and closure complications accounted for most of the morbidity. The presence of another major anomaly and the development of necrotizing enterocolitis were associated with increased mortality. The type of delivery (i.e. vaginal or by cesarean section) did not influence either morbidity or mortality. **III B**

8 Kamata S, Ishikawa S, Usui N *et al.* (1996) Prenatal diagnosis of abdominal wall defects and their prognosis. *J Pediatr Surg* **31**, 267–271. The authors reviewed 43 fetuses with an abdominal wall defect – 31 with an omphalocele and 12 with gastroschisis. 10 of the 12 fetuses with gastroschisis survived. 9 of 12 with a small omphalocele survived. 10 of 12 fetuses with a giant omphalocele survived. However, 6 of the 7 fetuses with a ruptured omphalocele died of pulmonary hypoplasia. Poor prognostic signs associated with an omphalocele include deformity of the spine and rupture of the covering membrane with an exposed liver. With advanced surgical techniques and medical management, most patients with abdominal wall defects who do not have other lethal malformations or chromosomal abnormalities will survive. **III B**

9 Shaw KS, Filiatrault D, Yazbeck S *et al.* (1994) Improved survival for congenital diaphragmatic hernia based on prenatal ultrasound diagnosis and referral to a combined obstetric-pediatric surgical center. *J Pediatr Surg* **29**, 1268–1269. A review of 36 cases of antenatally (19) or postnatally (17) diagnosed congenital diaphragmatic hernia (CDH) referred to a single unit over a 3-year period from 1990–93. 4 (11%) had spontaneous miscarriage. 5 died prior to surgery (14%), one was a false positive of CDH. Of the 26 who underwent surgery, 23 survived (66% overall, 74% live births and 89% postoperatively). Only one survivor had extracorporeal membrane oxygenation. Ultrasound diagnosis prior to 25 weeks and polyhydramnios separately resulted in a perinatal survival of only 50%. Antenatal diagnosis (19) was associated with increased neonatal morbidity (lower Apgar scores, premature delivery, lower birthweight). Survival for inborn and transferred cases was similar. **III B**

20.2 Gastroschisis

Bryan Beattie

Management option		Quality of evidence	Strength of recommendation	References
Prenatal	Increased surveillance			
	❑ Risk of death	III	B	1,2
	❑ Risk prematurity	III	B	3,4
	❑ Risk small for gestational age (intestinal atresia with gastroschisis protects against growth abnormalities)	III	B	2,3,5
	Sonography can predict postnatal outcome			
	❑ Yes	III	B	6,7
	❑ No	III	B	8,9

Management option		Quality of evidence	Strength of recommendation	References
Delivery	Mode of delivery does not affect outcome	III	B	10,11
	Surveillance for intrapartum fetal distress	III	B	1
Neonatal care	Primary closure minimizes morbidity	III	B	12
	Vigilance at surgery for associated bowel malformations	III	B	4,8,13

References

1 Burge DM, Ade-Ajaji N (1997) Adverse outcome after prenatal diagnosis of gastroschisis: the role of fetal monitoring. *J Pediatr Surg* **32**, 441–444. This is a retrospective review of 57 fetuses with gastroschisis between 1982 and 1995. Introduction of routine fetal monitoring from 32 weeks gestation in 1990 increased the ability to detect fetal distress twofold. The authors concluded that pregnancies associated with gastroschisis should be considered at significant risk of fetal distress, which might culminate in a late intrauterine demise, neonatal death or an adverse neurological outcome. **III B**

2 Crawford RA, Ryan G, Wright VM *et al.* (1992) The importance of serial biophysical assessment of fetal wellbeing in gastroschisis. *Br J Obstet Gynaecol* **99**, 899–902. A total of 24 consecutive cases of gastroschisis between 1986 and 1991 were retrospectively reviewed. The mean gestational age at sonographic diagnosis was 20.3 weeks and the mean gestational age was 36.5 weeks. There were 21 live births, who had a good surgical outcome. 16 of the deliveries were vaginal and 8 were by cesarean section. 46% of the study group were growth-restricted. In this study there was a 12.5% stillbirth rate even when the fetuses were appropriately grown. The authors therefore concluded that antenatal surveillance of fetal wellbeing was indicated in cases of gastroschisis. **III B**

3 Calzolari E, Bianchi F, Dolk H *et al.* and the Eurocat Working Group (1995) Omphalocele and gastroschisis in Europe: a survey of 3 million births 1980–1990. *Am J Med Genet* **58**, 187–194. A total of 732 cases of omphalocele and 274 cases of gastroschisis were registered in 21 regional registers in Europe during the period 1980–90. Omphalocele was an isolated malformation in 46% of cases; gastroschisis was isolated in 79% of cases. The average birthweight and gestational age of both isolated and multiply malformed cases of both omphalocele and gastroschisis were low. Isolated gastroschisis is associated with a significantly younger age than isolated omphalocele. Omphalocele is associated with a high association of other malformations and chromosomal abnormalities (21.0% vs 7.3% for gastroschisis cases). **III B**

4 Mayer T, Black R, Matlak ME *et al.* (1980) Gastroschisis and omphalocele. An eight-year review. *Ann Surg* **192**, 783–787. This was an 8-year review of 75 fetuses with gastroschisis and omphalocele. The authors found that gastroschisis occurred approximately twice as often as omphalocele and was increasing in frequency. Prematurity occurred in 65% of the fetuses with gastroschisis. Although the incidence of malformations associated with gastroschisis was 23%, the vast majority of these were due to jejunoileal or colonic atresias. The mortality rate for fetuses with gastroschisis was 12.7%. Omphalocele was associated with a 23% prematurity rate and an associated anomaly rate of 66%. Major cardiac malformations and chromosomal defects were quite common in fetuses with omphalocele. The mortality rate with omphalocele (34%) was primarily due to major cardiac malformations or chromosomal anomalies. The survival rate in fetuses with omphalocele who did not have either a cardiac malformation or a chromosomal defect was 94%. **III B**

5 Dixon JC, Penman DM, Soothill PW (2000) The influence of bowel atresia in gastroschisis on fetal growth, cardiotocography abnormalities and amniotic fluid staining. *Br J Obstet Gynaecol* **107**, 472–475. This was an observational study of 115 cases of gastroschisis between 1980 and 1996. Patent bowel gastroschisis was associated with significantly more fetal heart rate abnormalities and intrauterine growth restriction than cases within intestinal atresia. The authors concluded that bowel vomiting may be an important cause of amniotic fluid staining. They hypothesize that bowel atresia protects against the increased incidence of fetal heart rate abnormalities and growth restriction found in cases of gastroschisis. **III B**

6 Pryde PG, Bardicef M, Treadwell MC *et al.* (1994) Gastroschisis: can antenatal ultrasound predict infant outcomes? *Obstet Gynecol* **84**, 505–510. This study retrospectively reviewed 30 consecutive cases of gastroschisis. Bowel dilatation of more than 17 mm on antenatal sonography appeared to be associated with an increased short- and long-term infant morbidity. These studies did not permit the authors to determine whether intervention in the preterm gastroschisis-affected pregnancy should occur when substantial bowel dilatation is documented sonographically. **III B**

7 Bond SJ, Harrison MR, Filly RA *et al.* (1988) Severity of intestinal damage in gastroschisis: correlation with prenatal sonographic findings. *J Pediatr Surg* **23**, 520–525. This was a retrospective review of 26 abdominal wall

defects between 1982 and 1986. There were 15 fetuses with gastroschisis and 11 with omphalocele. In the fetuses with gastroschisis the size of the defect in the abdominal wall did not correlate with eventual clinical outcome. However, the presence of small-bowel dilatation and mural thickening on prenatal sonography correlated with intestinal damage and poor clinical outcome. The authors confirmed that gastroschisis appears to be more common than omphalocele. The authors found an association between omphaloceles and allantoic cysts. In the authors' experience with over 100 cases there has not been any damage that could be ascribed to vaginal rather than cesarean delivery. As a result, the authors do not advocate routine cesarean delivery for fetuses with prenatally diagnosed abdominal wall defects. **III B**

8 Haddock G, Davis CF, Raine PA *et al.* (1997) Gastroschisis in the decade of prenatal diagnosis: 1983–1993. *Eur J Pediatr Surg* **12**, 276–282. 50 cases of gastroschisis were reviewed between January 1983 and October 1993. The mean birth weight was 2.17 kg and the mean gestational age was 35.8 weeks. Associated bowel problems were noted in 22% of cases. Primary closure was achieved in 84%; there were five deaths. Spontaneous vaginal delivery occurred in 46%; the remaining 54% were delivered by cesarean section. Prenatal diagnosis and the mode of delivery did not show any direct correlation with mortality. **III B**

9 Babcook C, Hedrick MH, Goldstein RB *et al.* (1994) Gastroschisis: can sonography of the fetal bowel accurately predict postnatal outcome? *J Ultrasound Med* **13**, 701–706. This was a retrospective review of 24 fetuses with prenatally detected gastroschisis. Significantly more fetuses with a maximum small-bowel diameter greater than 11 mm (7/12) had bowel complications than did fetuses with a maximum small-bowel diameter less than 11 mm (2/12, $p < 0.05$). However, maximum bowel diameter was not a highly reproducible measurement between observers. The authors concluded that prenatal sonography could not accurately predict impending bowel damage. As a result, it should not be used to make a decision concerning delivery prior to term. **III B**

10 Kirk EP, Wah RM (1983) Obstetric management of the fetus with omphalocele or gastroschisis. A review of one-hundred and twelve cases. *Am J Obstet Gynecol* **146**, 512–518. Review of 112 cases with anterior abdominal wall defects admitted to a neonatal surgical unit prior to 1983. No cesarean sections were performed because of the antenatal diagnosis of an anterior abdominal wall defect (only made in four cases). The overall cesarean section rate was 16%. Decisions about delivery were made in the absence of the existence of the condition in 118 (97%) cases and there were no adverse effects on outcome from vaginal delivery. **III B**

11 Moretti M, Khoury A, Rodriquez J *et al.* (1990) The effect of mode of delivery on the perinatal outcome in fetuses with abdominal wall defects. *Am J Obstet Gynecol* **163**, 833–838. Review of 56 cases with gastroschisis and 69 cases of omphalocele. There were no significant differences between the groups in terms of cesarean section rate (26% vs 22%) and prematurity rate (30% vs 26%). There was a lower incidence of infant deaths (7% vs 22%), associated congenital abnormalities (5% vs 29%) and long-term infant morbidity (8.9% vs 14.5%). In either group there was no difference in infant mortality, acute or long-term infant outcome or frequency of associated major abnormalities between those delivered vaginally and those delivered by cesarean section. **III B**

12 Blakelock RT, Harding JE, Kolbe A *et al.* (1997) Gastroschisis: can the morbidity be avoided? *Pediatr Surg* **12**, 276–282. This study evaluated 44 cases of gastroschisis that were treated between 1969 and 1995; there were 6 deaths. Mode of delivery did not influence subsequent neonatal morbidity. Mode of delivery, gestational age, complications of surgery, admission temperature and a need for postoperative ventilation were not independently associated with any of the measures of morbidity. It was concluded that a term delivery with primary closure was likely to minimize the morbidity associated with gastroschisis. **III B**

13 Moore TC, Nur K (1986) An international survey of gastroschisis and omphalocele (490 cases). I. Nature and distribution of additional malformations. *Pediatr Surg Int* **1**, 46–50. This is an international survey of 16 pediatric surgery centers on four continents. In 203 cases of gastroschisis, additional malformations were infrequent and were primarily restricted to bowel atresias or stenosis. In 287 cases of omphalocele 14% were classified as syndromes. Additional malformations were found in approximately 74% of fetuses; approximately 5% of the fetuses had a karyotypic abnormality. **III B**

20.3 Congenital diaphragmatic hernia

Bryan Beattie

Management option		Quality of evidence	Strength of recommendation	References
Prenatal diagnosis	Survival poorer with: ❑ Liver herniation ❑ Small right lung ❑ Earlier gestational age at diagnosis ❑ Associated anomalies, particularly cardiac ❑ Chromosome abnormalities	III	B	1–3
	❑ Intrathoracic stomach	III	B	4,5

Management option		Quality of evidence	Strength of recommendation	References
Prenatal diagnosis (cont'd)	Survival poorer with (cont'd):			
	❑ Polyhydramnios			
	– Yes	III	B	4,5
	– No	III	B	3
	❑ Right lung to head circumference ratio of 0.6 between 24 and 26 weeks in fetuses with liver herniation	III	B	3,6
	❑ Posterior intrathoracic stomach associated with liver herniation	III	B	7
	Survival better with:			
	❑ Late herniation, normal ultrasound 15–23 weeks	III	B	8
	❑ Small volume of herniated viscera	III	B	8
	❑ Normal amniotic fluid volume	III	B	8
	❑ Stomach in abdomen, i.e. association with small defect	III	B	9
	❑ Right lung:head circumference ratio >1.35 at 24–26 weeks in fetuses with liver herniation	III	B	3,6
	Right lung:head circumference ratio is not predictive of outcome for bowel-only congenital diaphragmatic hernias	III	B	6
Prenatal repair	Hysterotomy with tracheal plug placement results in improved lung growth *in utero*; limited survival precludes recommendation of technique	III	B	10
	In-utero surgical repair; limited survival precludes recommendation of technique	III	B	11
	In-utero videofetoscopic tracheal occlusion without hysterotomy appears to improve survival in fetuses with worst prognosis (i.e. liver herniation, early diagnosis, low liver:head circumference ratio)	III	B	12
Neonatal treatment	Extracorporeal membrane oxygenation (ECMO) decreases mortality in infants with large defects or early respiratory distress	III	B	13,14
	No advantage to using ECMO prior to repair of congenital diaphragmatic hernia	III	B	14
	No clear support for either early (<24 h) or delayed (>24 h) repair	IIb	B	15

References

1 Wilson JM, Lund DP, Lillehei CW *et al.* (1994) Antenatal diagnosis of isolated congenital diaphragmatic hernia is not an indicator of outcome. *J Pediatr Surg* **29**, 815–819. The authors reviewed 173 infants with congenital diaphragmatic hernia. 77 cases were diagnosed antenatally and 96 cases were diagnosed postnatally. Among the 114 patients with an isolated congenital diaphragmatic hernia, the survival rate was 59% in those diagnosed antenatally in contrast to 63% in the postnatal group – a difference that was not significant. Of the 59 patients with other life-threatening anomalies, there was one survivor among the 34 in the antenatal group and only 2 among the 25 in the postnatal group. **III B**

2 Nakayama DK, Harrison MR, Chinn DH *et al.* (1985) Prenatal diagnosis and natural history of the fetus with a congenital diaphragmatic hernia: initial clinical experience. *J Pediatr Surg* **20**, 118–124. This study reviewed 9 babies born at one institution and 6 of 11 babies referred to the same institution over a 3-year period. The mortality rate was 75% – all the infants had pulmonary hypoplasia. 40% had associated malformations or chromosomal abnormalities. Polyhydramnios was present in all 9 cases diagnosed antenatally. **III B**

3 Metkus AP, Filly RA, Stringer MD *et al.* (1996) Sonographic predictors of survival in fetal diaphragmatic hernia. *J Pediatr Surg* **31**, 148–152. A review of 55 cases of prenatally diagnosed isolated congenital diaphragmatic hernia delivered prior to 1996 and managed in an extracorporeal membrane oxygenation center. Survival was correlated with various ultrasound features. There was no correlation between polyhydramnios, abdominal circumference, stomach position and survival. Survival was, however, poorer in cases with liver herniation (56% vs 100%), small right lung size (lung:head ratio <0.6 61% vs 100%) and lower gestation at diagnosis (<25 weeks 56% vs 100%). The overall survival rate was 65%. All cases with very small right lung size died. **III B**

4 Adzick NS, Shamberger RC, Winter HS *et al.* (1989) Fetal diaphragmatic hernia: ultrasound diagnosis and clinical outcome in 38 cases. *J Pediatr Surg* **24**, 654–658. This is a report of 38 cases of congenital diaphragmatic hernia diagnosed *in utero* and treated by the same surgical team. The authors concluded that: (1) survival was poor despite optimal postnatal therapy, including extracorporeal membrane oxygenation; (2) polyhydramnios is a common prenatal marker for congenital diaphragmatic hernia; (3) polyhydramnios is a predictor for poor clinical outcome; (4) amniocentesis is indicated to rule out chromosomal abnormalities (a chromosomal abnormality was found in 16% of the fetuses in this series); and (5) diagnosis prior to 25 weeks gestation was a poor prognostic sign. **III B**

5 Dommergues M, Louis-Sylvestre C, Mandelbrot L *et al.* (1996) Congenital diaphragmatic hernia: can prenatal ultrasonography predict outcome? *Am J Obstet Gynecol* **174**, 1377–1381. This is a retrospective multicenter cohort study of 135 patients with congenital diaphragmatic hernia. None of the 44 fetuses or infants with multiple malformations survived. Of the 91 cases of isolated congenital diaphragmatic hernia, 67% died in the neonatal period. The authors found a statistically significant relation between mortality and polyhydramnios, intrathoracic stomach and a major mediastinal shift. Mortality was found to increase along with the number of prognostic factors. **III B**

6 Sbragia L, Paek BW, Filly RA *et al.* (2000) Congenital diaphragmatic hernia without herniation of the liver: does the lung-to-head ratio predict survival? *J Ultrasound Med* **19**, 845–848. The authors reviewed 20 fetuses with isolated left congenital diaphragmatic hernia without herniation of the liver into the chest. The lung-to-head ratio was obtained in each of these fetuses. The fetuses were then subdivided into two groups depending upon the lung-to-head ratio – those with a ratio less than 1.4 and those with a ratio more than 1.4. Although the study population was limited, there was no difference noted in the need for extracorporeal membrane oxygenation support or survival between the two groups. Fetuses with a prenatally diagnosed left congenital diaphragmatic hernia without herniation of the liver into the chest had a favorable prognosis even with a low lung-to-head ratio. The authors therefore concluded that the lung-to-head ratio was not effective in predicting survival in fetuses with congenital diaphragmatic hernia without herniation of the liver. **III B**

7 Bootstaylor BS, Filly RA, Harrison MR *et al.* (1995) Prenatal sonographic predictors of liver herniation in congenital diaphragmatic hernia. *J Ultrasound Med* **14**, 515–520. This was a retrospective review of 25 fetuses with a left-sided congenital diaphragmatic hernia undergoing *in-utero* surgical repair. 16 fetuses were analyzed in order to determine predictors of liver herniation. The authors found that the stomach position was a good predictor if it was in the posterior or midthoracic location. However, this occurred in only 44% of cases. Bowing of the umbilical segment of the portal vein to the left of the midline and coursing of portal branches to the lateral segment of the left hepatic lobe toward or above the diaphragmatic ridge were the best predictors for liver herniation into the fetal thorax. **III B**

8 Adzick NS, Vacanti JP, Lillehei CW *et al.* (1985) Diaphragmatic hernia in the fetus; prenatal diagnosis and outcome in 94 cases. *J Pediatr Surg* **20**, 357–361. 94 cases of fetal congenital diaphragmatic hernia were reviewed from the USA and Canada. The authors found that the antenatal diagnosis of congenital diaphragmatic hernia was accurate. Despite optimal conventional therapy, most fetuses with a detected congenital diaphragmatic hernia died in the neonatal period (80% mortality). Polyhydramnios is a common prenatal marker for congenital diaphragmatic hernia and a predictor of poor outcome. Nonsurvivors tend to have larger defects and may have more viscera displaced into the chest at an earlier gestational age. **III B**

9 Goodfellow T, Hyde I, Burge DM *et al.* (1987) Congenital diaphragmatic hernia: the prognostic significance of the site of the stomach. *Br J Radiol* **60**, 993–995. The authors reviewed 50 consecutive cases of left-sided diaphragmatic hernia. The site of the stomach was found to be related to subsequent outcome. An abdominal site was associated with an excellent prognosis (6.2% mortality), while an intrathoracic stomach was associated with a 58.8% mortality. **III B**

10 Harrison MR, Adzick NS, Flake AW *et al.* (1996) Correction of congenital diaphragmatic hernia in utero. VIII: Response of the hypoplastic lung to tracheal occlusion. *J Pediatr Surg* **31**, 1339–1348. A review of 8 cases of congenital diaphragmatic hernia with liver herniation between 25 and 28 weeks treated with tracheal occlusion. 2 had an internal plug and 6 an external clip and more recently a technique has been developed to unplug them at delivery (*ex-utero* intrapartum tracheoplasty, EXIT). In most cases there was evidence of improved lung growth *in utero* with reversal of pulmonary hypoplasia documented before birth but limited survival (50% and 0%, although nonpulmonary deaths) precludes the recommendation of these techniques for treating pulmonary hypoplasia at present. **III B**

11 Harrison MR, Adzick NS, Flake AW *et al.* (1993) Correction of congenital diaphragmatic hernia in utero: VI Hard-earned lesions. *J Pediatr Surg* **28**, 1411–1417. A review of 61 further cases considered suitable for *in-utero* repair of congenital diaphragmatic hernia since their last report (1989–91). Fetal repair was attempted in 14 cases with severe isolated left CDH diagnosed before 24 weeks. 5 died intraoperatively because of technical reasons such as premature labour and incarcerated liver. 4 survived initially but 2 delivered prematurely and died. 3 died within 48 h of fetal surgery *in utero*. The main problems that the authors claim they have overcome are postoperative physiological management of the maternal–fetal unit and effective tocolysis. The overall survival was 33%. **III B**

12 Harrison MR, Mychaliska GB, Albanese CT *et al.* (1998) Correction of congenital diaphragmatic hernia in utero IX: Fetuses with poor prognosis (liver herniation and low lung-to-head ratio) can be saved by fetoscopic temporary tracheal occlusion. *J Pediatr Surg* **33**, 1017–1023. This study evaluated 13 fetuses with congenital diaphragmatic hernia who met the authors' conclusions for poor prognosis. Of these 34 fetuses, 13 underwent postnatal treatment with extracorporeal membrane oxygenation, 13 underwent open fetal tracheal occlusion and 8 underwent fetoscopic tracheal occlusion. The survival rate was 38% in the group treated by standard postnatal therapy, 15% in the open tracheal occlusion group and 75% in the 8 fetuses who underwent fetoscopic tracheal occlusion. The authors concluded that fetuses with a congenital diaphragmatic hernia with liver herniation appear to benefit from temporary tracheal occlusion when performed fetoscopically but not when performed by open fetal surgery. The authors considered fetuses with a congenital diaphragmatic hernia to have a 'poor prognosis' on the basis of liver herniation, early diagnosis before 25 weeks gestation and a low lung-to-head ratio. The lung-to-head circumference ratio was calculated between 24 and 26 weeks gestation. When the lung-to-head circumference ration was below 1.0 there were no survivors. All patients with a lung-to-head circumference ratio greater than 1.4 survived. **III B**

13 D'Agostino JA, Bernbaum JC, Gerdes M *et al.* (1995) Outcome for infants with congenital diaphragmatic hernia requiring extracorporeal membrane oxygenation: the first year. *J Pediatr Surg* **30**, 10–15. A review of 30 cases of neonates with congenital diaphragmatic hernia admitted over a 2-year period from 1990–92. 20 were treated with extracorporeal membrane oxygenation (ECMO) and this group were followed up at 3, 6 and 12 months for both medical and neuro-developmental outcome. 13 (65%) of these had a primary repair, 5 had a Gore-Tex® graft reconstruction and 2 did not have repair. The overall survival rate was 16 (80%). The overall survival rate increased from 31% in the 5 years prior to ECMO compared to 63% when ECMO became available. Common sequelae include gastroesophageal reflux (81%), need for tube feeding (69%), chronic lung disease (62%). At 12 months old, while cognitive skills were average, motor skills were borderline (Bayley Scales of Infant Development) and hypotonia was common (77%). **III B**

14 Lessin MS, Klein MD (1995) Congenital diaphragmatic hernia with or without extracorporeal membrane oxygenation: are we making progress? *J Am Coll Surg* **181**, 65–71. 123 newborns with congenital diaphragmatic hernia from 1972–94 were retrospectively reviewed. The overall survival rate was 41%. Patients who did not receive extracorporeal membrane oxygenation (ECMO) had a 27% survival rate in contrast to 39% (preoperative ECMO) and 45% (postoperative ECMO). The authors concluded that ECMO improved survival in newborns with congenital diaphragmatic hernia. However, there did not appear to be any advantage or disadvantage to using ECMO prior to repair of the hernia. **III B**

15 Moyer V, Moya F, Tibboel R *et al.* (2001) Late versus early surgical correction for congenital diaphragmatic hernia in newborn infants (Cochrane review). In: *The Cochrane library*, issue 3. Oxford: Update Software. The Cochrane review found two small studies ($n < 90$) which compared early (< 24 h) versus late (> 24 h) surgical correction for cases of congenital diaphragmatic hernia and found no difference in mortality as the main outcome. Meta-analysis was not performed because of significant clinical heterogeneity between the trials. The authors conclude that there is no clear support for either early or delayed repair of congenital diaphragmatic hernia and that a large multicenter randomized trial would be required to answer the question. **IIb B**

20.4 Esophageal atresia (± fistula)

David James

Management option		Quality of evidence	Strength of recommendation	References
Prenatal	Diagnosis by ultrasound during pregnancy is uncommon; raised alpha-fetoprotein is a reported association	III	B	1,2
	Hydramnios is common	III	B	1,2
	Examine for associated abnormalities with ultrasound and karyotype	III	B	1,2
	Interdisciplinary counseling	–	✔	–
Labor and delivery	Normal management but in tertiary center with facilities for advanced neonatal resuscitation, intensive care and surgery	–	✔	–
Postnatal	Remove excess secretions at birth; place esophageal tube to maintain low-pressure suction	–	✔	–

➡

Management option		Quality of evidence	Strength of recommendation	References
Postnatal (cont'd)	Early diagnostic imaging	III	B	1
	Avoid feeding	–	✓	–
	Check for other abnormalities	–	✓	–
	Small risk of recurrence	–	✓	–

References

1 Satoh S, Takashima T, Takeuchi HP *et al.* (1995) Antenatal sonographic detection of the proximal esophageal segment: specific evidence for congenital esophageal atresia. *J Clin Ultrasound* **23**, 419–423. Prospective study of 10 cases presenting both polyhydramnios and an unusually small stomach size due to a decrease in fetal stomach fluid. There were 8 cases with a transient anechoic area in the fetal neck, all of which were diagnosed as having congenital esophageal atresia (CEA) postnatally by plain X-ray, neonatal surgery or autopsy findings. The remaining 2 cases had no CEA; one had Nager syndrome and the other a disorder involving neuronal migration in the central nervous system. These results suggest that an anechoic area in the middle of the fetal neck can be used as an indication of CEA and also for differentiating this condition from diseases with possible swallowing impairment. **III B**

2 Chodirker BN, Chudley AE, MacDonald KM *et al.* (1994) MSAFP levels and oesophageal atresia. *Prenat Diagn* **14**, 1086–1089. This study was undertaken to evaluate the relationship between maternal serum alpha-fetoprotein (MSAFP) levels and esophageal atresia (OA). OA occurred in 16 fetuses of mothers who had an MSAFP test in the study interval. The multiple of the median (MOM) value for MSAFP averaged 1.54 ± 0.65 (range 0.5–2.9 MOM), which was significantly higher than the value seen in controls. The median MOM was 1.35. Using a cut-off of 2.5 MOM, the sensitivity of MSAFP for detecting OA was 19%. Although OA should be considered in the differential diagnosis of an elevated MSAFP level, MSAFP cannot be considered an appropriate screening test for OA, given the low sensitivity. **III B**

20.5 Duodenal atresia

Bryan Beattie

Management option		Quality of evidence	Strength of recommendation	References
Prenatal diagnosis	Double-bubble with dilated stomach and proximal duodenum (usually detected latter part of second or third trimester)	III	B	1,2
	Associated with: ❑ Polyhydramnios ❑ Annular pancreas ❑ Preterm labor	III	B	3
	❑ 20–30% incidence of Down syndrome	III	B	4–6
	❑ Higher incidence of other structural malformations	III	B	4,3
Neonatal	Antenatal detection results in earlier surgery	III	B	2
	Preoperative morbidity is higher with neonatal rather than antenatal diagnosis	III	B	7
	Antenatal detection does not affect long-term outcome	III	B	2

References

1 Nelson LH, Clark CE, Fishburne JI *et al.* (1982) Value of serial sonography in the in-utero detection of duodenal atresia. *Obstet Gynecol* **59**, 657–660. Serial ultrasound examinations were obtained on two patients. However, duodenal atresia was not detected until 29 and 32 weeks gestation, respectively. The authors concluded that early prenatal diagnosis by ultrasound and subsequent amniocentesis plays an important role in the antenatal and postpartum counseling and management of these patients. **III B**

2 Hancock BJ, Wiseman NE (1989) Congenital duodenal obstruction: The impact of an antenatal diagnosis. *J Pediatr Surg* **24**, 1027–1031. The authors reviewed a series of 34 infants with duodenal obstruction. 15 were diagnosed antenatally. The overall survival for the entire series was 88%. Definitive surgery was performed earlier when the diagnosis was made antenatally. However, long-term outcome was not affected by providing an antenatal diagnosis. Associated anomalies were present in 64.7% of patients with duodenal obstruction. Polyhydramnios was present in 50% of the patients. **III B**

3 Dalla Vecchia LK, Book BK, Milgrom ML *et al.* (1998) Intestinal atresia and stenosis. *Arch Surg* **33**, 490–497. A review of 277 neonates with intestinal atresia or stenosis over a 25-year period from 1972–97 managed in a single tertiary care center in Indianapolis, IN, USA. The major causes of morbidity and mortality were associated cardiac abnormalities (with duodenal atresia) and short bowel syndrome (12% of infants had less than 40cm of bowel remaining) requiring total parenteral nutrition, which can cause liver disease. Duodenal atresia was found in 138 infants and was usually treated by duodenoduodenostomy (86%). It was associated with prematurity (46%), associated polyhydramnios (33%), Down syndrome (24%), annular pancreas (33%) and malrotation (28%). Overall survival was 86%. Jejunoileal atresia was usually treated by resection (76%). It was associated with intrauterine volvulus (27%), gastroschisis (16%) and meconium ileus (11.7%). Overall survival was 84%. Colonic atresia was usually treated by initial ostomy and delayed anastomosis (86%). Overall survival was 100%. **III B**

4 Fonakalsrud EW, DeLorimier AA, Hays DM *et al.* (1969) Congenital atresia and stenosis of the duodenum. A review compiled from the members of the surgical section of the American Academy of Pediatrics. *Pediatrics* **43**, 79–83. This is a review of 503 patients with a congenital diaphragmatic obstruction. More than half of the infants with duodenal atresia had associated malformations. 30% of the patients had Down syndrome. **III B**

5 Nicolaides KH, Snijders RJ, Cheng HH *et al.* (1992) Fetal gastro-intestinal and abdominal wall defects: associated malformations and chromosomal abnormalities. *Fetal Diagn Ther* **7**, 102–115. This study reviewed the karyotypes of 235 fetuses with abdominal wall or gastrointestinal tract defects. The fetal karyotype was abnormal in 10 (43%) of the 23 fetuses with duodenal atresia. **III B**

6 Miro J, Bard H (1988) Congenital atresia and stenosis of the duodenum. The impact of a prenatal diagnosis. *Am J Obstet Gynecol* **158**, 555–559. The authors reviewed 46 cases of either atresia or stenosis of the small bowel. 12 fetuses had duodenal atresia. Prenatal diagnosis resulted in earlier surgical intervention. Neonatal complications were also less frequent when the diagnosis was made antenatally. **III B**

7 Romero R, Ghidini A, Costigan K *et al.* (1988) Prenatal diagnosis of duodenal atresia: does it make a difference. *Obstet Gynecol* **71**, 739–741. This study evaluated 11 cases of antenatally diagnosed duodenal atresia and compared the outcome with 7 cases in which the diagnosis was made during the neonatal period. Polyhydramnios was uniformly present in the antenatally diagnosed group. The authors found that the incidence of neonatal morbidity was higher and the preoperative condition of the neonate was poorer in the group in which the diagnosis was made neonatally. **III B**

20.6 Jejunoileal atresia

Bryan Beattie

Management option		Quality of evidence	Strength of recommendation	References
Prenatal	Diagnosis: ❑ Multiple loops of overdistended small bowel (>7 mm) ❑ Vigorous peristalsis ❑ Polyhydramnios ❑ Ascites	III	B	1,2
	Associated with: ❑ Volvulus ❑ Gastroschisis ❑ Meconium ileus	III	B	3
	Vigilance for prematurity	III	B	4

References

1 Langer JC, Adzick NS, Filly RA *et al.* (1989) Gastrointestinal tract obstruction in the fetus. *Arch Surg* **124**, 1183–1187. This study reviewed 17 cases of a gastrointestinal tract obstruction. 8 of the cases were due to duodenal obstruction; 7 of the 8 did well after transport and neonatal surgery. 6 fetuses had distal obstruction with dilated bowel and increased peristalsis. The authors suggest that: (1) polyhydramnios may not be present early in gestation or with distal obstruction; (2) there is an increased frequency of other anomalies when a gastrointestinal tract obstruction is detected; (3) dilated fetal bowel with increased peristalsis is diagnostic of a fetal gastrointestinal tract obstruction; (4) prenatal diagnosis with a planned delivery at a tertiary center followed by prompt resuscitation should improve neonatal outcome. **III B**

2 Corteville JE, Gray DL, Langer JC (1996) Bowel abnormalities in the fetus: correlation of prenatal ultrasonographic findings with outcome. *Am J Obstet Gynecol* **175**, 724–729. This study reviewed 16471 consecutive fetuses who were scanned in the second trimester or later. 22 fetuses had dilated bowel distal to the duodenum. 11 of these had a normal postnatal outcome and 11 cases had an abnormal outcome. The authors found that a bowel diameter greater than 10mm after 26 weeks gestation, increasing bowel diameter in the third trimester, an upper midabdominal loop of dilated bowel, hyperperistalsis and increased amniotic fluid volume were all more common in the abnormal group. However, there was no sonographic finding that was able to discriminate between the two groups in all cases. The positive predictive value of an ultrasound examination in the detection of small bowel obstruction was 72.7%. **III B**

3 Dalla Vecchia LK, Vecchia LK, Grosfeld JL *et al.* (1998) Intestinal atresia and stenosis. *Arch Surg* **133**, 490–497. A review of 277 neonates with intestinal atresia or stenosis over a 25-year period from 1972–97 managed in a single tertiary care center in Indianapolis, IN, USA. The major causes of morbidity and mortality were associated cardiac abnormalities (with duodenal atresia) and short bowel syndrome (12% infants had less than 40cm remaining bowel) requiring total parenteral nutrition which can cause liver disease. Duodenal atresia found in 138 infants and was usually treated by duodenoduodenostomy (86%). It was associated with prematurity (46%), associated polyhydramnios (33%), Down syndrome (24%), annular pancreas (33%) and malrotation (28%). Overall survival was 86%. Jejunoileal atresia was usually treated by resection (76%). It was associated with intrauterine volvulus (27%), gastroschisis (16%) and meconium ileus (11.7%). Overall survival was 84%. Colonic atresia was usually treated by initial colostomy and delayed anastomosis (86%). Overall survival was 100%. **III B**

4 Heij HA, Ekkelkamp S, Vos A (1990) Atresia of jejunum and ileum: is it the same disease? *J Pediatr Surg* **25**, 635–637. This is a retrospective analysis of 21 patients with jejunal atresia and 24 with ileal atresia. The authors found that antenatal perforation occurred more frequently with ileal in contrast to jejunal atresia; however, mortality was higher in jejunal atresia. The authors hypothesize that the differences observed between the two atresias was due to differences in bowel compliance – the compliant jejunal wall allows for massive dilatation with subsequent loss of peristaltic activity. It was therefore considered that jejunal and ileal atresia should be considered to be separate diseases. Patients with jejunal atresia had a significantly lower gestational age and birthweight than children with ileal atresia. The longer postoperative course in jejunal atresia could be explained by the difference in bowel wall compliance. Since the jejunum was more dilated it had lost its peristaltic activity and required a longer time period to regain function. In ileal atresia, since the bowel distension was less, function returned more quickly. **III B**

20.7 Large-bowel obstruction, anal atresia, imperforate anus

David James

Management option		Quality of evidence	Strength of recommendation	References
Prenatal	Vigilance for hydramnios (rare)	III	B	1,2
	Interdisciplinary counseling	IV	C	3,4
	Careful ultrasound examination for other abnormalities	III	B	2
Postnatal	Do not give baby anything by mouth	III IV	B C	3 4
	Pediatric assessment and management	III IV	B C	3 4

References

1 Yoo SJ, Park KW, Cho SY *et al.* (1999) Definitive diagnosis of intestinal volvulus in utero. *Ultrasound Obstet Gynecol* **13**, 200–203. Midgut volvulus with or without intestinal malrotation can occur in fetal life. Several reports have described congenital midgut volvulus showing nonspecific sonographic findings of intestinal obstruction and perforation *in utero*. None of the previously reported cases, however, were definitively diagnosed as midgut volvulus by fetal sonography. Two cases are reported, both exhibiting the sonographic 'whirlpool' sign *in utero*. Color Doppler interrogation provided a clue to the viability of the involved intestinal segment. **III B**

2 Bronshtein M, Zimmer EZ (1996) Early sonographic detection of fetal intestinal obstruction and possible diagnostic pitfalls. *Prenat Diagn* **16**, 203–206. Report of five fetuses at 15–17 weeks gestation with a sonographic diagnosis of intestinal obstruction. Dilation of the intestine was the presenting sonographic finding in fetuses with a volvulus and/or anal atresia. Two of the fetuses also had other abnormalities. Intestinal peristalsis may be observed in early pregnancy as transient dilation of intestinal segments. Sonographers are cautioned about a false-positive diagnosis of intestinal obstruction in such cases. **III B**

3 Gaillard D, Bouvier R, Scheiner C *et al.* (1996) Meconium ileus and intestinal atresia in fetuses and neonates. *Pediatr Pathol Lab Med* **16**, 25–40. Collaborative study to determine the different types and mechanisms of intestinal abnormalities during gestation. Cases had to fulfill one or more of the following: (1) meconium ileus, (2) intestinal stenosis/atresia, (3) meconium peritonitis. Esophageal atresia, anorectal atresia and abdominal wall defects were excluded. 102 cases were reviewed from autopsies of 42 induced abortions, 22 stillborns and surgical findings in 38 neonates. Meconium ileus was detected mainly during the second trimester (28/38) and was associated with cystic fibrosis (15), fetal blood deglutition (4), infection (6) or multiple abnormalities (10), in which three chromosomal aberrations were found. Intestinal stenosis or atresia was more commonly detected during the third trimester (46/56). 16 of the 30 duodenal malformations were associated with trisomy 21; in the 26 small-intestine atresias, signs of distress or ischemia were most frequently detected. Only 8 of 25 meconium peritonitis cases were isolated. 20 cases of cystic fibrosis could be proved. Functional abnormalities were observed predominantly in the second trimester and were associated mainly with cystic fibrosis or amniotic fluid abnormalities. Anatomical lesions were commonly detected later on and were associated with ischemic conditions, chromosomal aberrations and even cystic fibrosis. **III B**

4 Prasad TR, Bajpai M (2000) Intestinal atresia. *Indian J Pediatr* **67**, 671–678. Intestinal atresia accounts for about one third of all cases of neonatal intestinal obstruction. The survival rate has improved to 90% in most of the series with the operative mortality being less than 1%. The survival rate improves with distal atresias. An increased mortality is observed in multiple atresias (57%), apple peel atresia (71%) and when atresia is associated with meconium ileus (65%), meconium peritonitis (50%) and gastroschisis (66%). Although appearance of echogenic bowel on prenatal ultrasonography is suggestive of atresia, it is confirmed in only 27% cases. Prenatal ultrasonography is more reliable in detection of duodenal atresia than more distal lesions. Short bowel syndrome is the major impediment in the management of jejunoileal atresia. Although total parenteral nutrition (TPN) is the main adjunctive treatment, it delays intestinal adaptation and may cause cholestasia and subsequent liver damage. Graduated enteric feedings, use of growth hormone, glutamine and modified diets containing low fat, complex carbohydrates and protein supplements have been used in adults with short bowel syndrome to successfully diminish TPN requirements and enhance nutrient absorption in nearly half of the patients. Use of growth factors to facilitate intestinal adaptation and advances in small bowel transplant may improve the long-term outcomes in future. **IV C**

20.8 Meconium ileus/peritonitis

David James

Management option		Quality of evidence	Strength of recommendation	References
Prenatal	Diagnosis by ultrasound	III	B	1,2
	Consider diagnosis of cystic fibrosis and parvovirus	III	B	2–4
	Lack of data about value of drainage or delivery if ascites or hydramnios develops	III	B	2
	Interdisciplinary counseling	III	B	1,2
Labor and delivery	Timing depends on: ❑ Obstetric factors ❑ Ascites/hydramnios	III	B	1,2
	Delivery in a tertiary center	III	B	1,2

➡

Management option		Quality of evidence	Strength of recommendation	References
Postnatal	Outcome dependent upon: ❑ Surgical feasibility of repair ❑ Associated abnormalities ❑ Perforation ❑ Gestation	III	B	1,2
See also Section 20.10.				

References

1 Dirkes K, Crombleholme TM, Craigo SD *et al.* (1995) The natural history of meconium peritonitis diagnosed in utero. *J Pediatr Surg* **30**, 979–982. Case series of meconium peritonitis (MP) diagnosed *in utero* to define criteria for prenatal and postnatal management. Prenatal diagnosis was made by identifying abdominal calcification on serial ultrasound examinations in 9 fetuses between 18 and 37 weeks gestation. Cases without associated bowel abnormalities were considered 'simple MP' and those with bowel abnormalities were considered 'complex MP.' 5 cases of simple MP were identified at 18, 23, 30, 34 and 37 weeks gestation. These 5 fetuses were delivered at term and had normal abdominal examinations. Abdominal radiographs were obtained in 3 showing normal bowel gas patterns, and abdominal calcifications in only 2. All 5 patients were fed uneventfully. 4 cases of complex MP were identified at 26, 26, 31 and 31 weeks gestation. All 4 fetuses had dilated loops of bowel. 2 of the 4 had meconium cysts, one of which was associated with ascites and the other with polyhydramnios. Shortly after birth both infants with meconium cysts required ileal resection and ileostomy for ileal atresia and ileal perforation respectively. The remaining 2 infants had no evidence of dilated bowel, meconium cyst or ascites on postnatal radiograph and were fed uneventfully. These data suggest that only 22% of fetuses with a prenatal diagnosis of MP develop complications that require postnatal operation. Gestational age at diagnosis does not correlate with postnatal outcome. Fetuses with complex MP are at increased risk for postnatal bowel obstruction and perforation. **III B**

2 Konje JC, de Chazal R, MacFadyen U *et al.* (1995) Antenatal diagnosis and management of meconium peritonitis: a case report and review of the literature. *Ultrasound Obstet Gynecol* **6**, 66–69. Case report and review of the literature. The case was one of meconium peritonitis that was associated with a short bowel and complicated by progressive bowel distension and difficulty in making a definitive diagnosis of cystic fibrosis. Treatment was by bowel resection and an ileostomy (and later bowel anastomosis), followed by parenteral nutrition, which was complicated by hepatitis. The literature is reviewed and management dilemmas and options are discussed. **III B**

3 Caspi B, Elchalal U, Lancet M *et al.* (1988) Prenatal diagnosis of cystic fibrosis: ultrasonographic appearance of meconium ileus in the fetus. *Prenat Diagn* **8**, 379–382. Four of 10 fetuses carrying a risk of 1:4 for cystic fibrosis were found to have low levels of microvillar enzymes in the amniotic fluid obtained between 17 and 18 weeks gestation. On sonography performed prior to the amniocentesis, 3 fetuses showed enlarged bowel loops. At autopsy, meconium ileus was detected. Enlarged bowel loops are a sign that has not been described previously so early in pregnancies. **III B**

4 Zerbini M, Gentilomi GA, Gellinella G *et al.* (1998) Intra-uterine parvovirus B19 infection and meconium peritonitis. *Prenat Diagn* **18**, 599–606. Report of 4 cases of meconium peritonitis in hydropic fetuses with laboratory diagnosis of B19 infection. Parvovirus B19 DNA was detected by *in-situ* hybridization both in cord blood and in amniotic cells in 3 fetuses, while in one case only cord blood was available and proved positive. Signs of active or recent B19 infection in maternal serum samples were documented only in 2 cases, which proved positive for specific IgM antibodies anti-B19. Maternal B19 infections were asymptomatic and fetal anomalies were observed during a routine ultrasound scan. A common feature of the hydropic fetuses was the presence of abdominal ascites concomitant with or preceding alterations, suggesting meconium peritonitis. The 4 pregnancies had a preterm outcome: in 2 cases infants recovered following surgical treatment, in one case spontaneously, and the other one was stillborn. Since vascular inflammation has been documented in B19 infection and congenital bowel obstruction results from vascular damage during fetal life, our observation suggests the need for investigating B19 infection in the presence of meconium peritonitis for a better understanding of the pathogenetic potential of parvovirus B19 in intrauterine infection. **III B**

20.9 Intra-abdominal echolucent ('cystic') structures

David James

Management option		Quality of evidence	Strength of recommendation	References
Prenatal	Determine the organ of origin and diagnosis: ❑ Omental cysts ❑ Mesenteric cysts ❑ Ovarian cysts ❑ Urachus ❑ Liver cysts ❑ Choledochal cysts ❑ Bowel duplication cysts ❑ Retroperitoneal cysts	–	✔	–
	Exclude other fetal abnormalities	–	✔	–
Postnatal	Pediatric assessment and management	–	✔	–

20.10 Echogenic bowel and liver

David James

Management option		Quality of evidence	Strength of recommendation	References
Prenatal	Use strict criteria for diagnosis ('bone-white')	III	B	1, 2
	Make diagnosis if possible: ❑ Cystic fibrosis ❑ Viral infection (cytomegalovirus, parvovirus) ❑ Aneuploidy ❑ Intestinal obstruction (meconium ileus) ❑ Intra-amniotic bleeding ❑ Risk of placental bleed, intrauterine growth restriction and fetal death	III	B	3–6
Labor and delivery	Delivery in tertiary center with full pediatric resources	III	B	3,4
Postnatal	Pediatric assessment and management	III	B	3,4

References

1 Harrison KL, Martines D, Mason G (2000) The subjective assessment of echogenic fetal bowel. *Ultrasound Obstet Gynecol* **16**, 524–529. 87 women attending for their antenatal scan were selected in a random prospective manner over a 9-month period. Images of the fetal bowel were taken and evaluated by 10 sonographers, one consultant obstetrician and one consultant radiologist. Images from a further 13 fetuses, in which the subjective assessment of echogenic bowel was made, were also included. All ultrasound images were acquired on a dedicated ultrasound scanner, with a standard transducer, thermal paper printer and single operator using standardized equipment settings and reproducible image sections. Questionnaires with 100 sets of images of fetal bowel were distributed to the participants. Performance was assessed by means of percentage agreement and levels of chance-corrected agreement (Kappa). The subjective assessment of fetal bowel echogenicity was very variable. Intra- and interobserver variation discrepancies in the assessment of bowel echogenicity compared to bone were demonstrated between the sonographers. Good agreement was identified between the consultants with good to almost perfect intraobserver agreement. Overall, only moderate agreement was observed between the sonographers and the consultants. **III B**

2 Slotnick RN, Abuhamad AZ (1996) Prognostic implications of fetal echogenic bowel. *Lancet* **347**, 85–87. The authors report an ultrasonic grading system in which echogenicity was quantified by linear gain reduction and

comparison with fetal iliac crest. From 7400 second-trimester ultrasound referrals, 145 patients were identified as having a fetus with abnormally echogenic bowel. They were offered genetic counseling, parental and (if appropriate) cystic fibrosis (CF) carrier testing, and amniocentesis for karyotype and CF status if parents were informative. Follow-up was to 4 months of age. Of 40 fetuses with mild increase in bowel sonodensity (grade 1), none had CF or aneuploidy. Of 81 patients identified with a moderate increase (grade 2), 2 had trisomy 21 and 2 had CF, and of 24 pregnancies with a pronounced increase (grade 3), 5 had CF and 6 had trisomy 21. Parental CF carrier testing and amniocentesis to identify aneuploidy or fetal CF status has a high positive ascertainment rate in fetuses with echogenic bowel grades 2 and 3.
III B

3 Yaron Y, Hassan S, Geva E *et al.* (1999) Evaluation of fetal echogenic bowel in the second trimester. *Fetal Diagn Ther* **14**, 176–180. Previous studies cite different possible etiologies for fetal echogenic bowel (FEB). The purpose of this study was to evaluate the possible etiologies for second-trimester FEB and to provide clinical guidelines for evaluation of this finding. The study included 79 patients diagnosed with FEB in the second trimester. 15 cases (19%) were associated with maternal vaginal bleeding. Of these, 12 patients underwent amniocentesis, 9 of whom had visible blood products in the amniotic fluid. 7 cases (8.9%) had associated severe malformation. 7 other cases (8.9%) were noted in multifetal pregnancies. 5 fetuses (6.3%) had evidence of bowel obstruction or perforation not associated with cystic fibrosis (CF). Chromosomal aberrations were found in 5 fetuses (6.3%). Intrauterine infection with cytomegalovirus, herpes simplex virus, varicella-zoster virus or parvovirus B-19 was documented in 5 patients (6.3%). 3 cases (3.8%) were associated with subsequent unexplained stillbirth. 2 fetuses (2.5%) were found to be affected by CF. Finally, in 30 cases (38%) no obvious reason for FEB was found. Conclusion: the evaluation of second-trimester FEB should include targeted ultrasound for associated malformations, infectious studies, DNA analysis for CF mutations, amniocentesis for chromosomal analysis and evaluation of the amniotic fluid for degraded blood products, and an autopsy in cases of stillbirth. Even when no apparent reason is found, pregnancies should be considered at high risk for poor outcome.
III B

4 Lince DM, Pretorius DH, Manco-Johnson ML *et al.* (1985) The clinical significance of increased echogenicity in the fetal abdomen. *AJR Am J Roentgenol* **145**, 683–686. A total of 7 cases of increased echogenicity in the fetal abdomen detected on prenatal sonography were reviewed for findings and causes. In 4 cases, the findings corresponded to calcification secondary to meconium peritonitis, infection or unknown cause. One infant with meconium ileus had inspissated but noncalcified meconium corresponding to the increased echoes. In 2 cases, follow-up prenatal sonography was normal, and the neonate was also normal. 8 cases from the literature with increased echogenicity in the fetal abdomen were also reviewed: 2 cases were secondary to meconium ileus and 6 were caused by meconium peritonitis. Increased abdominal echogenicity on prenatal sonography may result from various processes that may affect obstetric and neonatal management.
III B

5 Strocker AM, Snijders RJ, Carlson DE *et al.* (2000) Fetal echogenic bowel: parameters to be considered in differential diagnosis. *Ultrasound Obstet Gynecol* **16**, 519–523. Observational study of the medical history, obstetric records and outcome details in 131 consecutive pregnancies with fetal hyperechogenic bowel. In 62 (47%) cases, there were no visible anomalies other than hyperechogenic bowel and no evidence of growth restriction. This group included 4 (7%) pregnancies with Down syndrome, 15 (24%) with infection or a recent episode of influenza and 8 (13%) with blood staining of amniotic fluid. In the remaining 69 (53%) cases, hyperechogenic bowel was accompanied by hydrops or nuchal edema (n = 16, 12.2%), growth restriction (n = 9, 6.9%), other markers for chromosome anomalies (n = 33, 25.2%) or multiple structural anomalies (n = 11, 8.4%). In this group, the prevalence of Down syndrome was 12%, infection or influenza was reported in 14 (20%) cases and there was blood staining of amniotic fluid in 7 (10%). Cystic fibrosis screening was performed in 65 (50%) pregnancies; the results were negative in all cases and clinical assessment did not indicate cystic fibrosis in any of the 91 infants who were born alive. Maternal serum screening was performed in 41 (31%) pregnancies. High alpha-fetoprotein levels were associated with multiple abnormalities or severe growth restriction. Conclusions: in many pregnancies with fetal hyperechogenic bowel, there are multiple factors that may explain these findings. Thus identification of one potential underlying cause should not preclude further testing. Once chromosome defects, cystic fibrosis, structural abnormalities, infection and growth restriction have been excluded, parents can be counseled that the prognosis is good, irrespective of the presence or absence of blood-stained amniotic fluid.
III B

6 Berlin BM, Norton ME, Sugarman EA *et al.* (1999) Cystic fibrosis and chromosome abnormalities associated with echogenic fetal bowel. *Obstet Gynecol* **94**, 135–138. Observational study. Fetal or parental samples obtained after a second-trimester sonographic finding of echogenic fetal bowel were submitted to a referral diagnostic laboratory during a 2-year period. Results of DNA testing and karyotyping on these samples were analyzed to determine the prevalence of cystic fibrosis transmembrane reductase gene mutations and chromosome abnormalities. Of 244 cases tested, 2 fetuses were positive for two cystic fibrosis mutations. This rate (0.8% or 2/244) is 20 times higher than the general white population rate of 1/2500. In a third case, both parents were carriers but the fetus was not tested. 9 (8%) of 113 fetuses tested had one cystic fibrosis mutation. Of 106 fetuses for whom chromosome results were available, 3 (2.8%) fetuses had a chromosomal abnormality: 2 had trisomy 21 and one had Klinefelter syndrome. A fourth fetus carried a *de-novo*, apparently balanced, 5;12 translocation. Conclusion: when a second-trimester sonographic diagnosis of fetal echogenic bowel is made, fetal testing for both cystic fibrosis and chromosome abnormalities is warranted.
III B

Chapter 21

Skeletal abnormalities

21.1 Skeletal abnormalities

David James

Management option		Quality of evidence	Strength of recommendation	References
Prepregnancy	Ensure accuracy of diagnosis before counseling	–	✔	–
	Counseling (possibly interdisciplinary) about recurrence risks and prenatal diagnostic options	–	✔	–
Prenatal	Careful ultrasonography by experienced sonographer, including general examination of fetus for other anomalies	–	✔	–
	Consider a karyotype or other additional tests if other anomalies or suspicion of genetic condition with DNA probe	–	✔	–
	Interdisciplinary discussion before counseling parents (differential diagnosis rather than definitive diagnosis may be all that is possible)	–	✔	–
	Ongoing review of sonographic findings if pregnancy continues (further features may develop allowing definitive diagnosis)	–	✔	–
	Psychological support of parents	–	✔	–
Labor/delivery	Consider pregnancy termination with severe and/or lethal anomalies	–	✔	–
	Psychological support of parents	–	✔	–
	Cesarean section for normal obstetric indications, although severe forms of arthrogryposis may only deliver safely with cesarean section	–	✔	–
Postnatal	If lethal, encourage post-mortem by experienced perinatal pathologist	–	✔	–
	Detailed postnatal examination including radiography	–	✔	–
	Tissue for karyotyping and other tests if not performed prenatally	–	✔	–
	Ensure accuracy of diagnosis before counseling	–	✔	–
	Counseling (possibly interdisciplinary) about recurrence risks and future prenatal diagnostic options	–	✔	–

Chapter 22

Fetal endocrinology

22.1 Fetal hyperthyroidism

Jane Rutherford

Management option		Quality of evidence	Strength of recommendation	References
Prepregnancy	Consider measurement of thyroid stimulating hormone (TSH) receptor immunoglobulins (TBII and TSI) in women with known autoimmune thyroid disease	–	✔	–
	Check maternal thyroid function tests – optimize thionamide therapy	III	B	1,2
	Consider changing to propylthiouracil in preference to carbimazole/methimazole	III	B	3
Prenatal	Monitor maternal thyroid function tests every 4–6 weeks – aim to keep free thyroxine at the upper end of the normal range on the minimum dose of thionamide	–	✔	–
	Sonographic fetal surveillance after 24 weeks ❑ Goiter ❑ Cardiac hypertrophy ❑ Tachycardia ❑ Intrauterine growth restriction ❑ Hydrops ❑ Oligohydramnios/polyhydramnios	III IV	B C	2 4,5
	Measure fetal thyroid function by fetal blood sampling if persistent tachycardia or goiter (poor correlation between maternal and fetal thyroid function tests)	IV	C	6
	If fetal hyperthyroidism confirmed adjust maternal thionamide dose to optimize maternal control	III	B	1,2
	Consider maternal beta-blockers if fetal tachycardia persists	IV	C	7
	Fetal thyroid assessment can be followed with color Doppler → reduced vascularization under appropriate therapy	IV	C	8
Postnatal	Measure free thyroxine and TSH in cord blood and at 7 days of age, and manage appropriately	–	✔	–
	Propylthiouracil if breastfeeding	IV	C	9

References

1 Davis LE, Lucas MJ, Hankins GD *et al.* (1989) Thyrotoxicosis complicating pregnancy. *Am J Obstet Gynecol* **160**, 63–70. Retrospective observational case review. 60 women. Women with actual thyrotoxicosis; those euthyroid on treatment excluded. Reduced maternal and fetal morbidity with good control. **III B**

2 Millar LK, Wing DA, Leung AS *et al.* (1994) Low birthweight and preeclampsia in pregnancies complicated by hyperthyroidism. *Obstet Gynecol* **84**, 946–949. Retrospective case review. 223 women. Increased risks of PET, intrauterine growth restriction, preterm labour with poor thyroid control in mother. **III B**

3 Mujtaba Q, Burrow GN (1975) Treatment of hyperthyroidism in pregnancy with propylthiouracil and methimazole. *Obstet Gynecol* **46**, 282–286. Study of 21 women who received propylthiouracil or methimazole during 26 pregnancies. The authors point out that the major difficulty with regard to therapy of hyperthyroidism in pregnancy is the possibility of fetal goiter with resulting hypothyroidism. **III B**

4 Hatjis CG (1993) Diagnosis and successful treatment of fetal goitrous hyperthyroidism caused by maternal Graves' disease. *Obstet Gynecol* **81**, 837–839. Case report of a fetal goitrous hyperthyroidism caused by maternal Graves' disease. It was diagnosed and treated in the second trimester. High concentrations of thyroid stimulatory Ig and thyrotropin binding inhibitory Igs were detected in fetal blood. Maternal propylthiouracil treatment resulted in normalization of fetal thyroid function and a decrease in the size of the fetal thyroid goiter. **IV C**

5 Wenstrom KD, Weiner CP, Williamson RA *et al.* (1990) Prenatal diagnosis of fetal hyperthyroidism using funipuncture. *Obstet Gynecol* **76**, 513–517. Report of two cases of fetal hyperthyroidism. The authors found fetal blood sampling to be useful not only to assist in making a diagnosis but also to manage the fetuses therapeutically. **IV C**

6 Vanderpump MP, Ahlquist JA, Franklyn JA *et al.* (1996) Consensus statement for good practice and audit measures in the management of hypothyroidism and hyperthyroidism. The Research Unit of the Royal College of Physicians of London, the Endocrinology and Diabetes Committee of the Royal College of Physicians of London, and the Society for Endocrinology. *Br Med J* **313**, 539–544. Consensus statement on an acceptable standard of care for patients with thyroid disease. Screening of the healthy adult population is not justified. Serum TSH should be obtained yearly to ensure compliance with treatment of hypothyroidism. Patients with hypothyroidism should be referred to a specialist. In Graves' disease, carbimazole is the treatment of choice. Patients treated with radioiodine or partial thyroidectomy should have a yearly check of thyroid function. **IV C**

7 American College of Obstetricians and Gynecologists (1993) *Thyroid disease in pregnancy*. ACOG Technical Bulletin no. 181. Washington, DC: ACOG. This bulletin addresses the effects of thyroid disorders and their treatment during pregnancy in the postpartum period. **IV C**

8 Luton D, Fried D, Sibony D *et al.* (1997) Assessment of fetal thyroid function by colored Doppler echography. *Fetal Diagn Ther* **12**, 24–27. Case report of a euthyroid patient with Graves' disease who is carrying a hyperthyroid fetus. Cordocentesis was performed in order to confirm the diagnosis of fetal hyperthyroidism. Fetal thyroid assessment was performed by color Doppler. After appropriate treatment the dense vascularization of the thyroid regressed. **IV C**

9 Cooper DS (1987) Antithyroid drugs: to breast-feed or not to breast-feed. *Am J Obstet Gynecol* **157**, 234–235. Review of antithyroid drugs and breast feeding. Propylthiouracil drug of choice but methimazole in small doses probably also safe. **IV C**

22.2 Fetal hypothyroidism

Jane Rutherford

Management option		**Quality of evidence**	**Strength of recommendation**	**References**
Prepregnancy	Genetic counseling if previous inborn errors of thyroid hormone biosynthesis that result in dyshormonogenesis	III	B	1
	Iodine supplementation in areas of iodine deficiency	IV	C	2
	In women with known hypothyroidism check maternal thyroid function and optimize thyroxine replacement	III	B	3,4
Prenatal	In at-risk fetus surveillance for: ❑ Reduced movements ❑ Cardiomegaly ❑ Bradycardia; heart block ❑ Growth restriction ❑ Goiter ❑ Polyhydramnios	IV	C	5

➡

Management option		Quality of evidence	Strength of recommendation	References
Prenatal (cont'd)	Amniotic fluid thyroxine concentration does not correlate with fetal serum thyroxine	IV	C	6
	Measure fetal thyroid function by fetal blood sampling if there is goiter or if there is growth restriction with bradycardia and/or reduced fetal movements in a fetus at risk	IV	C	5,7,8
	If fetal hypothyroidism confirmed – intra-amniotic thyroxine (T_4) with confirmation of response by repeat fetal blood sampling	IV	C	7,8
	Reappraise T_4 replacement in women with hypothyroidism at booking and once during the second and third trimesters	III	B	3,4
Postnatal	Measure free T_4 and thyroid stimulating hormone in cord blood in at-risk fetuses	–	✔	–
	Replace thyroxine to infants confirmed to be hypothyroid	IIa	B	9
	Where necessary reduce maternal dose of T_4 to prepregnancy levels	III	B	3
	Sequelae of congenital hypothyroidism, including intellectual impairment, can be prevented with prompt treatment	III	B	1

References

1 Fisher DA, Dussault JH, Foley TP *et al.* (1979) Screening for congenital hypothyroidism: results of screening one million North American infants. *J Pediatr* **94**, 700–705. Review of a regional screening program of newborn infants for congenital hypothyroidism. 1 046 362 infants were screened. A total of 277 infants with congenital hypothyroidism were detected; 7 neonates were missed. Preliminary evidence suggests that infants treated in the program have normal developmental testing scores at 18 months of age. **III B**

2 Glinoer D (1997) Maternal and fetal impact of chronic iodine deficiency. *Clin Obstet Gynecol* **40**, 102–116. Review of the effects of maternal iodine deficiency. In areas where dietary iodine levels are sufficient there is no need to give supplementary iodine. However, in areas where iodine is deficient inadequate physiological adaptation to pregnancy occurs with relative hypothyroidism and goiter. Supplementary iodine improves maternal and fetal thyroid function. **IV C**

3 Kaplan MM (1992) Monitoring thyroxine treatment during pregnancy. *Thyroid* **2**, 153–154. Retrospective observational cohort study of 77 pregnancies in 65 women with hypothyroidism, 36 women with previous thyroid ablation (group 1) and 29 women with Hashimoto's thyroiditis (group 2). Mean serum thyroxine values decreased significantly during pregnancy in both groups. Serum TSH rose above normal in 76% of women in group 1 and 47% of women in group 2. Elevated TSH values were detected early in pregnancy. **III B**

4 McDougall IR, Maclin N (1995) Hypothyroid women need more thyroxine when pregnant. *J Family Pract* **41**, 238–240. Prospective observational cohort study of 20 pregnant women with hypothyroidism. Women were followed with measurement of free thyroxine and TSH. There was an average increase of 36 μg in the required dose of thyroxine during pregnancy, which returned to prepregnancy levels post-partum. **III B**

5 Noia G, De Santis M, Tocci A *et al.* (1992) Early prenatal diagnosis and therapy of fetal hypothyroid goiter. *Fetal Diagn Ther* **7**, 138–143. Case report of an iodide-induced fetal hypothyroidism that was detected sonographically at 22 weeks gestation. A single injection of intra-amniotic levothyroxine resulted in a resolution of the fetal goiter. Cordocentesis was utilized to assess fetal thyroid status prior to treatment. **IV C**

6 Abuhamad AZ, Fisher DA, Warsof SL *et al.* (1995) Antenatal diagnosis and treatment of fetal goitrous hypothyroidism: case report and reviewing the literature. *Ultrasound Obstet Gynecol* **6**, 368–371. This is a case of fetal goiter diagnosed by ultrasound in the second trimester of pregnancy. Cordocentesis at 28 weeks gestation confirmed the presence of fetal hypothyroidism. Fetal therapy was then begun with weekly intra-amniotic injections of thyroxine. A repeat cordocentesis at 35 weeks showed normalization of fetal thyroid function. **IV C**

7 Bruner JP, Dellinger EH (1997) Antenatal diagnosis and treatment of fetal hypothyroidism: a report of 2 cases. Fetal Diagn Ther 12, 200–204. Two cases of fetal goiter in the presence of maternal Graves disease treated with propylthiouracil. Amniocentesis and fetal blood sampling were performed, which both diagnosed fetal hypothyroidism. Weekly intra-amniotic injections of thyroxine were given with subsequent fetal blood sampling. Blood sampling showed the fetus to be euthyroid and amniotic fluid TSH dropped to normal levels although more slowly than the blood levels. Both neonates had no goiter and were euthyroid. **IV C**

8 Hadi HA, Strickland D (1995) In utero treatment of fetal goitrous hypothyroidism caused by maternal Graves disease. *Am J Perinatol* **12**, 455–458. Two cases of fetal goiter in the presence of maternal Graves disease. Diagnosis of fetal hypothyroidism was made by cordocentesis. Serial intra-amniotic injections of thyroxine were performed. Both neonates had normal thyroid size at birth and normal thyroid function. **IV C**

9 Dubuis JM, Glorieux J, Richer F *et al.* (1996) Outcome of severe congenital hypothyroidism: closing the developmental gap with early high dose levothyroxine treatment. *J Clin Endocrinol Metab* **81**, 222–227. Case control study of 45 infants with permanent congenital hypothyroidism not due to maternal transfer of antibodies or antithyroid drugs. Patients were divided into those with moderate (n = 35) and severe (n = 10) hypothyroidism. Infants were treated with high-dose thyroxine from a median age of 14 days. Mean developmental quotients in both groups were similar at 18 months of age and were within normal range. **IIa B**

21.3 Congenital adrenal hyperplasia

Jane Rutherford

Management option		Quality of evidence	Strength of recommendation	References
Prepregnancy	Identify enzymatic and, where possible, DNA basis of disorder	IV	C	1
	Counsel families regarding risks and options for prenatal diagnosis and treatment	–	✔	–
Prenatal	Start maternal oral dexamethasone 0.5 mg thrice daily once pregnancy confirmed	IIa III	B B	2 3
	Chorionic villus sampling at 11 weeks for karyotype and DNA analysis	III	B	4,5
	Male fetus or unaffected female fetus – stop maternal dexamethasone	IV	C	1
	Measure maternal serum estriol levels every 6–8 weeks to confirm compliance and adrenal suppression	–	✔	–
	Ultrasonographic assessment of external genitalia – if there is evidence of virilization consider measurement of amniotic fluid 17-hydoxyprogesterone and androstenedione and, if elevated, increasing the dose of dexamethasone	III	B	6
	Monitor for maternal side-effects (hyperglycemia, hypertension, edema and excessive weight gain) and if necessary reduce dose of dexamethasone	IIa	B	2
Postnatal	Examine child carefully after birth for evidence of virilization and salt-wasting form of disease	–	✔	–
	Corticosteroid/ mineralocorticoid replacement	–	✔	–
	Long-term developmental follow-up	–	✔	–

References

1 American College of Obstetricians and Gynecologists (1995) *Hyperandrogenic chronic anovulation*. ACOG Technical Bulletin no. 202. Washington, DC: ACOG. This technical bulletin discusses congenital adrenal hyperplasia as a unique group of genetic disorders that can appear identical to hyperandrogenic chronic anovulation. **IV C**

2 Lajic S, Wedell A, Bui TH *et al.* (1998) Long term somatic follow-up of prenatally treated children with congenital adrenal hyperplasia. *J Clin Endocrinol Metab* **83**, 3872–3880. Retrospective case-review of 44 at-risk pregnancies. Treated mothers and children were compared to matched controls. Compared to their elder affected sisters, all five cases of severe congenital adrenal hyperplasia whose mothers were treated until term showed little virilization. There was normal growth in treated pregnancies. Treated mothers reported more side effects during pregnancy than controls. **IIa B**

3 Mercado AB, Wilson RC, Cheng KC *et al.* (1995) Prenatal treatment and diagnosis of congenital adrenal hyperplasia owing to steroid 21-hydroxylase deficiency. *J Clin Endocrinol Metab* **80**, 2014–2020. Retrospective case review of 239 pregnancies at risk of congenital adrenal hyperplasia. 37 affected cases, 21 of which were female; 13 treated prenatally with dexamethasone. Dexamethasone administered at or before 10 weeks was effective in reducing virilization. No significant side effects in mothers or infants. **III B**

4 Speiser PW, New MI (1994) Prenatal diagnosis of congenital adrenal hyperplasia due to 21-hydroxylase deficiency by allele-specific hybridization and Southern blot. *Hum Genet* **93**, 424–428. Feasibility study of identification of gene-specific molecular diagnosis for congenital adrenal hyperplasia in 24 pregnancies with 25% risk of affected fetus. Mutations identified in 95% of chromosomes examined. Molecular diagnosis accurate in 96% of infants confirmed on postnatal examination. **III B**

5 Rumsby G, Honour JW, Rodeck C (1993) Prenatal diagnosis of CAH by direct detection of mutations in the steroid-21 hydroxylase gene. *Clin Endocrinol* **38**, 421–425. Chorionic venous samples taken from three women carrying fetuses at risk of congenital adrenal hyperplasia. Blood samples taken from parents and index case. Three common mutations in the 21-hydroxylase B gene were detected. Prenatal diagnosis was successful in all three cases. **III B**

6 Mandell J, Bromley B, Peters CA *et al.* (1995) Prenatal sonographic detection of genital malformations. *J Urol* **153**, 1994–1996. Retrospective case review. 17 fetuses identified antenatally to have genital abnormalities. Postnatal outcome compared to antenatal findings. All were confirmed to have some abnormality. **III B**

Chapter 23

Fetal tumors

23.1 Fetal tumors

Jane Rutherford

Intracranial teratoma

Management option	Quality of evidence	Strength of recommendation	References
Vigilance for respiratory compromise, preterm labor, premature rupture of membranes and abruption in the presence of hydramnios, preeclampsia or hydrops	–	✔	–
Counsel about poor prognosis. Most reported cases have been lethal. Consider termination. Ongoing pregnancies should be managed with the goal of reducing maternal morbidity. Avoid cesarean section. Cephalocentesis may allow vaginal delivery despite significant ventriculomegaly	IV	C	1,2

References

1 Ten Broeke ED, Verdonk GW, Roumen FJ (1992) Prenatal ultrasound diagnosis of an intracranial teratoma influencing management: a case report and review of the literature. *Eur J Obstet Gynaecol Reprod Biol* **45**, 210–214. Review of the literature of 17 cases of prenatally diagnosed intracranial teratoma. 14 were delivered by cesarean section. All babies died before or shortly after delivery. **IV C**

2 Ferreira J, Eviatar L, Schneider S *et al.* (1993) Prenatal diagnosis of intracranial teratoma. *Pediatr Neurosurg* **19**, 84–88. Case report and literature review. Case of survivor of intracranial malignant teratoma after resection. Infant survived for 1 month. No other cases in the literature report survival for as long as 1 month. **IV C**

Other intracranial tumors

Management option	Quality of evidence	Strength of recommendation	References
Manage as for teratoma	–	✔	–
Fetal prognosis difficult to estimate. Magnetic resonance imaging may be helpful to further delineate intracranial anatomy. Large tumors associated with hydrocephalus or hemorrhage are likely to be lethal. In this situation termination or avoidance of cesarean section can be considered. Some tumors, however have a fairly good prognosis. Choroid plexus tumors have 52% survival rate. Meningeal tumors have a survival rate approaching 25% if the tumor can be completely resected	IV	C	1
The prognosis of tumors associated with genetic syndromes depends on the syndrome itself	–	✔	–

Reference

1 Wienk MA, Van Geijn HP, Copray FJ *et al.* (1990) Prenatal diagnosis of fetal tumors by ultrasonography. *Obstet Gynecol Surv* **45**, 639–653. Review of the recent literature on fetal tumors detected between 1982 and 1988. The authors have compartmentalized the fetal body areas into the head and neck region, the thorax and the abdomen.

Polyhydramnios was frequently associated with fetal tumors; premature labor, or premature rupture of the membranes was also common. The authors concluded from their review that, for tumors located intracranially, the chances for the fetus are very poor. The prognosis for tumors at other locations is variable and may be determined by such factors as the size of the tumor, involvement of other organs, other associated malformations, or mechanical obstruction during the birth process. **IV C**

Orbital tumors

Management option	Quality of evidence	Strength of recommendation	References
Fetal risk is difficult to estimate. Tumor histology, the size of the mass and the degree of involvement of other structures all influence the prognosis. Small orbital tumors have a good prognosis as they are usually benign; successful resection has been reported	–	✔	–
Prognosis for orbital retinoblastoma depends on tumor stage, which cannot be determined antenatally. Parents should be counseled that neonatal management of retinoblastoma includes enucleation as well as radiotherapy and chemotherapy. With current treatment, survival may exceed 90%	IV	C	1–3
There is a high incidence of second malignancy, particularly if the disease is bilateral	––	✔	–
Pregnancy termination can be offered if legal. Otherwise, pregnancy management is routine. Cesarean delivery is reserved for obstetric indications, or for those cases where a large tumor is likely to cause dystocia	IV	C	1,2
DNA-based prenatal diagnosis is available for hereditary retinoblastoma	IV	C	3

References

1 Zwaan CM, de Waal FC, Koole FD *et al.* (1994) A giant congenital orbital tumor: an unusual presentation of retinoblastoma. *Med Pediatr Oncol* **3**, 507–511. Case report of a giant tumor presenting in a newborn infant as a large exophytic mass emerging from the left orbit. After enucleation, orbital recurrence developed within 14 days. No antitumor treatment was given and the child died at the age of 4 weeks. The diagnosis was of a retinoblastoma, although a neuroblastoma could not be excluded. **IV C**

2 Spinelli HM, Criscuolo GR, Tripps M *et al.* (1993) Massive orbital teratoma in the newborn. *Ann Plast Surg* **31**, 453–458. Case report of a newborn girl with a massive orbital teratoma that caused significant orbital enlargement with inferior and lateral displacement of the zygoma and thinning of the orbital roof. Recommendations for definitive treatment and a review of the literature are presented. **IV C**

3 Maat-Kievit JA, Oepkes D, Hartwig NG *et al.* (1993) A large retinoblastoma detected in a fetus at 21 weeks of gestation. *Prenat Diagn* **13**, 377–384. Case report of a retinoblastoma detected in a fetus at 21 weeks gestation. **IV C**

Nasal and oral tumors

Management option	Quality of evidence	Strength of recommendation	References
Vigilance for maternal risks from hydramnios	IV	C	1
Prognosis depends on the type of tumor, the size and the degree of involvement of other structures. Most nasal/oral tumors are benign and successful neonatal resection of several types is described. About 10% of affected fetuses have other anomalies caused by the deforming effects of the tumor (cleft palate, facial hemangioma and heart defects)	–	✔	–

➡

Management option	Quality of evidence	Strength of recommendation	References
Greatest risk to the fetus is severe respiratory compromise at delivery. Coordination of delivery with appropriate consultants can significantly improve outcome. If tracheal occlusion is anticipated, delivery should be by cesarean section in cooperation with pediatric and surgical consultants to assure prompt intubation, tracheostomy or tracheoplasty	–	✔	–
In some perinates, an ex-utero intrapartum tracheoplasty (EXIT procedure) may be required. This procedure allows fetal/neonatal oxygenation via the placental circulation to continue while an airway is secured. If this is not possible, immediate initiation of extracorporeal membrane oxygenation may be the only option	IV	C	2

References

1 Wienk MA, Van Geijn HP, Copray FJ *et al.* (1990) Prenatal diagnosis of fetal tumors by ultrasonography. *Obstet Gynecol Surv* **45**, 639–653. Review of the recent literature on fetal tumors detected between 1982 and 1988. The authors have compartmentalized the fetal body areas into the head and neck region, the thorax and the abdomen. Polyhydramnios was frequently associated with fetal tumors; premature labor, or premature rupture of the membranes was also common. The authors concluded from their review that, for tumors located intracranially, the chances for the fetus are very poor. The prognosis for tumors at other locations is variable and may be determined by such factors as the size of the tumor, involvement of other organs, other associated malformations, or mechanical obstruction during the birth process. **IV C**

2 Liechty KW, Crombleholme TM, Flake AW *et al.* (1997) Intrapartum airway management for giant fetal neck masses: the exit (ex utero intrapartum treatment) procedure. *Am J Obstet Gynecol* **177**, 870–874. Review of the *ex-utero* intrapartum treatment procedure in the management of 5 cases with life-threatening fetal neck masses. This procedure provided up to 1 h of *in-utero* placental support so that an airway could be secured in fetuses with large neck masses. The 5 cases included 3 cervical teratomas and 2 lymphangiomas. **IV C**

Neck teratoma

Management option	Quality of evidence	Strength of recommendation	References
Sonographic findings:			
❑ Calcifications in a neck mass suggest cervical teratoma	IV	C	1
❑ Polyhydramnios due to esophageal obstruction	IV	C	2
❑ Assess tumor for rapid growth			
❑ Associated congenital anomalies are rare	IV	C	1
Cesarean section may be necessary if extreme dorsiflexion of fetal head or dystocia caused by large tumor	–	✔	–
Ex-utero intrapartum treatment (EXIT procedure) may provide up to 1 h of uteroplacental support to provide time to secure an airway	IV	C	3
Plans for intrapartum intubation, *ex-utero* tracheoplasty or extracorporeal membrane oxygenation should be coordinated with pediatric and surgical specialists as described for oral tumors. Surgical resection is usually performed as soon as possible after stabilization to avoid loss of secure airway	III	B	4
❑ Prognosis is poor – 50% of fetuses die *in utero* ❑ Some cases are surgically inoperable	IV	C	2
❑ Prompt surgery for appropriate cases after delivery has reduced the mortality to 15%	IV	C	1

References

1 Gundry SR, Wesley JR, Klein MD (1983) Cervical teratomas in the newborn. *J Pediatr Surg* **8**, 382–386. Review of 6 newborns who were diagnosed with cervical teratomas. In 4 infants, calcifications were seen on X-ray. 4 patients required intubation within the first hours of life for respiratory distress. The tumors were well incapsulated and were removed by performing a total thyroid lobectomy. **IV C**

2 Trecet JC, Claramunt V, Larraz J *et al.* (1984) Prenatal ultrasound diagnosis of fetal teratoma of the neck. *J Clin Ultrasound* **12**, 509–511. Case report of a fetal neck teratoma that was initially visualized sonographically at 16 weeks gestation. **IV C**

3 Liechty KW, Crombleholme TM, Flake AW *et al.* (1997) Intrapartum airway management for giant fetal neck masses: the exit (ex utero intrapartum treatment) procedure. *Am J Obstet Gynecol* **177**, 870–874. Review of the *ex-utero* intrapartum treatment procedure in the management of 5 cases with life-threatening fetal neck masses. This procedure provided up to 1 h of *in-utero* placental support so that an airway could be secured in fetuses with large neck masses. The 5 cases included 3 cervical teratomas and 2 lymphangiomas. **IV C**

4 Azizkhan RG, Haase GM, Applebaum H *et al.* (1995) Diagnosis, management and outcome of cervicofacial teratomas in neonates: a Children's Cancer Group study. *J Pediatr Surg* **30**, 312–316. Multicenter retrospective case review. 20 neonates presenting from 1971–94 with cervicofacial teratomas. Life-threatening airway obstruction in the early postnatal period occurred in 7. 2 died in the delivery room without having an airway secured. 2 had tracheostomies performed in the delivery room.18 had the primary tumor excised. 3 required tracheostomy. Survival rate 85%. 70% good functional and cosmetic outcome. **III B**

Cystic hygroma

Management option	Quality of evidence	Strength of recommendation	References
Manage as for fetal hydrops (see Section 14.1)	–	✔	–
Mortality high because of associated nonimmune hydrops and associated chromosomal defects	III	B	1
Prognosis for isolated (euploid) hygromas without hydrops is dependent on whether or not the hygroma resolves	III	B	2
Surviving fetuses should be evaluated with a detailed fetal anatomical survey including echocardiography at 20–22 weeks	III	B	1

References

1 Langer JC, Fitzgerald PG, Desa D *et al.* (1990) Cervical cystic hygroma in the fetus: clinical spectrum and outcome. *J Pediatr Surg* **25**, 58–62. Langer and co-workers reported 27 cases of cystic hygroma diagnosed prior to 30 weeks gestation; all but 2 fetuses died. Of the 25 fetuses that did not survive, nonimmune hydrops developed in 21. The only 2 survivors had spontaneous regression of their cystic hygromas and were subsequently diagnosed with Noonan's syndrome at birth. **III B**

2 Bronshtein M, Bar-Hava I, Blumenfeld I *et al.* (1993) The difference between septated and nonseptated nuchal cystic hygroma in the early second trimester. *Obstet Gynecol* **81**, 683–687. Case review of 125 cases of nonseptated cystic hygroma and 25 cases of septated cystic hygroma. 98% of nonseptated cystic hygromas were transient compared to 44% of the septated type. There was a higher rate of aneuploidy, hydrops and associated anomalies in the septated group. The live birth rate in the nonseptated type was 94% compared to 12% in the septated type. **III B**

Lung tumors

Management option	Quality of evidence	Strength of recommendation	References
Vigilance for hydramnios and hydrops	IV	C	1
Delivery should be in a tertiary care center with appropriate specialist consultants standing by	–	✔	–

Reference

1 Wienk MA, Van Geijn HP, Copray FJ *et al.* (1990) Prenatal diagnosis of fetal tumors by ultrasonography. *Obstet Gynecol Surv* **45**, 639–653. Review of the recent literature on fetal tumors detected between 1982 and 1988. The authors have compartmentalized the fetal body areas into the head and neck region, the thorax and the abdomen. Polyhydramnios was frequently associated with fetal tumors; premature labor, or premature rupture of the membranes was also common. The authors concluded from their review that, for tumors located intracranially, the chances for the fetus are very poor. The prognosis for tumors at other locations is variable and may be determined by such factors as the size of the tumor, involvement of other organs, other associated malformations, or mechanical obstruction during the birth process. **IV C**

Cystic adenomatous malformation

Management option	Quality of evidence	Strength of recommendation	References
Exclude other malformations	–	✔	–
Vigilance for hydramnios and hydrops	III	B	1,2
Cyst aspiration or placement of a cystoamniotic shunt may relieve intrathoracic pressure and reverse hydropic changes. However, these procedures do not always provide long-term benefit. The place of antenatal fetal surgery is not clear	III	B	1,2

References

1 Adzick NS, Harrison MR, Crombleholme TM *et al.* (1998) Fetal lung lesions: management and outcome. *Am J Obstet Gynecol* **179**, 884–889. Retrospective review of 175 fetal lung lesions diagnosed antenatally at two centers between 1983 and 1997. 134 congenital cystic adenomatoid malformations (CCAM) and 41 pulmonary sequestrations. All CCAM that were not associated with hydrops survived. Of the fetuses with CCAM, 14 had termination of pregnancy, 101 were managed expectantly. Fetal surgery was performed in 13 fetuses at 21–29 weeks gestation and 8 fetuses continued in pregnancy with resolution of hydrops and neonatal survival. 6 fetuses with solitary large cyst had thoracoamniotic shunting and 5 survived. Of 41 pulmonary sequestrations, 28 dramatically regressed antenatally and did not require postnatal resection, 2 had termination of pregnancy, 7 were resected after birth with survival, one hydropic fetus died and 3 had an associated tension hydrothorax with secondary hydrops that was successfully treated with fetal thoracocentesis or shunting. **III B**

2 Dommergues M, Louis-Sylvestre C, Mandelbrot LM *et al.* (1997) Congenital adenomatoid malformation of the lung: when is active fetal therapy indicated? *Am J Obstet Gynecol* **177**, 953–958. Prospective cohort study of 33 cases of prenatally diagnosed congenital cystic adenomatoid malformation. Thoracoamniotic shunting offered in 9 macrocystic cases with acute polyhydramnios or hydrops. 4 cases were postnatally diagnosed as sequestrations. Of 12 cases complicated by hydramnios or hydrops, 5 survived. 17 uncomplicated cases were managed conservatively and survived. **III B**

Pulmonary sequestration

Management option	Quality of evidence	Strength of recommendation	References
Vigilance for hydramnios and hydrops	III	B	1,2
Antenatal thoracoamniotic catheter placement to relieve pleural effusion and correct hydrops has been described, with mixed results	III	B	1–3
Postnatal survival is possible if the mass is resectable and enough normal pulmonary tissue remains. Prognosis depends on the size and location of the mass as well as the existence of other malformations and their severity	III	B	1,3
Pregnancy termination may be offered if legal and gestational age permits	–	✔	–

References

1 Adzick NS, Harrison MR, Crombleholme TM *et al.* (1998) Fetal lung lesions: management and outcome. *Am J Obstet Gynecol* **179**, 884–889. Retrospective review of 175 fetal lung lesions diagnosed antenatally at two centers between 1983 and 1997. 134 congenital cystic adenomatoid malformation (CCAM) and 41 pulmonary sequestrations. All CCAM that were not associated with hydrops survived. Of the fetuses with CCAM, 14 had termination of pregnancy, 101 were managed expectantly. Fetal surgery was performed in 13 fetuses at 21–29 weeks gestation and 8 fetuses continued in pregnancy with resolution of hydrops and neonatal survival. 6 fetuses with solitary large cyst had thoracoamniotic shunting and 5 survived. Of 41 pulmonary sequestrations, 28 dramatically regressed antenatally and did not require postnatal resection, 2 had termination of pregnancy, 7 were resected after birth with survival, one hydropic fetus died and 3 had an associated tension hydrothorax with secondary hydrops that was successfully treated with fetal thoracocentesis or shunting. **III B**

2 Dommergues M, Louis-Sylvestre C, Mandelbrot L *et al.* (1997) Congenital adenomatoid malformation of the lung: when is active fetal therapy indicated? *Am J Obstet Gynecol* **177**, 953–958. Prospective cohort study of 33 cases of prenatally diagnosed congenital cystic adenomatoid malformation. Thoracoamniotic shunting offered in 9 macrocystic cases with acute polyhydramnios or hydrops. 4 cases were postnatally diagnosed as sequestrations. Of 12 cases complicated by hydramnios or hydrops, 5 survived. 17 uncomplicated cases were managed conservatively and survived. **III B**

3 Becmeur F, Horta-Geraud P, Donato L *et al.* (1998) Pulmonary sequestrations: prenatal ultrasound diagnosis, treatment and outcome. *J Pediatr Surg* **33**, 492–496. Case review of 10 cases of antenatally diagnosed pulmonary sequestration. 2 fetuses required treatment either paracentesis and amniocentesis or thoracoamniotic shunt. In 5 there was regression of the mass size during pregnancy. All 10 had surgery after birth. **III B**

Cardiac tumors

Management option	Quality of evidence	Strength of recommendation	References
Determine the tumor type and likely diagnosis. Echocardiography may help to fully delineate lesion(s)	–	✔	–
Because the most common fetal cardiac tumor is rhabdomyoma, the diagnosis of tuberous sclerosis must be strongly considered. Linkage studies may help to confirm a familial case but no genetic test is available to diagnose cases due to a new mutation. Counseling is difficult. Fetal magnetic resonance imaging may detect brain abnormalities that are not visible by ultrasonography. Referral to a geneticist for counseling is suggested	IV	C	1,2
Development of hydrops before fetal viability should prompt counseling and consideration of pregnancy termination	–	✔	–

References

1 Krapp M, Baschat AA, Gembruch U *et al.* (1999) Tuberous sclerosis with intracardiac rhabdomyoma in a fetus with trisomy 21: case report and review of the literature. *Prenat Diagn* **19**, 610–613. A case of a prenatally ultrasound diagnosed cardiac rhabdomyoma. Left ventricular outflow was excluded by Doppler echocardiography. Autopsy after termination confirmed tuberous sclerosis. Review of the literature suggests that the association is strong and the diagnosis of cardiac rhabdomyoma should raise the suspicion. Trisomy 21 appears to be incidental in this case. **IV C**

2 Wienk MA, Van Geijn HP, Copray FJ *et al.* (1990) Prenatal diagnosis of fetal tumors by ultrasonography. *Obstet Gynecol Surv* **45**, 639–653. Review of the recent literature on fetal tumors detected between 1982 and 1988. The authors have compartmentalized the fetal body areas into the head and neck region, the thorax and the abdomen. Polyhydramnios was frequently associated with fetal tumors; premature labor, or premature rupture of the membranes was also common. The authors concluded from their review that, for tumors located intracranially, the chances for the fetus are very poor. The prognosis for tumors at other locations is variable and may be determined by such factors as the size of the tumor, involvement of other organs, other associated malformations, or mechanical obstruction during the birth process. **IV C**

Neuroblastoma

Management option	Quality of evidence	Strength of recommendation	References
Vigilance for hydramnios, hydrops	IV	C	1
If maternal symptoms occur in association with a fetal tumor, measurement of maternal urinary catecholamines may help confirm diagnosis	IV	C	2
Delivery may be the only effective treatment. The decision to deliver must include consideration of gestational age, the likelihood of fetal viability and the condition of the mother	–	✔	–
Maternal risks include hydramnios, uterine distension, premature rupture of membranes and preterm labor	–	✔	–
A very large renal mass may cause dystocia necessitating cesarean delivery	–	✔	–
Prognosis is based on tumor stage. Most cases of fetal neuroblastoma are in Stage I or II. Prognosis is generally good in these early stages	III	B	3

References

1 Jaffa AJ, Many A, Hartoov J et al. (1993) Prenatal sonographic diagnosis of metastatic neuroblastoma: report of a case and review of the literature. *Prenat Diagn* **13**, 73–77. Case report of metastatic neuroblastoma. **IV C**

2 Wienk MA, Van Geijn HP, Copray FJ *et al.* (1990) Prenatal diagnosis of fetal tumors by ultrasonography. *Obstet Gynecol Surv* **45**, 639–653. Review of the recent literature on fetal tumors detected between 1982 and 1988. The authors have compartmentalized the fetal body areas into the head and neck region, the thorax and the abdomen. Polyhydramnios was frequently associated with fetal tumors; premature labor, or premature rupture of the membranes was also common. The authors concluded from their review that, for tumors located intracranially, the chances for the fetus are very poor. The prognosis for tumors at other locations is variable and may be determined by such factors as the size of the tumor, involvement of other organs, other associated malformations, or mechanical obstruction during the birth process. **IV C**

3 Ho PT, Estroff JA, Kozakewich H *et al.* (1993) Prenatal detection of neuroblastoma: a ten year experience from the Dana-Farber Cancer Institute and Children's Hospital. *Pediatrics* **92**, 358–364. Retrospective case review of cases of antenatally diagnosed neuroblastoma in one center between 1982 and 1992. 11 cases: 9 adrenal, 2 thoracic paraspinal. All patients treated postnatally by surgical resection. One patient required additional chemotherapy. No deaths at mean follow up of 37 months. **III B**

Kidney tumors

Management option	Quality of evidence	Strength of recommendation	References
Polyhydramnios is frequently present with large tumors	IV	C	1
Wilms tumor and renal hamartomas are both solid with cystic areas	IV	C	1

Reference

1 Wienk MA, Van Geijn HP, Copray FJ *et al.* (1990) Prenatal diagnosis of fetal tumors by ultrasonography. *Obstet Gynecol Surv* **45**, 639–653. Review of the recent literature on fetal tumors detected between 1982 and 1988. The authors have compartmentalized the fetal body areas into the head and neck region, the thorax and the abdomen. Polyhydramnios was frequently associated with fetal tumors; premature labor, or premature rupture of the membranes was also common. The authors concluded from their review that, for tumors located intracranially, the chances for the fetus are very poor. The prognosis for tumors at other locations is variable and may be determined by such factors as the size of the tumor, involvement of other organs, other associated malformations, or mechanical obstruction during the birth process. **IV C**

Liver tumors

Management option	Quality of evidence	Strength of recommendation	References
Vigilance for hydramnios and hydrops	–	✔	–
Cesarean section may be considered for large tumors with possibility of dystocia or tumor rupture	IV	C	1
Metastatic lesions more common than primary tumors	IV	C	2
Hemangiomas: ❑ Most common benign neoplasm of the liver ❑ If large may be associated with: – high output failure – disseminated intravascular coagulation ❑ Other congenital anomalies occur in association with hemangiomas ❑ Involution accelerated by corticosteroid therapy	IV	C	3,4

References

1 Garmel SH, Crombleholme TM, Semple JP *et al.* (1994) Prenatal diagnosis and management of fetal tumors. *Sem Perinatol* **18**, 350–365. Review of the prenatal diagnosis and management of the following tumors: cervical teratoma, hepatic tumors, neuroblastoma, neoblastic nephroma and sacrococcygeal teratomas. **IV C**

2 Jaffa AJ, Many A, Hartoov J *et al.* (1993) Prenatal sonographic diagnosis of metastatic neuroblastoma: report of a case and review of the literature. *Prenat Diagn* **13**, 73–77. Case report of metastatic neuroblastoma. **IV C**

3 Abuhamad AZ, Lewis D, Inati MN *et al.* (1993) The use of color flow Doppler in the diagnosis of fetal hepatic hemangioma. *J Ultrasound Med* **12**, 223–226. Case report of fetal hepatic hemangioma first detected at 18 weeks gestation. The hemangioma increased significantly in size, compressing the chest contents and resulting in cardiac dextroposition and pulmonary hypoplasia. **IV C**

4 Mejides AA, Adra AM, O'Sullivan MJ *et al.* (1995) Prenatal diagnosis and therapy for a fetal hepatic vascular malformation. *Obstet Gynecol* **85**, 850–853. Case report of the antenatal diagnosis of a fetal hepatic hemangioma. Hydrocortisone injection directly into the umbilical vein and the amniotic cavity resulted in appreciable improvement in hemodynamic and hematologic indices. **IV C**

Intra-abdominal cysts

Management option	Quality of evidence	Strength of recommendation	References
Rarely, an ovarian cyst impinges on other organs, causes an ovarian torsion or results in dystocia. Transabdominal aspiration and decompression may be preferable to cesarean delivery. Fluid unlikely to be irritant or malignant (see below)	–	✔	–
Most cysts do not require intrauterine intervention	–	✔	–
Delivery should be in a tertiary center since neonatal surgery may be required	–	✔	–

Sacrococcygeal teratoma

Management option	Quality of evidence	Strength of recommendation	References
Vigilance for hydramnios and hydrops – predicts poor prognosis. Cystic tumors have a better prognosis	III IV	B C	1,2 3
Delivery usually has to be cesarean to avoid damage to tumor	–	✔	–
Fetal surgery has been attempted because of the lethality of cases identified before 30 weeks but without success	–	✔	–

References

1 Flake AW, Harrison MR, Adzick NS *et al.* (1986) Fetal sacrococcygeal teratoma. *J Pediatr Surg* **21**, 563–566. Retrospective case review of 6 cases of sacrococcygeal teratoma and literature review. Most present at 22–34 weeks with enlarged uterus due to tumor or polyhydramnios. Presentation after 30 weeks is good prognostic sign: fetal survival in 6 of 8 cases after planned cesarean section. Hydrops is poor prognostic sign: 7 out of 7 fetuses died *in utero*. **III B**

2 Chisholm CA, Heider AL, Kuller JA *et al.* (1999) Prenatal diagnosis and perinatal management of fetal sacrococcygeal teratoma. *Am J Perinatol* **16**, 89–92. Retrospective case review of 9 cases of sacrococcygeal teratoma diagnosed antenatally. All 6 diagnosed after 20 weeks survived the neonatal period. Hydrops developed in 3, all of whom died as a consequence of delivery at extremely premature gestation. **III B**

3 Garmel SH, Crombleholme TM, Semple JP *et al.* (1994) Prenatal diagnosis and management of fetal tumors. *Sem Perinatol* **18**, 350–365. Review of the prenatal diagnosis and management of the following tumors: cervical teratoma, hepatic tumors, neuroblastoma, neoblastic nephroma and sacrococcygeal teratomas. **IV C**

Limb tumors

Management option	Quality of evidence	Strength of recommendation	References
Vigilance for hydrops	IV	C	1
Cesarean section may be necessary to avoid dystocia	IV	C	1

Reference

1 Wienk MA, Van Geijn HP, Copray FJ *et al.* (1990) Prenatal diagnosis of fetal tumors by ultrasonography. *Obstet Gynecol Surv* **45**, 639–653. Review of the recent literature on fetal tumors detected between 1982 and 1988. The authors have compartmentalized the fetal body areas into the head and neck region, the thorax and the abdomen. Polyhydramnios was frequently associated with fetal tumors; premature labor, or premature rupture of the membranes was also common. The authors concluded from their review that, for tumors located intracranially, the chances for the fetus are very poor. The prognosis for tumors at other locations is variable and may be determined by such factors as the size of the tumor, involvement of other organs, other associated malformations, or mechanical obstruction during the birth process. **IV C**

Placental and umbilical cord tumors

Management option	Quality of evidence	Strength of recommendation	References
Vigilance for hydramnios and hydrops	IV	C	1

Reference

1 Zoppini C, Acaia B, Lucci G *et al.* (1997) Varying clinical course of large placental chorioangiomas. Report of 3 cases. *Fetal Diagn Ther* **12**, 61–64. The authors report three cases of placental chorioangiomas. Fetal hydrops was present in one case, necessitating delivery. The other cases were managed conservatively. **IV C**

Fetal ovarian cyst

Management option	Quality of evidence	Strength of recommendation	References
Torsion reported in up to 40%; majority more than 5 cm – intracystic debris characteristic of torsion	III	B	1

Management option	Quality of evidence	Strength of recommendation	References
Gastrointestinal and urinary tract obstruction possible with larger cysts	III	B	2,3
Polyhydramnios may be present with large cysts	–	✔	–
Aspiration of fetal ovarian cysts larger than 4.0cm has been recommended. Since simple ovarian cysts may regress, this may not be justified in every case	III	B	2,4,5
Cesarean section should be performed for obstetrical indications only	III	B	3

References

1 Meizner I, Levy A, Katz M *et al.* (1991) Fetal ovarian cysts: prenatal ultrasonographic detection and postnatal evaluation and treatment. *Am J Obstet Gynecol* **164**, 874–878. Review of 15 fetuses between 19 and 37 weeks gestation with antenatally ovarian cysts. They noted intracystic dependent debris was a sign of ovarian torsion. The mean size of the cysts with evidence of torsion was 5.4cm. **III B**

2 Bagolan P, Rivosecchi M, Giorlandino C *et al.* (1992) Prenatal diagnosis and clinical outcome of ovarian cysts. *J Pediatr Surg* **27**, 879–881. Series of 26 cases of fetal ovarian cysts in 25 patients. 8 of the 26 cysts were complex – all required surgical intervention after birth. There were 5 cases of ovarian torsion. There were 2 cases of intestinal obstruction secondary to a fetal ovarian cyst. In this series 60% of newborns with ovarian cysts required oophorectomy. **III B**

3 Sakala EP, Leon ZA, Rouse GA (1991) Management of antenatally diagnosed fetal ovarian cysts. *Obstet Gynecol Surv* **46**, 407–414. Review of 65 sonographically diagnosed fetal ovarian cysts with a single case report added. Guidelines for antenatal, intrapartum and neonatal management were derived from these 66 cases. Polyhydramnios was present in 18% of the cases and was generally associated with larger ovarian cysts. Larger cysts also could result in bowel obstruction and renal compression. There were no cases of tissue dystocia in the 40 vaginally delivered patients. The authors therefore concluded that cesarean section should be performed for obstetrical indications only. **III B**

4 Brandt ML, Luks FI, Flilatrault D *et al.* (1991) Surgical indications in antenatally diagnosed ovarian cysts. *J Pediatr Surg* **26**, 276–282. Retrospective review of 29 ovarian cysts in 27 patients diagnosed by prenatal ultrasound between 28 and 36 weeks gestation. The authors also reviewed 230 cases of antenatally diagnosed ovarian cysts. They concluded that simple cysts of the ovary tend to resolve spontaneously and may be treated conservatively. Serial ultrasound examinations were recommended in order to appropriately assess either the resolution of a cyst or an increase in size or change in architectural configuration that would mandate surgery. The authors felt that cysts larger than 4cm may be candidates for percutaneous aspiration or removal. Complex cystic masses, as well as symptomatic ovarian cysts, should be removed. **III B**

5 Crombleholme TM, Craigo SD, Garmel S *et al.* (1997) Fetal ovarian cyst decompression to prevent torsion. *J Pediatr Surg* **32**, 1447–1449. This study reviews 7 patients with fetal ovarian cysts. The mean gestational age at presentation was 31.9 ± 3.6 weeks. All 7 cases involved isolated unilateral cysts without associated anomalies. Mean initial cyst diameter was 3.4 ± 1.7cm. One apparent 'ovarian cyst' was found to be a persistent cloaca. Two cysts with diameters of 6.1cm and 4.0cm were decompressed *in utero*. Neither cyst recurred. The authors hypothesize that fetal ovarian cyst decompression may reduce the likelihood of ovarian torsion. **III B**

INFECTION

Chapter 24

Infection

24.1 Measles (rubeola)

David Howe and Clare Tower

Management option		Quality of evidence	Strength of recommendation	References
Prepregnancy	Prevention by childhood vaccination	–	✔	–
	Serological evaluation and, if negative, vaccination of woman inquiring about status prepregnancy	–	✔	–
Prenatal	Treat acute infection symptomatically	–	✔	–
	Antibiotics if secondary bacterial infection suspected	–	✔	–
	Vigilance for uterine activity	–	✔	–
	Immunoglobulin should be considered for susceptible women exposed to infection	IV	C	1
	Accidental vaccination is not an indication for termination	–	✔	–
Labor, delivery and postnatal	Appropriate isolation precautions when in hospital	–	✔	–

Reference

1 Centers for Disease Control (CDC) (1991) Update on adult immunization: recommendations of the Immunization Practices Advisory Committee (ACIP). *Morbid Mortal Wkly Rep* **40** (RR-12), 48. Overview on immunization for adults containing specific recommendations. Information is provided on vaccine-preventable diseases; indications for use of vaccines, toxoids and immune globulins recommended for adults; and specific side effects, adverse reactions, precautions and contraindications associated with their use. It also gives immunization recommendations for adults in specific risk groups. This section specifically deals with measles. **IV C**

24.2 Rubella

David Howe and Clare Tower

Management option		Quality of evidence	Strength of recommendation	References
Prepregnancy	Prevention by childhood vaccination	III	B	1
	Vaccination programs for girls in their early teens contribute to prevention	III	B	1
	Assess serological status and offer vaccination in susceptible women: ❑ who inquire prepregnancy ❑ who are receiving infertility treatment	IV	C	2
	❑ after delivery	IIa	B	3

➡

Management option		Quality of evidence	Strength of recommendation	References
Prenatal	Routine check of rubella immunity status at first visit for all women is standard practice in many centers	–	✔	–
	Accidental vaccination in early pregnancy is not an indication for termination	IV	C	4
	If suspected exposure in woman with 'immunity': ❑ Confirm presence of rubella-specific IgG (if immediately after exposure) ❑ Confirm failure of appearance of IgM (acute phase) antibodies with two serum samples 2–3 weeks apart ❑ Reassure	–	✔	–
	If suspected exposure in susceptible woman: ❑ Establish validity of diagnosis serologically in index case if possible ❑ Check for appearance of IgM (acute phase) antibodies ❑ If no serological evidence of infection, reassure patient ❑ If maternal infection confirmed serologically, options will depend on gestation at time of infection: – In early pregnancy, termination should be discussed; either immediately or only after confirmation by invasive procedure – In late pregnancy, confirmation of fetal infection by invasive procedure can be considered; fetal growth and health should be monitored if infection suspected or confirmed	III	B	5
Labor, delivery and postnatal	If fetal infection suspected, cord blood should be sent for serological confirmation	–	✔	–
	If fetal infection confirmed, careful pediatric assessment and follow-up	–	✔	–

References

1 Chu SY, Bernier RH, Stewart JA *et al.* (1988) Rubella antibody persistence after immunization. Sixteen-year follow-up in the Hawaiian islands. *JAMA* **259**, 3133–3136. Follow up study of 1290 individuals 16 years after receiving rubella vaccine. Vaccine-induced rubella antibodies persisted in 92–96%. **III B**

2 Centers for Disease Control (1991) Update on adult immunization: recommendations of the Immunization Practices Advisory Committee (ACIP). *Morbid Mortal Wkly Rep* **40** (No. RR-12), 24–26.
Overview on immunization for adults containing specific recommendations. Information is provided on vaccine-preventable diseases; indications for use of vaccines, toxoids and immune globulins recommended for adults; and specific side effects, adverse reactions, precautions and contraindications associated with their use. This section specifically deals with rubella. **IV C**

3 Black NA, Parsons A, Kurtz JB *et al.* (1983) Post-partum rubella immunisation: a controlled trial of two vaccines. *Lancet* **2**, 990–992. Trial comparing the effectiveness of two rubella vaccines given post-partum in 298 women. The two vaccines were given in alternate months. Cendehill gave higher geometric mean titers (43.6 vs 17.0) and was significantly more effective at producing seroconversion than RA 27/3 (97.6% vs 82.2%). **IIa B**

4 Centers for Disease Control (1989) Rubella vaccination during pregnancy – United States, 1971–1988. *Morbid Mortal Wkly Rep* **38**, 289–291.
Review of outcome of vaccination during pregnancy over 18 years. No evidence of adverse fetal outcome. Recommendation that vaccination is not an indication for termination. **IV C**

5 Tanemura M, Suzumori K, Yagami Y *et al.* (1996) Diagnosis of fetal rubella infection with reverse transcription and nested polymerase chain reaction: a study of 34 cases diagnosed in fetuses. *Am J Obstet Gynecol* **174**, 578–582. Descriptive study of the use of reverse transcription polymerase chain reaction to detect rubella RNA in chorionic villi, amniotic fluid and fetal blood. The test was carried out on 34 women with suspected primary rubella infection. 8 of 34 cases were positive. 24 of the 26 remaining cases delivered a healthy fetus, one was electively aborted and one was an unexplained intrauterine death at 36 weeks. **III B**

24.3 Varicella-zoster virus

David Howe and Clare Tower

Management option		Quality of evidence	Strength of recommendation	References
Prepregnancy	Availability of vaccination programs in infancy/childhood is variable	IV	C	1,2
Prenatal	If mother exposed to varicella-zoster virus, check immunity status (serially if susceptible)	–	✔	–
	If patient develops chickenpox:			
	❏ Counsel about risks	–	✔	–
	❏ Policies over use of varicella-zoster immunoglobulin vary (e.g. 'only give to immunosuppressed patient, in first trimester, in last 4 weeks')	IV	C	3
	❏ Monitor for dissemination to severe systemic form of illness	–	✔	–
	❏ Consider acyclovir with severe illness	IV	C	4
	❏ Vigilance for preterm uterine activity	–	✔	–
Labor, delivery and postnatal	Appropriate infection control measures	–	✔	–
	Evaluate newborn clinically and serologically	–	✔	–
	Prophylactic measures if not infected (e.g. passive or active immunization, aciclovir)	–	✔	–
	Aciclovir and supportive therapy if infected	–	✔	–

References

1 Krause PR, Klinman DM (1995) Efficacy, immunogenicity, safety, and use of live attenuated chickenpox vaccine. *J Pediatr* **127**, 518–525. Review article. **IV C**

2 Lieu TA, Cochi SL, Black SB *et al.* (1994) Cost-effectiveness of a routine varicella vaccination program for US children. *JAMA* **271**, 375–381. An assessment of economic consequences of vaccinating healthy children using decision analysis and a mathematical model of efficacy. Concludes that routine vaccination would be beneficial from a societal perspective, and would be cost effective compared with other prevention programs. **IV C**

3 Rouse DJ, Gardner M, Allen SJ *et al.* (1996) Management of the presumed susceptible varicella (chickenpox)-exposed gravida: a cost-effectiveness/cost-benefit analysis. *Obstet Gynecol* **87**, 932–936. Assessment of cost effectiveness of three strategies of managing susceptible pregnant women exposed to varicella: do nothing, assess immune status before administration of immunoglobulin, and a universal administration strategy. The testing immune status prior to treatment was concluded to be most cost-effective. **IV C**

4 Eder SE, Apuzzio JJ, Weiss G (1988) Varicella pneumonia during pregnancy. Treatment of two cases with acyclovir. *Am J Perinatol* **5**, 168. Report of the use of aciclovir for the treatment of varicella pneumonia in pregnancy. Both mothers and infants survived and no adverse fetal effects were observed. **IV C**

24.4 Cytomegalovirus

David Howe and Clare Tower

Management option		Quality of evidence	Strength of recommendation	References
Prepregnancy	Advice about risks for women working in high-risk environment (e.g. child care)	–	✔	–
	Counseling about planning pregnancy in women with history of proven cytomegalovirus (CMV) infection is difficult; establishing their 'shedding status' may help	–	✔	–
Prenatal	Advice about risks for women working in high-risk environment (e.g. child care)	–	✔	–
	If patient is diagnosed to have CMV infection in pregnancy: ❑ Careful counseling about fetal risks ❑ Consider invasive procedure to establish fetal risk ❑ Check fetal growth and health ❑ Consider pregnancy termination (if early gestational age) ❑ No effective treatment ❑ ?Ganciclovir for patients positive for human immunodeficiency virus	–	✔	–
Labor, delivery and postnatal	If patient is diagnosed to have CMV infection in pregnancy: ❑ Infection control measures ❑ Clinical and serological evaluation of the newborn with pediatric follow-up if infection confirmed	–	✔	–

24.5 Parvovirus B19

David Howe and Clare Tower

Management option		Quality of evidence	Strength of recommendation	References
Prepregnancy	If diagnosis confirmed before pregnancy, pregnancy should be avoided until clinical cure and antibody response	–	✔	–
Prenatal	If infection is diagnosed: ❑ Symptomatic treatment of patient ❑ Screen serially for fetal hydrops ❑ Tertiary center management	III IV	B C	1,2 3
	If hydrops develops, consider fetal blood transfusion	III IV	B C	2 3,4

References

1 Public Health Laboratory Service Working Party on Fifth Disease (1990) Prospective study of human parvovirus (B19) infection in pregnancy. *Br Med J* **300**, 1166–1170. Prospective study of 190 pregnant women with serologically confirmed parvovirus B19 infection. 186 continued the pregnancy. 84% delivered a normal baby and transplacental transmission rate was 33%. Overall fetal loss rate was similar to an uninfected sample, although there was an increased fetal loss rate in the second trimester of 11%. Based on virological findings, the risk of fetal death in an infected pregnancy was 9%. **III B**

2 Fairley CK, Smoleniec JS, Caul OE *et al.* (1995) Observational study of effect of intrauterine transfusions on outcome of fetal hydrops after parvovirus B19 infection. *Lancet* **346**, 1335–1337. This observational study examined the outcome of fetuses found to be hydropic after maternal parvovirus B19 infection. 66 cases were identified and in 29 the fetus was dead at presentation or therapeutic abortion was performed. In the 38 fetuses alive at presentation 12 received transfusions, of whom 3 died. Of those not transfused 13 of 26 died. The odds of death were significantly lower amongst those who received an intrauterine transfusion, after adjustment for the severity of hydrops at presentation. **III B**

3 Peters MT, Nicolaides KH (1990) Cordocentesis for the diagnosis and treatment of human fetal parvovirus infection. *Obstet Gynecol* **75**, 501–504. Report of two cases of B19 infection in hydrops fetuses at 22 and 26 weeks gestation. Both fetuses were IgM-negative and anemic. Both were treated with blood transfusions and hydrops resolved. **IV C**

4 Pryde PG, Nugent CE, Pridjian G *et al.* (1992) Spontaneous resolution of nonimmune hydrops fetalis secondary to human parvovirus B19 infection. *Obstet Gynecol* **79**, 859–861. Case report of two parvovirus-related hydropic infants. The hydrops resolved without intervention in both and full-term healthy infants were delivered. **IV C**

24.6 Herpes simplex virus (genital)

David Howe and Clare Tower

Management option		Quality of evidence	Strength of recommendation	References
Prenatal	Symptomatic treatment of infections (primary and recurrent); hospitalization for severe cases	–	✔	–
	Vigilance for dissemination	–	✔	–
	Vigilance for uterine activity	–	✔	–
	Aciclovir (oral and topical) has been used in pregnancy without adverse outcome, although not generally advocated unless disseminated disease	–	✔	–
	Serial viral cultures in the last trimester for patients who are asymptomatic are no longer recommended; culture only to document a new case	III	B	1–3
	Consider delivery with septicemic cases	–	✔	–
Labor and delivery	Inspect perineum, vagina, cervix of women with history of herpes simplex virus at onset of labor	–	✔	–
	Allow vaginal delivery if no active lesions and no prodromal symptoms at time of labor	–	✔	–
	Active lesion at time of labor is considered by most obstetricians to be an indication for cesarean section, although the risk of fetal infection is less with recurrent disease	–	✔	–
	Counseling about the benefits of cesarean section in preventing fetal infection with membrane rupture is difficult	–	✔	–
	Avoid fetal electrodes if possible	IV	C	4

➡

Management option		Quality of evidence	Strength of recommendation	References
Postnatal	Infection control measures with active lesions	–	✔	–
	Clinical, microbiological and serological evaluation of the newborn with active maternal lesions	–	✔	–
	Treatment of infection reduces dissemination and morbidity	III	B	5

References

1 Tookey P, Peckham CS (1996) Neonatal herpes simplex virus infection in the British Isles. *Paediatr Perinat Epidemiol* **10**, 432–442. This study aimed to establish the incidence of neonatal herpes simplex virus (HSV) infection in the UK by obtaining notification through the monthly reporting scheme of the British Paediatric Association Surveillance Unit. Over 5.5 years 76 infected children were reported, an incidence of 1.65/100000 livebirths. 25% died neonatally and a further 33% died subsequently or had long-term sequelae. There was rarely a history of maternal HSV infection and routine screening for genital herpes infection was not thought to be justified. **III B**

2 Garland SM (1992) Neonatal herpes simplex: Royal Women's Hospital 10-year experience with management guidelines for herpes in pregnancy. *Aust N Z J Obstet Gynecol* **32**, 331–334. Report of the outcome of six cases of neonatal herpes that occurred in a 10-year period (1982–91) in a single hospital and provides a protocol for management of herpes in pregnancy. None of the mothers had an overt recent or past history of genital infection and two infections were acquired *in utero*. Routine screening for viral shedding in the last trimester in women with a history of genital herpes was not recommended. **III B**

3 Boehm FH, Estes W, Wright PF *et al.* (1981) Management of genital herpes simplex virus infection occurring during pregnancy. *Am J Obstet Gynecol* **141**, 735–740. Prospective observational study cultured 120 pregnant women with genital lesions suspicious of herpes simplex virus (HSV) infection. 80 were negative and 40 positive for HSV. The authors conclude that the use of HSV culture to determine mode of delivery limits the incidence of cesarean section and neonatal infection. **III B**

4 Goldkrand JW (1982) Intrapartum inoculation of herpes simplex virus by fetal scalp electrode. *Obstet Gynecol* **59**, 263–265. Case report of transmission of herpes simplex virus (HSV) from a mother with no past history of HSV infection to the infant via a fetal scalp electrode. **IV C**

5 Whitley RJ (1986) Neonatal herpes simplex virus infections. Presentation and management. *J Reprod Med* **31**, 426–432. Review of the evidence from several studies performed by the National Institute of Allergy and Infectious Diseases Collaborative Antiviral Study Group. It reported the presentation, natural history, disease outcome and value of antiviral therapy in infants developing neonatal herpes simplex virus infections. Infections were classified into local – either central nervous system (CNS) or skin, eye, mouth (SEM) – or disseminated. CNS infections affected 35%, SEM 41% and disseminated 24%. Without treatment there is high mortality and morbidity after CNS or disseminated infections, and significant morbidity following SEM infections. Antiviral treatment with vidarabine reduced the progression from SEM to CNS or disseminated disease and reduced morbidity and mortality from all forms of infection. **III B**

24.7 Hepatitis B virus

David Howe and Clare Tower

Management option		Quality of evidence	Strength of recommendation	References
Prepregnancy	In known hepatitis-B-virus-positive patients, risks for fetus and preventive measures after birth should be discussed	–	✔	–
	Vaccinate health-care workers	Ia	A	1

Management option		Quality of evidence	Strength of recommendation	References
Prenatal	**Acute disease:** ❑ Supportive care ❑ Dietary advice ❑ Monitor liver function ❑ Assess fetal growth and health ❑ Vigilance for uterine activity ❑ Infection control measures ❑ Contact tracing, testing and vaccination where appropriate	–	✔	–
	Chronic carriers: ❑ Assessment of carrier status varies (some perform screening on all women, others only on those 'at risk' – US recommendations below) ❑ Infection control measures with body products ❑ At-risk seronegative women: offer vaccination	III IV	B C	2 3
Labor, delivery and postnatal	Infection control measures	–	✔	–
	Advice about breastfeeding is controversial	–	✔	–
	Newborn should receive passive (HBIg) and active immunization	Ib	A	4–8
	Thereafter repeat vaccination not required for more than 10 years	IIb	B	9

Recommendations for hepatitis B screening during pregnancy

(quality IV, strength C, reference 3)

- ❑ Screen all pregnant women for hepatitis B surface antigen (HB_SAg) at the same time as other routine screening
- ❑ Health-care personnel should be informed of a HB_SAg-positive mother
- ❑ In special circumstances (e.g. exposure to HBV, acute hepatitis or high-risk behavior), additional testing may be warranted later in pregnancy
- ❑ Unscreened women presenting for delivery should be screened with 24 h results
- ❑ Newborns of HB_SAg-positive mothers should receive HBIG (0.5 ml intramuscularly) within 12 h of birth and an initial dose of HBV vaccine (5 mg of recombinant vaccine intramuscularly) within 7 days
- ❑ Infants should receive the second and third doses of vaccine at 1 and 6 months and be tested for HB_SAg at 12–15 months.
- ❑ Family members of HB_SAg-positive women (and infants) should be counseled appropriately

References

1 Jefferson T, Demicheli V, Deeks J *et al.* (2000) Vaccines for preventing hepatitis B in health workers. In: *Cochrane database of systematic reviews*, issue 4. Oxford: Update Software. Cochrane meta-analysis review of trials of hepatitis B vaccination in health-care workers. Only four trials met the selection criteria, and all compared plasma-derived vaccines with placebo. In health workers in high-risk situations, e.g. dialysis units, the odds risk for infection was lowered by vaccination (OR 0.34, 95% CI 0.21–0.53). There was a nonsignificant trend towards benefit in low-risk workers. **Ia A**

2 Gonzalez L, Roses A, Alomar P *et al.* (1988) The maternal–infant center in the control of hepatitis B. *Acta Obstet Gynecol Scand* **67**, 421–427. Observational study of 864 pregnant women and their infants and 783 health services personnel found the carriage rate of HB_SAg to be 0.9% in pregnant women and 1.5% in health workers. Of those pregnant women who were chronic carriers of HB_SAg, 11% of their children and 2.1% of their husbands were also HB_SAg positive. 67 newborns of HB_SAg carrier mothers received one dose of Hep B immunoglobulin and 3 doses of Hep B vaccine. Seroconversion rate was 98.5% and one child became a chronic carrier. The authors conclude that maternity hospitals provide an ideal opportunity for Hep B screening of patients and their contacts. **III B**

3 American College of Obstetricians and Gynecologists (1992) *Viral hepatitis in pregnancy.* ACOG Education Bulletin, no. 248. Washington, DC: ACOG. All pregnant women should be screened. Women in high-risk groups who are negative for hepatitis B should be vaccinated. The CDC recommends universal active immunization of all infants. **IV C**

4 Ip HM, Lelie PN, Wong VC *et al.* (1989) Prevention of hepatitis B carrier status in infants according to maternal levels of HBV DNA. *Lancet* **1**, 406–410. Randomized placebo-controlled trial in which 235 infants of mothers positive for the hepatitis B e antigen (Hb_eAg) were allocated to treatment with placebo, vaccination alone, or vaccination and hepatitis B immunoglobulin (HBIg). All treated groups were significantly protected against infection, with the highest protection afforded in those receiving both vaccine and immunoglobulin. In those not given HBIg the infants of mothers with higher hepatitis B virus (HBV) DNA levels were more likely to become HBV carriers. Infants given repeated doses of HBIg were significantly less likely to become carriers than those receiving vaccine alone. Infants given HBIg who did not develop active immunity to HB vaccine became susceptible once the passive immunity had worn off. The authors recommend that HBIg be given to all infants of Hb_eAg-positive mothers. **Ib A**

5 Zanetti AR, Dentico P, Del Vecchio Blanco C *et al.* (1986) Multicenter trial on the efficacy of HBIG and vaccine in preventing perinatal hepatitis B. Final report. *J Med Virol* **18**, 327–334. Study of 92 babies born to mothers positive for the hepatitis B e antigen were treated with hepatitis B immunoglobulin (HBIg) at birth and 1 month of age, and given HB vaccine at 3, 4 and 9 months. 3 infants became infected, 2 by 6 months of age, presumably through infection prior to vaccination, and one at 9 months in spite of a response to previous vaccination. The authors conclude that a combination of HBIg and vaccine is effective at preventing transmission of hepatitis B virus. **Ib A**

6 Xu ZY, Liu CB, Francis DP *et al.* (1985) Prevention of perinatal acquisition of hepatitis B virus carriage using vaccine: preliminary report of randomized double-blind placebo-controlled and comparative trial. *Pediatrics* **76**, 713–718. Randomized placebo-controlled trial comparing two hepatitis B vaccines (National Institute of Allergy and Infectious Disease, NIAID, versus Beijing Institute of Vaccine and Serum, BIVS) with placebo in 180 infants born to mothers positive for the hepatitis B surface antigen. Infants were vaccinated at birth, 1 month and 6 months. The NIAID vaccine was more effective than the BIVS vaccine (efficacy 88% vs 51%). An additional 28 children were given hepatitis B immunoglobulin at birth in combination with BIVS vaccine, resulting in 83% efficacy. **Ib A**

7 Beasley RP, Hwang LY, Lee GC *et al.* (1983) Prevention of perinatally transmitted hepatitis B virus infections with hepatitis B immune globulin and hepatitis B vaccine. *Lancet* **2**, 1099–1102. Randomized blind controlled trial in which 172 infants of mothers positive for the hepatitis B e antigen were randomized to receive hepatitis B immunoglobulin (HBIg) at birth plus hepatitis B vaccine in one of three schedules, and 84 infants received no prophylaxis. There was no difference in efficacy between the three schedules, whose combined efficacy was 94%. The combination of HBIg and vaccine was more effective than HBIg alone (71% efficacy) or vaccine alone (75% efficacy). The authors conclude that HBIg should be given immediately at birth but need not be given again provided that vaccination is carried out. **Ib A**

8 Beasley RP, Hwang LY, Lin CC *et al.* (1983) Efficacy of hepatitis B immune globulin for prevention of perinatal transmission of hepatitis B virus carrier state: final report of a randomized double-blind, placebo-controlled trial. *Hepatology* **3**, 135–141. Randomized double blind placebo-controlled trial in which 185 infants of mothers positive for the hepatitis B e antigen were given either hepatitis B immunoglobulin (HBIg) or placebo at birth and were followed for 15 months. Treated infants were given either 1.0 ml of HBIg as a single dose at birth or 0.5 ml at birth, 3 months and 6 months. Efficacy was highest in those infants treated with repeat doses of HBIg. Some infants who became carriers were probably infected as HBIg protection waned and the authors concluded that higher efficacy would be likely if HBIg was combined with active vaccination. **Ib A**

9 Huang LM, Chiang BL, Lee CY *et al.* (1999) Long term response to hepatitis B vaccination and response to booster in children born to mothers with hepatitis B e-antigen. *Hepatology* **29**, 954–959. The study examined the humoral and cellular immune response at age 10 in 118 children born to hepatitis-B-positive mothers. The children had been given HB immunization in infancy. Immunological memory was found in all children, including those who had lost their seropositivity, suggesting that repeat vaccination was not required before age 10. **IIb B**

24.8 Human immunodeficiency virus

David Howe and Clare Tower

Management option		Quality of evidence	Strength of recommendation	References
Prepregnancy	Careful counseling and offer of screening for at-risk women	–	✔	–
	In human immunodeficiency virus (HIV)-positive women, careful counseling of risks and prognosis for the patient and fetus/baby, and consideration of whether pregnancy should be avoided	–	✔	–
Prenatal	Screening practices vary – options: ❑ Many centers offer screening to *all* women ❑ Counseling and offer of selective screening for at-risk women; most centers require informed consent before testing can occur	–	✔	–
	All unscreened at-risk women should be managed as if they were HIV-positive in terms of infection control measures with blood and other body products (preventative measures should be employed when handling blood from all women in pregnancy)	–	✔	–
	For HIV-positive women:			
	❑ Interdisciplinary care with HIV specialist	–	✔	–
	❑ Counseling and support	–	✔	–
	❑ Consideration of termination of pregnancy			
	❑ Screen for other sexually transmitted diseases	–	✔	–
	❑ Baseline serology for cytomegalovirus and *Toxoplasma*	–	✔	–
	❑ Oral zidovudine (100 mg) 3–5 times/day during prenatal period	Ia	A	1
	❑ Monitor $CD4^+$ counts serially: – If less than 200 cells/mm^3, commence antibiotic prophylaxis and intensive antiviral therapy (zidovudine) – If less than 500 cells/mm^3, liaise with HIV specialist to individualize therapy and treat opportunistic infection	IV	C	2
Labor, delivery and postnatal	Intravenous zidovudine for labor/delivery	Ia	A	1
	Cesarean section reduces vertical transmission	Ia	A	1
	Oral zidovudine for newborn for 6 weeks	Ib	A	3
	Dosage of antibiotic, antiviral and immunosupportive therapy may need review after delivery	–	✔	–
	Contraceptive advice	–	✔	–
	Advise against breastfeeding (just in developed countries?)	–	✔	–

References

1 Brocklehurst P (2000) Interventions aimed at reducing the mother to child transmission of HIV. In: *Cochrane database of systematic reviews*, issue 4. Oxford: Update Software. Cochrane meta-analysis of trials investigating methods of reducing mother-to-child transmission of human immunodeficiency virus. Significant reductions in transmission rates were found with the use of zidovudine, nevirapine and delivery by cesarean section. Four trials compared zidovudine with placebo and found a relative risk of transmission of 0.54 (95% CI 0.42–0.69). One trial compared nevirapine with zidovudine and found a lower transmission rate with nevirapine: RR 0.58 (95%CI 0.4–0.83). One trial compared cesarean section with anticipated vaginal delivery. The relative risk of transmission with cesarean section was 0.17 (95% CI 0.05–0.55). One trial investigated the use of hyperimmune immunoglobulin plus zidovudine with nonspecific immunoglobulin plus zidovudine and found no advantage. **Ia A**

2 American College of Obstetricians and Gynecologists (1992) Human immunodeficiency virus infections. ACOG Technical Bulletin, no. 169. Washington, DC: ACOG. An outline of the pathophysiology of HIV and the role of the OB/Gyn in managing both obstetrical and gynecologic patients with HIV. **IV C**

3 Connor EM, Sperling RS, Gelber R *et al.* (1994) Reduction of maternal–infant transmission of human immunodeficiency virus type 1 with zidovudine treatment. *N Engl J Med* **331**, 1173–1180. Randomized, double-blind placebo-controlled trial investigating the efficacy of a combination of antenatal, intrapartum and neonatal zidovudine treatment to reduce vertical transmission of human immunodeficiency virus (HIV). There were 363 patients who took part (180 in the zidovudine group, 183 in the placebo group) for whom neonatal HIV status was available. The proportion of infants infected in the zidovudine group infected at 18 months was 8.3% compared with 25.5% in the placebo group. This corresponded to a 67% reduction in risk for the treated group ($p < .05$). Although infants in the zidovudine group had a significantly lower hemoglobin, this corrected by 12 weeks. **Ib A**

24.9 Listeriosis

David Howe and Clare Tower

Management option		Quality of evidence	Strength of recommendation	References
Prenatal, labor, delivery and postnatal	Preventative measures with food handling (see below)	IV	C	1
	Vigilance for diagnosis	–	✔	–
	Antibiotics (penicillins)	IV	C	2–5
	Fetal health assessment during pregnancy	–	✔	–

Dietary recommendations for preventing foodborne *Listeria monocytogenes* infection (quality IV, strength C, reference 1)

For all patients:

- ❑ Thoroughly cook raw food from animal sources
- ❑ Thoroughly wash raw vegetables before eating
- ❑ Keep uncooked meats separate from other foods
- ❑ Avoid consumption of raw milk or food made from it
- ❑ Wash hands, knives and cutting boards after handling uncooked foods

For high-risk patients:

- ❑ Avoid soft cheeses (avoidance of hard cheeses not necessary)
- ❑ Reheat leftover or ready-to-eat foods until steaming hot

The risk of listeriosis associated with delicatessens is low; however, pregnant women and immunosuppressed patients may choose to avoid foods from such outlets, or at least reheat them as noted above

Adapted from Centers for Disease Control 1992[1]

References

1 Centers for Disease Control (1992) Update: foodborne listerosis – United States, 1988–1990. *Morbid Mortal Wkly Rep* **41**(15), 251–258. **IVC**

2 Hume OS (1976) Maternal *Listeria monocytogenes* septicemia with sparing of the fetus. *Obstet Gynecol* **48**(suppl), 33S–34S. Single case report of successful treatment with antibiotics of a *Listeria monocytogenes* septicemia that developed at 19 weeks gestation. The fetus was unaffected at delivery. **IV C**

3 Fleming AD, Ehrlich DW, Miller NA *et al.* (1985) Successful treatment of maternal septicemia due to *Listeria monocytogenes* at 26 weeks gestation. *Obstet Gynecol* **66**(suppl), 52S–53S. Single case report of successful treatment of *Listeria* septicemia that developed at 26 weeks. **IV C**

4 Cruikshank DP, Warenski JC (1989) First-trimester maternal *Listeria monocytogenes* sepsis and chorioamnionitis with normal neonatal outcome. *Obstet Gynecol* **73**, 469–471. Single case report of a successfully treated *Listeria* infection in pregnancy. **IV C**

5 Katz VL, Weinstein L (1982) Antepartum treatment of *Listeria monocytogenes* septicemia. *South Med J* **75**, 1353–1354. This is a further single case report of a woman who delivered prematurely at 27 weeks as a result of a *Listeria* septicemia. The paper contains a summary of outcome of 11 previously reported cases. **IV C**

24.10 Toxoplasmosis

David Howe and Clare Tower

Management option		Quality of evidence	Strength of recommendation	References
Prevention	Cook meat to well done (industrial deep-freezing also seems to destroy parasites efficiently)	–	✔	–
	When handling raw meat, avoid touching mouth and eyes	–	✔	–
	Wash hands thoroughly after handling raw meat, or vegetables soiled by earth	–	✔	–
	Wash kitchen surfaces that come into contact with raw meat	–	✔	–
	Wash fruit and vegetables before consumption	–	✔	–
	Avoid contact with things that are potentially contaminated with cat feces	–	✔	–
	Wear gloves when gardening or handling cat litter box	–	✔	–
	Disinfect cat litter box for 5 min with boiling water	–	✔	–
Treatment	With spiramycin, pyrimethamine and sulfonamides	III IV	B C	1 2

References

1 Hohlfeld P, Daffos F, Thulliez P *et al.* (1989) Fetal toxoplasmosis: outcome of pregnancy and infant follow-up after in utero treatment. *J Pediatr* **115**, 75–79. Pregnancy outcome of 89 fetuses proven to have an *in-utero* toxoplasmosis infection, and postnatal follow-up of the 54 surviving infants. In mothers who developed toxoplasmosis in pregnancy the transmission rate to the fetus was 7%. Termination was performed in 34 pregnancies, in 27 of which there were ultrasound abnormalities, and in 7 where infection occurred very early in pregnancy. 54 surviving infants received postnatal treatment and were followed up. 76% had subclinical infections. One, who did not receive pyrimethamine/sulfonamides in pregnancy, developed hydrocephalus. The remaining 53 had normal neurological development, but 5 of these developed peripheral chorioretinitis without visual impairment. **III B**

2 Wong S-Y, Remington JS (1994) Toxoplasmosis in pregnancy. *Clin Infect Dis* **18**, 853–852. Review article describing the transmission, pathogenesis and clinical manifestations of toxoplasmosis infection. It goes on to discuss

the diagnosis of *Toxoplasma* infection in pregnancy and the diagnosis of infection in the fetus. The article recommends treatment with spiramycin and with combined pyrimethamine and sulfadiazine where fetal infection is documented. The recommendations for treatment are based on the previous article from Hohlfeld et al. The article ends by discussing methods of prevention of congenital toxoplasmosis infection. **IV C**

24.11 Urinary tract infections

Ed Howarth

Management option		Quality of evidence	Strength of recommendation	References
Prepregnancy	Investigate renal function	IV	C	1
	Treat and eliminate asymptomatic bacteriuria	Ia	A	2,3
Prenatal – screening	Regular surveillance for asymptomatic bacteria	–	✔	–
Prenatal – treatment	Treat asymptomatic bacteria	Ia	A	2,3
	Acute cystitis: 7–14 day course of antibiotics may be too long	Ib Ia	A A	4 5
	Acute pyelonephritis: ❑ Hospitalization ❑ Intravenous hydration ❑ Intravenous antibiotics if bacteremia (change to oral when infection is under control) ❑ Monitor clinical condition, full blood count, urea, creatinine, electrolytes, urine and blood culture	Ib	A	6
	Frequent testing for recurrence of bacteriuria after treatment of any form of infection	IV	C	7
	Investigate renal function, renal ultrasound and even intravenous urogram if recurrent or resistant infections	IV	C	7
	Consider prophylaxis in all pregnancies with urological complications	IV	C	1
Postnatal	Investigate women with recurrent infection or pyelonephritis	IV	C	7

References

1 Van den Broek PJ, van Everdingen JJ (1999) 'Urinary tract infections'– revised CBO guideline. Dutch Institute for Quality Assurance. *Ned Tijdschr Geneeskd* **143**, 2461–2465. Guidelines with regard to the treatment of urinary tract infections in general. Investigations for anatomical abnormalities and impaired renal function are advocated in recurrent urinary tract infections. **IV C**

2 Romero R, Oyarzum E, Mazor M *et al.* (1989) Meta-analysis of the relationship between asymptomatic bacteriuria and pre-term delivery. *Obstet Gynecol* **73**, 576–582. Early meta-analysis, which could be criticized by present-day standards as no unpublished series were included. Otherwise, the search strategy and criteria for inclusion/exclusion are well described. Paper includes a meta-analysis of available randomized trials and additional meta-analysis of cohort studies. These meta-analyses demonstrate a clear relationship between asymptomatic bacteriuria and low birthweight (a surrogate for prematurity at the time of the original studies), and a clear reduction in this rate of low birthweight when these women were treated with antibiotics as opposed to placebo. **Ia A**

3 Smaill F (2001) Antibiotics for asymptomatic bacteriuria in pregnancy (Cochrane review). In: *Cochrane database of systematic reviews*, issue 2. Oxford: Update Software, CD000490 Meta-analysis of 14 randomized trials of antibiotics versus placebo. Antibiotics were effective in clearing asymptomatic bacteriuria (OR 0.07, 95% CI 0.05–0.10). There was a statistically significant reduction in pyelonephritis (OR 0.25, 95% CI 0.19 to 0.32), and in preterm delivery/low birthweight (OR 0.60, CI 95% 0.45–0.80). **Ia A**

4 Krcmery S, Hromec J, Demesova D (2001) Treatment of lower urinary tract infection in pregnancy. *Int J Antimicrob Agents* **17**, 279–282. Comparative study of single-dose treatment with 3 g fosfomycin–trometamol versus a 3-day course of 400 mg ceftibuten orally for acute cystitis, significant bacteriuria (≥10^3 CFU/ml) or pyuria during pregnancy. It was found that acute cystitis in pregnant women using a single-dose of fosfomycin–trometamol was equally effective as the 3-day course of oral ceftibuten. **Ib A**

5 Villar J, Lydon-Rochelle MT, Gulmezoglu AM *et al.* (2000) Duration of treatment for asymptomatic bacteriuria during pregnancy. In: *Cochrane database of systematic reviews*, issue 2. Oxford: Update Software, CD000491. Meta-analysis on the efficacy of single-dose versus conventional antibiotic treatment in pregnant women with asymptomatic bacteriuria. It comprises eight randomized and quasi-randomized trials involving over 400 women, comparing single dose treatment with 4–7-day treatments. It is noted that the trials were generally of poor quality with significant heterogeneity between the results. There was no difference in 'no-cure' rate between single-dose and short-course (4–7-day) treatment for asymptomatic bacteriuria in pregnant women, recurrent asymptomatic bacteriuria, preterm births and pyelonephritis. Longer-duration treatment was associated with an increase in reports of adverse effects (RR 0.53, 95% CI 0.31–0.91). It was concluded that, because single-dose treatment has lower cost and increases compliance, this should be explored in a properly sized RCT. **Ia A**

6 Angel JL, O'Brien WF, Finan MA *et al.* (1990) Acute pyelonephritis in pregnancy: a prospective study of oral versus intravenous antibiotic therapy. *Obstet Gynecol* **76**, 28–32. Prospective randomized trial of oral versus intravenous antibiotics in 90 pregnant women with acute pyelonephritis. Bacteremia mandated IV therapy in 13 women. There was no difference in outcome between the two groups. The study outcome was not analyzed by intention to treat. As such this study does not support the use of intravenous antibiotics as cited in the summary of management options; it does support the use of oral antibiotics for the treatment of pyelonephritis in pregnancy in the absence of bacteremia. **Ib A**

7 Patterson TF, Andriole VT (1997) Detection, significance, and therapy of bacteriuria in pregnancy. Update in the managed health care era. *Infect Dis Clin North Am* **11**, 593–608. Review on the management of pregnant women with asymptomatic bacteriuria. It is stated that all pregnant women should be screened at the first antenatal visit and short-course therapy should be given if positive. Clearance of bacteriuria should be documented after therapy is complete. All women with persistent bacteriuria or recurrent infection should have follow-up cultures and a urological evaluation after delivery. **IV C**

24.12 Intra-amniotic infections (chorioamnionitis)

Ed Howarth

Management option		Quality of evidence	Strength of recommendation	References
Prenatal, labor and delivery	Parenteral antibiotics (broad-spectrum or combination if severe sepsis)	III Ib	B A	1,2 3
	and Deliver (cesarean only for normal obstetric indications)	III	B	4
	No clear evidence whether a time limit for deliveries is advisable	III	B	3,5
Postnatal	Continue antibiotic therapy (duration determined by clinical course and severity)	Ib III	A B	4 2
	Practices vary with respect to newborn management (many would consider the minimum to be antibiotic therapy until negative swabs obtained)	–	✔	–

References

1 Gilstrap LC, Levani KJ, Cox SM *et al.* (1988) Intra-partum treatment of acute chorioamnionitis: impact on neonatal sepsis. *Am J Obstet Gynecol* **159**: 579–583. Observational study of 312 women with acute chorioamnionitis, 152 receiving antibiotics before delivery, 90 after and 70 not at all. In neonates of 35 weeks gestation or more, antibiotics reduced the incidence of positive neonatal blood cultures for group B streptococci (0/133 vs 8/140). Timing of antibiotic administration did not affect maternal outcome. **III B**

2 Sperling R S, Ramamurthy RS, Gibbs RS (1987) A comparison of intrapartum versus immediate postpartum

treatment of intra-amniotic infection. *Obstet Gynecol* **70**, 861–865. Observational study of 257 women with a clinically diagnosed intra-amniotic infection. All women received penicillin (or a first-generation cephalosporin if penicillin-allergic) and gentamicin. 82% received intrapartum treatment, 18% postpartum. The rate of neonatal sepsis was 2.8% in the intrapartum-treated group versus 19.6% in the postpartum-treated group, $p < 0.001$. Although neonatal mortality did not reach significance because of the small numbers, there was a relative risk of neonatal mortality of 5 in the postpartum-treated group. **III B**

3 Gibbs RS, Castillo MS, Rodgers PJ (1980) Management of acute chorioamnionitis. *Am J Obstet Gynecol* **136**, 709–713. Review article combined with a cohort study. Clinical acute chorioamnionitis occurred in 171 women with a perinatal mortality of 140 per 1000. Cesarean section (38%) did not show a clear perinatal benefit but had an increased maternal morbidity. No critical diagnosis-to-delivery interval could be identified. There was no long-term follow-up of the infants. **III B**

4 Gibbs RS, Dinsmoor MJ, Newton ER *et al.* (1988) A randomized trial of intrapartum versus immediate postpartum treatment of women with intra-amniotic infection. *Obstet Gynecol* **72**, 823–828. Randomized trial of 48 women with intra-amniotic infection to either intrapartum or postpartum penicillin and gentamicin. Exclusion criteria and method of randomization (sealed envelopes) are adequately described. There were 26 women in the intrapartum arm, 22 in the postpartum arm (3 of these were lost to protocol violations, leaving 19). Analysis not done on intention to treat, just those who had correct management. The study was stopped early by the Safety Committee. The rate of neonatal sepsis was 0% in the intrapartum group and 21% in the postpartum group. Maternal morbidity was significantly reduced in the intrapartum-treated group. **Ib A**

5 Garite TJ, Freeman RK (1982) Chorioamnionitis in the preterm gestation. *Obstet Gynecol* **59**, 539–545. Observational study of preterm premature rupture of the membranes in which 47 out of 251 (19%) cases developed chorioamnionitis. Length of fever did not correlate with neonatal outcome but onset of maternal pyrexia prior to labor was associated with worse outcomes than onset during labor. This study provides some observational evidence for performing amniocentesis for predicting subsequent chorioamnionitis, endometritis and neonatal infection. **III B**

24.13 Sexually transmitted diseases

Ed Howarth

Syphilis

Management option		Quality of evidence	Strength of recommendation	References
Prepregnancy	Identify and treat prior to pregnancy	III	B	1
	Contact tracing and treatment	IV	C	2
	Confirm response with serial serology	IV	C	3
Prenatal	Routine serological screening in early pregnancy	III	B	1,4
	Treat all with lesions positive for *Treponema pallidum* (rare)	–	✓	–
	Probably safer to treat all women with positive serology even if history suggests they have been treated in the past	–	✓	–
	Drug treatment	III IV	B C	5 6,7
	Consider desensitization for penicillin allergy	III IV	B C	5 6,7
	Contact tracing and treatment	IV	C	2
	Confirm response with serial serology	IV	C	2
Postnatal	Baby requires pediatric evaluation for evidence of infection	III	B	4
	Continued surveillance for maternal response to therapy	IV	C	2,3,6

References

1 Anonymous (2001) Congenital syphilis – United States, 2000. *Morb Mortal Wkly Rep* **50**, 573–577. Report on the effects of the National Syphilis Elimination Plan in the USA, initiated in 1999, to reduce the incidence of primary and secondary syphilis in adults to less than 0.4 cases per 100000 and congenital syphilis to less than 40 per 100000 live births in the year 2000. Between 1997 and 2000 the incidence of congenital syphilis declined substantially. It was concluded that elimination of congenital syphilis is feasible and to achieve this collaborative efforts are needed among health-care providers, health insurers, policymakers and the public. **III B**

2 Van Voorst Vader PC (1998) Syphilis management and treatment. *Dermatol Clin* **4**, 699–711. Review article on syphilis and human immunodeficiency virus infection. Laboratory tests for syphilis and false-positive and false-negative serological reactions are discussed. The diagnosis and management of neurosyphilis, ocular, cardiovascular and congenital syphilis are addressed, as well as management of syphilis patients allergic to penicillin and the Jarisch–Herxheimer reaction. Role of partner and contact tracing is discussed. **IV C**

3 Erbelding E, Quinn TC (1997) The impact of antimicrobial resistance on the treatment of sexually transmitted diseases. *Infect Dis Clin North Am* **4**, 889–903. Review article on antimicrobial resistance and sexually transmitted diseases. Although there is no evidence of such resistance in syphilis, intensive treatment and follow-up to ensure effectiveness is advocated. **IV C**

4 Martin D, Bertrand J, McKegney C *et al.* (2001) Congenital syphilis surveillance and newborn evaluation in a low-incidence state. *Arch Pediatr Adolesc Med* **155**, 140–144. Retrospective study on congenital syphilis and prenatal syphilis screening in 80 newborns who were at risk for congenital syphilis. It was concluded that standardized protocols should be adhered to in the evaluation and management of at-risk newborns. Prenatal screening and testing at delivery with adequate follow-up are critical to reduce congenital syphilis. **III B**

5 Wendel GD, Stark BJ, Janison RB *et al.* (1985) Penicillin allergy and desensitization in serious infections during pregnancy. *N Engl J Med* **312**, 1229–1232. Observational study of 15 penicillin-allergic women who had infections best treated by penicillin – 13 with syphilis, one with *Listeria* infection and one with *Streptococcus viridans* endocarditis. Oral desensitization was undertaken in all women successfully and no extracutaneous reactions were detected. All infections were cured, although the pregnancy complicated by *Listeria* infection resulted in first-trimester miscarriage. **III B**

6 Genc M, Ledger WJ (2000) Syphilis in pregnancy. *Sex Transm Infect* **76**, 73–79. Review on screening for syphilis, concluding that first-trimester screening with nontreponemal tests such as rapid plasma reagin (RPR) or the venereal disease research laboratory (VDRL) test, combined with further testing of positives with treponemal tests such as the fluorescent treponemal antibody absorption (FTA-ABS) assay, is cost-effective. Those at risk should be retested in the third trimester. Treatment during pregnancy should be with penicillin and desensitization of patients who are allergic to penicillin before treatment is advocated. Despite appropriate treatment, 14% will have a fetal death or deliver infected infants. Surveillance of treatment is important, as the Jarich–Herxheimer reaction may cause fetal distress and uterine contractions. **IV C**

7 CDC (1998) 1998 Guideline for treatment of sexually transmitted diseases. *Morbid Mortal Wkly Rep* **47** (No. RR-1), 1–116. Review article containing small section specific to syphilis in pregnancy, pp. 40–41. Recommendations based on expert committee consensus. Penicillin considered the only known safe treatment in pregnancy. Where penicillin-allergic, desensitization is recommended. **IV C**

Gonorrhea

Management option		Quality of evidence	Strength of recommendation	References
Prepregnancy	Identify and treat prior to pregnancy	–	✔	–
	Contact tracing and treatment	–	✔	–
	Confirm response with follow-up swabs	–	✔	–
Prenatal	Give antibiotics	IIa Ia	A A	1 2
	Contact tracing and treatment	–	✔	–
	Exclude *Chlamydia* infection	IIa	B	1,3
Postnatal	Screening of newborn for infection, although most units treat anyway	III	B	4
	Confirm cure with follow-up swabs	–	✔	–

References

1 Christmas JT, Wendel GD, Bawdon RE *et al.* (1989) Concomitant infection with *Neisseria gonorrhoeae* and *Chlamydia trachomatis* in pregnancy. *Obstet Gynecol* **74**, 295–298. Case-control study comparing the prevalence of endocervical chlamydial infections in pregnant women with gonorrhea against a control group of pregnant women without. The control group was not matched, and was older, more often married and more often Caucasian. The prevalence of chlamydial infection was 46% in the study group and 5% in the control group. Erythromycin 500 mg four times daily provided an excellent cure rate without intolerable side effects. **IIa B**

2 Brocklehurst P (2000) Interventions for treating gonorrhea in pregnancy. In: *Cochrane database of systematic reviews*, issue 4. Oxford: Update Software. Meta-analysis of two randomized trials of different antibiotic regimens for the treatment of gonorrhea in pregnancy. Amoxicillin with probenecid or spectinomycin or ceftriaxone had similar rates of microbiological cure. **Ia A**

3 Christmas JT, Wendel GD, Bawdon RE *et al.* (1989) Concomitant infection with *Neisseria gonorrhoeae* and *Chlamydia trachomatis* in pregnancy. *Obstet Gynecol* **74**, 295–298. Case-control study on concomitant infection with gonorrhea and chlamydial infection in pregnant patients. *C. trachomatis* in patients with gonorrhea occurred significantly more often than in the control population (46 vs 5%; $p < 0.001$). **IIa B**

4 Hammerschlag MR, Cummings C, Robin PM *et al.* (1989) Efficacy of neonatal ocular prophylaxis for the prevention of chlamydial and gonococcal conjunctivitis. *N Engl J Med* **320**, 769–772. Prospective comparative study on the efficacy of silver nitrate drops, erythromycin ophthalmic ointment or tetracycline ophthalmic ointment as prophylaxis against neonatal chlamydial and gonococcal conjunctivitis in 12431 infants. There was no significant difference between the groups in the prevention of gonococcal ophthalmia or chlamydial conjunctivitis. It is concluded that better management of maternal chlamydial infection is required to reduce chlamydial conjunctivitis in the newborn and that neonatal gonococcal ophthalmia could be better prevented by improved prenatal screening and treatment of maternal gonococcal infection. **III B**

Chlamydial infection

Management option		Quality of evidence	Strength of recommendation	References
Prepregnancy	Identify and treat with doxycycline or ofloxacin	III	B	1
	Contact tracing and treatment	III	B	2
Prenatal	If diagnosed, give antibiotics	Ia	A	3
	Contact tracing and treatment	IV	C	2
Postnatal	Prophylactic antibiotic eye ointment to newborn (erythromycin or tetracycline)	III	B	4

References

1 Catalan F, Milovanovic A, Prouteau C *et al.* (1998) Evaluation of in vitro activity of ofloxacin against 73 strains of *Chlamydia trachomatis* isolated from gynecologic infections. *Pathol Biol (Paris)* **46**, 144–146. *In-vitro* activity of ofloxacin, levofloxacin, ciprofloxacin, doxycycline, erythromycin and roxithromycin was determined against 73 strains of *Chlamydia trachomatis*. The MIC_{90} was 0.4, 0.1, 1.6, 0.2, 1.6 and 0.1 mg/l respectively. 100% of strains were susceptible to ofloxacin, roxithromycin and doxycycline. Erythromycin and ciprofloxacin had a lower *in-vitro* activity against *C. trachomatis*. **III B**

2 Jolly AM, Muth SQ, Wylie JL *et al.* (2001) Sexual networks and sexually transmitted infections: a tale of two cities. *J Urban Health* **78**, 433–445. A social network analysis on transmission of sexually transmitted infections comparing three different geographical areas in the USA. On the basis of the results it is suggested that small, loosely linked networks peripheral to the core group of people with high-risk behavior are responsible for *Chlamydia* remaining endemic. **III B**

3 Brocklehurst P, Rooney G (2000) Interventions for treating genital chlamydial trachomatis infection in pregnancy. In: *Cochrane database of systematic reviews*, issue 4. Oxford: Update Software. Review of 11 randomized trials comparing antibiotic regimens for the treatment of genital chlamydial infection in pregnancy. Amoxicillin appears as effective as erythromycin but is better tolerated. Clindamycin and azithromycin also appear to be effective, although the trials are small. **Ia A**

4 Hammerschlag MR, Cummings C, Robin PM *et al.* (1989) Efficacy of neonatal ocular prophylaxis for the prevention of chlamydial and gonococcal conjunctivitis. *N Engl J Med* **320**, 769–772. Prospective comparative

study on the efficacy of silver nitrate drops, erythromycin ophthalmic ointment or tetracycline ophthalmic ointment as prophylaxis against neonatal chlamydial and gonococcal conjunctivitis in 12431 infants. There was no significant difference between the groups in the prevention of gonococcal ophthalmia or chlamydial conjunctivitis. It is concluded that better management of maternal chlamydial infection is required to reduce chlamydial conjunctivitis in the newborn and that neonatal gonococcal ophthalmia could be better prevented by improved prenatal screening and treatment of maternal gonococcal infection. **III B**

Human papilloma virus

Management option		Quality of evidence	Strength of recommendation	References
Prepregnancy	Identify and treat lesions	–	✔	–
	Counseling about risks	IIa	B	1,2
Prenatal	Topical 80% trichloroacetic acid	III	B	3
	Cryotherapy	IV	C	4
	Electrodiathermy	IV	C	4
	Laser vaporization	III	B	3
	Excision	IV	C	4
	Contraindicated preparations: ❑ Podophyllum ❑ 5-fluorouracil ❑ Interferon	 IV – IV	 C ✔ C	 4 – 5
Labor and delivery	Avoid treatment at delivery	–	✔	–
	Cesarian section may be necessary	III	B	6
Postnatal	Vigilance for secondary infection	–	✔	–

References

1 Tenti P, Zappatore R, Migliora P *et al.* (1999) Perinatal transmission of human papillomavirus from gravidas with latent infections. *Obstet Gynecol* **93**, 475–479. Prospective study on perinatal human papilloma virus (HPV) transmission from mothers with latent infections to the oropharyngeal mucosa of their infants in 711 cases. The vertical transmission rate was 30% (95% CI 15.9–47). There was no transmission in all 11 cases, in which rupture of membranes (ROM) was less than 2 h before delivery. When ROM was 2–4 h and more than 4 h before delivery, transmission occurred in 7/21 and 4/5 cases. It was concluded that the time between ROM and delivery appears to be a critical factor in transmission. **III B**

2 Kjellberg L, Hallmars G, Ahren AM *et al.* (2000) Smoking, diet, pregnancy and oral contraceptive use as risk factors for cervical intra-epithelial neoplasia in relation to human papillomavirus infection. *Br J Cancer* **82**, 1332–1338. Case-control study on the effects of smoking, nutrition, parity and oral contraceptive use as independent cofactors of human papilloma virus (HPV) infection in cervical carcinogenesis in 137 women with high-grade cervical intraepithelial neoplasia and 253 healthy age-matched women. Pregnancy was found to be a risk factor in the multivariate analysis ($p < 0.0001$). Prolonged oral contraceptive use and sexual history were associated with cervical intraepithelial neoplasia (CIN) 2–3 in univariate analysis but not after taking HPV into account. Smoking was associated with CIN 2–3 (OR 2.6, 95% CI 1.7–4.0), and this was not affected by adjusting for HPV. **IIa B**

3 Schwartz DB, Greenberg MD, Daoud Y *et al.* (1988) Genital condylomas in pregnancy: use of trichloroacetic acid and laser therapy. *Am J Obstet Gynecol* **158**, 1407–1416. Describes itself as a case-control series, but this refers to pregnancy outcome only. Effectively a retrospective observational series concerning the treatment of 32 women with genital condylomas in pregnancy, with this combined therapy. 31/32 were controlled with this therapy. **III B**

4 Eskelinen A, Mashkilleyson N (1987) Optimum treatment of genital warts. *Drugs* **34**, 599–603. Review advocating podophyllin 20% as first-line treatment of condylomata acuminata, but mentions pregnancy as a contraindication for its use. Other treatment modalities addressed are surgical removal, electrocautery, cryosurgery, laser treatment, topical application of 5-fluorouracil and intralesional or systemic use of interferons. **IV C**

5 Piper JM, Wen TT, Xenakis EM (2001) Interferon therapy in primary care. *Prim Care Update Obstet Gynecol*

8, 163–169. Review on interferon therapy including a wide variety of malignancies, chronic granulomatous disease skin conditions (human-papilloma-virus-related and keloids), viral infections, multiple sclerosis and myeloproliferative disorders. Some use of interferon therapy during pregnancy without adverse maternal and neonatal outcomes is described. It is noted that interferon therapy during early pregnancy is not an indication for termination of pregnancy. **IV C**

6 Wang X, Zhu Q, Rao H (1998) Maternal–fetal transmission of human papillomavirus. *Chin Med J (Engl)* **111**, 726–727. Prospective study on the maternal–fetal transmission of human papilloma virus (HPV) in 73 third-trimester pregnancies. It was found that the maternal–fetal transmission rate of HPV was 50% (7/14) in spontaneous vaginal deliveries and 33.3% (4/12) in cesarean sections. It was concluded that HPV can be transmitted through the placenta during pregnancy and through the genital tract during delivery. **III B**

Trichomonal infection

Management option		Quality of evidence	Strength of recommendation	References
Prepregnancy and prenatal	Treat patient and partner systemically with a nitroimidazole antibiotic (metronidazole, ornidazole, tinidazole)	Ib	A	1

Reference

1 Gulmezoglu AM (2000) Interventions for trichomoniasis in pregnancy. In: *Cochrane database of systematic reviews*, issue 4. Oxford: Update Software. Analysis of a single randomized trial of metronidazole versus no treatment. Parasitological cure occurred in over 90% of the treated group; the relative risk of persistent infection was 0.11. No effect on pregnancy outcome can be identified from this trial. **Ib A**

24.14 Candidiasis

Ed Howarth

Management option		Quality of evidence	Strength of recommendation	References
Prepregnancy and prenatal	Treat topically with an imidazole (miconazole, clotrimazole, terconazole, butoconazole)	Ia	A	1
	Ketoconazole and fluconazole are best avoided in pregnancy except for severe systemic infection	-	✓	-
	However, fluconazole appears not to be teratogenic in the first trimester	IIa	B	2,3

References

1 Young GL, Jewell D (2000) Topical treatment for vaginal candidiasis in pregnancy. In: *Cochrane database of systematic reviews*, issue 4. Oxford: Update Software. 12 randomized trials for the treatment of vaginal candidiasis in pregnancy were included in this meta-analysis. Clotrimazole was more effective than both placebo, OR 0.14, and nystatin, OR 0.21. Treatment for 7 days was more effective than treatment for 3–4 days, which in turn was more effective than single-dose treatment. **Ia A**

2 Sorensen HT, Nielsen GL, Olesen C *et al.* (1999) Risk of malformations and other outcomes in children exposed to fluconazole in utero. *Br J Clin Pharmacol* **48**, 234–238. Retrospective study on the effect of fluconazole treatment on pregnancy outcome in 165 women compared to 13 327 women who did not take fluconazole. Malformations were seen in 3.3% (n = 4) of 121 women who had used fluconazole in the first trimester and 5.2% (697 cases) in the control group (OR 0.65, 95% CI 0.24–1.77). There was no elevated risk of preterm delivery or low birthweight. It was concluded that single-dose fluconazole treatment before conception or during pregnancy does not increase the risk of congenital malformations, low birthweight or preterm birth. **IIa B**

3 Jick SS (1999) Pregnancy outcomes after maternal exposure to fluconazole. *Pharmacotherapy* **19**, 221–222. Retrospective case-control study on the pregnancy outcome in 234 women exposed to fluconazole, 492 exposed to a topically administered azole preparation, 88 exposed to an oral azole preparation other than fluconazole and 1629 not exposed to any of these agents during the first trimester of pregnancy. It was found that fluconazole exposure in the first trimester of pregnancy does not increase the risk of congenital disorders in infants. **IIa B**

24.15 Group B streptococcal infection

Ed Howarth

Management option		Quality of evidence	Strength of recommendation	References
Prepregnancy	No benefit in treatment of group B streptococcus (GBS) carrier before pregnancy	–	✔	–
Prenatal, labor and delivery – screening-based approach	Universal GBS screening at 35–37 weeks gestation	IV	C	1
	Offer all colonized women intrapartum chemoprophylaxis (ICP)	Ia	A	2,3
	If screening results unknown, offer ICP if risk factors (intrapartum fever >38°C or rupture of membranes >18h, or anticipated delivery <37 weeks)	IV	C	1
	Also offer ICP if history of a previously infected infant, or GBS bacteriuria in the current pregnancy	IV	C	1
Prenatal, labor and delivery – risk-factor-based approach	Offer ICP only if risk factors are present:	Ib	A	4,5
	❑ Previously infected infant	IV	C	1
	❑ GBS bacteriuria in the current pregnancy	IV	C	1
	❑ Anticipated delivery before 37 weeks gestation	IV III	C B	1 6
	❑ Rupture of membranes more than18h	III Ib	B A	6 5
	❑ Intrapartum fever above 38°C	IV	C	1
Recommended prophylaxis regimens	Penicillin G: 5mU i.v. followed by 2.5mU i.v. every 4h	Ib	A	5
	or			
	Ampicillin: 2g i.v. every 6h	Ia	A	2
	Clindamycin 900mg i.v. every 8h	–	✔	–
	or			
	Erythromycin: 500mg i.v. every 6h	III	B	7
	Immunization against GBS needs to be further evaluated	–	✔	–
Postnatal	Chemoprophylaxis need not be continued after delivery	–	✔	–
	Diagnosis of postpartum endometritis in a GBS-positive woman should be treated with broad-spectrum antibiotics	–	✔	–

References

1 Centers for Disease Control (1996) Prevention of perinatal Group B streptococcal disease: a public health perspective. *Morbid Mortal Wkly Rep* **45** (No. RR-7), 1–24. Review article and guidelines offering alternate screening and management strategies. These strategies are based on either universal screening or treatment of defined at-risk groups. The use of one of two prevention strategies is advocated. In the first, intrapartum antibiotic prophylaxis is given to group-B-streptococcus (GBS) carriers detected through screening at 35–37 weeks gestation and to women who develop premature onset of labor or rupture of membranes at less than 37 weeks gestation. In the second strategy, intrapartum antibiotic prophylaxis is given to those who have one or more risk conditions at the time of labor or membrane rupture. Issues addressed include laboratory facilities, risk conditions indicating the need for intrapartum antibiotics and the management of newborns whose mothers receive intrapartum antibiotic prophylaxis for GBS disease. **IV C**

2 Allen UD, Navas L, King SM (1993) Effectiveness of intrapartum penicillin prophylaxis in preventing early-onset group B streptococcal infection: results of a meta-analysis. *Can Med Assoc J* **149**, 1659–1665. Meta-analysis combining four randomized trials and three cohort studies. Pooled data show a 30-fold risk reduction for early-onset neonatal group B streptococcal disease when penicillin/ampicillin prophylaxis used. Magnitude of reduction did not differ between those with risk factors and those without. **Ia A**

3 Smaill F (2000) Intrapartum antibiotics for Group B streptococcal disease. In: *Cochrane database of systematic reviews*, issue 4. Oxford: Update Software. Meta-analysis of five trials comparing intrapartum antibiotic treatment with no treatment. A statistically significant reduction in infant colonization and early onset group B streptococcal disease was observed in the treated group. The difference in mortality does not reach significance. **Ia A**

4 Boyer KM, Gotoff SP (1986) Prevention of early onset neonatal group B streptococcal disease with selective intrapartum chemoprophylaxis. *N Engl J Med* **314**, 1665–1669. Randomized trial of 180 women with prenatal group B streptococcal colonization and identified risk factors. Patients were randomized to either intravenous ampicillin or no treatment. Randomization adequately described – opaque sealed envelopes with assignments generated by random number tables. Subjects in the control group who developed intrapartum fever were dropped from the study and treated with ampicillin. Neonatal bacteremia occurred in none of 85 treated with ampicillin versus 5 of 79 in the control group, $p = 0.024$. **Ib A**

5 Tuppurainen N, Hallman M (1989) Prevention of neonatal group B streptococcal disease: intrapartum detection and chemoprophylaxis of heavily colonized parturients. *Obstet Gynecol* **73**, 583–587. Randomized study – method of randomization sequential sealed envelopes. Rapid latex agglutination test to detect heavy colonization of group B streptococcus (GBS). 199 test-positive women entered into study, 88 receiving intravenous penicillin and 111 receiving no treatment. GBS neonatal disease occurred in 1 (1.1%) in the treated group and 10 (9.0%) in the untreated group, $p < 0.01$. The incidence of GBS disease in the offspring of women with negative results was 0.07%. Of these 6 infants, 4 were premature and all had rupture of membranes greater than 24 h. Maternal outcomes not described. **Ib A**

6 Morales WJ, Lim D (1987) Reduction of group B streptococcal maternal and neonatal infections in preterm pregnancies with premature rupture of membranes through a rapid identification test. *Am J Obstet Gynecol* **157**, 13–16. Observational study comparing women admitted with preterm premature rupture of membranes, and identified as having group B streptococcus (GBS) colonization, treated with intravenous ampicillin or not. There were 260 women, 84 of whom were GBS-positive. Of the 36 who received antibiotics there were no cases of chorioamnionitis or neonatal sepsis. Of the 48 who were untreated there were 11 (23%) cases of chorioamnionitis and 13 (27%) of neonatal sepsis. Even light colonization resulted in significant rates of maternal and neonatal infection. **III B**

7 Garland SM, Fliegner JR (1991) Group B streptococcus (GBS) and neonatal infections: the case for intrapartum chemoprophylaxis. *Aust N Z J Obstet Gynecol* **31**, 119–122. Observational study comparing regimens in the public hospitals – screening for group B streptococcus (GBS) at 32 weeks and intrapartum intravenous penicillin, or erythromycin for those with penicillin allergy – with those in the private hospital – no screening. In the public hospital there were 16 cases of GBS neonatal infection and one death in 30197 live births, none occurring in women who were treated asymptomatic carriers. In the private hospitals there were 27 infections with 8 deaths in 26915 livebirths. Maternal outcomes were not reported. **III B**

24.16 Tuberculosis

Ed Howarth

Management option		Quality of evidence	Strength of recommendation	References
Prepregnancy	Screen those at increased risk	IV	C	1
	Treat those who are positive	IV III Ib	C B A	1 2 3
Prenatal	Confirm diagnosis with ❑ Tuberculin skin test (PPD) ❑ Chest radiograph ❑ Three sputum samples	 IV IV III	 C C B	 4 4 5

Management option		Quality of evidence	Strength of recommendation	References
Prenatal (cont'd)	If positive PPD, and clinically and radiologically positive, commence treatment	III	B	2
	Follow-up cultures and clinical monitoring for response to therapy	–	✔	–
	If PPD positive but negative clinically and radiologically, consider isoniazid prophylaxis (risk factors, age, liver function and medical history will influence decision)	IV	C	4
	Monitor liver function in patients taking isoniazid	III	B	6
Labor and delivery	Special anesthetic precautions if general anesthesia	–	✔	–
Postnatal	Continue treatment until course completed	–	✔	–
	Breastfeeding is not contraindicated	IV	C	7
	If mother has been treated, baby should receive isoniazid-resistant BCG and a course of prophylactic isoniazid	–	✔	–
	Some antituberculosis agents may reduce efficacy of oral contraceptives	–	✔	–

References

1 Davies PD (2001) Comparison of international guidelines on the control and prevention of tuberculosis. *Monaldi Arch Chest Dis* **56**, 74–78. Review on guidelines from several countries and organizations on the control of tuberculosis. All guidelines propagate identification and treatment of patients with disease, screening of high-risk groups and preventive therapy for selected individuals with latent tuberculosis infection. Guidelines only differ in practical details. **IV C**

2 Schaefer G, Zervoudakis IA, Fuchs FF *et al.* (1975) Pregnancy and pulmonary tuberculosis. *Obstet Gynecol* **46**, 706–715. Observational study, mixed with opinion, covering 1565 deliveries of 1588 infants at the New York Hospital from January 1933 through December 1972. There were no cases of congenital infection. Newer antituberculous drugs had slowed the number of women with progressive disease from 4% to less than 1%. Standard therapy was now isoniazid and ethambutol. Pregnant women did not fare any worse than their nonpregnant counterparts. **III B**

3 Mwandumba HC, Squire SB (2001) Fully intermittent dosing with drugs for treating tuberculosis in adults (Cochrane Review). In: *Cochrane database of systematic reviews*, issue 4. Oxford: Update Software, CD000970. Literature search for (quasi-)randomized trials comparing the effectiveness of intermittent versus continuous treatment with rifampicin in pulmonary tuberculosis aiming to perform a meta-analysis. Only one trial involving 399 patients was included. It was concluded that presently there is no evidence to prefer one regimen over the other and that larger randomized studies are required to establish the equivalence of fully intermittent, short-course chemotherapy with daily regimens. **Ib A**

4 Ortona L, Fantoni M (1998) Tuberculin skin test and chemoprophylaxis of tuberculosis. *Rays* **23**, 218–224. Review underlining the value of the tuberculin test for screening purposes. It is stated that prophylaxis is best performed with isoniazid (300 mg/daily for 12 months) in cases with a tuberculin test larger than 5 mm; recent contacts with patients with infective tuberculosis; chest X-ray indicative for old fibrotic lesions, human immunodeficiency virus (HIV) infection; subjects with a tuberculin test smaller than 10 mm who are HIV-negative; drug addicts; and in clinical conditions at high risk for tuberculosis (e.g. silicosis, hematological malignancy, immunosuppression). **IV C**

5 Palmer DL, Soo Hoo GH, Sopher RL (1981) Clinical determinants of tuberculosis screening. *South Med J* **74**, 170–174. Retrospective control study on screening methods for tuberculosis in 79 patients with active tuberculosis and 226 patients with negative cultures. Those variables that distinguished the active from the nonactive form were: history, abnormal pulmonary examination, abnormal chest X-ray, positive skin test (PPD). It was concluded that signs and symptoms are good screening variables and combined with chest X-rays may be followed by cultures as a confirmatory test. **III B**

6 Stuart RL, Wilson J, Grayson ML (1999) Isoniazid toxicity in health care workers. *Clin Infect Dis* **28**, 895–897. Prospective study on clinical and liver toxicity of isoniazid in 83 health-care workers receiving a 6-month course. In 26 cases (76%), toxicity required cessation of treatment. Liver function abnormalities occurred in 14 subjects, with 8 requiring cessation of therapy. Monthly liver function testing and frequent review in those receiving isoniazid prophylactic therapy is recommended. **III B**

7 Centers for Disease Control (1993) Initial therapy for tuberculosis in the era of multidrug resistance. Recommendations of the advisory council for the elimination of tuberculosis. *Morbid Mortal Wkly Rep* **42** (RR-7), 1–8. Review article covering tuberculosis and human immunodeficiency virus infection. Current recommended first-line therapy in pregnancy is isoniazid, rifampicin and ethambutol. The use of streptomycin is discouraged during pregnancy because of VIIIth nerve problems in the fetus. The use of pyrazinamide is discouraged in view of limited safety data in pregnancy. Safety of breastfeeding on therapy well-established. **IV C**

24.17 Malaria

Ed Howarth

Management option		Quality of evidence	Strength of recommendation	References
Prepregnancy	If possible, women trying to conceive should avoid travel to endemic areas	–	✔	–
	If such travel is unavoidable, prophylaxis should be taken	Ia	A	1
Prenatal – general	If possible, pregnant women should avoid travel to endemic areas, especially those with drug-resistant strains	–	✔	–
	If such travel is unavoidable, prophylaxis should be taken	Ia	A	1,2
Prenatal – treatment	Antimalarial agents	Ia IIa III	A B B	2 3 4
	Supportive therapy (fluids, blood, glucose, anticonvulsants) – although lack of evidence from small number of RCTs	Ia	A	5
	Monitor electrolytes, renal and liver function, hematology	–	✔	–
	Monitor fetal growth and health	III	B	6,7

References

1 Lengeler C (2000) Insecticide treated bednets and curtains for preventing malaria. In: *Cochrane database of systematic reviews*, issue 4. Oxford: Update Software. A total of 18 randomized or quasi-randomized trials were combined in a meta-analysis. Insecticide-treated nets reduced the risk of infection (RR 0.83) and also reduced child mortality. Extrapolating from this, the use of insecticide-treated nets should be recommended to pregnant women traveling to endemic areas in order to reduce their risk of acquiring infection. **Ia A**

2 Garner P, Gulmezoglu AM (2000) Prevention versus treatment for malaria in pregnant women. In: *Cochrane database of systematic reviews*, issue 2. Oxford: Update Software,CD000169. Meta-analysis of 15 (quasi-) randomized trials on the effects of antimalarial interventions in pregnant women. The routine use of antimalarials was associated with fewer episodes of fever, maternal anemia and a higher birthweight in infants, particularly in primigravidae. There was no difference in perinatal, neonatal and infant mortality. However it was concluded that, in view of the costs and inputs required to effectively deliver widescale prophylaxis programs, a large simple placebo-controlled trial testing the impact of drugs given routinely on pregnancy outcome and neonatal/infant survival is needed. **Ia A**

3 Wolfe MS, Cordero JF (1985) Safety of chloroquine in chemo-suppression of malaria during pregnancy. *Br Med J* **290**, 1466–1467. Case-control study comparing rates of teratogenicity in 169 births to women who took chloroquine 300 mg weekly throughout pregnancy against 454 controls. No excess of congenital malformations was detected. The size of the study necessitated a fivefold increase in congenital malformations to be significant and this

shortcoming is acknowledged by the authors. However the study does support the hypothesis that chloroquine is not a strong teratogen. **IIa B**

4 Nosten F, Vincenti M, Simpson J *et al.* (1999) The effects of mefloquine treatment in pregnancy. *Clin Infect Dis* **28**, 808–815. Observational study that appears to indicate that mefloquine therapy is associated with an increased risk of stillbirth compared with quinine, other anti-malarials and no treatment. This needs to be interpreted with caution as most of the stillbirths are related to obstetric factors. **III B**

5 Mermikwu M, Logan K, Garner P (2000) Antipyretic measures for treating fever in malaria. In: *Cochrane database of systematic reviews*, issue 4. Oxford: Update Software. Meta-analysis of three randomized trials amounting to 128 adults and children. No conclusive evidence found to confirm or refute an impact of antipyretic measures on parasitemia or malarial illness. **Ia A**

6 Steketee RW, Nahlen BL, Parise ME *et al.* (2001) The burden of malaria in pregnancy in malaria-endemic areas. *Am J Trop Med Hyg* **64**(1–2 suppl), 28–35. Review of studies published between 1985 and 2000 on malaria and pregnancy complications such as maternal anemia, prematurity, intrauterine growth restriction, congenital infection and infant mortality. The population attributable risk (PAR) was calculated, which accounts for both the prevalence of the risk factors in the population and the magnitude of the associated risk for anemia, low birthweight and infant mortality. These were 3–15%, 8–70% and 3–8% respectively. The authors estimate that each year 75 000–200 000 infant deaths are associated with malaria infection in pregnancy. **III B**

7 Menendez C, Ordi J, Ismail MR *et al.* (2000) The impact of placental malaria on gestational age and birth weight. *J Infect Dis* **181**, 1740–1745. Observational study on the effects of malaria-related placental changes on birthweight and gestational age at delivery in 1177 mothers in Tanzania. 75.5% of placentas were infected. Only massive mononuclear intervillous inflammatory infiltration was associated with increased risk of low birthweight. Premature delivery was associated with maternal infected red blood cells and perivillous fibrin deposition. It was concluded that even in endemic areas malaria is a cause of low birthweight and premature delivery. **III B**

24.18 Lyme disease

Ed Howarth

Management option		Quality of evidence	Strength of recommendation	References
Prepregnancy	Minimize exposure risks in endemic regions	III	B	1,2
	Serological testing for women with history of exposure and/or symptoms consistent with infection	III	B	1,2
	Antibiotic treatment when diagnosis confirmed	IV	C	3
Prenatal	Continue treatment course	–	✔	–
	Monitor response to therapy	IV	C	4
Postnatal	Breastfeeding not contraindicated	–	✔	–

References

1 Williams CL, Strobino B, Weinstein A *et al.* (1995) Maternal Lyme disease and congenital malformations: a cord blood serosurvey in endemic and control areas. *Paediatr Perinat Epidemiol* **9**, 320–330. Large hospital control cohort study on pregnancy outcome of Lyme disease in over 5000 infants and their mothers. The mothers in an endemic hospital were five to 20 times more likely to have been exposed to *Borrelia burgdorferi* than those in the control hospital. The incidence of congenital cardiac malformations was significantly higher in the endemic group (OR 2.40; 95% CI 1.25–4.59) and polydactyly was significantly more common in the control group. There was no difference in the rate of major or minor malformations or mean birthweight by category of possible maternal exposure to Lyme disease or cord blood serology in the endemic group. This study was hampered by the small number of women who were actually exposed either in terms of serology or clinical history. **III B**

2 Strobino BA, Williams CL, Abid S *et al.* (1993) Lyme disease and pregnancy outcome: a prospective study of two thousand prenatal patients. *Am J Obstet Gynecol* **69**, 367–374. Prospective study on some 2000 women in an endemic area with a questionnaire survey and antibody testing for *Borrelia burgdorferi* at their booking visit and at delivery. It was concluded that Lyme disease around the time of conception or during pregnancy is not associated

with fetal death, prematurity or congenital malformations. Tick bites less than 3 years before conception, however, were significantly related to an increased risk of congenital malformations (this finding needs to be interpreted with caution, as reporting bias can not be ruled out). Seroconversion at delivery was very low, suggesting awareness amongst the population and health-care workers. **III B**

3 Rahn DW (1992) Antibiotic treatment of Lyme disease. *Postgrad Med* **91**, 57–64. Review article. Recommended regimens include oral amoxicillin for localized early disease, parenteral penicillin or ceftriaxone for other manifestations. No supporting evidence is cited, and it should be noted that the treatment of Lyme disease is controversial. **IV C**

4 Kalish R (1993) Lyme disease. *Rheum Dis Clin North Am* **19**, 399–426. Review on Lyme disease highlighting the possible difficulties in clinical and serological diagnosis. Antibiotic treatment is discussed, discouraging multiple repeated courses in nonresponders. Further studies on treatment during pregnancy are warranted. Prevention of Lyme disease is discussed. **IV C**

MATERNAL PROBLEMS

Chapter 25

Smoking and drugs

25.1 Cigarette smoking

Doris Campbell

Management option		Quality of evidence	Strength of recommendation	References
Staff trained to give advice and support		III	B	1
Advice to be given	Women to be told smoking puts their baby at risk, although other confounders may also play a role	III	B	2,3
	Stopping smoking by mid pregnancy will improve the outcome	III	B	3
	Reducing smoking is better than not reducing but not as good as stopping	III	B	3
	Repeated encouragement and especially designed programs increase the chance of success and reduces relapse	Ia IIb	A B	4 5
Factors affecting success	Low-risk, more educated, lighter smoker is more likely to stop	III	B	6
	Specific targeted intervention programs do have benefit for mother and newborn	Ia	A	7,8
	Hypnosis is not an intervention with benefit	IIa	B	9
	Acupuncture is of no proven benefit	Ia	A	10
	Women will under-report failure to stop smoking and smoking relapse	IIa	B	11

References

1 Sidorov J, Christianson M, Girdami S *et al.* (1997) A successful tobacco cessation program led by primary care nurses in a managed care setting. *Am J Manag Care* **3**, 207–214. Descriptive study of a tobacco cessation program sponsored by a health maintenance organization (HMO) and led by primary-care nurses at 20 primary care-clinics in north-eastern and central Pennsylvania. Of 1695 patients enrolled in the program from July 1993 to March 1996, 1140 completed 1 year of follow-up. Of these, 348 (30.5%) reported that they had stopped using tobacco. Among the 810 HMO enrollees who participated in the program the quit rate was 280 (34.6%); among the 330 non-HMO participants the quit rate was 69 (20.9%), a statistically significant difference ($p < 0.001$). For all patients, keeping more than four appointments with the program nurse was associated with a significantly higher likelihood of stopping (317/751, 42.2% vs 32/389, 8.2%; $p < 0.001$). **III B**

2 Hulse GK, English DR, Milne E *et al.* (1997) Maternal cocaine use and low birth weight newborns: a meta-analysis. *Addiction* **92**,1561–1570. Meta-analyses using only studies that had adjusted for tobacco smoking to estimate more precisely the effect of maternal cocaine use on birthweight. Results suggest that more frequent cocaine exposure was associated with a higher relative risk for low birthweight. Data from studies on mean reduction in birthweight produced a pooled estimate of 112 g (95% CI 62–161 g). The study suggests that maternal cocaine use causes low birthweight and that the effect is greater with heavier use. However, despite the adjustment for tobacco and the adjustment by some studies for other confounders such as race, maternal age, gravidity and socioeconomic status, it could be argued that other lifestyle factors not controlled for might account for the observed effects. **III B**

3 Nordstrom ML, Cnattingius S (1994) Smoking habits and birth weights in 2 successive births in Sweden. *Early Hum Dev* **37**, 195–204. Swedish population-based study considered the change in smoking habits from one pregnancy

to the next and the effect on infant birthweight. 61% were nonsmokers and 18% smokers in both pregnancies. 6% stopped between first and second and 3% commenced smoking. Information was missing for 12%. Women who stopped smoking were different in terms of age, level of education and degree of smoking. With respect to birthweight, among the women who stopped smoking, the second birthweight was the same as among women who had never smoked, however the first infant of women who stopped smoking were heavier than those of women who continued to smoke. **III B**

4 Dollan-Mullen P, Ramirez G, Groff JY *et al.* (1994) A meta-analysis of randomized trials of prenatal smoking cessation interventions. *Am J Obstet Gynecol* **171**, 1328–1334.Meta-analysis comparing smoking cessation and low birthweight outcomes, including 11 randomized controlled trials with objective validation of smoking status, four of which also measured rate of low birthweight. The risk ratio for smoking cessation ranged from 0.9 to 7.1 with a combined risk ratio after excluding the one outlier of 1.5 (CI 1.22–1.86). The risk of low birthweight was reduced in two studies that achieved a 50% increase in smoking cessation. The authors concluded that intervention was effective in increasing rates of stopping smoking during pregnancy. **Ib A**

5 Secker-Walker RH, Solomon LJ, Flynn BS *et al.* (1995) Smoking relapse prevention counseling during prenatal and early postnatal care. *Am J Prevent Med* **11**, 86–93.Study looking at those women who had stopped smoking by the time of their first antenatal visit. They were randomly assigned to receive routine advice or routine advice plus individual relapse counseling. Smoking status was assessed both by self-reporting and urinary cotinine/creatinine ratio. The relapse rates during pregnancy were not significantly different between the two groups but those based on cotinine/creatinine ratios were higher than those based on self-reporting. Long-term relapses were not significantly different between the two groups either. **IIb B**

6 Mas R, Escriba V, Colomer C (1996) Who quits smoking during pregnancy? *Scand J Soc Med* **24**, 102–106.Study of approximately 600 women in Valencia, Spain. 62% smoked before pregnancy. 28% gave up during pregnancy. Results indicate that those who gave up were older, with a higher level of education and lighter smokers initially. **III B**

7 Lancaster T, Stead LF (2000) Individual behavioural counselling for smoking cessation. In: *Cochrane database of systematic reviews*, issue 4. Oxford: Update Software. Cochrane review: the selection criteria included randomized or quasi-randomized trials with at least one treatment arm of face-to-face individual counseling from a health-care worker over and above routine clinical care. The outcome was stopping smoking at follow-up period of 6 months minimum. 11 trials were included. The conclusion was that smoking cessation counseling can help smokers to quit. The study, however, was not specifically addressing cessation of smoking in pregnancy. **Ia A**

8 Lumley J, Oliver S, Waters C *et al.* (2000) Interventions for promoting smoking cessation during pregnancy. In: *Cochrane database of systematic reviews*, issue 4. Oxford: Update Software.Cochrane review: the objective was to assess the effect of stopping-smoking programs on the health of the fetus and infant, on the mother and the family. 44 randomized and quasi-randomized trials were identified. The conclusion was that smoking cessation programs in pregnancy appeared to reduce smoking, low birthweight and preterm birth but no effect was detected for very low birthweight or perinatal mortality. **Ia A**

9 Valbo A, Eide T (1996) Smoking cessation in pregnancy: the effect of hypnosis in a randomized study. *Addict Behav* **21**, 29–35.An intervention study concluded that using hypnosis aimed at smoking cessation was not effective, with 10% giving up smoking in both the intervention and control groups. **IIa B**

10 White A R, Rampes H, Ernst E *et al.* (2000) Acupuncture for smoking cessation. In: *Cochrane database of systematic reviews*, issue 4. Oxford: Update Software.Cochrane review: compared randomized trials of a form of acupuncture with either sham acupuncture, no intervention or no intervention for smoking cessation. Not specifically in pregnant women. The conclusion was there was no clear evidence that acupuncture was effective for smoking cessation. **Ia A**

11 Kendrick JS, Zahniser SC, Miller N *et al.* (1995) Integrating smoking cessation into routine public prenatal care – the smoking cessation in pregnancy project. *Am J Public Health* **85**, 217–222.Study that was part of the WIC program for women receiving prenatal care and services in public clinics in the state health departments of Colorado, Maryland and Missouri. Clinics were randomly allocated to intervention or control status and the method of intervention was low-intensity. Smoking was assessed by questionnaire and cotinine measurement in urine. Self-reported quitting was higher in clinics with intervention programs than in control clinics but the cotinine-verified quitting rates were not different between the two. **IIa B**

25.2 Alcohol

Doris Campbell

Management option	Quality of evidence	Strength of recommendation	References
Obstetrics risks are related to exposure as well as other associated social factors	III IIa	B B	1,2 3
Multidisciplinary approach is valuable in the care of these families	III	B	4
Cessation help should be given to all 'at risk' groups	III IIa	B B	5 6
Some heavy drinkers will require specific counseling with support from outside agencies	IIa III	B B	6 7,8
Dietary advice and vitamin supplementation should be given	-	✓	-
Breast-feeding can be allowed but it may not be possible	-	✓	-

References

1 Kaskutas LA, Graves K (2001) Pre-pregnancy drinking: how drink size affects risk assessment. *Addiction* **96**, 1199–1209. In-person hour-long interviews gathered cross-sectional retrospective data about drinking before an index pregnancy at public clinics in the USA involving 324 women, 102 Native Americans, 185 African Americans and 34 Caucasians. For most beverages, the difference in milliliters between self-selected drink size and a standard size drink was significant, with the mean self-selected drink sizes ranging from 49% above the standard size (for beer) to 307% above the standard size (for spirits). Results suggest that true risk levels may be higher than previously thought. Also, risk drinkers presenting at prenatal clinics may be missed if screening protocols do not ask about drink size. **III B**

2 Kesmodel U, Olsen SF, Secher NJ (2001) [Does alcohol increase the risk of preterm delivery?] *Ugeskr Laeger* **163**, 4578–4582. Descriptive study of women attending routine antenatal care at Aarhus University Hospital, Denmark, from 1989–91 and 1992–96. Analyses included 18228 singleton pregnancies. For women with an alcohol intake of 1–2, 3–4, 5–9 and 10 or more drinks/week, the risk ratio (RR) of preterm delivery was 0.91 (95% CI 0.76–1.08), 0.86 (0.64–1.15), 0.89 (0.52–1.52) and 2.93 (1.52–5.63) respectively, compared with an intake of less than 1 drink/week at about 16 weeks of gestation, and 0.69 (0.56–0.86), 0.82 (0.60–1.13), 0.97 (0.58–1.64) and 3.56 (1.78–7.13) at about 30 weeks. Adjustment for smoking habits, caffeine intake, age, height, prepregnant weight, marital status, occupational status, education, parity, chronic diseases, previous preterm delivery, mode of initiation of labor and sex of the child did not alter the conclusions, nor did restriction of the highest-intake group to women drinking 10–14 drinks/week (RR = 3.41, CI1.71–6.81 at 16 weeks and RR = 3.47, CI 1.64–7.35 at 30 weeks). The association between alcohol intake and preterm delivery appeared to be J-shaped, with a threshold for adverse effect at a level of about 10–14 drinks/week. **III B**

3 Yang Q, Witkiewicz BB, Olney RS *et al.* (2001) A case-control study of maternal alcohol consumption and intrauterine growth retardation. *Ann Epidemiol* **11**, 497–503. Case-control study, among 701 case and 336 control infants born during 1993–95 in Monroe County, New York. The results provide no evidence of an independent association between moderate maternal alcohol consumption (<14 drinks/week) and risk for intrauterine growth retardation (IUGR). The risk (OR) for IUGR among heavy drinkers (≥14 drinks/week) around the time of conception was 1.4 (95% CI 0.7–2.6) for IUGR ≤ 5th percentile and 1.4 (95% CI 0.7–2.8) for IUGR 5th–10th percentile. For heavy drinkers during the first trimester, the OR was 1.3 (95% CI 0.4–4.5) for IUGR ≤ 5th percentile and OR = 1.3 (95% CI 0.4–4.8) for IUGR 5th–10th percentile. **IIa B**

4 Handmaker NS, Miller WR, Manicke M (1999) Findings of a pilot study of motivational interviewing with pregnant women. *J Stud Alcohol* **60**, 285–287. Study of 42 pregnant women who reported alcohol consumption during their pregnancy. Participants were randomly assigned either to receive written information or to have a 1 h motivational interview. No control group was used. The authors concluded that motivational interviewing showed promise as a specific intervention for reduction in drinking among pregnant women who were at greatest risk. **III B**

5 Cornelius MD, Richardson GA, Day NL *et al.* (1994) A comparison of prenatal drinking in 2 recent samples of adolescents and adults. *J Stud Alcohol* **55**, 412–419. This was an observational study comparing pregnant teenagers with adults attending an antenatal clinic in Pittsburgh, PA, USA. While adults had a significantly higher intake of alcohol prior to pregnancy, there was no difference between the two groups during pregnancy. Binge drinking was commoner in the teenage sample, particularly among the white teenage group. **III B**

6 Reynolds K D, Coombs DW, Lowe JB et al. (1995) Evaluation of a self-help program to reduce alcohol

consumption among pregnant women. *Int J Addict* **30**, 427–443. Study of economically disadvantaged pregnant women attending public health maternity clinics who were assessed prior to intervention and then randomly allocated to self-help intervention or usual clinical care. Alcohol quitting rates were higher among the intervention participants (88%) than controls (69%). **IIa B**

7 Testa M, Reifman A (1996) Individual differences in perceived riskiness of drinking in pregnancy – antecedents and consequences. *J Stud Alcohol* **57**, 360–367. This sample of pregnant women who drank regularly before pregnancy was recruited both from clinics and by newspaper advertisement. The perceived riskiness of drinking during pregnancy was lower among women who had previously given birth to a healthy child and among women with greater numbers of previous alcohol problems. Adverse pregnancy experience before did not predict perceived risk. Perceived risk negatively predicted alcohol consumption during pregnancy. **III B**

8 Bolumar F, Rebagliato M, Hernandez-Aguado I *et al.* (1994) Smoking and drinking habits before and during pregnancy in Spanish women. *J Epidemiol Commun Health* **48**, 36–40. Cross-sectional survey of approximately 1000 pregnant women between 12 and 18 weeks gestation attending an antenatal clinic in Valencia, Spain. Refusal to participate in the survey was very low. A structured questionnaire was used to obtain information on both smoking and alcohol consumption. 60% of the women smoked and 72% drank alcohol before pregnancy. 48% of smokers stopped smoking and 37% of drinkers stopped drinking alcohol during pregnancy. Predictors for stopping included only the number of cigarettes and the amount of alcohol consumed during pregnancy. High levels of alcohol consumption were limited to a small group of pregnant women. **III B**

25.3 Drug abuse: general

Doris Campbell

Management option	Quality of evidence	Strength of recommendation	References
Provide accurate rather than alarmist information	–	✔	–
General guidelines include assessing living environment and whether the woman's partner uses drugs, getting her to take some responsibility for herself, making sure she understands what is expected of her, improving her general health and working towards achievable goals	–	✔	–
Multidisciplinary approach may be beneficial	III	B	1,2
Wear gloves to take blood from all patients (not just addicts)	–	✔	–
Increased risk of sexually transmitted disease, including human immunodeficiency virus, should be discussed	Ia	A	3
Screen for fetal normality and growth with ultrasonography and signs of neonatal withdrawal	IV III	C B	4 5

References

1 Waller CS, Zollinger TW, Saywell RW Jr *et al.* (1996) Indiana prenatal substance use prevention program: its impact on smoking cessation among high-risk pregnant women. *Indiana Med* **89**, 184–187. This program aims to help pregnant women give up cigarette smoking as well as alcohol and drugs. 80% of those surveyed stated that the knowledge they gained through the program was helpful with relation to tobacco use; only two thirds of the clients responded that they agreed with the statement that tobacco use causes babies to have a lower birthweight. The authors concluded that more attention needed to be placed in making women more aware of the risks involved in smoking during pregnancy. **III B**

2 Killeen TK, Brady KT, Thevos A (1995) Addiction severity, psychopathology and treatment compliance in cocaine-dependent mothers. *J Addict Dis* **14**, 75–84. This was a case review of 41 cocaine-dependent pregnant or postpartum women, 30 of whom were administered the structured clinical interview for DSM-III-R and screened for history of victimization during inpatient treatment. The authors concluded that the majority of women had psychiatric disorders as well as a history of victimization. **III B**

3 Prendergast ML, Urada D, Podus D (2001) Meta-analysis of HIV risk-reduction interventions within drug abuse treatment programs. *J Consult Clin Psychol* **69**, 389–405. Meta-analysis on studies using a treatment-comparison group design to evaluate HIV/AIDS risk-reduction interventions for clients enrolled in drug abuse treatment programs. Overall, the interventions studied were found to have a reliable positive (weighted) effect size (d = 0.31).

Effect sizes were negatively correlated with the presence of predominantly ethnic-minority samples and positively correlated with the number of intervention techniques used, the intensity of the intervention, intervention delivery at a later stage of drug treatment or within methadone treatment, and the presence of a number of specific intervention techniques. **Ia A**

4 Hepburn M (1993) Drug use in pregnancy. *Br J Hosp Med* **49**, 51–55. Review article of drug use in pregnancy and the management problems resulting by an expert in the UK. Of 200 babies, 9.5% were preterm, 12.5% were low-birthweight, 11% were small for gestational age. These figures are comparable to rates for non-drug-users from similar deprived backgrounds. **IV C**

5 Stevens SJ, Arbiter N (1995) A therapeutic community for substance abusing pregnant women and women with children, process and outcome. *J Psychoactive Drugs* **27**, 49–56. Descriptive study of a therapeutic community for women and children providing long-term residential treatment. 65 women and 30 children lived together on a single ranch. No controls involved. **III B**

25.4 Drug abuse: specific – heroin, cocaine, barbiturates etc.

Doris Campbell

Management option	Quality of evidence	Strength of recommendation	References
Multidisciplinary approach	IIb	B	1
Explain risks of low birthweight, intrauterine growth retardation (IUGR) and preterm labor and higher need for neonatal care, especially if withdrawal symptoms occur	III	B	2
Explain developmental abnormality in infants of such mothers	III IIb	B B	3 4
Encourage detoxification or methadone maintenance with heroin	III	B	3
Encourage cessation with cocaine and amphetamines	IIb	B	4
Avoid acute withdrawal from barbiturates in pregnancy	–	✓	–
Screen for fetal abnormality, growth and well being	III	B	2
Increased dose of narcotic analgesia (epidural preferable)	–	✓	–
Fetal monitoring if IUGR	–	✓	–
Breast-feeding is controversial – avoid if still current injecter	IV	C	5
Vigilance for baby withdrawal (from 3 days with heroin, cocaine and solvents; 7 days with methadone, barbiturates and amphetamines)	IV	C	5
Addiction team follow-up	IV	C	6

References

1 Wolff K, Hay AW, Vail A *et al.* (1996) Non-prescribed drug use during methadone treatment by clinic- and community-based patients. *Addiction* **91**, 1699–1704. Quasi-experimental study of methadone maintenance treatment in clinic-based (n = 10) and community-based (n = 10) patients. Clinic-based patients had significantly reduced odds of having a urine sample test positive for illicit drugs when compared to community-based patients (OR = 0.20, 95% CI 0.10–0.38, $p < 0.001$). There was no relationship between either methadone dose or plasma methadone concentration and testing positive for nonprescribed drugs (including cocaine, cannabis, amfetamine, Ecstasy, benzodiazepines). **IIb B**

2 Nair P, Rothblum S, Hebel R *et al.* (1994) Neonatal outcome in infants with evidence of fetal exposure to opiates, cocaine, and cannabinoids. *Clin Pediatr (Phila)* **33**, 280–285. Meconium from 141 infants admitted to the full-term nursery was analyzed for metabolites of opiates, cocaine and cannabinoids. The population was 72% African-American; 82% had medical assistance; history of drug use was reported in the medical records in 18%; mean

maternal age was 24.2 years; mean birthweight was 3234 ± 502 g; and neonatal abstinence syndrome was reported in 7%. Meconium analysis data showed the following: 52.5% were drug-free; cocaine was present in 31%, opiates in 18% (cocaine and/or opiates 39%) and cannabinoids in 17%. In 38 infants in whom urine toxicology was obtained for clinical indications, meconium was more sensitive than urine in detecting drug exposure (55.3% vs 31.5%). There was no significant difference between cocaine/opiate-exposed and drug-free infants in race, socioeconomic status, maternal age, birthweight, head circumference, length and Apgar score. Cocaine/opiate-exposed infants had greater length of stay and increased frequency of maternal sexually transmitted diseases during pregnancy, with a trend toward a higher percentage with fetal distress. **III B**

3 Soepatmi S (1994) Developmental outcomes of children of mothers dependent on heroin or heroin/methadone during pregnancy. *Acta Paediatr* **404**(suppl), 406–439. Study from Amsterdam of the developmental outcomes of infants of drug-dependent mothers who used heroin, either alone or in combination with methadone, during pregnancy. Outcomes in such infants were unfavorable compared with outcomes of infants who were not drug-dependent or those of the general population. Prenatal care with social support and methadone substitution were critical factors for such infants' outcome. **III B**

4 Eisen M, Keiser-Smith J, Dampeer J *et al.* (2000) Evaluation of substance use outcomes in demonstration projects for pregnant and postpartum women and their infants: findings from a quasi-experiment. *Addict Behav* **25**, 123–129. Study of the impact of nine community-based drug prevention education and treatment programs for pregnant and postpartum women (*n* = 370) and women who received no intervention (*n* = 288). No comment was given as to how the women were selected for the two groups. Although project clients had significantly lower use on four of the measures – alcohol, any listed drug, marijuana and crack – from intake to delivery, none of the results were maintained through to 6 months postpartum. **IIb B**

5 Marquet P, Chevrel J, Lavignasse P *et al.* (1997) Buprenorphine withdrawal syndrome in a newborn. *Clin Pharmacol Ther* **62**, 569–571. Case report of a pregnant woman who was addicted to heroin but rapidly withdrew from illicit drugs after the onset of a 4 mg/d buprenorphine treatment. In the newborn's blood, urine and meconium 20 h after birth, high concentrations of buprenorphine and its metabolite norbuprenorphine were detected, with a higher buprenorphine/norbuprenorphine ratio than in adults, possibly as a consequence of immature hepatic function; no illicit drugs were found. The child had a weak withdrawal syndrome on the second day of life and recovered rapidly. The measured daily dose of buprenorphine ingested by the newborn through mother's milk was very low (3.28 μg) and probably had little pharmacological effect because no withdrawal signs could be noted when maternal feeding was later abruptly interrupted. Further investigations are required to determine whether buprenorphine can be considered to be a good alternative to methadone in the treatment of pregnant heroin addicts to prevent marked withdrawal syndromes in newborns. **IV C**

6 Berkowitz G, Brindis C, Peterson S (1998) Substance use and social outcomes among participants in perinatal alcohol and drug treatment. *Women's Health* **4**, 231–254. Observational study of initially 591 women enrolled in a treatment program for pregnant and parenting women. 460 completed follow-up 6 months later. Results suggested that there had been reductions in alcohol and other drug usage and maintenance of some kind of treatment contact after discharge from the perinatal treatment program. There were however no controls in this study. **III B**

25.5 Medication during pregnancy

David James

Management option		Quality of evidence	Strength of recommendation	References
Inadvertent exposure to medication	Obtain accurate details of exposure, especially gestational age	–	✔	–
	Check for confounding family or medical history	–	✔	–
	Obtain up-to-date information regarding published risks of the specific drug in humans	–	✔	–
	Emphasize 'background' risks in counseling	–	✔	–
	Be clear about what is known, but do not assume that absence of data means no risk	–	✔	–

➡

➡

Management option		Quality of evidence	Strength of recommendation	References
Considering commencing or continuing medication	Medication should be used only if expected benefits (usually to mother) are greater than risks (usually to fetus)	–	✔	–
	Try and avoid first trimester	–	✔	–
	Use drugs that have been extensively used in pregnancy rather than new/untried drugs	–	✔	–
	Use minimum dose for desired effect	–	✔	–
	Absence of data does not imply safety	–	✔	–
Medications known or suspected of being human teratogens or having adverse fetal effects	Retinoids:			
	❑ High-dose vitamin A	IV	C	1
	❑ Isotretinoin	III	B	2
	❑ Etretinate	IV	C	3
	❑ Acitretin	III	B	4
	Hormones:			
	❑ Danazol and androgens	IV	C	5,6
	❑ Diethylstilbestrol	IIa	B	7
		III	B	8–10
	Anticoagulants:			
	❑ Warfarin and other coumarin anticoagulants	III	B	11
	Antineoplastics:			
	❑ Aminopterin and methylaminopterin	IV	C	12
	❑ Methotrexate	IV	C	12
	❑ Busulfan	IV	C	13
	❑ Cyclophosphamide	IV	C	14,15
	Anticonvulsants:	III	B	16
	❑ Phenytoin and other hydantoins	III	B	17
	❑ Carbamazepine	III	B	18
	❑ Valproic acid	III	B	19
	❑ Trimethadione and paramethadione	III	B	20
	Antibiotics:			
	❑ Tetracycline	III	B	21
	Others:			
	❑ Cocaine	IV	C	22
	❑ Lithium	III	B	23
	❑ Penicillamine	III	B	24
	❑ Thalidomide	III	B	25

References

1 Rothman KJ, Moore LL, Singer MR *et al.* (1995) Teratogenicity of high vitamin A intake. *N Engl J Med* **333**, 1369–1373. Case report. **IV C**

2 Dai WS, LaBraico JM, Stern RS (1992) Epidemiology of isotretinoin exposure during pregnancy. *J Am Acad Dermatol* **26**, 599–606. Observational study of 433 spontaneous reports of isotretinoin exposure in pregnancy. Timing of exposure was known for 396 women. Of these, 130 patients (33%) were already pregnant when they started isotretinoin. An additional 65 patients (16%) became pregnant in the first 3 weeks of isotretinoin use. Pregnancy outcomes were known for 409 pregnancies. Among these, 222 (54%) ended in elective abortion and 29 (7%) in spontaneous or missed abortion. Of 151 births, 72 (48%) were normal, 71 (47%) had congenital malformations and 8 (5%) had abnormalities other than malformations. Of 94 prospectively ascertained pregnancies that ended in births, 28% had congenital malformations (95% CI 19–37%). Exposure to isotretinoin during any time and as little as one capsule within the first trimester has been associated with congenital malformations. **III B**

3 Verloes A, Dodinval P, Koulischer L et al. (1990) Etretinate embryotoxicity 7 months after discontinuation of treatment. *Am J Med Genet* **37**, 437–438. Case report. **IV C**

4 Geiger JM, Baudin M, Saurat JH (1994) Teratogenic risk with etretinate and acitretin treatment. *Dermatology* **189**, 109–116. Review article. Etretinate are known teratogens. Pregnancy should be avoided during treatment and until 2 years after treatment discontinuation. A threshold dose in human therapy below which there is no risk of congenital malformation cannot be determined on the basis of animal experimental data. With regard to pharmacokinetics, there are currently no data suggesting that blood levels of the drug below the detection limit of 2 ng/ml are associated with a teratogenic risk. The most useful information is given by reports in women who were exposed to either retinoid before or during pregnancy, which indicate that the risk of spontaneous abortion or congenital malformation is high when the drug is administered during the first trimester of pregnancy. **III B**

5 Kingsbury AC (1985) Danazol and fetal masculinization: a warning. *Med J Aust* **143**, 410–411. Masculinization of a female fetus occurred during a pregnancy in which the mother received danazol for infertility due to endometriosis. The biochemical theories and the necessary treatment are outlined. Conception may occur before or during a course of danazol and patients should be made aware of the need for concomitant contraception. **IV C**

6 Quagliarello J, Greco MA (1985) Danazol and urogenital sinus formation in pregnancy. *Fertil Steril* **43**, 939–942. Case report. **IV C**

7 Robboy SJ, Noller KL, O'Brien P *et al.* (1984) Increased incidence of cervical and vaginal dysplasia in 3,980 diethylstilbestrol-exposed young women. Experience of the National Collaborative Diethylstilbestrol Adenosis Project. *JAMA* **252**, 2979–2983. The incidence rates of dysplasia and carcinoma-*in-situ* (CIS) of the cervix and vagina were determined in 3980 young women exposed prenatally to diethylstilbestrol. Strict criteria were developed to minimize selection bias among the subset of 744 pairs of matched exposed and unexposed (control) cohort participants, all of whom were identified through review of prenatal obstetric records. A high degree of compliance was achieved throughout the 7-year study period, since in each group about 90% of the women remained as active participants, kept 77% of the annual anniversary examinations and had separate Papanicolaou smears of the cervix and vagina performed in 99% of the anniversary examinations. The incidence rate for dysplasia and CIS was significantly higher in the women exposed to diethylstilbestrol than in those not exposed in the matched cohort (15.7 vs 7.9 cases per 1000 person-years of follow-up). The rates were higher in the exposed women if squamous metaplasia extended to the outer half of the cervix or on to the vagina. **IIa B**

8 Kaufman RH, Noller K, Adam E *et al.* (1984) Upper genital tract abnormalities and pregnancy outcome in diethylstilbestrol-exposed progeny. *Am J Obstet Gynecol* **148**, 973–984. In a collaborative study, 676 diethylstilbestrol-exposed women had hysterosalpingographic examinations, and the findings were related to the outcome of pregnancy in 327 of these women. The findings revealed that: (1) there is a considerable variation of frequency of different types of upper genital tract anomaly in women from different sources and with different motivations for enrollment in the study; (2) the presence of structural cervical changes and vaginal epithelial changes are markers for the likelihood of abnormalities in the uterine fundus; (3) women with upper genital tract abnormalities have increased odds for poor pregnancy outcome compared to women with normal hysterosalpingographic findings; and (4) although some abnormalities were most often or consistently associated with poor pregnancy outcome, no specific changes could be related to specific types of pregnancy outcome. **III B**

9 Herbst AL (1981) Clear cell adenocarcinoma and the current status of DES-exposed females. *Cancer* **48**, 484–488. Over 400 cases of clear-cell adenocarcinoma of the vagina and cervix occurring in females born after 1940 have been accessioned into the Registry for Research on Hormonal Transplacental Carcinogenesis. Intrauterine exposure to diethylstilbestrol (DES) and similar nonsteroidal estrogens have been uncovered in about two thirds of the cases with an available maternal history. A peak in the age incidence curve of the DES-related cases has been observed at about 19 years, with the age range being 7–30 years. The 5-year survival for 400 patients has been 80%. Numerous nonmalignant epithelial changes have been observed. It appears that there has not been an increase in the occurrence of premalignant or malignant squamous cell lesions among the DES-exposed. Premature birth has been more common among DES-exposed women. For those in whom there is evidence of a midpregnancy loss or premature ripening of the cervix during pregnancy, a cerclage procedure has been effective in producing a desirable outcome. **III B**

10 Barnes AB, Colton T, Gundersen J *et al.* (1980) Fertility and outcome of pregnancy in women exposed in utero to diethylstilbestrol. *N Engl J Med* **302**, 609–613. Fertility and outcome of pregnancy were examined in women participating in the National Cooperative Diethylstilbestrol Adenosis (DESAD) Project. We compared 618 subjects who had prenatal exposure to diethylstilbestrol (DES) with 618 control subjects. Fertility, measured in terms of pregnancies achieved, did not differ between the women exposed to DES and the controls. An increased risk of unfavorable outcome of pregnancy was associated with DES exposure (the relative risk of any unfavorable outcome of pregnancy was 1.69; $p < 0.001$). Among DES-exposed women who became pregnant, 81% had at least one full-term live birth. **III B**

11 Hall JG, Pauli RM, Wilson KM (1980) Maternal and fetal sequelae of anticoagulation during pregnancy. *Am J Med* **68**, 122–140. Review of published cases of pregnancies in which coumarin derivatives or heparin were administered demonstrates that use of either class of anticoagulant carries substantial risks. Of 418 reported pregnancies in which coumarin derivatives were used, one sixth resulted in abnormal liveborn infants, one sixth in abortion or stillbirth and, at most, two thirds in apparently normal infants. In addition to the expected hemorrhagic complications, fetal effects of coumarin-derivative administration include a specific embryopathy and central nervous system abnormalities. **III B**

12 Warkany J (1978) Aminopterin and methotrexate: folic acid deficiency. *Teratology* **17**, 353–357. Case report. **IV C**

13 Diamond I (1960) Transplacental transmission of busulphan (Myleran) in a mother with leukemia. Production of fetal malformations and cytomegaly. *Pediatrics* **25**, 85–90. Case report. **IV C**

14 Kirshon B, Wasserstrum N, Willis R *et al.* (1988) Teratogenic effects of first-trimester cyclophosphamide therapy. *Obstet Gynecol* **72**, 462–464. Case report: intravenous cyclophosphamide was administered for severe exacerbation of systemic lupus erythematosus to a patient not known to be in the first trimester of pregnancy. The patient received no other medication except prednisone. Her neonate was born with multiple anomalies, including absent thumbs, cleft palate, low-set ears and multiple eye abnormalities. These anomalies probably reflect the teratogenic effects of cyclophosphamide. **IV C**

15 Murray CL, Reichert JA, Anderson J *et al.* (1984) Multimodal cancer therapy for breast cancer in the first trimester of pregnancy. A case report. *JAMA* **252**, 2607–2608. Case report. **IV C**

16 Kelly TE (1984) Teratogenicity of anticonvulsant drugs. I: Review of the literature. *Am J Med Genet* **19**, 413–434. Review of the literature. **III B**

17 Strickler SM, Dansky LV, Miller MA *et al.* (1985) Genetic predisposition to phenytoin-induced birth defects. *Lancet* **2**, 746–749. To find out whether arene oxide metabolites of phenytoin and a genetic defect in arene oxide detoxification contribute to susceptibility to phenytoin-induced birth defects, lymphocytes from 24 children exposed to phenytoin throughout gestation and from their families were challenged in a blind protocol with phenytoin metabolites generated by a murine hepatic microsomal drug-metabolizing system. 14 of the children had a 'positive' assay result, i.e. a significant increase in cell death associated with phenytoin metabolites. Each child with a positive result had one parent whose cells also were positive. A positive *in-vitro* challenge was highly correlated with major birth defects, including congenital heart disease, cleft lip/palate, microcephaly and major genitourinary, eye and limb defects. There was no difference between children with positive and negative results in the number or distribution of minor birth defects, including stigmata of the fetal hydantoin syndrome. Although many factors contribute to the outcome of pregnancies in epileptic women treated with phenytoin, a genetic defect in arene oxide detoxification seems to increase the risk of the baby having major birth defects. **III B**

18 Jones KL, Lacro RV, Johnson KA *et al.* (1989) Pattern of malformations in the children of women treated with carbamazepine during pregnancy. *N Engl J Med* **320**, 1661–1666. Study of eight children whom we identified retrospectively as having had prenatal exposure to carbamazepine alone or in combination with a variety of anticonvulsants other than phenytoin. In addition, a prospective study documented the outcome of the pregnancies of 72 women exposed in early pregnancy to carbamazepine. A pattern of malformation, the principal features of which are minor craniofacial defects and fingernail hypoplasia, and of developmental delay was identified in the eight children retrospectively ascertained to have been exposed to carbamazepine *in utero*; this pattern was subsequently confirmed through the evaluation of 48 children born alive to the women in the prospective study. That carbamazepine itself is teratogenic is indicated by the incidence of craniofacial defects (11%), fingernail hypoplasia (26%) and developmental delay (20%) in the 35 live-born children of the women in the prospective study who were exposed prenatally to carbamazepine alone. The similarity between the children exposed prenatally to carbamazepine and those with the fetal hydantoin syndrome is probably related to the fact that both drugs are metabolized through the arene oxide pathway and raises the possibility that it is the epoxide intermediate rather than the specific drug itself that is the teratogenic agent. **III B**

19 DiLiberti JH, Farndon PA, Dennis NR *et al.* (1984) The fetal valproate syndrome. *Am J Med Genet* **19**, 473–481. Study of 7 children exposed to sodium valproate (or valproic acid) *in utero*. A consistent facial phenotype was observed in all 7 in addition to other birth defects in 4. The facial changes consisted of epicanthal folds that continued inferiorly and laterally to form a crease or groove just under the orbit, flat nasal bridge, small upturned nose, long upper lip with a relatively shallow philtrum, a thin upper vermillion border and downturned angles of the mouth. Hypospadias, strabismus and psychomotor delay were found in 2 males; 2 children had nystagmus and 2 had low birthweight. **III B**

20 Zackai EH, Mellman WJ, Neiderer B *et al.* (1975) The fetal trimethadione syndrome. *J Pediatr* **87**, 280–284. Study of three families in which each of the mothers took trimethadione during pregnancy. From a comparison of siblings in each family and of others exposed to trimethadione *in utero*, a specific phenotype is delineated. Features included in the fetal trimethadione syndrome are developmental delay, speech difficulty, V-shaped eyebrows, epicanthus, low-set ears with anteriorly folded helix, palatal anomaly and irregular teeth. Additional anomalies in some of the patients include intrauterine growth restriction, short stature, microcephaly, cardiac anomaly, ocular anomaly, hypospadias, inguinal hernia and simian creases. **III B**

21 Genot MT, Golan HP, Porter PJ *et al.* (1970) Effect of administration of tetracycline in pregnancy on the primary dentition of the offspring. *J Oral Med* **25**, 75–79. Review article. **III B**

22 Jick H, Holmes LB, Hunter JR *et al.* (1981) First-trimester drug use and congenital disorders. *JAMA* **246**, 343–346. Review article. **IV C**

23 Cohen LS, Friedman JM, Jefferson JW *et al.* (1994) A reevaluation of risk of in utero exposure to lithium. *JAMA* **271**, 146–150. Review of all published literature. In the 1970s a very strong association was suggested between maternal lithium treatment during pregnancy and Ebstein's anomaly of the heart in the offspring. The relative risk for Ebstein's anomaly among such children was estimated to be 400 on the basis of data collected from a registry of voluntarily submitted cases. More recent controlled epidemiological studies have consistently shown a lower risk. No women who took lithium during pregnancy were found among four case-control studies of Ebstein's anomaly involving

25, 34, 59 and 89 affected children respectively. In two cohort studies, risk ratios of 3.0 (95% CI 1.2–7.7) and 1.5 (95% CI 0.4–6.8) for all congenital anomalies have been observed. The risk ratios for cardiac malformations in these studies were 7.7 (95% CI 1.5–41.2) and 1.2 (95% CI 0.1–18.3) respectively. **III B**

24 Rosa FW (1986) Teratogen update: penicillamine. *Teratology* **33**, 127–131. Review article. **III B**

25 McBride WG (1977) Thalidomide embryopathy. *Teratology* **16**, 79–82. Review article. **III B**

Chapter 26

Hypertension, preeclampsia and eclampsia

26.1 Chronic hypertension

Margaret Ramsay

Management option		Quality of evidence	Strength of recommendation	References
Prepregnancy	Establish etiology, if possible, and severity of hypertension	–	✔	–
	Evaluate renal function	–	✔	–
	In those with mild–moderate hypertension, stop medication or switch to medication with few fetal side effects	–	✔	–
	Those with severe or difficult-to-control hypertension may need to stay on medication despite potential fetal risks	–	✔	–
	Encourage early prenatal care in an appropriate setting	–	✔	–
Prenatal	Early and frequent prenatal care	IV	C	1
	Discontinue antihypertensive medication unless maternal diastolic pressure exceeds 100–110 mmHg	Ia	A	2
	Use oral medication in severe hypertensives and in those with mild hypertension complicated by risk factors	Ia	A	3
	Fetal surveillance using serial ultrasound for growth, umbilical artery Doppler, biophysical profile testing: ❑ Start at 26 weeks in women with severe hypertension and/or risk factors ❑ Start later in women with mild uncomplicated hypertension	IV	C	1
	Be vigilant for superimposed preeclampsia	IV	C	1
Labor and delivery	Continuous electronic fetal monitoring	IV	C	1
	Use antihypertensives to maintain blood pressures below 160/110 mmHg	Ia	A	4
	Monitor for potential complications (e.g. abruption, superimposed preeclampsia)	IV	C	1
Postnatal	Monitor closely in first 48 h to anticipate hypertensive encephalopathy, pulmonary edema or renal failure	IV	C	1
	Use oral or intravenous medication to control hypertension	IV	C	1
	Evaluate for deterioration in cardiac or renal status	IV	C	1
	Most hypertensives are safe during lactation – avoid thiazide diuretics	IV	C	1

References

1 Sibai BM (1991) Diagnosis and management of chronic hypertension in pregnancy. *Obstet Gynecol* **78**, 451–461. Review article. Pregnancies complicated by chronic hypertension are at increased risk for the development of superimposed preeclampsia, abruptio placentae and poor perinatal outcome. The frequency of these complications is particularly increased in patients with severe hypertension and those with preexisting cardiovascular and renal disease. Such women should receive appropriate antihypertensive therapy and frequent evaluations of maternal and fetal wellbeing. In contrast, in patients with mild essential chronic hypertension, the maternal and perinatal benefits from antihypertensive medication are highly controversial. A review of the literature revealed two placebo-controlled studies, four trials comparing treatment versus no medication and three comparisons of methyldopa and oxprenolol. In only one of these studies were subjects randomized in the first trimester. No differences in pregnancy outcome were found with the use of antihypertensive drugs. Evaluation of the woman with chronic hypertension who is considering pregnancy should begin before conception to establish the cause and severity of the hypertension. Appropriate management should include frequent evaluation of maternal and fetal wellbeing; antihypertensive medications may be useful in patients with severe disease as well as in those with target organ involvement. **IV C**

2 Abalos E, Duley L, Steyn DW *et al.* (2001) Antihypertensive drug therapy for mild to moderate hypertension during pregnancy (Cochrane Review). In: *The Cochrane library*, issue 2. Oxford: Update Software. Systematic review of randomized trials evaluating any hypertensive drug treatment for mild to moderate hypertension during pregnancy. Forty studies were included, involving 3797 women. Twenty-four studies (2815 women) compared an antihypertensive drug with placebo or no drug. Antihypertensive drug treatment resulted in a halving of the risk of developing severe hypertension but little evidence of a difference in the incidence of preeclampsia (relative risk 0.99, 95% CI 0.84–1.18). There were no clear effects of treatment on the risk of preeclampsia, fetal or neonatal death, preterm birth, or small-for-gestational-age babies. In trials comparing one antihypertensive drug with another, there were no clear differences between any of these drugs in the risk of developing severe hypertension, and proteinuria/preeclampsia. Other antihypertensive agents appeared better than methyldopa for reducing the risk of the baby dying [14 trials, 1010 subjects, RR 0.49 (0.24 to 0.99)]. **Ia A**

3 Magee LA, Duley L (2001) Oral beta-blockers for mild to moderate hypertension during pregnancy (Cochrane Review). In: *The Cochrane library*, issue 2. Oxford: Update Software. Systematic review of 27 randomized trials comparing beta-blockers with placebo/no therapy, or other antihypertensive agents, for women with mild–moderate pregnancy hypertension (i.e. blood pressure less than 170 mmHg systolic or 110 mmHg diastolic). Oral beta-blockers decreased the risk of severe hypertension (14 trials, 1516 women; RR 0.37, 95% CI 0.26–0.53) and the need for additional antihypertensive drugs. Insufficient data prevented firm conclusions about the effect on perinatal mortality or preterm delivery. Beta-blockers appeared to be associated with an increase in small-for-gestational-age infants (RR 1.34, 95% CI 1.01–1.79). In 11 trials (787 women) comparing beta-blockers with methyldopa, there was no evidence of any differences between the drugs in efficacy or safety (either maternal or fetal). **Ia A**

4 Duley L, Henderson-Smart DJ (2001) Drugs for rapid treatment of very high blood pressure during pregnancy (Cochrane Review). In: *The Cochrane library*, issue 2. Oxford: Update Software. Systematic review of 14 randomized trials of intravenous drugs for severe hypertension in pregnancy. Ketanserin was found to be less effective than hydralazine in reducing blood pressure. Diazoxide was associated with profound hypotension requiring treatment. Otherwise, there was no evidence that any one of the other antihypertensive agents was better than another. **Ia A**

26.2 Preeclampsia

Margaret Ramsay

Management option		Quality of evidence	Strength of recommendation	References
Prepregnancy	Advise early prenatal care	–	✔	–
	Prepregnancy diabetic control	–	✔	–
	Prepregnancy hypertension control	–	✔	–
	Good nutrition for those at risk	–	✔	–
Prenatal – prediction	Increased risk and hence vigilance with: ❑ Preexisting hypertension ❑ Renal disease ❑ Connective tissue disorders ❑ Diabetes mellitus ❑ Previous preeclampsia	–	✔	–

Management option		Quality of evidence	Strength of recommendation	References
Prenatal – prevention	Calcium supplements result in a modest reduction in risk and severity	Ia	A	1
	No apparent benefit from magnesium supplements	Ia	A	2
	No clear benefit from dietary sodium restriction	Ia	A	3
	Diuretics therapy may reduce blood pressure but no benefit in terms of perinatal mortality	Ia	A	4
	Antihypertensives for mild to moderate hypertension reduces severity of preeclampsia	Ia	A	5
	Low-dose aspirin results in a significant reduction in risk in women at high risk of early preeclampsia	Ia	A	6
Prenatal – early detection/ prediction	Roll-over test has a poor predictive value	III	B	7
	Plasma cellular fibronectin is increased in pregnancy with pregnancy-induced hypertension but is not a predictor	III	B	8
	Platelet angiotensin II receptors are a poor predictor for preeclampsia	III	B	9
	Low urinary calcium excretion has poor predictive value	III	B	10
	Elevated mean arterial pressure poor predictor of preeclampsia	IIb	B	11
	Value of isometric exercise test inconsistent	III	B	12,13
	Serum uric acid is an unreliable predictor	III	B	14
	Microalbuminuria is raised in women who develop preeclampsia but its predictive value is poor	III	B	15
	Corrected platelet aggregability may have a good predictive value	III	B	16
	Doppler velocimetry of uterine artery has good potential as an early predictor	III	B	17
Prenatal – management	Diagnosis at term mandates delivery	–	✔	–
	Mild preeclampsia remote from term can be managed conservatively	Ib	A	18
	Expectant management of severe preeclampsia or eclampsia is controversial	III	B	19
	Laboratory studies used during expectant management: ❑ 24h urine collections for quantitative protein and creatinine clearance ❑ Platelet count ❑ Liver function tests ❑ Serum fibrinogen ❑ Clotting studies (PT and PTT)	–	✔	–

Management option		Quality of evidence	Strength of recommendation	References
Labor and delivery	Judicious use of fluid therapy	–	✔	–
	Frequent assessment of maternal vital signs	–	✔	–
	Continuous electronic fetal heart rate monitoring	–	✔	–
	Magnesium sulfate for seizure prophylaxis	Ia	A	20
	Antihypertensive medication to maintain blood pressures below 160/110 mmHg	Ia	A	21
	Potential complications include oliguria, pulmonary edema, HELLP syndrome, seizures	–	✔	–
	Invasive monitoring infrequently needed (use in unstable patients or where volume status is uncertain)	III	B	22
Postnatal	Continue seizure prophylaxis for approximately 24 h post-partum	–	✔	–
	In patients with severe disease, close monitoring and seizure prophylaxis should continue for 2–4 days, until resolution of disease process	–	✔	–
	Patients still requiring antihypertensive medication on discharge from the hospital should remain under surveillance	–	✔	–
	Further investigations should be done for those persistently hypertensive at or more than 6 weeks post-partum	–	✔	–

References

1 Atallah AN, Hofmeyr GJ, Duley L *et al.* (2001) Calcium supplementation during pregnancy for preventing hypertensive disorders and related problems (Cochrane Review). In: *The Cochrane library*, issue 2. Oxford: Update Software.Systematic review of 10 randomized trials comparing at least 1 g daily of calcium during pregnancy with placebo. Calcium supplementation resulted in a modest reduction in high blood pressure (RR 0.81, 95% CI 0.74–0.89) and in risk of preeclampsia (RR 0.70, 95% CI 0.58–0.83). These effects were most marked in women at high risk of hypertension and in those with low baseline dietary calcium. The optimal dosage requires further study. **Ia A**

2 Makrides M, Crowther CA (2001) Magnesium supplementation in pregnancy (Cochrane Review). In: *The Cochrane library*, issue 2. Oxford: Update Software.Systematic review of six randomized and quasi-randomized trials of dietary magnesium supplementation during pregnancy, involving 2637 women. There was no apparent effect of magnesium treatment on blood pressure during pregnancy or preeclampsia. **Ia A**

3 Duley L, Henderson-Smart D (2001) Reduced salt intake compared to normal dietary salt, or high intake, in pregnancy (Cochrane Review). In: *The Cochrane library*, issue 2. Oxford: Update Software.Systematic review including two randomized trials of advice to reduce dietary salt during pregnancy or continue a normal diet. Data were reported for 603 women and all the confidence intervals for outcome measures were wide. The relative risk for preeclampsia was 1.11 (95% CI 0.44–2.78). Only quasi-randomized trials evaluated the effects of a high salt diet; no firm conclusions could be drawn from these. Overall, there is no good evidence from which to make recommendations to pregnant women about dietary salt intake. **Ia A**

4 Collins R, Yusuf F, Peto R (1985) Overview of randomised trials of diuretics in pregnancy. *Br Med J* **290**, 17–23. Review of nine randomized trials (nearly 7000 women) showing that diuretics significantly reduced the incidence of 'preeclampsia', defined mostly as an increase in blood pressure. There was no significant effect of diuretic use on perinatal mortality. **Ia A**

5 Abalos E, Duley L, Steyn DW *et al.* (2001) Antihypertensive drug therapy for mild to moderate hypertension during pregnancy (Cochrane Review). In: *The Cochrane library*, issue 2. Oxford: Update Software.Systematic

review of randomized trials evaluating any hypertensive drug treatment for mild to moderate hypertension during pregnancy. Forty studies were included, involving 3797 women. Twenty-four studies (2815 women) compared an antihypertensive drug with placebo or no drug. Antihypertensive drug treatment resulted in a halving of the risk of developing severe hypertension but little evidence of a difference in the incidence of preeclampsia (relative risk 0.99, 95% CI 0.84–1.18). There were no clear effects of treatment on the risk of preeclampsia, fetal or neonatal death, preterm birth, or small-for-gestational-age babies. In trials comparing one antihypertensive drug with another, there were no clear differences between any of these drugs in the risk of developing severe hypertension, and proteinuria/preeclampsia. Other antihypertensive agents appeared better than methyldopa for reducing the risk of the baby dying [14 trials, 1010 subjects, RR 0.49 (0.24 to 0.99)]. **Ia A**

6 Knight M, Duley L, Henderson-Smart DJ *et al.* (2001) Antiplatelet agents for preventing and treating pre-eclampsia (Cochrane Review). In: *The Cochrane library*, issue 2. Oxford: Update Software. Systematic review of 42 trials involving over 32 000 women. There was a 15% reduction in the risk of preeclampsia associated with the use of antiplatelet agents (32 trials with 29 331 women; RR 0.85, 95% CI 0.78–0.92). The reduction in preeclampsia was regardless of risk status at trial entry or whether a placebo was used, and was irrespective of the dose of aspirin or gestation at randomization. **Ia A**

7 Mahomed K, Lasiende OO (1990) The roll over test is not of value in predicting pregnancy induced hypertension. *Paediatr Perinat Epidemiol* **4**, 71–75. As a predictor of pregnancy-induced hypertension (PIH) the roll-over test has conflicting predictive values in the literature, possibly as a result of sample size, composition or methodology. In this study the roll-over test was performed on 600 African women in their first pregnancy and at 26–32 weeks. The test was positive in 15% of women and had a positive predictive value of only 20%. It is concluded that the roll-over test is of no value in the prediction of PIH. **III B**

8 Islami D, Shoukir Y, Dupont P *et al.* (2001) Is cellular fibronectin a biological marker for pre-eclampsia? *Eur J Obstet Gynecol Reprod Biol* **97**, 40–45. Cellular fibronectin (cFn) appears to be an important factor in the regulation of cell–cell interactions. This study measured cFn longitudinally in 198 consecutive pregnant patients, with or without pathologies associated to pregnancy. The values of cFn increased throughout the normal pregnancy but a significant increase was observed only after the 36th week of pregnancy ($p < 0.0001$). The values of doubling time of cFn gradually decreased, being inverse to cFn concentrations. The values of cFn were significantly higher (3.53 μg/ml; $p = 0.0009$) in the third trimester in the group of women who developed preeclampsia, as compared to normals (2.23 μg/ml). cFn could not be used as a predictor of preeclampsia because the clinical symptoms of this pathology were already present at the time of measurement. **III B**

9 Masse J, Forest JC, Moutquin JM *et al.* (1998) A prospective longitudinal study of platelet angiotensin II receptors for the prediction of preeclampsia. *Clin Biochem* **3**, 251–255. This substance was prospectively evaluated in 801 women attending for routine prenatal care. A specimen was obtained at each trimester of pregnancy whenever possible. Diagnosis of preeclampsia was done postnatally by an experienced obstetrician. No differences in mean maximum binding were observed between normal and affected pregnancies at either trimester. Even when the results were analyzed longitudinally, using the change in maximum binding between two trimesters for each patient, no significant increase could be documented in preeclamptic pregnancies. **III B**

10 Suarez VR, Trelles JG, Miyahira JM (1996) Urinary calcium in asymptomatic primigravidas who later developed preeclampsia. *Obstet Gynecol* **87**, 79–82. This study involved young healthy primigravidas from the prenatal clinic and the collection of a 24-h urine sample at 17–20 weeks gestation from 69 patients. A low urinary excretion of calcium per kilogram of body weight per 24 h before the end of the first half of gestation is a risk factor for preeclampsia, with an acceptable sensitivity and high negative predictive value but with a positive predictive value no better than chance. **III B**

11 Atterbury JL, Groome LJ, Baker SL (1996) Elevated midtrimester mean arterial blood pressure in women with severe preeclampsia. *Appl Nurs Res* **9**, 161–166. Although early identification of pregnant women who are at risk for severe preeclampsia may help reduce maternal–perinatal sequelae, an adequate screening test for this disorder has not been described. The purpose of this study was to determine if a group of women ($n = 57$) who developed severe preeclampsia had a higher midtrimester mean arterial pressure (MAP-2) than a matched group of women ($n = 57$) who remained normotensive throughout pregnancy and the puerperium. It was found that women who developed severe preeclampsia had a significantly higher MAP-2 than normotensive women and that significantly more preeclamptic subjects had an MAP-2 of 85 mmHg or more than did control subjects. Thus, an elevated MAP-2 may help to identify women who are at risk for the development of severe preeclampsia. **IIb B**

12 Tomoda S, Kitanaka T, Ogita S *et al.* (1994) Prediction of pregnancy-induced hypertension by isometric exercise. *Asia Oceania J Obstet Gynaecol* **20**, 249–255. The purpose of this study was to evaluate an isometric exercise (hand-grip test) as a method of predicting pregnancy-induced hypertension (PIH). 125 pregnant women were given the test before the 15th gestational week. The test was rated positive when the systolic blood pressure increased by 15 mmHg or more during isometric exercise or decreased 14 mmHg or more immediately after isometric exercise. As a result, the hand-grip test had the highest sensitivity (81.8%) and specificity (68.4%) for predicting PIH, compared to other risk factors. The positive predictive value was 20% (second highest among risk factors, the actual incidence of hypertension was 8.8%), and the negative predictive value was 97.5% (highest). In conclusion, by use of a very simple hand-grip test early in gestation, the authors can predict PIH with the highest sensitivity. **III B**

13 Watson WJ, Katz VL, Caprice PA *et al.* (1995) Pressor response to cycle ergometry in the midtrimester of pregnancy: can it predict preeclampsia? *Am J Perinatol* **12**, 265–267. A total of 97 primigravid patients were prospectively studied to assess the predictive value of the pressor response to aerobic exercise as a screening test for preeclampsia. The blood pressure response to cycle ergometry exercise to a maternal pulse of 140 beats/min was recorded on each subject. Each subject was studied in the second trimester of pregnancy at a mean gestational age of 23 weeks (range 18–27). 3 of the study subjects developed hypertension with proteinuria in the third trimester. A rise in systolic blood pressure of at least 30 mmHg occurred in 29 patients but this did not predict third-trimester preeclampsia ($p = 0.21$). A rise in diastolic blood pressure of 20 mmHg was observed in 18 patients, 2 of whom developed preeclampsia ($p = 0.08$). An increase of diastolic pressure of 20 mmHg with moderate cycle ergometry exercise in the second trimester may predict a subset of patients at elevated risk of preeclampsia in the third trimester. However, the positive predictive value of this 20 mmHg pressor increase (11%) limits its applicability as a screening test. Thus the use of an exercise screening test cannot be recommended. **III B**

14 Redman CW, Williams GF, Jones DD *et al.* (1977) Plasma urate and serum deoxycytidylate deaminase measurements for the early diagnosis of pre-eclampsia. *Br J Obstet Gynaecol* **84**, 904–908. The value of measuring plasma urate and serum deoxycytidylate deaminase (dCMP deaminase) for the early diagnosis of preeclampsia was investigated in 45 patients. A combination of increased blood pressure and increased plasma urate identified 19 patients with a high incidence of fetal and maternal morbidity ascribable to preeclampsia. 17 of the 19 patients also had an increased serum dCMP deaminase. Serial antenatal observations for a mean period of 104 days (36–179 days) on 33 of the patients demonstrated that plasma urate and serum dCMP deaminase increased together as early changes in the development of preeclampsia. In 6 patients, blood pressure, plasma urate and serum dCMP deaminase all increased but in only one was the rise in blood pressure the first change. Elevations of plasma urate and serum dCMP deaminase are therefore both early features of preeclampsia. Serial measurements can give warning of the disorder before the appearance of other clinical features. The change in dCMP deaminase is probably another reflection of early renal involvement in the preeclamptic process. **III B**

15 Shaarawy M, Salem ME (2001) The clinical value of microtransferrinuria and microalbuminuria in the prediction of pre-eclampsia. *Clin Chem Lab Med* **39**, 29–34. The aim of this study was to determine whether the presence of microtransferrinuria and microalbuminuria detected in pregnant women who were free of symptoms could predict the subsequent development of preeclampsia. 155 pregnant women were successfully followed from 10 weeks gestation to delivery. Preeclampsia developed in 31 women (17 mild and 12 severe preeclampsia) and eclampsia developed in 2 cases, whereas 124 women remained normotensive (controls). First morning urine specimens were collected during 10–12 weeks gestation and were analyzed for microalbuminuria by a specific immunochemical test strip method. Mid-trimester mean arterial blood pressure (MAP) was also measured. Urinary microtransferrin levels in pregnant women who subsequently developed severe preeclampsia and eclampsia were significantly higher than those of pregnant women who remained normotensive. Microtransferrinuria as a predictor for preeclampsia had a sensitivity of 93.5%, specificity 65%, positive predictive value 83% and negative predictive value 98.4%, whereas these values for microalbuminuria were: 50%, 58%, 50% and 91% respectively. Urinary microtransferrin levels were significantly elevated in women with elevated MAP and in women who delivered low-birthweight and low-Apgar-score babies. In conclusion, microtransferrinuria is a potentially more sensitive predictor of preeclampsia than microalbuminuria. Moreover, microtransferrinuria in early pregnancy might be a negative marker of fetal outcome in preeclampsia. **III B**

16 Felfernig-Boehm D, Salat A, Vogl SE *et al.* (2000) Early detection of preeclampsia by determination of platelet aggregability. *Thromb Res* **98**, 139–146. Investigation of the suitability of corrected whole-blood impedance aggregometry as an early predictor of preeclampsia in 71 consecutive, high-risk pregnancies. According to the occurrence of preeclampsia, defined post-partum by an independent investigator, and the stage of pregnancy (early and late; cutoff 25 weeks), four study groups were defined. Platelet aggregation data were corrected for the influence of hematocrit and platelet count by a special-purpose software package. Women developing preeclampsia showed significantly higher platelet aggregation response than controls in early and late pregnancy. In early pregnancy, all women developing preeclampsia had aggregation responses to collagen higher than the highest responses among the controls. Hence, this test had a 100% positive predictive value of subsequent preeclampsia. Despite being significantly increased, platelet aggregability was of minor predictive value in late pregnancy. We conclude that preeclampsia is accompanied by exaggerated platelet aggregability, particularly perceptible early in the course of pregnancy. We propose collagen-induced whole-blood platelet aggregation with correction for the influence of hematocrit and platelet count for early detection of preeclampsia. **III B**

17 Coleman MA, McCowan LM, North RA (2000) Mid-trimester uterine artery Doppler screening as a predictor of adverse pregnancy outcome in high-risk women. *Placenta* **21**, 115–121. A total of 116 pregnancies in 114 women at high risk of preeclampsia and/or small-for-gestational-age (SGA) babies had uterine artery Doppler screening performed as part of clinical practice between 22 and 24 weeks gestation. 32 (27.5%) women developed preeclampsia, 31 (26.7%) had SGA babies, 23 (20%) were delivered at less than 34 weeks because of pregnancy complications and there were 3 (2.6%) placental abruptions and 3 (2.6%) perinatal deaths. The sensitivity of any RI of more than 0.58 for preeclampsia, SGA, 'all' outcomes and 'severe' outcome was 91%, 84%, 83% and 90%, respectively. The specificity of any RI of more than 0.58 for these outcomes was 42%, 39%, 47% and 38% respectively. The positive predictive value of any RI of more than 0.58 for the same outcomes was 37%, 33%, 58% and 24% respectively. Among women with both RI values of 0.7 or more, 58%, 67%, 85% and 58% developed preeclampsia, SGA, 'all' and 'severe' outcomes respectively. In women with bilateral notches, 47%, 53%, 76% and 65% developed the respective outcomes. Women with both RI values of 0.7 or more and women with bilateral notches had relative risks of 11.1

(95% CI 2.6–46.4) and 12.7 (95% CI 4.0–40.4) respectively for developing severe outcome. Only 5% of women with both RI values less than 0.58 developed a severe outcome. **III B**

18 Sibai BM, Gonzalez AR, Mabie WC *et al.* (1987) A comparison of labetalol plus hospitalization versus hospitalization alone in the management of preeclampsia remote from term. *Obstet Gynecol* **70**, 323–327. Randomized trial of 200 women at 26–35 weeks gestation. Patients receiving labetalol had significantly decreased blood pressure during treatment but in both groups there was deterioration in preeclampsia, as documented by worsening proteinuria, serum creatinine and urate levels. There was no difference in the mean prolongation of pregnancy between groups. The incidence of small-for-gestational-age infants was increased in the labetalol-treated group. **Ib A**

19 Hall DR, Odendaal HJ, Steyn DW (2001) Expectant management of severe pre-eclampsia in the mid-trimester. *Eur J Obstet Gynecol Reprod Biol* **96**, 168–172. Prospective case series; 39 women admitted between 24 and 27 weeks gestation with severe preeclampsia, whose pregnancies were otherwise stable, were managed expectantly with careful clinical and biochemical monitoring of maternal and fetal status, together with careful blood pressure control, in a high-care obstetric ward. The aim was to safely prolong the pregnancies and thereby improve perinatal outcome. Gestation was prolonged by a median of 12 (range 3–47) days, with greater periods gained at earlier gestations. The overall perinatal loss was 26% and the neonatal loss 17%. The rates of significant maternal complications were low. **III B**

20 Duley L, Gulmezoglu AM, Henderson-Smart DJ (2000) Anticonvulsants for women with pre-eclampsia (Cochrane Review). In: *The Cochrane library*, issue 2. Oxford: Update Software. Systematic review of nine randomized trials of anticonvulsant usage in women with preeclampsia. In trials comparing magnesium sulfate with placebo/no anticonvulsant the relative risk of eclampsia was 0.33, 95% CI 0.11–1.02. Magnesium sulfate was better than phenytoin at reducing the risk of eclampsia (RR 0.05, 95% CI 0.00–0.84). Studies comparing magnesium sulfate and diazepam were too small for any reliable conclusions. Overall, there was not enough evidence to establish the benefits and hazards of anticonvulsants for women with preeclampsia but magnesium sulfate appeared to be the best choice. **Ia A**

21 Duley L, Henderson-Smart DJ (2001) Drugs for rapid treatment of very high blood pressure during pregnancy (Cochrane Review). In: *The Cochrane library*, issue 2. Oxford: Update Software. Systematic review of 14 randomized trials of intravenous drugs for severe hypertension in pregnancy. Ketanserin was found to be less effective than hydralazine in reducing blood pressure. Diazoxide was associated with profound hypotension requiring treatment. Otherwise, there was no evidence that any one of the other antihypertensive agents was better than another. Ia A

22 Clark SL, Greenspoon JS, Aldahl D (1986) Severe pre-eclampsia with persistent oliguria: management of hemodynamic subsets. *Am J Obstet Gynecol* **154**, 490–494. Study of nine patients with severe preeclampsia or eclampsia who had persistent oliguria unresponsive to fluid challenge. Pulmonary artery catheterization was performed to allow study of central hemodynamic function (pulmonary capillary wedge pressure, central venous pressure, systemic vascular resistance, cardiac output, mean arterial pressure). This information allowed selective treatment with either volume infusion or reduction of cardiac preload and/or afterload. **III B**

26.3 Severe/acute hypertension

Margaret Ramsay

Management option		Quality of evidence	Strength of recommendation	References
Prepregnancy	Counsel those women at risk	–	✔	–
Prenatal – prediction	Increased risk and vigilance with: ❑ Preexisting hypertension ❑ Renal disease ❑ Connective tissue disorders ❑ Diabetes mellitus ❑ Previous preeclampsia	–	✔	–
Prenatal – prevention	No evidence of benefit from fish liver oil	Ib	A	1,2
	Some reduction in those at high risk of early-onset disease from use of low-dose aspirin	Ia	A	3
	Calcium supplements have some beneficial effect	Ia	A	4
	Antioxidants – vitamin C and E supplements appear to be of benefit in those at high risk	Ib	A	5

➡

Management option		Quality of evidence	Strength of recommendation	References
Prenatal – early detection	Doppler velocimetry of uterine artery has good potential as an early predictor	III	B	6
Prenatal – management	High-dependency care with appropriately trained staff and support	–	✔	–
	Reduce blood pressure	IV Ia	C A	7 8,9
	Prevent convulsions	Ia	A	10
	Assess/monitor renal function and fluid balance	–	✔	–
	Selective use of invasive monitoring (central venous pressure, pulmonary capillary wedge pressure)	III	B	11
	Careful use of intravenous fluids to avoid fluid overload	–	✔	–
	Assess clotting status	–	✔	–
	Assess liver function	–	✔	–
	Fetal assessment	–	✔	–
	Give steroids if preterm	Ia	A	12
	Consider *in utero* transfer if neonatal facilities not appropriate	–	✔	–
	Timing of delivery depends on gestation, steroid administration, fetal status, maternal complications	–	✔	–
	Mode of delivery depends on maternal and fetal factors	–	✔	–
Labor and delivery	If allowed to labor, closely monitor progress	–	✔	–
	Monitor maternal condition	–	✔	–
	Continuous electronic fetal monitoring	–	✔	–
	Avoid fluid overload	–	✔	–
	Epidural frequently advocated but there is no evidence of benefit and care is needed to avoid fluid overload	IIb	B	13
	Consider assisted second stage	–	✔	–
	Oxytocin for third stage	–	✔	–
Postnatal	Early: confirm resolution by monitoring ❑ Blood pressure ❑ Fluid balance ❑ Renal function ❑ Pulmonary function ❑ Neurological status ❑ Coagulation status	–	✔	–
	Late: investigate for underlying cause	–	✔	–

References

1 Onwude JL, Lilford RJ, Hjartardottir H *et al.* (1995) A randomised double-blind placebo-controlled trial of fish oil in high-risk pregnancy. *Br J Obstet Gynaecol* **102**, 95–100. Trial involved 233 women at high risk of developing hypertension. The active treatment was 2.7 g of MaxEpa daily (1.62 g eicosapentaenoic acid and 1.08 g docosahexaenoic acid). Dietary supplements with ω-3 fatty acids did not affect the frequency of proteinuric or nonproteinuric hypertension, the proportion of babies with birthweight below the 3rd centile nor the duration of pregnancy. **Ib A**

2 Bulstra-Ramakers MT, Huisjes HJ, Visser GH *et al.* (1995) The effects of 3 g eicosapentaenoic acid on recurrence of intrauterine growth retardation and pregnancy-induced hypertension. *Br J Obstet Gynaecol* **102**, 123–126. Randomized, double-blind trial of 3 g eicosapentaenoic acid or placebo in 63 women with a history of birthweight below the 10th centile or pregnancy-induced hypertension in the previous pregnancy. There were no differences between the groups in incidence of hypertension or low-birthweight babies. **Ib A**

3 Knight M, Duley L, Henderson-Smart DJ *et al.* (2001) Antiplatelet agents for preventing and treating pre-eclampsia (Cochrane Review). In: *The Cochrane library*, issue 2. Oxford: Update Software. Systematic review of 42 trials involving over 32 000 women. There was a 15% reduction in the risk of preeclampsia associated with the use of antiplatelet agents (32 trials with 29 331 women; RR 0.85, 95% CI 0.78–0.92). The reduction in preeclampsia was regardless of risk status at trial entry or whether a placebo was used, and was irrespective of the dose of aspirin or gestation at randomization. **Ia A**

4 Atallah AN, Hofmeyr GJ, Duley L *et al.* (2001) Calcium supplementation during pregnancy for preventing hypertensive disorders and related problems (Cochrane Review). In: *The Cochrane library*, issue 2. Oxford: Update Software. Systematic review of 10 randomized trials comparing at least 1 g daily of calcium during pregnancy with placebo. Calcium supplementation resulted in a modest reduction in high blood pressure (RR 0.81, 95% CI 0.74–0.89) and in risk of preeclampsia (RR 0.70, 95% CI 0.58–0.83). These effects were most marked in women at high risk of hypertension and in those with low baseline dietary calcium. The optimal dosage requires further study. **Ia A**

5 Chappell LC, Seed PT, Briley AL *et al.* (1999) Effect of antioxidants on the occurrence of pre-eclampsia in women at increased risk: a randomised trial. *Lancet* **354**, 810–816. Randomized trial of 1000 mg/day vitamin C and 400 IU/day vitamin E or placebo in women at high risk of preeclampsia (identified from previous history or by uterine artery Doppler velocimetry). There were fewer cases of preeclampsia in the vitamin-treated cohort compared to placebo, whether analyzed by intention to treat or by those who completed the study. **Ib A**

6 Coleman MA, McCowan LM, North RA (2000) Mid-trimester uterine artery Doppler screening as a predictor of adverse pregnancy outcome in high-risk women. *Placenta* **21**, 115–121. A total of 116 pregnancies in 114 women at high risk of preeclampsia and/or small-for-gestational-age (SGA) babies had uterine artery Doppler screening performed as part of clinical practice between 22 and 24 weeks gestation. 32 (27.5%) women developed preeclampsia, 31 (26.7%) had SGA babies, 23 (20%) were delivered at less than 34 weeks because of pregnancy complications and there were 3 (2.6%) placental abruptions and 3 (2.6%) perinatal deaths. The sensitivity of any RI of more than 0.58 for preeclampsia, SGA, 'all' outcomes and 'severe' outcome was 91%, 84%, 83% and 90%, respectively. The specificity of any RI of more than 0.58 for these outcomes was 42%, 39%, 47% and 38% respectively. The positive predictive value of any RI of more than 0.58 for the same outcomes was 37%, 33%, 58% and 24% respectively. Among women with both RI values of 0.7 or more, 58%, 67%, 85% and 58% developed preeclampsia, SGA, 'all' and 'severe' outcomes respectively. In women with bilateral notches, 47%, 53%, 76% and 65% developed the respective outcomes. Women with both RI values of 0.7 or more and women with bilateral notches had relative risks of 11.1 (95% CI 2.6–46.4) and 12.7 (95% CI 4.0–40.4) respectively for developing severe outcome. Only 5% of women with both RI values less than 0.58 developed a severe outcome. **III B**

7 Sibai BM (1991) Diagnosis and management of chronic hypertension in pregnancy. *Obstet Gynecol* **78**, 451–461. Review article. Pregnancies complicated by chronic hypertension are at increased risk for the development of superimposed preeclampsia, abruptio placentae and poor perinatal outcome. The frequency of these complications is particularly increased in patients with severe hypertension and those with preexisting cardiovascular and renal disease. Such women should receive appropriate antihypertensive therapy and frequent evaluations of maternal and fetal wellbeing. In contrast, in patients with mild essential chronic hypertension, the maternal and perinatal benefits from antihypertensive medication are highly controversial. A review of the literature revealed two placebo-controlled studies, four trials comparing treatment versus no medication and three comparisons of methyldopa and oxprenolol. In only one of these studies were subjects randomized in the first trimester. No differences in pregnancy outcome were found with the use of antihypertensive drugs. Evaluation of the woman with chronic hypertension who is considering pregnancy should begin before conception to establish the cause and severity of the hypertension. Appropriate management should include frequent evaluation of maternal and fetal wellbeing; antihypertensive medications may be useful in patients with severe disease as well as in those with target organ involvement. **IV C**

8 Magee LA, Duley L (2001) Oral beta-blockers for mild to moderate hypertension during pregnancy (Cochrane Review). In: *The Cochrane library*, issue 2. Oxford: Update Software. Systematic review of 27 randomized trials comparing beta-blockers with placebo/no therapy, or other antihypertensive agents, for women with mild–moderate pregnancy hypertension (i.e. blood pressure less than 170 mmHg systolic or 110 mmHg diastolic). Oral beta-blockers

decreased the risk of severe hypertension (14 trials, 1516 women; RR 0.37, 95% CI 0.26–0.53) and the need for additional antihypertensive drugs. Insufficient data prevented firm conclusions about the effect on perinatal mortality or preterm delivery. Beta-blockers appeared to be associated with an increase in small-for-gestational-age infants (RR 1.34, 95% CI 1.01–1.79). In 11 trials (787 women) comparing beta-blockers with methyldopa, there was no evidence of any differences between the drugs in efficacy or safety (either maternal or fetal). **Ia A**

9 Duley L, Henderson-Smart DJ (2001) Drugs for rapid treatment of very high blood pressure during pregnancy (Cochrane Review). In: *The Cochrane library*, issue 2. Oxford: Update Software. Systematic review of 14 randomized trials of intravenous drugs for severe hypertension in pregnancy. Ketanserin was found to be less effective than hydralazine in reducing blood pressure. Diazoxide was associated with profound hypotension requiring treatment. Otherwise, there was no evidence that any one of the other antihypertensive agents was better than another. **Ia A**

10 Duley L, Gulmezoglu AM, Henderson-Smart DJ (2000) Anticonvulsants for women with pre-eclampsia (Cochrane Review). In: *The Cochrane library*, issue 2. Oxford: Update Software. Systematic review of nine randomized trials of anticonvulsant usage in women with preeclampsia. In trials comparing magnesium sulfate with placebo/no anticonvulsant the relative risk of eclampsia was 0.33 (95% CI 0.11–1.02). Magnesium sulfate was better than phenytoin at reducing the risk of eclampsia (RR 0.05, 95% CI 0.00–0.84). Studies comparing magnesium sulfate and diazepam were too small for any reliable conclusions. Overall, there was not enough evidence to establish the benefits and hazards of anticonvulsants for women with preeclampsia but magnesium sulfate appeared to be the best choice. **Ia A**

11 Clark SL, Greenspoon JS, Aldahl D (1986) Severe pre-eclampsia with persistent oliguria: management of hemodynamic subsets. *Am J Obstet Gynecol* **154**, 490–494. Study of nine patients with severe preeclampsia or eclampsia who had persistent oliguria unresponsive to fluid challenge. Pulmonary artery catheterization was performed to allow study of central hemodynamic function (pulmonary capillary wedge pressure, central venous pressure, systemic vascular resistance, cardiac output, mean arterial pressure). This information allowed selective treatment with either volume infusion or reduction of cardiac preload and/or afterload. **III B**

12 Crowley P (2001) Prophylactic corticosteroids for preterm birth (Cochrane Review). In: *The Cochrane library*, issue 2. Oxford: Update Software. Systematic review (of 18 trials including more than 3700 babies) of the effects of corticosteroids administered to pregnant women to accelerate fetal lung maturity prior to preterm delivery. Antenatal administration of 24 mg betamethasone, 24 mg dexamethasone, or 2 g hydrocortisone to women expected to give birth preterm was associated with a significant reduction in mortality (OR 0.60, 95% CI 0.48–0.75), respiratory distress syndrome (OR 0.53, 95% CI 0.44–0.63) and intraventricular hemorrhage in preterm infants. No adverse consequences of prophylactic corticosteroids for preterm birth were identified. **Ia A**

13 Hogg B, Hauth JC, Caritis SN *et al.* (1999) Safety of labor epidural anesthesia for women with severe hypertensive disease. National Institute of Child Health and Human Development Maternal–Fetal Medicine Units Network. *Am J Obstet Gynecol* **181**, 1096–1101. Retrospective analysis of a subgroup population within a multicenter double-blind trial of low-dose aspirin therapy for women at high risk for development of preeclampsia. Subjects in whom severe hypertensive disease developed were selected. The primary outcomes were the overall frequencies of cesarean delivery among women with severe hypertensive disease who had labor with and without epidural anesthesia. Other maternal and neonatal outcomes were also compared between women who did and did not receive epidural anesthesia. Among the women with severe hypertensive disease ($n = 444$) 327 had labor. Among the women with severe disease who had labor there was no difference in either the overall cesarean delivery rate (32.1% vs 28.0%; $p = 0.44$) or the rate of cesarean delivery for fetal distress or failure to progress (27.8% vs 22.0%; $p = 0.26$) between women who did and did not receive epidural analgesia. Women with chronic hypertension were more likely to have a cesarean delivery overall if they received epidural anesthesia but there was otherwise no difference in the frequencies of cesarean delivery for these indications between women with and without epidural anesthesia within each of the high-risk groups. Pulmonary edema was rare and acute renal failure did not develop in any women. Conclusion: epidural anesthesia use did not increase the frequencies of cesarean delivery, pulmonary edema and renal failure among women with severe hypertensive disease. **IIb B**

26.4 Eclampsia

Margaret Ramsay

Management option		Quality of evidence	Strength of recommendation	References
Prepregnancy	Discuss relatively low recurrence risk	–	✔	–
	Counsel regarding prevention	–	✔	–
Prenatal – prediction	Maintain vigilance with preeclampsia, previous eclampsia, hypertension	–	✔	–

Management option		Quality of evidence	Strength of recommendation	References
Prenatal – prevention	Low-dose aspirin as for preeclampsia but no direct evidence of benefit	–	✔	–
	Antihypertensive therapy	–	✔	–
	Prompt action with warning clinical features	–	✔	–
	No evidence of benefit from prophylactic anticonvulsants in preeclampsia	Ia	A	1
Prenatal – management	General measures: resuscitation, maintain airway, give oxygen, nurse semi-prone	–	✔	–
	Transfer to high-dependency area	–	✔	–
	Control and prevent further convulsions using magnesium sulfate (some use diazepam for immediate control of convulsions)	III	B	2–4
	Control blood pressure	Ia	A	5–7
	Assess renal function and fluid balance; avoid fluid overload	–	✔	–
	Assess liver function	–	✔	–
	Assess clotting status	–	✔	–
	Assess pulmonary function	–	✔	–
	Assess fetal health	–	✔	–
	Deliver when stable	–	✔	–
Labor and delivery	Mode of delivery will depend on maternal status and fetal viability	–	✔	–
	If patient labors: ❑ Continuous fetal heart rate monitoring ❑ Assisted second stage ❑ Oxytocin for third stage ❑ Avoid prolonged labor	–	✔	–
	Regional analgesia contraindicated if clotting abnormality	–	✔	–
Postnatal	Maintain high-dependency care for 24–48 h	–	✔	–
	Stop anticonvulsants 24 h after last fit	–	✔	–
	Use antihypertensives as necessary (oral after 24 h)	–	✔	–
	Reduce intensive monitoring when recovery noted	–	✔	–
	Counsel about risks of recurrence	–	✔	–
	Long-term follow up: ❑ Neurological assessment if atypical fits ❑ Monitor blood pressure and proteinuria and consider investigation if they remain abnormal	–	✔	–

References

1 Duley L, Gulmezoglu AM, Henderson-Smart DJ (2000) Anticonvulsants for women with pre-eclampsia (Cochrane Review). In: *The Cochrane library*, issue 2. Oxford: Update Software. Systematic review of nine randomized trials of anticonvulsant usage in women with preeclampsia. In trials comparing magnesium sulfate with placebo/no anticonvulsant the relative risk of eclampsia was 0.33 (95% CI 0.11–1.02). Magnesium sulfate was better than phenytoin at reducing the risk of eclampsia (RR 0.05, 95% CI 0.00–0.84). Studies comparing magnesium sulfate and diazepam were too small for any reliable conclusions. Overall, there was not enough evidence to establish the benefits and hazards of anticonvulsants for women with preeclampsia but magnesium sulfate appeared to be the best choice. **Ia A**

2 Watson WJ, Katz VL, Caprice PA *et al.* (1995) Pressor response to cycle ergometry in the midtrimester of pregnancy: can it predict preeclampsia? *Am J Perinatol* **12**, 265–267. A total of 97 primigravid patients were prospectively studied to assess the predictive value of the pressor response to aerobic exercise as a screening test for preeclampsia. The blood pressure response to cycle ergometry exercise to a maternal pulse of 140 beats/min was recorded on each subject. Each subject was studied in the second trimester of pregnancy at a mean gestational age of 23 weeks (range 18–27). 3 of the study subjects developed hypertension with proteinuria in the third trimester. A rise in systolic blood pressure of at least 30 mmHg occurred in 29 patients but this did not predict third-trimester preeclampsia ($p = 0.21$). A rise in diastolic blood pressure of 20 mmHg was observed in 18 patients, 2 of whom developed preeclampsia ($p = 0.08$). An increase of diastolic pressure of 20 mmHg with moderate cycle ergometry exercise in the second trimester may predict a subset of patients at elevated risk of preeclampsia in the third trimester. However, the positive predictive value of this 20 mmHg pressor increase (11%) limits its applicability as a screening test. Thus the use of an exercise screening test cannot be recommended. **III B**

3 Redman CW, Williams GF, Jones DD *et al.* (1977) Plasma urate and serum deoxycytidylate deaminase measurements for the early diagnosis of pre-eclampsia. *Br J Obstet Gynaecol* **84**, 904–908. The value of measuring plasma urate and serum deoxycytidylate deaminase (dCMP deaminase) for the early diagnosis of preeclampsia was investigated in 45 patients. A combination of increased blood pressure and increased plasma urate identified 19 patients with a high incidence of fetal and maternal morbidity ascribable to preeclampsia. 17 of the 19 patients also had an increased serum dCMP deaminase. Serial antenatal observations for a mean period of 104 days (36–179 days) on 33 of the patients demonstrated that plasma urate and serum dCMP deaminase increased together as early changes in the development of preeclampsia. In 6 patients, blood pressure, plasma urate and serum dCMP deaminase all increased but in only one was the rise in blood pressure the first change. Elevations of plasma urate and serum dCMP deaminase are therefore both early features of preeclampsia. Serial measurements can give warning of the disorder before the appearance of other clinical features. The change in dCMP deaminase is probably another reflection of early renal involvement in the preeclamptic process. **III B**

4 Shaarawy M, Salem ME (2001) The clinical value of microtransferrinuria and microalbuminuria in the prediction of pre-eclampsia. *Clin Chem Lab Med* **39**, 29–34. The aim of this study was to determine whether the presence of microtransferrinuria and microalbuminuria detected in pregnant women who were free of symptoms could predict the subsequent development of preeclampsia. 155 pregnant women were successfully followed from 10 weeks gestation to delivery. Preeclampsia developed in 31 women (17 mild and 12 severe preeclampsia) and eclampsia developed in 2 cases, whereas 124 women remained normotensive (controls). First morning urine specimens were collected during 10–12 weeks gestation and were analyzed for microalbuminuria by a specific immunochemical test strip method. Mid-trimester mean arterial blood pressure (MAP) was also measured. Urinary microtransferrin levels in pregnant women who subsequently developed severe preeclampsia and eclampsia were significantly higher than those of pregnant women who remained normotensive. Microtransferrinuria as a predictor for preeclampsia had a sensitivity of 93.5%, specificity 65%, positive predictive value 83% and negative predictive value 98.4%, whereas these values for microalbuminuria were: 50%, 58%, 50% and 91% respectively. Urinary microtransferrin levels were significantly elevated in women with elevated MAP and in women who delivered low-birthweight and low-Apgar-score babies. In conclusion, microtransferrinuria is a potentially more sensitive predictor of preeclampsia than microalbuminuria. Moreover, microtransferrinuria in early pregnancy might be a negative marker of fetal outcome in preeclampsia. **III B**

5 Sibai BM (1991) Diagnosis and management of chronic hypertension in pregnancy. *Obstet Gynecol* **78**, 451–461. Review article. Pregnancies complicated by chronic hypertension are at increased risk for the development of superimposed preeclampsia, abruptio placentae and poor perinatal outcome. The frequency of these complications is particularly increased in patients with severe hypertension and those with preexisting cardiovascular and renal disease. Such women should receive appropriate antihypertensive therapy and frequent evaluations of maternal and fetal wellbeing. In contrast, in patients with mild essential chronic hypertension, the maternal and perinatal benefits from antihypertensive medication are highly controversial. A review of the literature revealed two placebo-controlled studies, four trials comparing treatment versus no medication and three comparisons of methyldopa and oxprenolol. In only one of these studies were subjects randomized in the first trimester. No differences in pregnancy outcome were found with the use of antihypertensive drugs. Evaluation of the woman with chronic hypertension who is considering pregnancy should begin before conception to establish the cause and severity of the hypertension. Appropriate management should include frequent evaluation of maternal and fetal wellbeing; antihypertensive medications may be useful in patients with severe disease as well as in those with target organ involvement. **IV C**

6 Magee LA, Duley L (2001) Oral beta-blockers for mild to moderate hypertension during pregnancy (Cochrane

Review). In: *The Cochrane library*, issue 2. Oxford: Update Software. Systematic review of 27 randomized trials comparing beta-blockers with placebo/no therapy, or other antihypertensive agents, for women with mild–moderate pregnancy hypertension (i.e. blood pressure less than 170 mmHg systolic or 110 mmHg diastolic). Oral beta-blockers decreased the risk of severe hypertension (14 trials, 1516 women; RR 0.37, 95% CI 0.26–0.53) and the need for additional antihypertensive drugs. Insufficient data prevented firm conclusions about the effect on perinatal mortality or preterm delivery. Beta-blockers appeared to be associated with an increase in small-for-gestational-age infants (RR 1.34, 95% CI 1.01–1.79). In 11 trials (787 women) comparing beta-blockers with methyldopa, there was no evidence of any differences between the drugs in efficacy or safety (either maternal or fetal). **Ia A**

7 Duley L, Henderson-Smart DJ (2001) Drugs for rapid treatment of very high blood pressure during pregnancy (Cochrane Review). In: *The Cochrane library*, issue 2. Oxford: Update Software. Systematic review of 14 randomized trials of intravenous drugs for severe hypertension in pregnancy. Ketanserin was found to be less effective than hydralazine in reducing blood pressure. Diazoxide was associated with profound hypotension requiring treatment. Otherwise, there was no evidence that any one of the other antihypertensive agents was better than another. **Ia A**

Chapter 27

Diabetes

27.1 Diabetes

Robert Fraser

Management option		Quality of evidence	Strength of recommendation	References
Prepregnancy	Explain general risks and management of diabetes in pregnancy	IV	C	1
	Evaluate any additional risks with appropriate specialist referral (e.g. renal, ophthalmological)	III Ib	B A	2 3
	Optimize blood glucose control	III	B	4
	Discuss effective contraception until good glucose control (avoid estrogen-containing preparations with vascular disease)	–	✔	–
	Folate supplementation (4–5 mg daily) for at least 2 months before and during first trimester	Ib	A	5
Prenatal	Screen for gestational diabetes, ideally in all pregnancies	IV	C	6
	Regular capillary glucose series	Ia	A	7
	Avoid oral hypoglycemic agents	–	✔	–
	Appropriate diet	IV	C	8
	Amend insulin regimen to keep capillary glucose values as normal as possible, though limited evidence to support this approach	Ia III	A B	7 9
	Insulin pump does not confer advantage over conventional insulin treatment	Ib	A	10
	Instruct partners/relatives in glucagon use for hypoglycemic attacks	–	✔	–
	Baseline renal and possibly cardiac function	–	✔	–
	Randomized trials of low-dose aspirin in women with vascular disease are awaited	–	✔	–
	Regular ophthalmological review	Ib	A	3
	Monitor for hypertensive disease	III	B	2
	Fetal surveillance; limited evidence for value of these tests in diabetic pregnancies: ❑ Normality ❑ Growth ❑ Wellbeing ❑ Umbilical artery blood flow	 III III Ia IIb III III	 B B A B B B	 11 12–14 15,16 17 18,19 20,21

Management option		Quality of evidence	Strength of recommendation	References
Prenatal (cont'd)	Gestational diabetics: initially try to control with diet rather before insulin; otherwise manage as for established diabetics (evidence supporting this approach is limited)	IV Ia Ib	C A A	22 23 24–29
Labor and delivery	Timing: can be delayed until term if diabetes is well-controlled and pregnancy uncomplicated. Limited evidence on the value of induction of labour to prevent complications of macrosomia	Ib	A	30
	Use of tests of lung maturity is controversial	III	B	31
	Method: will depend on complications in mother (e.g. hypertension, ophthalmic) and/or fetus (e.g. macrosomia, acute fetal compromise) when cesarean section more likely	III	B	12,13,14
	Maintain good perinatal glucose control	III	B	32
Postnatal	Reduced insulin requirements	–	✓	–
	Continue capillary glucose monitoring	–	✓	–
	Encourage breastfeeding	–	✓	–
	Give contraceptive advice	–	✓	–

References

1 Elixhauser A, Weschler JM, Kitzmiller JL *et al.* (1993) Cost benefit analysis of pre-conception care for women with established diabetes mellitus. *Diabetes Care* **16**, 1146–1157. Literature review, consensus statements and surveys used to obtain cost benefits of preconceptional care and antenatal care compared to antenatal care alone. Preconceptional care estimated to save US $1720 per subject enrolled in the hypothetical program. **IV C**

2 Gordon M, Landon MB, Samuels P *et al.* (1996) Perinatal outcome and long term follow-up associated with modern management of diabetic nephropathy. *Obstet Gynecol* **87**, 401–409. Retrospective analysis of single units case series of 46 pregnancies in White's class F diabetics. Mean GA 36 weeks, birthweight 2623g with 100% perinatal survival. Most complications seen with initial creatinine above 1.5mg/dl or urinary protein above 3g/ml. **III B**

3 Laatikainen L, Teramo K, Hieta-Heikurainen H *et al.* (1987) A controlled study of the influence of CSII treatment of diabetic retinopathy in pregnancy. *Acta Med Scand* **221**, 367–376. A total of 40 type I diabetics were randomized to conventional or continuous subcutaneous insulin infusion (CSII) treatment at end of 1st trimester. 9 in the CSII group refused treatment. The proportion of patients whose retinopathy deteriorated was similar: 2/18 control, 5/13 CSII, but 2 subjects in the CSII group developed acute ischemic retinopathy. They progressed to proliferative retinopathy despite laser treatment. **Ib A**

4 Kitzmiller JL, Gavin LA, Gin GD *et al.* (1991) Preconception care of diabetes. Glycemic control prevents congenital anomalies. *JAMA* **265**, 731–736. A total of 84 type I diabetics entered into a preconceptional program of enhanced control had one (1.2%) major congenital malformation. In 110 women already pregnant at registration there were 12 anomalies (10.9%). **III B**

5 MRC Vitamin Study Research Group (1991) Prevention of neural tube defects: results of the Medical Research Council Vitamin Study. *Lancet* **338**, 131–137. RCT demonstrating significant reduction in recurrence of neural tube defects in women who took periconceptional folic acid supplements. No reference to diabetes in this paper, although maternal diabetes was not an exclusion factor. **Ib A**

6 Carpenter MW, Coustan DR (1982) Criteria for screening tests for gestational diabetes. *Am J Obstet Gynecol* **144**, 768–773. Review of O'Sullivan GDM screening criteria in light of changes in laboratory technology. Suggested plasma glucose value below 135mg/dl after 50g oral glucose challenge test associated with less than 1% gestational diabetes mellitus (GDM) by ADA criteria, value below182mg/dl 95% probability of GDM, intermediate group 135–142 12.9%. More than 142 83% sensitivity, 87% specificity. Low groups on glucose challenge test not offered oral glucose tolerance test, so calculations not valid (272 /381 subjects). **IV C**

7 Walkinshaw SA (2000) Very tight versus tight control for diabetes in pregnancy. In: *Cochrane database of systematic reviews*, issue 4. Oxford: Update Software. Two unsatisfactory studies compared. No benefit of enhanced control seen in perinatal outcome. Episodes of maternal hypoglycemia a disadvantage. **Ia A**

8 Nuttal FQ, Brunzell DJ (1979) Principles of nutrition and dietary recommendation for individuals with diabetes mellitus. *Diabetes* **28**, 1027–1030. Consensus statement on nutrition guidelines for diabetics by American Diabetes Association Committee on Food and Nutrition. **IV C**

9 Anonymous (1991) Multicentre study of diabetic pregnancy in France. Gestation and Diabetes in France Study Group. *Diabetes Care* **14**, 994–1000. Prospective study in 46 centers using HbA_{1c} analysis to reflect quality of glycemic control. 487 pregnancies, 232 type I, 78 type II, 173 gestational diabetes mellitus. Results 1.8% perinatal mortality (1.2% – nondiabetics), 3% congenital malformations. High rates of preterm birth and cesarian section. Higher than average birthweights. Poor control associated with miscarriage and malformations. **III B**

10 Coustan DR, Reese EA, Sherwin RS *et al.* (1986) A randomized clinical trial of the insulin pump vs intensive conventional therapy in diabetic pregnancies. *JAMA* **255**, 631–636. RCT of 22 type I diabetic women to conventional (II) or insulin pump therapy (II). There were no differences in mean glucose levels, symptomatic hypoglycemia or glycated hemoglobin levels. There were no significant differences in mode of delivery or neonatal outcome. **Ib A**

11 Greene MF, Benacerraf BR (1991) Prenatal diagnosis in diabetic gravidas: utility of ultrasound and maternal serum alpha-fetoprotein screening. *Obstet Gynecol* **77**, 520–524. In a series of 432 type I/II diabetics, maternal serum alpha-fetoprotein ascertained in 393 did not increase the sensitivity of ultrasound scanning for congenital malformations performed between 12 and 23 weeks. Sensitivity of ultrasound 56% and specificity 99.5%, PPV 90%. **III B**

12 Acker DB, Sachs B, Friedman EA (1985) Risk factors for shoulder dystocia. *Obstet Gynecol* **66**, 762–768. Retrospective analysis of shoulder dystocia in 144 diabetics (all types) and 14577 non-diabetic women delivering vaginally. Shoulder dystocia (diagnosed by individual conducting delivery) rates were 10% over 4.0kg and 22.6% over 4.5kg in normals and 23% and 50% in diabetics respectively. **III B**

13 Tamaura RK, Sabbagha RE, Depp R *et al.* (1986) Diabetic macrosomia: accuracy of third trimester ultrasound. *Obstet Gynecol* **67**, 828–832. In a series of 147 diabetics (all types) sensitivity of late pregnancy ultrasound examination for identification of macrosomia (birthweight > 90th centile for gestational age) was biparietal diameter 13.4%, head circumference 50%, but abdominal circumference was 78% with specificity at 76.7% and PPV at 79.4%. **III B**

14 Landon MB, Mintz MC, Gabbe SG (1989) Sonographic evaluation of fetal abdominal growth: predictor of the large-for-gestational age infant in pregnancies complicated by diabetes mellitus. *Am J Obstet Gynecol* **160**, 115–121. Longitudinal study of ultrasound measurements of abdominal circumference, head circumference and femur length in 79 diabetic women (type II, $n = 24$; type I, $n = 55$). Among large-for-gestational-age fetuses there was no difference in rates of growth of head circumference and femur length compared to average-for-gestational-age. Abdominal circumference increased at 1.36 ± 0.16 cm/week in the large-for-gestational-age group and 0.90 ± 0.21 cm/week in the average-for-gestational-age group, the difference emerging only at 32 weeks onwards. **III B**

15 Alfirevic Z, Nielson JP (2000) Biophysical profile for fetal assessment in high risk pregnancies. In: *Cochrane database of systematic reviews*, issue 4. Oxford: Update Software. There is not enough evidence from RCT to evaluate the use of biophysical profile as a test of fetal wellbeing in high-risk pregnancies. Two studies in meta-analysis included diabetics; two did not. **Ia A**

16 Pattison N, McCowan L (2000) Cardiotocography for antepartum fetal assessment. In: *Cochrane database of systematic reviews*, issue 4. Oxford: Update Software. Antenatal cardiotocography had no significant effect on perinatal mortality or morbidity. Of four papers included, three excluded diabetes. **Ia A**

17 Golde SH, Montoro M, Good-Anderson B *et al.* (1984) The role of nonstress tests, fetal biophysical profile and contraction stress tests in the outpatient management of insulin-requiring diabetic pregnancies. *Am J Obstet Gynecol* **148**, 269–273. Observational study of twice-weekly contraction stress tests from 34 weeks in 107 type I diabetics compared with once-weekly tests in 140 historical controls. No excess mortality in either group. **III B**

18 Landon MB, Langer O, Gabbe SG *et al.* (1992) Fetal surveillance in pregnancies complicated by insulin-dependent diabetes mellitus. *Am J Obstet Gynecol* **167**, 617–621. Observational study of abnormal CTG in relation to blood glucose control in 114 type I diabetic women. 8% nonreactive tests but no relationship to quality of diabetic control. **III B**

19 Johnson JM, Lange IR, Harman CR *et al.* (1988) Biophysical profile scoring in the management of the diabetic pregnancy. *Obstet Gynecol* **72**, 841–846. Evaluation of biophysical profiles in 50 type I and 188 gestational diabetes (GDM) pregnancies. 8 subjects had abnormal biophysical profiles and were delivered electively as a result. None had a perinatal death, or respiratory distress syndrome, or 5 min Apgar less than 7. In the normal biophysical profile group, labor was awaited until 40 weeks in type I and 42 weeks in GDM with no intrauterine fetal distress recorded. **III B**

20 Landon MB, Gabbe SG, Bruner JP *et al.* (1989) Doppler umbilical artery flow velocitometry in pregnancy complicated by insulin dependent diabetes mellitus. *Obstet Gynecol* **73**, 961–965. Umbilical artery peak systolic to end diastolic (S/D) ratio performed in 35 type I diabetics between 18–38 weeks. No evidence of Doppler abnormalities except in those with established vascular disease – (White's class F/R), 4 of 5 abnormal S/D ratios associated with intrauterine growth restriction, 5 of 5 normal S/D ratios associated with appropriately grown infants. **III B**

21 Johnstone FD, Steel JM, Haddad NG *et al.* (1992) Doppler umbilical artery flow velocity waveforms in diabetic pregnancy. *Br J Obstet Gynecol* **99**, 135–140. 128 Insulin-treated diabetic studied every 2 weeks compared with cross-sectional study of 170 nondiabetics for abnormal umbilical artery resistance index (RI). Normal range for diabetics without vasculopathy similar to nondiabetics. No relationship between RI and glycemic control. 3 of 7 pregnancies with antenatal fetal compromise (variously defined) had abnormal RI. 9 subjects with abnormal RI were more likely to show antenatal fetal compromise and birthweight below the 50th centile. **III B**

22 O'Sullivan J (1991) Summary and recommendations of the Third International Workshop-Conference on Gestational Diabetes Mellitus. *Diabetes* **40**(suppl 2), 197–201. Consensus statements on diagnosis, perinatal implications and long term implications from workshop on gestational diabetes mellitus. **IV C**

23 Walkinshaw SA (2000) Dietary regulation for 'gestational diabetes'. In: *Cochrane database of systematic reviews*, issue 4. Oxford: Update Software. No evidence of benefit from diet therapy versus no therapy for birthweight above 4.0kg or cesarean section rate. **Ia A**

24 Hopp H, Leis R, Albus C (1990) Indications and results of insulin therapy for gestational diabetes mellitus. *J Perinat Med* **24**, 521–530. 123 women with gestational diabetes mellitus were randomized to conventional insulin therapy, based on maternal mean blood glucose levels, or target-orientated insulin therapy based on levels of liquor insulin after amniocentesis performed at 28 and 32 weeks gestation (AFI). No difference in severe preeclampsia, urinary tract infection, preterm labour or delivery. AFI group had higher insulin dose (59U/day vs 42U/day) and significantly lower rate of cesarian section (8/61 vs 17/62). Birthweight above the 95% centile occurred in 3/61 and 22/62 respectively and neonatal hypoglycemia in 8/61 vs 17/62. **Ib A**

25 Buchanan TA (1994) Use of fetal ultrasound to select metabolic therapy for pregnancies complicated by mild gestational diabetes. *Diabetes Care* **17**, 275–283. RCT of Hispanic women with diet-treated gestational diabetes (n = 29) or diet and insulin (n = 30) identified by ultrasound detection of abdominal circumference above the 75th centile between 29 and 33 weeks. GA at delivery was 39.6 in insulin-treated and 39.5 in diet-treated groups. Birthweight and large-for-gestational-age rates were 3647g and 3878g and 13% vs 45%. Neonatal hypoglycemia rates were not significantly different (14% vs 18%). **Ib A**

26 Bancroft K, Tuffnell DJ, Mason GC *et al.* (2000) A randomised controlled pilot study of the management of gestational impaired glucose tolerance. *Br J Obstet Gynaecol* **107**, 959–963. 68 women with impaired glucose tolerance by World Health Organization criteria were randomized to monitor plasma glucose, or not, in late pregnancy. Monitoring group had 19% rate of insulin prescription but no statistically significant differences emerged in perinatal outcomes – cesarian section 10/32 monitored 11/36 unmonitored; special care baby unit admission 6% vs 17%; hypoglycemia 6% vs 17%; gestation at delivery 39 weeks vs 39 weeks; birthweight 3580g vs 3620g; birthweight above the 90th centile 25% vs 19%. **Ib A**

27 Garner P, Okun N, Keely E *et al.* (1997) A randomized controlled trial of strict glycemic control and tertiary level obstetric care vs routine obstetric care in the management of gestational diabetes: a pilot study. *Am J Obstet Gynecol* **177**, 190–195. Pilot study designed to assess feasibility of larger scale study. RCT in 300 women in gestational diabetes mellitus by World Health Organization criteria. Trial group referred to tertiary care for detailed blood glucose monitoring and diet and insulin to maintain glycemic levels below 7.8 1h postprandial. Controls monitored glucose twice a week but care givers unaware of their test results. If fasting plasma glucose above 7.8 or 1h above 11.1mmol/l , controls were revealed (16/150 – 10.6%). No difference in length of gestation; cesarian section rates 20% treated, 18% controls; mean birthweight 3437g vs 3544g; birthweight over 4000g 16.1% treated 18.7% controls. No perinatal mortality or birth trauma; neonatal hypoglycemia 14.1% treated, 8.7% controls. **Ib A**

28 Langer O, Conway DL, Berkus MD *et al.* (2000) A comparison of glyburide and insulin in women with gestational diabetes mellitus. *N Engl J Med* **343**, 1134–1138. 404 women with gestational diabetes mellitus by American Diabetes Association criteria randomized to glyburide (glibenclamide) or insulin for hypoglycemic therapy in pregnancy. No difference in HbA_{1c}, large-for-gestational-age, RDS/TTN, hypoglycemia, admission to special care baby unit, congenital anomalies. **Ib A**

29 Persson B, Stangenberg M, Hansson U *et al.* (1985) Gestational diabetes mellitus (GDM). Comparative evaluation of two treatment regimens, diet versus insulin and diet. *Diabetes* **34**, 101–105. 302 women with gestational diabetes mellitus based on 50g oral glucose tolerance test randomized to diet and insulin or diet alone. Insulin was given to 14% of diet alone group when fasting levels of blood glucose exceeded 7mmol/l or postprandial 9mmol/l. No difference in gestational age, birthweight, large-for-gestational-age, skinfold thickness in newborn, hypoglycemia or neonatal respiratory problems. **Ib A**

30 Kjos SL, Henry OA, Montoro M *et al.* (1993) Insulin-requiring diabetes in pregnancy: a randomized trial of active induction of labour and expectant management. *Am J Obstet Gynecol* **169**, 611–615. RCT in 200 women with insulin-requiring gestational diabetes or class B type I diabetes, of active induction within 5 days of 38 completed weeks gestation or expectant management until spontaneous labor, monitored by twice-weekly nonstress tests and ultrasound amniotic fluid volume estimation weekly. Cesarian section rates not significantly different, 31% expectant, 25% active. Birthweights and macrosomia rates (birthweight above the 90th centile for gestational age) higher in expectant group (3672g vs 3466g) and 23% vs 10% large for gestational age. Shoulder dystocia 0% in active, 3% in expectant group. **Ib A**

31 Kjos SL, Walther FJ, Montoro M *et al.* (1990) Prevalence and etiology of respiratory distress in infants of diabetic mothers: predictive value of fetal lung maturation tests. *Am J Obstet Gynecol* **163**, 898–903. Comparison of three diagnostic tests for respiratory distress syndrome in newborns of 526 diabetic women delivered within 5 days of test – lecithin/sphingomyelin ratio, positive phosphatidylglycerol, or optical density at 650nm ≥0.150. Each test had 100% sensitivity and specificity by limited positive predictive values, 15%, 9% and 3% respectively. **III B**

32 McManus RM, Ryan EA (1992) Insulin requirements in insulin-dependent and insulin-requiring women during final months of pregnancy. *Diabetes Care* **15**, 1323–1327. Observational study to identify significance of falling insulin requirements after 36 weeks gestation in type I and gestational diabetes mellitus insulin-requiring diabetic women. 62% of women had a reduction in insulin requirements but this was not an adverse prognostic index for either maternal or fetal complications. **III B**

Chapter 28

Cardiac disease

28.1 Cardiac disease: general

Catherine Nelson-Piercy

Management option		Quality of evidence	Strength of recommendation	References
Prepregnancy	Obstetrician and cardiologist in collaboration	IV	C	1
	Discussion of maternal/fetal risks	IV	C	1
	Discussion of effective/safe contraception	–	✔	–
	Obtain update on cardiac status	III	B	2
	Optimize medical and surgical management	III	B	3
	Advise against pregnancy with certain conditions	III	B	4
Prenatal	Assess functional class of heart disease	III	B	2
	Termination is an option with a few conditions	III	B	4–7
	Joint management with a cardiologist	IV	C	1
	Optimize medical management	IV	C	1
	Avoid/minimize aggravating factors	IV	C	1
	Anticoagulation for certain conditions (stop warfarin and change to subcutaneous heparin)	IIb	B	8
	Prophylactic antibiotics with certain conditions	IV	C	9
	Fetal surveillance: ❑ Growth and umbilical artery Doppler (especially if left-to-right shunt) ❑ Detailed fetal cardiac ultrasonography if maternal congenital heart disease	III	B	2
Labor and delivery	Elective induction may be necessary for maternal and/or fetal indications	IIb III	B B	8 7
	Prophylactic antibiotics with certain conditions	IV	C	9
	Avoid mental and physical stress (epidural?)	III	B	7
	Labor in left lateral or upright position	III	B	3
	Monitor electrocardiogram; more invasive monitoring with certain conditions	–	✔	–
	Administer extra oxygen with certain conditions	–	✔	–

Management option		Quality of evidence	Strength of recommendation	References
Labor and delivery (cont'd)	Full resuscitation facilities available	–	✔	–
	Continuous fetal heart rate monitoring	–	✔	–
	Assisted second stage with certain conditions	–	✔	–
	Avoid ergometrine for third stage	–	✔	–
Postnatal	Vigilance for cardiac failure	–	✔	–
	Avoid fluid overload	IV	C	1
	Continued high-dependency care	–	✔	–
	Discuss effective/safe contraception	–	✔	–

References

1 Tan J, de Swiet M (1998) *Cardiac disease in pregnancy*. PACE review no. 98/02. London: Royal College of Obstetricians and Gynaecologists. Review of cardiac disease in pregnancy. **IV C**

2 McCaffrey FM, Sherman FS (1995) Pregnancy and congenital heart disease: the Magee Women's Hospital. *J Matern Fetal Med* **4**, 152–159. Retrospective single-institution review of 111 pregnancies in 61 women with significant congenital heart disease. The data show that the hemodynamic significance of any lesion predicts maternal morbidity and functional class deterioration as well as being inversely related to the percentage of term live births. Women who are in a poor functional status (New York Heart Association III or IV), regardless of their specific lesion, do not do well. Cyanotic women may have successful pregnancies provided they do not have Eisenmenger physiology or poor functional class. The authors recommend that the patient's functional state is the single best variable to follow during pregnancy. **III B**

3 Desai DK, Adanlawo M, Naidoo DP *et al.* (2000) Mitral stenosis in pregnancy: a four-year experience at King Edward VIII Hospital Durban, South Africa. *Br J Obstet Gynaecol* **107**, 953–958. Observational study of 128 women with mitral stenosis, of whom 42% were diagnosed for the first time in pregnancy. 51% developed maternal complications, most commonly in the third trimester or early post-partum. The commonest complication was pulmonary edema, which could be predicted by: severity of mitral stenosis as assessed by mitral valve area; late antenatal presentation; moderate to severe symptoms prior to pregnancy; diagnosis during pregnancy. 20 women had a balloon mitral valvulotomy with good effect. Other persistently symptomatic women were managed conservatively with good outcome. **III B**

4 Yentis SM, Steer PJ, Plaat F (1998) Eisenmenger's syndrome in pregnancy: maternal and fetal mortality in the 1990s. *Br J Obstet Gynaecol* **105**, 921–922. Questionnaire study of all obstetric units in the UK, which identified 15 pregnancies progressing into the second trimester in women with Eisenmenger syndrome. The maternal mortality rate was 40% (a figure that has remained unchanged over 50 years), and fetal loss 8%. Only 15% of infants were born at term. The authors reiterate previous advice that such women should be strongly advised against pregnancy or offered therapeutic termination in the event of pregnancy. **III B**

5 Elkayam U, Tummala PP, Rao K *et al.* (2001) Maternal and fetal outcomes of subsequent pregnancies in women with peripartum cardiomyopathy. *N Engl J Med* **344**, 1567–1571. Retrospective cohort study of 44 women identified by a questionnaire survey as having subsequent pregnancies after previous peripartum cardiomyopathy. These pregnancies were associated with a reduction in the mean left ventricular (LV) ejection fraction from 49 ± 12% to 42 ± 13%. In the 28 pregnancies occurring in women whose LV function had returned to normal, 21% were associated with symptoms of heart failure and LV ejection fraction reduced from 56 ± 7% to 49 ± 10%. In the 16 pregnancies occurring in women with persistent LV dysfunction, 44% of the women had symptoms of heart failure, the LV ejection fraction reduced from 36 ± 9% to 32 ± 11%, and maternal mortality was 19%. The authors conclude that subsequent pregnancy in women with previous peripartum cardiomyopathy causes significant reduction in LV function and possibly death. As in previous studies, the risks are higher for those whose LV function does not recover after the initial episode. **III B**

6 Avila, WS, Grinberg M, Snitcowsky R *et al.* (1995) Maternal and fetal outcome in pregnant women with Eisenmenger's syndrome. *Eur Heart J* **16**, 460–464. Series of women with Eisenmenger syndrome who continued with pregnancies despite recommendation for therapeutic abortion. There were 13 pregnancies in 12 women. There were 3 maternal deaths at 23 weeks, 27 weeks and 4 weeks postpartum. The successful pregnancies were with admission for bed rest from the end of the second trimester, heparin and oxygen therapy. **III B**

7 Lipscomb KJ, Smith JC, Clarke B *et al.* (1997) Outcome of pregnancy in women with Marfan's syndrome. *Br J Obstet Gynaecol* **104**, 201–206. Retrospective series of 91 pregnancies in 36 women with Marfan syndrome. It demonstrates that there is a significant risk of aortic dissection (and death) in women with Marfan during pregnancy. Progressive aortic root dilation and an aortic root dimension of 4 cm or more suggest an increased risk. The authors recommend (1) monthly echocardiography, (2) vaginal delivery with epidural for those with stable measurements, (3) elective cesarean section with epidural for those with aortic roots 4 cm or more or increases during pregnancy and (4) beta-blockers for hypertension and possibly from the second trimester in those with aortic dilation. **III B**

8 Chan WS, Anand S, Ginsberg JS (2000) Anticoagulation of pregnant women with mechanical heart valves. *Arch Intern Med* **160**, 191–196. Systematic review of the literature from 1966–97 including 28 articles (6 cohort studies and 22 case series; 8 prospective longitudinal follow-up) and 1234 pregnancies in 976 women. Fetal and maternal outcomes were analyzed according to three broad anticoagulation regimes: oral anticoagulants throughout pregnancy; replacement with heparin for the first trimester; or heparin throughout pregnancy. Warfarin use throughout pregnancy is associated with warfarin embryopathy in 6.4% of cases. This risk is eliminated if heparin is substituted at or before 6 weeks and until 12 weeks. Risks for fetal wastage (miscarriage, stillbirths and neonatal deaths) were similar in all three groups (33.6%, 26.5%, 42.9%) but thromboembolic complications and maternal death are more common with low-dose heparin throughout (60%, 40%), adjusted-dose heparin throughout (25%, 6.7%) and heparin substitution in the first trimester (9.2%, 4.2%) than with the maintenance of oral anticoagulants throughout pregnancy (3.9%, 1.8%). **IIb B**

9 Dajani AS, Taubert KA, Wilson W *et al.* (1997) Prevention of bacterial endocarditis. Recommendations by the American Heart Association. *JAMA* **277**, 1794–1801. Consensus statement. Useful stratification of cardiac conditions associated with high, medium and low risk of endocarditis. High risk: prosthetic valves; previous bacterial endocarditis; complex cyanotic congenital heart disease, e.g. Fallot's; surgically constructed systemic pulmonary shunts, e.g. Fontan. Difference from UK guidelines = use clindamycin instead of erythromycin for penicillin-allergic patients. **IV C**

28.2 Cardiac disease: specific

Catherine Nelson-Piercy

Management option		Quality of evidence	Strength of recommendation	References
Cardiac murmur	Echocardiography for significant history or pathological murmur (late systolic, pansystolic, diastolic)	III	B	1
	Cardiological referral if abnormal echocardiography	–	✔	–
Mitral valve prolapse	Cardiological and echocardiographic evaluation prenatally for mitral regurgitation	–	✔	–
	Surveillance and treatment of arrhythmias in pregnancy	–	✔	–
	Antibiotic prophylaxis for delivery if regurgitation present	–	✔	–
Atrial septal defect	**Prepregnancy**: screen for arrhythmias and/or pulmonary hypertension (PH); manage accordingly both before and during pregnancy	III	B	2
	Prenatal: routine except if arrhythmias and/or PH	III	B	2
	Labor/delivery: screen for arrhythmias, monitor blood pressure (BP), avoid fluid overload	III	B	2
	Postnatal: encourage early mobilization	III	B	2

Management option		Quality of evidence	Strength of recommendation	References
Patent ductus arteriosus	**Prepregnancy**: screen for pulmonary hypertension and manage accordingly before and during pregnancy (risks related to degree of PH)	III	B	2
	Prenatal: screen for PH	III	B	2
	Labor/delivery/postnatal: monitor BP, attention to normal fluid balance, antibiotic prophylactics except for normal deliveries	III	B	2
Coarctation of the aorta	**Prepregnancy**: screen for aneurysms and/or aortic valve disease and manage appropriately prior to conception, including surgical repair	IV	C	3
	Prenatal: consider termination with severe uncorrected disease	IV	C	3
	Labor/delivery/postnatal: avoid hypertension, antibiotic prophylaxis except for normal delivery, screen newborn for congenital heart disease (CHD)	IV	C	3
Ventricular septal defect	**Prepregnancy**: screen for PH and manage accordingly, consider repair of uncorrected lesions, counseling about CHD risks	III	B	2
	Prenatal: serial echocardiography and manage accordingly	III	B	2
	Labor/delivery: avoid hypertension, antibiotic prophylaxis except for normal delivery	III	B	2
	Postnatal: careful fluid balance, early ambulation	III	B	2
Primary pulmonary hypertension	**Prepregnancy**: counsel against pregnancy because of high maternal mortality, sterilization if requested	III	B	4–6
	Prenatal: consider termination, obstetric and cardiological joint care, early anesthesiologist consultation, thromboembolism prophylaxis, consider hospital admission, monitor arterial oxygen saturation (S_aO_2), fetal surveillance	III	B	4–6
	Labor/delivery: high-dependency setting (degree of invasive monitoring varies); dilemma over induction (end pregnancy) versus spontaneous (shorter labor) onset of labor, oxytocic or E series prostaglandins safe, O_2 at 5–6 l/min, monitor S_aO_2 continuously, monitor BP, maintain fluid balance, epidural analgesic, reduce/stop anticoagulant for a few hours for delivery	III	B	4–6
	Postnatal: maintain high-dependency monitoring, O_2 therapy and thromboembolism prophylaxis, vigilance for fluid retention and consequences, consider sterilization	III	B	4–6

➡

Management option		Quality of evidence	Strength of recommendation	References
Eisenmenger complex	As for primary pulmonary hypertension (NB: high maternal mortality)	III	B	4–6
	Echocardiography may be helpful	III	B	4–6
Tetralogy of Fallot	**Prepregnancy**: surgical correction; evaluation of cardiac status after corrective surgery (risks dependent on success of repair)	III	B	2,7
	Prenatal: consider termination with uncorrected lesions, monitor maternal S_aO_2 and exercise tolerance, consider rest and supplemental O_2, fetal surveillance	III	B	2,7
	Labor/delivery: careful fluid management, monitor BP, electrocardiogram (ECG). Epidural use requires careful preloading, need to shorten second stage, fetal monitoring	III	B	2,7
	Postnatal: maintain maternal monitoring, discuss effective contraception	III	B	2,7
Rheumatic heart disease: general	**Principles**: ❑ Prevent heart failure ❑ Prevent bacterial endocarditis	–	✔	–
Mitral stenosis	**Prepregnancy**: assess cardiac function, optimize medical therapy, consider surgical correction	III	B	8,9
	Prenatal: avoid excess weight gain, tachycardia, serial echocardiography, treat tachycardia/arrhythmias, surgery for symptomatic severe disease, fetal surveillance	III	B	8,9
	Labor/delivery: high-dependency/intensive-care setting, consider central invasive monitoring, epidural analgesia has benefits, antibiotic prophylaxis for complicated deliveries, fetal surveillance	III	B	8,9
Mitral regurgitation	**Prepregnancy**: as for stenosis (although condition has many causes, not just rheumatic disease)	IV	C	10
	Prenatal: restrict activity, serial echocardiography, adjust medical control, consider surgery for symptomatic severe disease, fetal surveillance (although fetal risk not high)	IV	C	10
	Labor/delivery/postnatal: avoid fluid overload and hypertension, maternal cardiac monitoring, endocarditis prophylaxis for complicated deliveries	IV	C	10
Aortic regurgitation	**Prepregnancy**: as for mitral disease	IV	C	10
	Prenatal: surveillance for cardiac failure, surgery for failed medical therapy, fetal surveillance	IV	C	10
	Labor/delivery/postnatal: avoid fluid overload, invasive monitoring usually unnecessary, epidural beneficial, fetal surveillance	IV	C	10

➡

Management option		Quality of evidence	Strength of recommendation	References
Prosthetic valves	**Prepregnancy**: assess cardiac status, counseling about valve function and warfarin risks	IIb	B	11–13
	Prenatal: biosynthetic valves – vigilance for deterioration, mechanical valves, adequate anticoagulation	IIb	B	11
	Labor/delivery: adjust anticoagulation, endocarditis prophylaxis	IIb	B	11,12
	Postnatal: readjust anticoagulation	IIb	B	11–13
Marfan syndrome	**Prepregnancy**: genetic counseling, echocardiography (especially aortic root), counsel against pregnancy	III	B	14
	Prenatal: serial aortic root. echocardiography, beta-blocker, avoid hypertension, encourage rest, surgery in extreme cases	III Ia	B A	14 15
	Labor/delivery/postnatal: epidural beneficial, avoid hypertension, ensure adequate oxygenation, short second stage, vigilance for aortic root dissection for at least 8 weeks postnatally	III	B	14
Dilated cardiomyopathy	**Prepregnancy**: counsel against pregnancy, if history of peripartum cardiomyopathy	III	B	16,17
	Prenatal: termination of pregnancy with abnormal echocardiogram, medical therapy if symptomatic, anticoagulation	III	B	16–18
	Labor/delivery: monitor for heart failure, avoid fluid overload, care with invasive monitoring	III	B	16–18
	Postnatal: avoid fluid overload, discuss contraception	III	B	16–18
Cardiac arrhythmias	**Prepregnancy**: investigate and rest	IIa III	B B	19 20,21
	Prenatal/labor/delivery/postnatal: maintenance of therapy to control arrhythmia, cardioconversion can be used	IIa III	B B	19 20,21
Myocardial infarction	**Prepregnancy**: assess cardiac function (especially echocardiography and stress test), counsel for pregnancy on basis of results, low-dose aspirin; look for underlying conditions (e.g. antiphospholipid syndrome)	III Ib	B A	22 23
	Prenatal: avoid strenuous activity, surveillance for failure and arrhythmias, management as for nonpregnant, surgery can be carried out in pregnancy, thrombolytic therapy	III Ib IV	B A C	22 23 24–29
	Labor/delivery: monitor ECG, supplementary oxygen, epidural beneficial	III Ib IV	B A C	22 23 24–29
	Postnatal: avoid fluid overload and exertion, discuss contraception (avoid combination oral preparations)	III	B	22

Management option		Quality of evidence	Strength of recommendation	References
Idiopathic hypertrophic subaortic stenosis	**Prepregnancy**: genetic counseling if parents have condition	III	B	30
	Prenatal: limit activity, beta-blockers for symptomatic parents	III	B	30
	Labor/delivery/postnatal: avoid dehydration/hypotension, beta-blockers for tachycardia, endocarditis prophylaxis for complicated pregnancies	III	B	30

References

1 Tan J, de Swiet M (1998) Prevalence of heart disease diagnosed de novo in pregnancy in a West London population. *Br J Obstet Gynaecol* **105**, 1185–1188. Population study showing that it was unusual to find new heart disease except in immigrants. **III B**

2 McCaffrey FM, Sherman FS (1995) Pregnancy and congenital heart disease: the Magee Women's Hospital. *J Matern Fetal Med* **4**, 152–159. Retrospective single-institution review of 111 pregnancies in 61 women with significant congenital heart disease. The data show that the hemodynamic significance of any lesion predicts maternal morbidity and functional class deterioration as well as being inversely related to the percentage of term live births. Women who are in a poor functional status (New York Heart Association III or IV), regardless of their specific lesion, do not do well. Cyanotic women may have successful pregnancies provided they do not have Eisenmenger physiology or poor functional class. The authors recommend that the patient's functional state is the single best variable to follow during pregnancy. **III B**

3 Barash PG, Hobbins JC, Hook R *et al.* (1975) Management of coarctation of the aorta during pregnancy. *J Thorac Cardiovasc Surg* **69**, 781–784. Case report of fetal heart rate monitoring at 24 weeks gestation during resection of coarctation. **IV C**

4 Smedstad KG, Cramb R, Morison DH *et al.* (1994) Pulmonary hypertension and pregnancy: a series of eight cases. *Can J Anaesth* **41**, 502–512. Case series of 8 women with primary or secondary pulmonary hypertension between 1978 and 1987 delivered in one unit. Maternal death = 1/8. The remaining 7 had assisted vaginal deliveries using epidural analgesia. The authors recommend elective admission, oxygen and anticoagulation. Intrapartum monitoring was with arterial and central venous but not pulmonary artery lines. **III B**

5 Avila, WS, Grinberg M, Snitcowsky R *et al.* (1995) Maternal and fetal outcome in pregnant women with Eisenmenger's syndrome. *Eur Heart J* **16**, 460–464. Series of women with Eisenmenger syndrome who continued with pregnancies despite recommendation for therapeutic abortion. There were 13 pregnancies in 12 women. There were 3 maternal deaths at 23 weeks, 27 weeks and 4 weeks postpartum. The successful pregnancies were with admission for bed rest from the end of the second trimester, heparin and oxygen therapy. **III B**

6 Yentis SM, Steer PJ, Plaat F (1998) Eisenmenger's syndrome in pregnancy: maternal and fetal mortality in the 1990s. *Br J Obstet Gynaecol* **105**, 921–922. Questionnaire study of all obstetric units in the UK, which identified 15 pregnancies progressing into the second trimester in women with Eisenmenger syndrome. The maternal mortality rate was 40% (a figure that has remained unchanged over 50 years), and fetal loss 8%. Only 15% of infants were born at term. The authors reiterate previous advice that such women should be strongly advised against pregnancy or offered therapeutic termination in the event of pregnancy. **III B**

7 Singh H, Bolton PJ, Oakley CM (1982) Pregnancy after surgical correction of tetralogy of Fallot. *Br Med J Clin Res Ed* **285**, 168–170. Review of reported literature of 40 pregnancies in 27 women after surgically corrected Fallot's. Pregnancy was well tolerated and no serious cardiac complications. One out of 31 babies had congenital heart disease (pulmonary atresia). **III B**

8 Desai DK, Adanlawo M, Naidoo DP *et al.* (2000) Mitral stenosis in pregnancy: a four-year experience at King Edward VIII Hospital Durban, South Africa. *Br J Obstet Gynaecol* **107**, 953–958. Observational study of 128 women with mitral stenosis, of whom 42% were diagnosed for the first time in pregnancy. 51% developed maternal complications, most commonly in the third trimester or early post-partum. The commonest complication was pulmonary edema, which could be predicted by: severity of mitral stenosis as assessed by mitral valve area; late antenatal presentation; moderate to severe symptoms prior to pregnancy; diagnosis during pregnancy. 20 women had a balloon mitral valvulotomy with good effect. Other persistently symptomatic women were managed conservatively with good outcome. **III B**

9 Al Kasab SM, Sabag T, al Zaibag M *et al.* (1990) Beta-adrenergic receptor blockade in the management of pregnant women with mitral stenosis. *Am J Obstet Gynecol* **163**, 37–40. Case series of 25 women with symptomatic mitral stenosis. 92% improved with propranolol or atenolol and the incidence of pulmonary edema was reduced. **III B**

10 Tan J, de Swiet M (1998) *Cardiac disease in pregnancy*. PACE review no. 98/02. London: Royal College of Obstetricians and Gynaecologists. Review of cardiac disease in pregnancy. **IV C**

11 Chan WS, Anand S, Ginsberg JS (2000) Anticoagulation of pregnant women with mechanical heart valves. *Arch Intern Med* **160**, 191–196. Systematic review of the literature from 1966–97 including 28 articles (6 cohort studies and 22 case series; 8 prospective longitudinal follow-up) and 1234 pregnancies in 976 women. Fetal and maternal outcomes were analyzed according to three broad anticoagulation regimes: oral anticoagulants throughout pregnancy; replacement with heparin for the first trimester; or heparin throughout pregnancy. Warfarin use throughout pregnancy is associated with warfarin embryopathy in 6.4% of cases. This risk is eliminated if heparin is substituted at or before 6 weeks and until 12 weeks. Risks for fetal wastage (miscarriage, stillbirths and neonatal deaths) were similar in all three groups (33.6%, 26.5%, 42.9%) but thromboembolic complications and maternal death are more common with low-dose heparin throughout (60%, 40%), adjusted-dose heparin throughout (25%, 6.7%) and heparin substitution in the first trimester (9.2%, 4.2%) than with the maintenance of oral anticoagulants throughout pregnancy (3.9%, 1.8%). **IIb B**

12 Vitale N, De Feo M, De Santo LS *et al.* (1999) Dose-dependent fetal complications of warfarin in pregnant women with mechanical heart valves. *J Am Coll Cardiol* **33**, 1637–1641. Seminal study demonstrating that the adverse fetal effects of warfarin are dose-dependent (not simply dependent on the international normalized ratio, INR) a logical finding considering the immature fetal liver and the importance of the dose received by the fetus versus the degree of anticoagulation of the mother. This was a prospective study of 58 pregnancies in 43 women. Of the 33 pregnancies in women who required 5 mg or less of warfarin to maintain an INR of 2.5–3.5, there were 5 fetal complications (4 spontaneous miscarriages and one intrauterine growth restriction). However in the 25 pregnancies in women requiring more than 5 mg of warfarin, there were 22 fetal complications, including 2 warfarin embryopathies, 18 miscarriages, one stillbirth and one ventricular septal defect. There were 2 cases of valve thrombosis, but no embolic or bleeding events. **IIb B**

13 Sadler L, McCowan L, White H *et al.* (2000) Pregnancy outcomes and cardiac complications in women with mechanical, bioprosthetic and homograft valves. *Br J Obstet Gynaecol* **107**, 245–253. Retrospective cohort study of 147 pregnancies in 79 women. It highlights the high pregnancy loss rate in women with mechanical mitral valves (59%) compared to bioprosthetic valves (7%). The fetal loss was related to warfarin use and those maintained throughout pregnancy on warfarin suffered a 70% loss rate compared to 25% for those who switched to heparin. Furthermore all the fetal losses in the heparin group occurred in the first trimester whereas there were 4 stillbirths in the group who continued warfarin. No dose-dependent effect of warfarin was demonstrated. The risk with mitral bioprosthetic valves is valve deterioration, which occurred in 10%. This study confirms the substantial risk of thromboembolic complications in women with mechanical valves treated with heparin (4/14, 29%) but it is noteworthy that all these women had Starr–Edwards valves. **IIb B**

14 Lipscomb KJ, Smith JC, Clarke B *et al.* (1997) Outcome of pregnancy in women with Marfan's syndrome. *Br J Obstet Gynaecol* **104**, 201–206. Retrospective series of 91 pregnancies in 36 women with Marfan syndrome. It demonstrates that there is a significant risk of aortic dissection (and death) in women with Marfan during pregnancy. Progressive aortic root dilation and an aortic root dimension of 4 cm or more suggest an increased risk. The authors recommend (1) monthly echocardiography, (2) vaginal delivery with epidural for those with stable measurements, (3) elective cesarean section with epidural for those with aortic roots 4 cm or more or increases during pregnancy and (4) beta-blockers for hypertension and possibly from the second trimester in those with aortic dilation. **III B**

15 Shores J, Berger KR, Murphy EA *et al.* (1994) Progression of aortic dilation and the benefit of long-term beta-adrenergic blockade in Marfan's syndrome. *N Engl J Med* **330**, 1335–1341. RCT of propranolol in 70 nonpregnant patients with Marfan syndrome. Rate of aortic root dilation was lower in the treated group. Beta-blockers also reduced development of aortic complications in some patients. **Ib A**

16 Elkayam U, Tummala PP, Rao K *et al.* (2001) Maternal and fetal outcomes of subsequent pregnancies in women with peripartum cardiomyopathy. *N Engl J Med* **344**, 1567–1571. Retrospective cohort study of 44 women identified by a questionnaire survey as having subsequent pregnancies after previous peripartum cardiomyopathy. These pregnancies were associated with a reduction in the mean left ventricular (LV) ejection fraction from 49 ± 12% to 42 ± 13%. In the 28 pregnancies occurring in women whose LV function had returned to normal, 21% were associated with symptoms of heart failure and LV ejection fraction reduced from 56 ± 7% to 49 ± 10%. In the 16 pregnancies occurring in women with persistent LV dysfunction, 44% of the women had symptoms of heart failure, the LV ejection fraction reduced from 36 ± 9% to 32 ± 11%, and maternal mortality was 19%. The authors conclude that subsequent pregnancy in women with previous peripartum cardiomyopathy causes significant reduction in LV function and possibly death. As in previous studies, the risks are higher for those whose LV function does not recover after the initial episode. **III B**

17 Witlin AG, Mabie WC, Sibai BM *et al.* (1997) Peripartum cardiomyopathy: a longitudinal echocardiographic study. *Am J Obstet Gynecol* **177**, 1129–1132. Serial echocardiography on nine women with peripartum cardiomyopathy concluding that those with severe myocardial dysfunction, defined as left-ventricular end-diastolic dimension 6 cm or more and fractional shortening 21% or less, are unlikely to regain normal cardiac function on follow-up. **III B**

18 Felker GM, Thompson RE, Hare JM *et al.* (2000) Underlying causes and long-term survival in patients with initially unexplained cardiomyopathy. *N Engl J Med* **342**, 1077–1084. Cohort of 1230 patients with unexplained cardiomyopathy, all of whom underwent endomyocardial biopsy. There were 51 cases of peripartum cardiomyopathy. These women had better survival than patients with heart failure due to other causes (idiopathic, ischemic, infiltrative, connective tissue disease) with a 94% survival at 5 years. Contrary to previous studies, 50% had histological evidence of myocarditis on endomyocardial biopsy. **III B**

19 Shotan A, Ostrzega E, Mehra A *et al.* (1997) Incidence of arrhythmias in normal pregnancy and relation to palpitations, dizziness and syncope. *Am J Cardiol* **79**, 1061–1064. Case control study of 110 women with palpitations, dizziness and syncope and 52 women with asymptomatic precordial murmur. Both groups had a high incidence of atrial premature complexes (56% and 58%) and ventricular complexes (59% and 50%). There was no correlation between premature complexes and symptoms and most symptomatic episodes were not accompanied by arrhythmias. **IIa B**

20 Lee SH, Chen SA, Wu TJ *et al.* (1995) Effects of pregnancy on first onset and symptoms of paroxysmal supraventricular tachycardia. *Am J Cardiol* **76**, 675–678. Questionnaire study of 207 women prior to catheter ablation or electrophysiological studies. First onset of supraventricular tachycardia (SVT; both accessory-pathway-mediated and atrioventricular-nodal reentrant) is rare. 22% of 63 women with SVT had exacerbation of symptoms in pregnancy. **III B**

21 Magee LA, Downar ES, Sermer M *et al.* (1995) Pregnancy outcome after gestational exposure to amiodarone. *Am J Obstet Gynecol* **172**, 1307–1311. Historic cohort of 12 cases, 6 first trimester. One case of hypothyroidism, one of hyperthyroidism, 3 fetuses with bradycardia (but one also exposed to beta-blockers). **III B**

22 Roth A, Elkayam U (1996) Acute myocardial infarction associated with pregnancy. *Ann Intern Med* **125**, 751–757. Review of 125 reported cases of myocardial infarction (MI) in pregnancy or the early postpartum period. The incidence is highest in the third trimester and in multigravid women over 33 years. Infarction is most commonly in the anterior wall. Maternal death rate was 21%, most commonly at the time of acute MI or within 2 weeks and usually related to labor and delivery. Underlying etiologies (ascertained in 54%) were: coronary atherosclerosis (± thrombus) 43%; coronary thrombus (without atheroma) 21%; coronary dissection 16%; normal coronaries 29%. **III B**

23 CLASP Collaborative Group (1995) Low-dose aspirin in pregnancy and early childhood development: follow-up of the collaborative low-dose aspirin study in pregnancy. *Br J Obstet Gynaecol* **102**, 861–868. Almost 10000 women were randomized to low-dose aspirin or placebo for preeclampsia intrauterine growth restriction prophylaxis. No increase in adverse fetal/neonatal/childhood outcomes in aspirin group. Low-dose aspirin is safe in pregnancy. **Ib A**

24 Schumacher B, Belfort MA, Card RJ (1997) Successful treatment of acute myocardial infarction during pregnancy with tissue plasminogen activator. *Am J Obstet Gynecol* **176**, 716–719. Case report of acute myocardial infarction at 21 weeks gestation successfully treated with intravenous tissue plasminogen activator. **IV C**

25 Ascarelli MH, Grider AR, Hsu HW (1996) Acute myocardial infarction during pregnancy managed with immediate percutaneous transluminal coronary angioplasty. *Obstet Gynecol* **88**, 655–657. Case report of anterior myocardial infarction in the third trimester successfully treated with immediate percutaneous transluminal coronary angioplasty. **IV C**

26 Eickman FM (1996) Acute coronary artery angioplasty during pregnancy. *Cathet Cardiovasc Diagn* **38**, 369–372. Case report of acute inferior/lateral myocardial infarction at 30 weeks gestation treated with percutaneous transluminal coronary angioplasty. **IV C**

27 Webber MD, Halligan RE, Schumacher JA (1997) Acute infarction, intracoronary thrombolysis, and primary PTCA in pregnancy. *Cathet Cardiovasc Diagn* **42**, 38–43. Case report of acute myocardial infarction in third trimester successfully treated with intracoronary thrombolysis and percutaneous transluminal coronary angioplasty of an occluded left anterior descending artery. **IV C**

28 Silberman S, Fink D, Berko RS *et al.* (1996) Coronary artery bypass surgery during pregnancy. *Eur J Cardiothorac Surg* **10**, 925–926. Case report of acute myocardial infarction followed by angina at 22 weeks gestation. Cardiac catheterization revealed dissection of the left anterior descending artery. Coronary artery bypass graft was performed without bypass with good maternal and fetal outcome. **IV C**

29 Garry D, Leikin E, Fleisher AG *et al.* (1996) Acute myocardial infarction in pregnancy with subsequent medical and surgical management. *Obstet Gynecol* **87**, 802–804. Case report of anterior myocardial infarction in the third trimester in a patient with severe coronary artery disease. Treatment included defibrillation, intra-aortic balloon pump, coronary artery bypass graft using bypass. Good outcome for mother and baby. **IV C**

30 Oakley GD, McGarry K, Limb DG *et al.* (1979) Management of pregnancy in patients with hypertrophic cardiomyopathy. *Br Med J* **1**, 749–750. Case series of 54 pregnancies in 23 patients with hypertrophic cardiomyopathy. 6 women needed diuretics for dyspnea. Beta-blockers were used in 18 pregnancies and, of these, 3 infants were small-for-dates and 2 had fetal bradycardia. **III B**

Chapter 29

Thyroid disease

29.1 Hyperthyroidism

Robert Fraser

Management option		Quality of evidence	Strength of recommendation	References
Prepregnancy	Establish the diagnosis of hyperthyroidism prior to pregnancy so that a complete diagnostic workup can be performed and therapy instituted	III	B	1
	Counsel regarding the need to continue therapy during pregnancy, the potential perinatal risks and the need for serial thyroid function studies	III	B	2–4
Prenatal	Continue thioamide therapy to maintain the patient clinically euthyroid and ensure that the laboratory parameters remain in the acceptable ranges for pregnancy	III	B	2,4
	Use beta-blockers for symptomatic complaints (i.e. tachycardia, palpitations)	III	B	5
	Thyroid function studies should be obtained every 1–3 months	III	B	5
	Serial ultrasonography of the fetus should be obtained to rule out fetal growth restriction and/or fetal goiter	III	B	5
	Recognition and management of thyroid storm	III	B	6
Postnatal	Watch for worsening of symptoms if autoimmune etiology is suspected	III	B	6,7
	Adjust thioamide therapy according to laboratory parameters and symptoms	–	✔	–
	Complete the diagnostic evaluation of hyperthyroidism and, when, appropriate institute definitive therapy	III	B	8
	Evaluate the newborn for evidence of goiter and transient hyperthyroidism	III	B	9

References

1 Sherif IH, Oyan WT, Bosairi S *et al.* (1991) Treatment of hyperthyroidism in pregnancy. *Acta Obstet Gynecol Scand* **70**, 461–463. Observational study of 75 pregnancies in women on treatment before conception for hyperthyroidism and 30 in whom diagnosis was made after conception. No congenital defects associated with universal carbimazole therapy, but high miscarriage rate in those treated with propranolol as well. **III B**

2 Wing DA, Millar LK, Koonings PP *et al.* (1994) A comparison of propylthiouracil versus methimazole in the treatment of hyperthyroidism in pregnancy. *Am J Obstet Gynecol* **170**, 90–95. Retrospective analysis of 135 hyperthyroid patients treated in pregnancy with propylthiouracil (99) or methimazole (35). No differences detected in

time to achieve euthyroid status (7–8 weeks) or in recorded congenital anomalies (3.0% vs 2.7%) between the two drugs. **III B**

3 Momotani N (1984) Maternal hyperthyroidism and congenital malformation in the offspring. *Clin Endocrinol* **20**, 695–700. Major congenital malformations sought in the offspring of 643 women with Graves disease in pregnancy. Reported in relation to treatment mode and thyroid states. Hyperthyroid and not on methimazole 6% (3/50), euthyroid and not on methimazole 0.3% (1/350), hyperthyroid on methimazole 1.7% (2/117), euthyroid on methimazole 0% (0/126). No dose-related effect of methimazole on congenital malformation detected. **III B**

4 Momotani N, Noh J, Oyanagi H *et al.* (1986) Antithyroid drug therapy for Graves disease during pregnancy. Optimal regimen for fetal thyroid status. *N Engl J Med* **315**, 24–28. Observational study of 70 women with Graves disease treated with propylthiouracil. Recommended maintaining maternal free thyroxine index in the mildly thyrotoxic range to reduce risk of neonatal hypothyroidism. **III B**

5 Vanderpump MP, Ahlquist JA, Franklyn JA *et al.* (1996) Consensus statement for good practice and audit measure in the management of hypothyroidism and hyperthyroidism. *Br Med J* **313**, 539–544. Consensus statement on good practice in management of hypothyroidism and hyperthyroidism. **IV C**

6 Nelson NC, Becker WFL (1969) Thyroid crisis: diagnosis and treatment. *Ann Surg* **170**, 263–273. Case series of 21 subjects with thyroid crisis (storm) from 2329 subjects with hyperthyroidism collected over a 20-year period in the USA (1949–68). Mortality was 16; none of the subjects was pregnant. **III B**

7 Fung HY, Kologlu M, Collison K *et al.* (1988) Postpartum thyroid dysfunction in Mid Glamorgan. *Br Med J* **296**, 241–244. 13% of 901 unselected pregnant women with no relevant history were found to have thyroid autoantibodies. 16% of women had postpartum thyroiditis, of whom 25% had no thyroid autoantibodies. **III B**

8 Pekonen F, Teramo K, Ikonen E *et al.* (1984) Women on thyroid hormone therapy: pregnancy course, fetal outcome, and amniotic hormone level. *Obstet Gynecol* **63**, 635–638. Case series of 37 pregnancies in hypothyroidism and 19 in women on thyroid suppression after surgery for primary thyroid carcinoma. 23% required alteration in thyroxine dose, usually an increase, to maintain euthyroidism in pregnancy. **III B**

9 Kriplani A, Buckshee K, Bhargava VL *et al.* (1994) Maternal and perinatal outcome in thyrotoxicosis complicating pregnancy. *Eur J Obstet Gynecol Reprod Biol* **54**, 159–163. In 32 pregnancies in India complicated by maternal hyperthyroidism there was an excess of preterm labor and pregnancy-induced hypertension. 3 women experienced thyroid crisis during pregnancy, one of whom died of thyroid storm. 3 newborns had thyroid-related complications: hypothyroidism in 2 cases and hyperthyroidism with goiter in one. **III B**

29.2 Hypothyroidism

Robert Fraser

Management option		Quality of evidence	Strength of recommendation	References
Prepregnancy	Consider hypothyroidism in differential diagnosis of infertility and/or menstrual disorders	–	✔	–
	Delay pregnancy until maintenance drug levels are achieved	III	B	1
Prenatal	Continue until full thyroid hormone replacement levels are achieved	III	B	1,2
	Serial (every trimester) thyroid function studies	III	B	1
	Watch for evidence of myxedema	III	B	1
Postnatal	Watch for exacerbation of subclinical thyroid disease, which may present with transient hyperthyroidism	IV	C	3

References

1 Pekonen F, Teramo K, Ikonen E *et al.* (1984) Women on thyroid hormone therapy: pregnancy course, fetal outcome, and amniotic hormone level. *Obstet Gynecol* **63**, 635–638. Case series of 37 pregnancies in hypothyroidism and 19 in women on thyroid suppression after surgery for primary thyroid carcinoma. 23% required alteration in thyroxine dose, usually an increase, to maintain euthyroidism in pregnancy. **III B**

2 Mandel SJ, Larsen PR, Seely EW *et al.* (1990) Increased need for thyroxine in pregnancy in women with primary hypothyroidism. *N Engl J Med* **323**, 91–96. Basing therapy on levels of thyroid-stimulating hormone, 9 of 12 hypothyroid subjects required an increased dose of replacement therapy during pregnancy. **III B**

3 Vanderpump MP, Ahlquist JA, Franklyn JA *et al.* (1996) Consensus statement for good practice and audit measure in the management of hypothyroidism and hyperthyroidism. *Br Med J* **313**, 539–544. Consensus statement on good practice in management of hypothyroidism and hyperthyroidism. **IV C**

29.3 Thyroid nodule in pregnancy

Robert Fraser

Management option		Quality of evidence	Strength of recommendation	References
Diagnostic evaluation	Ultrasonography is the preferred mode for evaluating a thyroid nodule in pregnancy	IV	C	1
	Cystic lesions are usually benign	IV	C	1
	Fine needle aspiration of a suspicious solitary thyroid nodule is indicated and can be performed safely in pregnancy with a high sensitivity and specificity	IV	C	1

Reference

1 Vanderpump MP, Ahlquist JA, Franklyn JA *et al.* (1996) Consensus statement for good practice and audit measure in the management of hypothyroidism and hyperthyroidism. *Br Med J* **313**, 539–544. Consensus statement on good practice in management of hypothyroidism and hyperthyroidism. **IV C**

Chapter 30

Pituitary and adrenal disease

30.1 Pituitary disorders

Janet Cresswell

Prolactin-producing adenomas

Management option		Quality of evidence	Strength of recommendation	References
Prepregnancy	Treatment (bromocriptine, surgery, radiotherapy depending on tumor size)	III	B	1,2
	Advise against pregnancy until 'cured'	III	B	3
Prenatal	Bromocriptine is probably safe for fetus	III	B	1,3,4
	Screening/monitoring for recurrence or exacerbation is best undertaken by vigilance for clinical features (headaches, visual disturbance) and prompt investigation. Some advocate visual field testing every trimester	III	B	1–3,5,6
	Interdisciplinary management	III	B	1–3,5,6
	If enlargement/recurrence, bromocriptine if fetus not mature (possibly surgery in extreme cases); delivery and definitive management if fetus mature	III	B	1,6
Postnatal	Can breastfeed	III	B	1
	Monitor symptoms, prolactin (can be difficult to interpret in breastfeeding mothers), tumor size	III	B	2

References

1 Zarate A, Canales ES, Alger M *et al.* (1979) The effect of pregnancy and lactation on pituitary prolactin-secreting tumors. *Acta Endocrinol* **92**, 407–412. 14 women with prolactin-secreting adenomas treated with bromocriptine were observed through pregnancy. All 14 women conceived within 6 months and had uneventful term pregnancies with no evidence of tumor enlargement. They all lactated for at least 6 months without problems. **III B**

2 Wallace EA, Holdaway IM (1995) Treatment of macroprolactinomas at Auckland Hospital 1975–91. *N Z Med J* **108**, 50–52. Retrospective review of 34 cases of macroprolactinoma in New Zealand between 1974 and 1993. Treatment responses and major treatment complications were similar in both medically and surgically treated groups. However, only a third of patients had normal serum prolactin at last follow-up. **III B**

3 Jewelewicz R, Vande Wiele RL (1980) Clinical course and outcomes of pregnancy in twenty-five patients with pituitary microadenomas. *Am J Obstet Gynecol* **136**, 339–343. 25 women with pituitary microadenoma were treated with bromocriptine until conception. All women had successful pregnancies without neurological or visual symptoms. **III B**

4 Turkalj I, Braun P, Krupp P (1982) Surveillance of bromocriptine in pregnancy. *JAMA* **247**, 1589–1591. Study of 1410 pregnancies between 1973 and 1980 in which bromocriptine had been given. Bromocriptine was stopped in most cases with confirmation of pregnancy. The miscarriage rate was 11% and the congenital anomaly rate was 3.5%. Data suggest that the intake of bromocriptine during pregnancy is not associated with increased risk to the fetus. **III B**

5 Divers WA Jr, Yen SS (1983) Prolactin-producing microadenomas in pregnancy. *Obstet Gynecol* **62**, 425–429.

Review of 54 patients with a prolactin-secreting pituitary microadenoma through pregnancy and 15 controls. 4 women developed visual field defects and 4 developed headaches. Prolactin levels did not increase in pregnancy. Pregnancy appears to be safe in women with microadenoma. **III B**

6 Gsponer J, De Tribolet N, Deruaz JP *et al.* (1999) Diagnosis, treatment and outcome of pituitary tumors and other abnormal intrasellar masses. Retrospective analysis of 353 patients. *Medicine* **78**, 236–269. Retrospective review of 353 patients with a presumed diagnosis of pituitary tumor between 1984 and 1997 in Switzerland. 322 abnormal pituitary masses were found, of which prolactinomas and nonsecreting adenomas were the most frequent tumor types. Medical treatment usually resulted in satisfactory control of prolactin levels and tumor shrinkage and progressively replaced surgery as a primary treatment for prolactinomas throughout the study period. **III B**

Acromegaly

Management option		Quality of evidence	Strength of recommendation	References
Prepregnancy	Definitive surgical management before conception	–	✔	–
Prenatal	Screen for diabetes, hypertension and cardiomyopathy	–	✔	–
	Vigilance for tumor expansion (headaches, visual disturbance)	–	✔	–

Diabetes insipidus

Management option		Quality of evidence	Strength of recommendation	References
Prepregnancy	Vigilance for tumor expansion (headaches, visual disturbance)	–	✔	–
Prenatal	Continue supplementation with synthetic vasopressin; dose may need to be increased	IV	C	1,2
	Monitor disease control with clinical features and specific gravity of urine	IV	C	1,2
Labor and delivery	Vigilance for dysfunctional labor (minority of cases)	IV	C	1
Postnatal	Vigilance for poor lactation (minority of cases)	IV	C	1

References

1 Burrow GN, Wassenaar W, Robertson GL *et al.* (1981) DDAVP treatment of diabetes insipidus during pregnancy and the post-partum period. *Acta Endocrinol* **97**, 23–25. Case report on a 23-year-old woman with diabetes insipidus. She was treated with 1-desamino-8-D-arginine vasopressin (DDAVP). Pregnancy was uneventful and successful. Low levels of DDAVP assayed in breast milk suggest that breastfeeding could be recommended in these women. **IV C**

2 Jin-no Y, Kamiya Y, Okada M *et al.* (1998) Pregnant woman with transient diabetes insipidus resistant to 1-desamino-8-D-arginine vasopressin. *Endocrine J* **45**, 693–696. Case report in Japan of a pregnant women with transient diabetes insipidus during the third trimester. She was managed conservatively and the pregnancy progressed normally to term. The abnormality in the posterior pituitary gland (which was noted on magnetic resonance imaging in pregnancy) disappeared post-partum, suggesting that subclinical diabetes insipidus was exacerbated by pregnancy. **IV C**

Pituitary insufficiency

Management option		Quality of evidence	Strength of recommendation	References
Prepregnancy and prenatal	Give appropriate replacement hormones (usually thyroxine and corticosteroids)	–	✔	–
	Monitor clinical feature and levels of thyroid-stimulating hormone	–	✔	–
Labor and delivery	Increase dose of glucocorticoids	–	✔	–
Postnatal	Readjust dose of drugs if necessary	–	✔	–

30.2 Adrenal disease

Janet Cresswell

Cushing's syndrome

Management option		Quality of evidence	Strength of recommendation	References
Prepregnancy	Investigate and treat before conception	–	✔	–
Prenatal	If diagnosed in pregnancy, identify and treat cause (usually by surgery; only possible exception is diagnosis in third trimester, where delivery and subsequent definitive management may be an option	III	B	1

Reference

1 Buescher MA, McClamrock HD, Adashi EY (1992) Cushing syndrome in pregnancy. *Obstet Gynecol* **79**, 130–137. Review of 65 cases of Cushing syndrome in pregnancy in the literature. Maternal morbidity is high through hypertension, congestive cardiac failure and poor tissue healing. Perinatal mortality was 15.4%, mostly due to prematurity and *in-utero* growth restriction. Surgical treatment during pregnancy is described and usually uneventful. Vaginal delivery is recommended because of the tendency towards poor tissue healing. Cushing syndrome should be treated in pregnancy because otherwise it is associated with poor outcome. **III B**

Primary aldosteronism

Management option		Quality of evidence	Strength of recommendation	References
Prenatal	If diagnosed in pregnancy, options are medical (antihypertensives and spironolactone) or surgery	IV	C	1
NB: Spironolactone is an antiandrogen				

Reference

1 Lotgering FK, Derkx FM, Wallenburg HC (1986) Primary hyperaldosteronism in pregnancy. *Am J Obstet Gynecol* **155**, 986–988. Case report of a primigravid woman who presented in mid pregnancy with primary hyperaldosteronism. Medical treatment enabled the pregnancy to progress to 36 weeks and a live infant was delivered. Post-partum, an adrenal adenoma was removed. **IV C**

Adrenal insufficiency

Management option		Quality of evidence	Strength of recommendation	References
Prenatal	Continue glucocorticoid and mineralocorticoid supplementation	IV	C	1
	Vigilance for fluid overload and electrolyte disturbance	IV	C	1
	Vigilance for adrenal crisis (treat with i.v. hydrocortisone, i.v. fluids and medical supportive therapy)	IV	C	1
Labor and delivery	Increase glucocorticoid supplementation	IV	C	1

Reference

1 O'Shaughnessy RW, Hackett KJ (1984) Maternal Addison's disease and fetal growth retardation. A case report. *J Reprod Med* **29**, 752–756. Case report of a 40-year-old woman who presented at 34 weeks gestation with Addison's disease. Steroid replacement therapy was commenced and the pregnancy progressed to term but the fetus was growth-restricted. **IV C**

Pheochromocytoma

Management option		Quality of evidence	Strength of recommendation	References
Prepregnancy	Avoid pregnancy until definitive treatment implemented and 'cured'	–	✔	–
Prenatal	If suspected clinically, establish diagnosis and location of tumor	IV	C	1
	Medical stabilization and control of blood pressure prior to and during surgery	IV	C	1
Labor and delivery	Cesarean section preferable once medical stabilization established	IV	C	1
	Concomitant surgery at time of cesarean section is debatable	IV	C	1
Postnatal	Monitor for recurrence	IV	C	1

Reference

1 Venuto R, Burstein P, Schneider R (1984) Pheochromocytoma: antepartum diagnosis and management with tumor resection in the puerperium. *Am J Obstet Gynecol* **150**, 431–432. Case report of a 27-year-old primigravida who presented with severe hypertension at 32 weeks gestation. Pheochromocytoma was diagnosed. She was treated with antihypertensives. Pregnancy progressed to term, when a live infant was born by cesarean section. Successful removal of the pheochromocytoma was performed a few weeks later. **IV C**

Chapter 31

Hematological disease

31.1 Iron- and folate-deficiency anemia

Janet Cresswell

Management option		Quality of evidence	Strength of recommendation	References
Prepregnancy	Dietary advice and iron therapy in order to ensure satisfactory hemoglobin status prior to pregnancy	III	B	1
	Public health measures to prevent periconceptual folate deficiency	Ia	A	2
	Folic acid periconceptually reduces risk of neural tube defect	Ia	A	2
Prenatal	Prophylactic iron/folate controversial in industrialized countries but important for pregnant women in developing countries to maintain or raise predelivery hemoglobin	Ia	A	3–5
	Where iron/folate is prescribed selective use better than routine if women can have their hemoglobin status assessed and followed up reliably	Ia	A	3–5
	Oral preparation preferred – different compounds used to minimize side effects	IV	C	6
	Slow-release preparations used to reduce gastrointestinal complaints	Ib	A	7
	Side effects related to dose and weekly oral iron may be an alternative to improve compliance without losing efficacy	Ib	A	8,9
	Parenteral iron if oral iron fails from noncompliance, poor follow-up or poor absorption	IIa	B	10
	In resistant cases recombinant human erythropoietin may be used in addition to iron	IIa	B	11
	Blood transfusion may be considered with severe symptomatic anemia close to delivery	–	✔	–
	Where malaria is a problem antimalarial prophylaxis is recommended	Ia	A	12

References

1 Harrison KA (1985) Child-bearing, health and social priorities: a survey of 22 774 consecutive hospital births in Zaria, Northern Nigeria. *Br J Obstet Gynaecol* **92**, 1–119. Large prospective descriptive study that showed some possible advantage in improvement of adolescents' anthropometry with iron treatment in a socioeconomically deprived population in Africa. Has not been confirmed again. **III B**

2 Lumley J, Watson L, Watson M et al. (2001) Periconceptional supplementation with folate and/or

multivitamins for preventing neural tube defects. In: *Cochrane database of systematic reviews*, issue 3. Oxford: Update Software. In this systematic review four trials of supplementation involving 6425 women were included. Periconceptional folate supplementation reduced the incidence of neural tube defects (relative risk 0.28, 95% CI 0.13–0.58). Folate supplementation did not significantly increase miscarriage, ectopic pregnancy or stillbirth, although there was a possible increase in multiple gestation. Multivitamins alone were not associated with prevention of neural tube defects and did not produce additional preventive effects when given with folate. **Ia A**

3 Mahomed K (2000) Iron supplementation in pregnancy. In: *Cochrane database of systematic reviews*, issue 4. Oxford: Update Software. Systematic review that included 20 trials. Iron supplementation raised or maintained the serum ferritin above 10mg/l. It resulted in a substantial reduction of women with a hemoglobin level below 10 or 10.5g in late pregnancy. Iron supplementation, however, had no detectable effect on any substantive measures of either maternal or fetal outcome. One trial, with the largest number of participants of selective versus routine supplementation, showed an increased likelihood of cesarean section and post-partum blood transfusion, but a lower perinatal mortality rate (up to 7 days after birth). **Ia A**

4 Mahomed K (2001) Folate supplementation in pregnancy. In: *Cochrane database of systematic reviews*, issue 3. Oxford: Update Software. Meta-analysis of 21 trials of folate supplementation in pregnancy or placebo or no supplementation. Folate supplementation was associated with a reduction in the proportion of women with low hemoglobin in late pregnancy. No other benefits or harm were found for mothers or babies from folate supplementation. **Ia A**

5 Mahomed K (2001) Iron and folate supplementation in pregnancy. In: *Cochrane database of systematic reviews*, issue 3. Oxford: Update Software. Meta-analysis of eight trials of 5449 women receiving or not either iron and folate supplementation during pregnancy. Routine supplementation did elevate serum iron and folate levels but had no effect on maternal or fetal outcome. **Ia A**

6 World Health Organization (1998) *Expert committee document on anaemia in developing countries*. Geneva: WHO. Paper produced as a consensus statement of a working party discussing problems of anemia in pregnancy in developing countries with emphasis on diagnosis and prevention as well as treatment. **IV C**

7 Simmons WK, Cook JD, Bingham KC *et al.* (1993) Evaluation of a gastric delivery system for iron supplementation in pregnancy. *Am J Clin Nutr* **58**, 622–626. RCT to assess the efficacy of oral iron supplementation during pregnancy by using a gastric delivery system (GDS). 376 pregnant women between 16 and 35 years of age and 14 and 22 weeks gestation were selected if mild anemia was present (hemoglobin concentration 80–110g/l). The participants were randomly assigned to one of three study groups given no iron, two $FeSO_4$ tablets (100mg Fe) daily, or one GDS capsule (50mg Fe) daily. Blood was obtained initially and after 6 and 12 weeks for measurement of red blood cell and iron indices, including serum transferrin receptor. There was a significant and comparable improvement in hematologic and iron-status measurements in the two groups of women given iron, whereas iron deficiency evolved in women given no iron supplement. We conclude that by eliminating gastrointestinal side effects and reducing the administration frequency of an iron supplement to once daily, a GDS offers significant advantages for iron supplementation of pregnant women. **Ib A**

8 Young MW, Lupafya E, Kapenda E *et al.* (2000) The effectiveness of weekly iron supplementation in pregnant women of rural northern Malawi. *Trop Doctor* **30**, 84–88. Randomized trial to compare 60mg iron/0.25mg folate per day ($n = 211$) or 120mg iron/0.50mg folate once a week ($n = 202$). Supplementation was continued for a minimum of 8 weeks (10 weeks on average) and was self-administered by the women at home. Initial hemoglobin values for the daily (mu = 105.7g/l) and weekly (mu = 104.4g/l) groups as well as final hemoglobin values (107.5g/l and 105.6g/l respectively) did not differ significantly between the two groups. Hemoglobin values increased by similar levels in both groups, with the subset of anemic women increasing by an average of 6.3g/l in the daily group ($n = 70$) and 5.9g/l in the weekly group ($n = 66$) for all women. Reported side effects were significantly reduced in the weekly group (6% compared with 17%, $p < 0.05$). **Ib A**

9 Lopes MC, Ferreira LO, Batista-Filho M *et al.* (1999) Use of daily and weekly ferrous sulfate to treat anemic childbearing-age women. *Cad Saude Publica* **15**, 799–808. Blinded randomized trial conducted in a low-income community in a city in Brazil, with 193 anemic (Hb < 12mg/dl) and 'menstruating' women (age range: 15–45 years) to compare daily and weekly doses of ferrous sulfate (60mg elemental iron). After 12 weeks' follow-up, 150 women completed the trial, 79 on the alternative weekly regimen and 71 on the conventional daily regimen. Mean corpuscular hemoglobin concentrations prior to treatment were 10.52g/dl (DP = 1.13) and 10.72g/dl (DP = 0.92), respectively, for the alternative and conventional regimens. After the intervention they were 11.83g/dl (DP = 0.97) for the weekly regimen and 11.62g/dl (DP = 1.39) for the daily one. The alternative regimen was better accepted than the conventional one. **Ib A**

10 Singh K, Fong YF, Kuperan P (1998) A comparison between intravenous iron polymaltose complex (Ferrum Hausmann) and oral ferrous fumarate in the treatment of iron deficiency anaemia in pregnancy. *Eur J Haematol* **60**, 119–124. Study comparing the efficacy of Ferrum Hausmann with oral ferrous fumarate therapy in the treatment of iron deficiency anemia in pregnancy. Intravenous Ferrum Hausmann (iron dextrin) resulted in a significantly better level and rate of increase of hemoglobin ($p < 0.001$). Serum ferritin was significantly higher ($p < 0.001$) in the intravenous group. There were also no reports of any adverse reactions with intravenous iron dextrin, whereas a considerable proportion of women on oral iron therapy reporteded side effects. **IIa A**

11 Breymann C, Zimmermann R, Huch R *et al.* (1996) Use of recombinant human erythropoietin in combination with parenteral iron in the treatment of postpartum anaemia. *Eur J Clin Invest* **26**, 123–130. 90 patients (30 patients/group) received either recombinant human erythropoietin (rhEPO; 300 U/kg, i.v. or s.c., once) and iron (parenteral and oral), or iron therapy only. Erythropoiesis was assessed by hemoglobin and hematocrit increase, absolute reticulocyte counting and reticulocyte flow cytometry. There was no difference before therapy for baseline hematological values or iron status. Patients with endogenous EPO levels below 145 mU/ml had a significant benefit from intravenous rhEPO administration with highest hematocrit and hemoglobin levels 4 and 14 days after therapy. rhEPO-treated groups showed a higher absolute reticulocyte count 1 and 4 days after therapy and an elevated percentage of high fluorescent reticulocytes. Parenteral iron therapy caused a significant increase of ferritin and transferrin saturation, while transferrin concentration decreased. Ferritin and transferrin levels were lowest after intravenous administration of rhEPO, 1 and 4 days after therapy. A single dose of rhEPO in combination with iron was more effective in treating postpartum anemia than iron therapy only, in patients who had low EPO levels despite peripartum blood loss. **IIa A**

12 Garner P, Gulmezoglu AM (2001) Prevention versus treatment for malaria in pregnant women. In: *Cochrane database of systematic reviews*, issue 4. Oxford: Update Software. Review of 15 randomized or quasi-randomized studies of antimalarial prophylaxis (drugs or vector control measures) in pregnancy. Drug prophylaxis reduced antenatal anemia but did not affect maternal or perinatal mortality. Bednets (insecticide-impregnated or not) did not appear to affect outcome. Women living in malarious areas need access to prompt treatment from malaria and anemia as a priority over prophylaxis regimes. **Ia A**

31.2 Sickle-cell anemia

Janet Cresswell

Management option	Quality of evidence	Strength of recommendation	References
Pregnancy has a deleterious effect on maternal wellbeing and is associated with poor fetal outcome	III	B	1,2
Use of blood transfusion should be limited but data are few	Ib	A	3

References

1 Tuck SM, Studd JW, White JM (1983) Pregnancy in sickle cell disease in the United Kingdom. *Br J Obstet Gynaecol* **90**, 112–117. Review of a 125 pregnancies with sickle-cell disease and 717 controls (same racial group with no hemoglobinopathy) between 1975 and 1981 in the UK. There were no maternal deaths but the perinatal mortality rate was 48/1000 in the sickle-cell group and 9/1000 in the controls. Maternal complications included sickling crises (38%) and infections (61%). In the sickle-cell group the preterm delivery rate was 13%, and it was 6% in the control group. **III B**

2 Howard RJ, Tuck SM, Person TC *et al.* (1995) Pregnancy in sickle cell disease in the UK: results of a multicentre survey of the effect of prophylactic blood transfusion on maternal and fetal outcome. *Br J Obstet Gynaecol* **102**, 947–951. An observation on a multicenter study of 81 sickle-cell disease pregnancies and 100 black African pregnancies without hemoglobinopathy in England and Wales between 1991 and 1993. Within the sickle-cell group there were 2 maternal deaths and the perinatal mortality rate was 60/1000 births. Antenatal sickling complications occurred in 46%; this did not significantly reduce with prophylactic transfusion. **III B**

3 Mahomed K (2001) Prophylactic versus selective blood transfusion for sickle cell anaemia during pregnancy In: *Cochrane database of systematic reviews*, issue 3. Oxford: Update Software. One trial involving 72 women was included. Half the women received a blood transfusion only if hemoglobin fell below 6 g/dl and the other half received two units of blood every week for 3 weeks, or until hemoglobin level was 10–11 g/dl. A policy of selective transfusion reduced the number of transfusions required at the expense of more frequent pain crises. There is not enough evidence at present to draw conclusions about the prophylactic use of blood transfusion for sickle cell anemia during pregnancy. **Ia A**

31.3 Thrombocytopenia

Clare Tower

Gestational thrombocytopenia

Management option	Quality of evidence	Strength of recommendation	References
Exclude pathological causes	IV	C	1
Monitor platelet count	IV	C	2
Fetal blood sampling not indicated	III	B	3
Observe if platelet count over 100 000/ml. If rapid fall or less than 50 000/ml, reevaluate	III IIb	B B	4,5 6
Cord blood at delivery	III	B	4,5
Check maternal count post-delivery	III	B	4,5

References

1 Faridi A, Rath W (2001) Differential diagnosis of thrombocytopenia in pregnancy. *Zentralbl Gynakol* **123**, 80–90. Review article highlighting the differential diagnosis of thrombocytopenia in pregnancy. Occurs in 7–8% of pregnancies. Gestational thrombocytopenia poses no maternal or fetal risks. **IV C**

2 Letsky EA, Greaves M (1996) Guidelines on the investigation and management of thrombocytopenia in pregnancy and neonatal alloimmune thrombocytopenia. *Br J Haematol* **95**, 21–26. Review of management guidelines for gestational thrombocytopenia, autoimmune thrombocytopenia (ITP), thrombocytopenia due to preeclampsia, disseminated intravascular coagulation, thrombotic thrombocytopenic purpura, hemolytic uremic syndrome and neonatal alloimmune thrombocytopenia. **IV C**

3 Aster RH (1990) 'Gestational' thrombocytopenia – a plea for conservative management. *N Engl J Med* **323**, 264–266. Observational study conducted over 11 years, which found that, out of 162 women identified as having thrombocytopenia in pregnancy, 88 had a previous history of idiopathic thrombocytopenic purpura. Of the 38 babies born with thrombocytopenia, 35 were babies of mothers with a history of ITP. The mothers of these 35 babies all had platelet-binding IgG in their plasma. The authors conclude that women with a history of previous ITP and the presence of plasma platelet-binding IgG are likely to deliver a baby with thrombocytopenia. **III B**

4 Burrows RF, Kelton JG (1988) Incidentally detected thrombocytopenia in healthy mothers and their infants. *N Engl J Med* **319**, 142–145. Prospective observational study of maternal and fetal platelet counts in otherwise normal pregnant women. Of the 1357 normal women, mild thrombocytopenia (97–150 000 × 10^9/l) was identified in 112 (8.3%). Neonatal thrombocytopenia found in 4.3% of babies born to thrombocytopenic mothers and this was no different from babies born to mothers with normal platelet counts. No mothers or babies suffered complications attributable to thrombocytopenia. Therefore, obstetric intervention due to maternal thrombocytopenia is not justified. **III B**

5 Ruggeri M, Schiavotto C, Castaman G *et al.* (1997) Gestational thrombocytopenia: a prospective study. *Haematologica* **82**, 341–342. Observational study following 37 consecutive patients with gestational thrombocytopenia. Newborn platelet count was performed within 24 h of birth: 2 had mild thrombocytopenia (75 and 80 × 10^9/l) and one had severe thrombocytopenia (12 × 10^9/l). All recovered spontaneously and no episodes of neonatal bleeding were observed. 28 women were followed postnatally for 12 months and 5 women still had a low platelet count at 12 months. 4 women had a second pregnancy and thrombocytopenia recurred in all of them. The possibility that some of the women had idiopathic thrombocytopenic purpura cannot be excluded. **III B**

6 Copplestone JA (1992) Asymptomatic thrombocytopenia developing during pregnancy (gestational thrombocytopenia) – a clinical study. *Q J Med* **84**, 593–601. Observational study comparing maternal and fetal outcomes in 31 women with asymptomatic (gestational) thrombocytopenia, 12 women with preeclampsia-associated thrombocytopenia and 34 normal pregnant controls. Women with preeclampsia had more maternal bleeding but there was no difference between the gestational thrombocytopenic group and the controls. Only one baby in the asymptomatic thrombocytopenia group had mild thrombocytopenia and platelet counts were not statistically different from the controls. Data also presented on 1469 platelet counts in normal pregnant women, suggesting that the lower limit of normal (2 SD of mean) for pregnancy is 120 × 10^9/l. **IIb B**

Autoimmune thrombocytopenia

Management option		Quality of evidence	Strength of recommendation	References
Prepregnancy	Optimize management and consider need for splenectomy/azathioprine	–	✔	–
	Discuss risks in pregnancy if not responsive to all therapy	–	✔	–
Prenatal	Monitor platelet count	IV	C	1
	Treat if symptoms and platelet count less than 20 000/ml at any stage in pregnancy Treat if less than 50 000/ml in late pregnancy even if asymptomatic complications and keep level above 50 000/ml for delivery	IV	C	2,3
	Prednisolone may help to sustain level above 50 000/ml	IV III	C B	1,3 4
	High-dose intravenous IgG as first line or if patient fails to respond/needs high doses of steroids	IV Ib	C A	3,5,6 7
	Splenectomy may be performed in refractory cases in the second trimester and occasionally in third trimester at time of cesarian section	IV	C	3,8
	Azathioprine in nonresponsive cases – safe in pregnancy but beware of intrauterine growth restriction	III	B	9
Labor and delivery	Platelets available if count below 50 000/ml	IV	C	1,2
	Avoid epidural if platelets below 80 000/ml	IV	C	1,2
	Avoid traumatic delivery, fetal scalp electrodes and fetal blood sampling	IV III	C B	1,2,10 11
	Cesarean section has no benefit over vaginal delivery	III	B	11,12
Postnatal	Because of risk of bleeding prompt repair of any perineal trauma	–	✔	–
	Cord blood platelet count	IV	C	1,2
	Daily platelet if initial low for a few days	IV	C	1,2
	If count below 20 000/ml or symptomatic, perform ultrasound scan of brain and treat with intravenous IgG	IV III	C B	1,2 10
	Platelets if bleeding life-threatening	IV	C	1,2

References

1 Letsky EA, Greaves M (1996) Guidelines on the investigation and management of thrombocytopenia in pregnancy and neonatal alloimmune thrombocytopenia. *Br J Haematol* **95**, 21–26. Review of management guidelines for gestational thrombocytopenia, autoimmune thrombocytopenia (ITP), thrombocytopenia due to preeclampsia, disseminated intravascular coagulation, thrombotic thrombocytopenic purpura, hemolytic uremic syndrome and neonatal alloimmune thrombocytopenia. **IV C**

2 Bussel, J, Kaplan C, McFarland J (1991) Recommendations for the evaluation and treatment of neonatal autoimmune and alloimmune thrombocytopenia. *Thromb Haemost* **65**, 631–634. Management guidelines from the Working Party on Neonatal Thrombocytopenia of the Neonatal Hemostasis Subcommittee of the Scientific and Standardization Committee of the ISTH. **IV C**

3 George, JN, Woolf SH, Raskob GE *et al.* (1996) Idiopathic thrombocytopenic purpura: a practice guideline developed by explicit methods for the American Society of Hematology. *Blood* **88**, 3–40. Evidence-based practice guidelines. Comments that many management points cannot be addressed through evidence-based recommendations as evidence is scanty. **IV C**

4 Kaplan C, Daffos F, Forestier F *et al.* (1990) Fetal platelet counts in thrombocytopenic pregnancy. *Lancet* **336**, 979–982. Prospective observational study of 33 pregnancies with chronic immune thrombocytopenia and 31 pregnancies with asymptomatic thrombocytopenia. 11/33 and 4/31 fetuses were found to be thrombocytopenic by percutaneous umbilical blood sampling. No correlation between maternal antiplatelet antibodies and fetal thrombocytopenia. Maternal treatment with corticosteroids (4 cases) or immunoglobulins (3 cases) did not improve fetal platelet counts. **III B**

5 Crowther MA, Burrows RF, Ginsberg J *et al.* (1996) Thrombocytopenia in pregnancy: diagnosis, pathogenesis and management. *Blood Rev* **10**, 8–16. Maternal thrombocytopenia is a common finding during pregnancy. The majority of patients with thrombocytopenia in pregnancy will have incidental thrombocytopenia of pregnancy, which is of no clinical significance. **IV C**

6 Clark AL, Gall SA (1997) Clinical uses of intravenous immunoglobulin in pregnancy. *Am J Obstet Gynecol* **176**, 241–253. Review article on the use of immunoglobulin in pregnancy. Highlights the fact that much of the evidence in the treatment of thrombocytopenia in pregnancy is based on case reports. **IV C**

7 Godeau B, Lesage S, Divine M *et al.* (1993) Treatment of adult chronic autoimmune thrombocytopenic purpura with repeated high-dose intravenous immunoglobulin. *Blood* **82**, 1415–1421. Small (n = 9 in each group) prospective randomized study comparing two doses of IgG in nonpregnant patients. No difference in the response of the platelet count was observed. **Ib A**

8 Martin JN Jr, Morrison JC, Files JC *et al.* (1984) Autoimmune thrombocytopenic purpura: current concepts and recommended practices. *Am J Obstet Gynecol* **150**, 86–96. Review of pathogenesis and management options. **IV C**

9 Alstead EM, Ritchie JK, Lennard-Jones JE *et al.* (1990) Safety of azathioprine in pregnancy in inflammatory bowel disease. *Gastroenterology* **99**, 443–446. A retrospective analysis of 16 pregnancies in which azathioprine was taken. The drug was stopped at 16 weeks gestation in 7 pregnancies and continued throughout gestation in 9. No congenital abnormalities or adverse neonatal effects were reported. **III B**

10 Silver RM, Branch DW, Scott JR (1995) Maternal thrombocytopenia in pregnancy: time for a reassessment. *Am J Obstet Gynecol* **173**, 479–482. Review article considering the role of cordocentesis, fetal blood sampling and cesarean section in the management of thrombocytopenia. Concludes that these are potentially risky and are ineffective in the prevention of neonatal bleeding complications. **IV C**

11 Burrows RF, Kelton JG (1993) Pregnancy in patients with idiopathic thrombocytopenic purpura: assessing the risks for the infant at delivery. *Obstet Gynecol Surv* **48**, 781–788. Meta-analysis of all English language publications from January 1980 to December 1990. Includes 885 pregnancies producing 893 infants. Risk of thrombocytopenia ($<50\times10^9$/l) in the infant was 10.1%, and the risk of severe thrombocytopenia was 4.2% ($<20\times10^9$/l). There was no major morbidity attributable to mode of delivery. Cordocentesis, fetal scalp sampling or umbilical cord sampling at birth did not affect the outcome of these infants. **III B**

12 Cook RL, Miller RC, Katz VL *et al.* (1991) Immune thrombocytopenic purpura in pregnancy: a reappraisal of management. *Obstet Gynecol* **78**, 578–583. An observational study of 31 pregnancies complicated by thrombocytopenia. 14 infants were delivered vaginally and 18 by cesarean section (most for obstetric indications, although in 4 cases the thrombocytopenia was cited as the only indication). 6 major complications were reported in those delivered by cesarean, compared to none of those delivered vaginally (p = 0.028). A literature review concluded that there was no significant association between intracranial hemorrhage and mode of delivery for moderately/severely thrombocytopenic infants. **III B**

Secondary autoimmune thrombocytopenia

Management option		Quality of evidence	Strength of recommendation	References
Antiphospholipid syndrome/ systemic lupus erythematosus	Manage thrombocytopenia as for autoimmune idiopathic thrombocytopenic purpura (ITP)	IV	C	1
HIV thrombo-cytopenia	Platelet count may be improved by use of intravenous IgG, zidovudine or steroids	III	B	2
	Cesarean section – consider platelet cover as with autoimmune ITP	–	✔	–

➡

Management option		Quality of evidence	Strength of recommendation	References
Drug-induced	Stop drug or use alternative (e.g. for heparin consider danaparoid; study cited was mainly in nonpregnant patients)	III	B	3

References

1 Galli M, Finazzi G, Barbui T (1996) Thrombocytopenia in the antiphospholipid syndrome. *Br J Haematol* **93**, 1–5. Review of the pathogenesis, clinical significance and treatment of thrombocytopenia in antiphospholipid syndrome, but not specific to pregnancy. **IV C**

2 Mandelbrot L, Schlienger I, Bongain A et al. (1994) Thrombocytopenia in pregnant women infected with human immunodeficiency virus: maternal and neonatal outcome. *Am J Obstet Gynecol* **171**, 252–257. Retrospective observational analysis of 890 pregnant women with human immunodeficiency virus infection. 29 (3.2%) women were thrombocytopenic ($<100\times10^9$/l). 16 of the 29 patients received treatment. 7 patients received zidovudine, 5 of whom showed an improved platelet count. Intravenous gammaglobulin was effective in 5 of 11 cases. 13 women were delivered by cesarean section and 5 had a hemorrhagic complication. Only one infant was thrombocytopenic at birth. **III B**

3 Magnani HN (1993) Heparin-induced thrombocytopenia (HIT): An overview of 230 patients treated with orgaran (Org10172). *Thromb Haemost* **70**, 554–561. Report on the use of a low-molecular-weight heparin, orgaran (Org10172), in 230 patients with heparin-induced thrombocytopenia. This included 4 pregnant patients. In 2 of the pregnant patients, treatment was considered successful. A failure (due to the development of cross-reactivity) was considered likely in one patient, and the fourth patient should not have been treated, as cross-reactivity was demonstrated *in vitro*. **III B**

Nonimmune platelet consumption

Management option		Quality of evidence	Strength of recommendation	References
Disseminated intravascular coagulation	See Section 31.9			
Thrombotic thrombocytopenic purpura	Plasma exchange is better than fresh frozen plasma (study cited was in non-pregnant patients)	Ib	A	1
	Avoid platelet transfusion	IV	C	2

References

1 Rock GA, Shumak KH, Buskard NA *et al.* (1991) Comparison of plasma exchange with plasma infusion in the treatment of thrombotic thrombocytopenic purpura. *N Engl J Med* **326**, 393–397. A prospective randomized trial comparing plasma exchange with infusion of fresh-frozen plasma in the treatment of thrombotic thrombocytopenic purpura in a nonpregnant group of 102 patients. All patients also received aspirin and dipyridamole. The plasma exchange therapy produced improved increase in platelet count (24/51 showed improvement, compared with 13/51, $p = 0.025$), and improved survival (2 deaths vs 8 deaths, $p = 0.035$). **Ib A**

2 Weiner CP (1987) Thrombotic microangiopathy in pregnancy and the postpartum period. *Semin Hematol* **24**, 119–129. Review of the three common thrombotic microangiopathies occurring in pregnancy: preeclampsia, thrombotic thrombocytopenic purpura and postpartum hemolytic uremic syndrome. **IV C**

31.4 Abnormalities in neutrophil count

Clare Tower

Management option		Quality of evidence	Strength of recommendation	References
Neutropenia	Consider prophylactic antibiotics for labor and delivery	IV	C	1
	Antibiotics for fever and antifungals if fever persists	–	✔	–
	For severe cases consider recombinant granulocyte-colony-stimulating factor (G-CSF). No experience in pregnancy	Ib	A	2

References

1 Polcz TE, Stiller RJ, Whetham JC (1993) Pregnancy in patients with cyclic neutropenia. *Am J Obstet Gynecol* **169**, 393–394. Case report of two successful pregnancies in a single patient suffering from this rare disorder. In both pregnancies, the disorder improved. In one pregnancy, the delivery was covered with prophylactic antibiotics. **IV C**

2 Dale DC, Bonilla MA, Davis MW *et al.* (1993) A randomized controlled phase III trial of recombinant human granulocyte colony-stimulating factor (filgrastim) for treatment of severe chronic neutropenia. *Blood* **81**, 2496–2502. RCT in 120 nonpregnant patients with cyclic, idiopathic or congenital neutropenia. One months treatment with recombinant human granulocyte colony-stimulating factor (filgrastim) compared with no treatment. The no-treatment group then went on to receive treatment. All patients had a pretreatment absolute neutrophil count of less than 0.5×10^9/l. In 108 patients, this increased to 1.5×10^9/l or more, and was accompanied by a decrease in infective episodes and antibiotic use. There was a statistically significant difference between treated and non-treated groups ($p < 0.001$). Mild side effects of bone pain, headache and rash were reported. **Ib A**

31.5 Coagulation disorders: congenital

Philip Owen

Von Willebrand's disease and carriers of hemophilia A and B

Management option		Quality of evidence	Strength of recommendation	References
Prepregnancy	Genetic counseling and evaluation	III	B	1
	Establish molecular genetic marker to aid prenatal testing	III	B	1
	Hepatitis immunization	III	B	1
	For type 1 von Willebrand disease (vWD) and carriers of hemophilia A with low factor VIII levels, perform desmopressin (DDAVP) trial to establish efficacy	IV	C	2
Prenatal	Combined/interdisciplinary team approach (obstetric/hemophilia team)	III	B	1
	Serial clotting factor levels in mother	III	B	1
	Offer prenatal diagnosis at 11–14 weeks (cover with factor concentrate if levels of factor VIII or IX are less than 50 IU/dl). Use recombinant products if available	IV	C	3

➡

Management option		Quality of evidence	Strength of recommendation	References
Prenatal (cont'd)	Fetal sexing by ultrasonography at 16–20 weeks if no invasive prenatal diagnosis	III	B	1
Labor and delivery	Consider further concentrate cover for labor and delivery for hemophilia carrier if factor VIII/IX less than 50 IU/dl and for vWD if hemostatic defect has not improved	III	B	4,1
	For vWD or hemophilia A carriers consider postpartum DDAVP alone if responsive, if normal vaginal delivery anticipated and coagulation defect is mild	IV	C	3
	If high-risk fetus aim for atraumatic delivery (vaginal if uncomplicated delivery anticipated but avoid fetal scalp electrode/ fetal scalp sampling)	III	B	1, 5
Postnatal	Cord blood for neonatal evaluation if risk of hemophilia A or B or type 3 vWD	III	B	1, 5
	Avoid neonatal intramuscular injections until status known	III	B	1
	Maternal hemostatic support for 3–4 days if vaginal delivery and for 4–5 days if cesarean section	IV	C	3

References

1 Kadir RA, Economides DL, Braithwaite J *et al.* (1997) The obstetric evidence of carriers of haemophilia. *Br J Obstet Gynaecol* **104**, 803–816. Retrospective review of 82 pregnancies among 24 hemophilia A carriers and 8 hemophilia B carriers attending one obstetric unit over a 10-year period. No adverse effects were encountered with the use of intrapartum fetal blood sampling or the application of fetal scalp electrodes. Knowledge of fetal gender considered valuable for intrapartum care. The incidence of primary and secondary postpartum hemorrhage was 22% and 11% respectively. **III B**

2 Rodeghiero F, Castaman G, Mannucci PM *et al.* (1991) Clinical indications for desmopressin (DDAVP) in congenital and acquired von Willebrand disease. *Blood Rev* **5**, 155–161. Literature review of the use of desmopressin (DDAVP) in congenital and acquired vWD. DDAVP is effective in achieving hemostasis at the time of major surgery and is the treatment of choice for achieving hemostasis in mild to moderate vWD. There are no comments specific to its use in pregnancy, cesarean section or in the puerperium. **IV C**

3 Walker ID, Walker JJ, Colvin BT *et al.* (1994) Investigation and management of haemorrhagic disorders in pregnancy. *J Clin Pathol* **47**, 100–108. Review of inherited and acquired coagulation disorders in pregnancy. Recommendations for practice based upon literature review and the opinions of the authors. The method of literature review is not described. **IV C**

4 Lubetsky A, Schulman S, Varon D *et al.* (1999) Safety and efficacy of continuous infusion of a combined factor VIII–von Willebrand factor (vWF) concentrate (Haemate-P) in patients with von Willebrand disease. *Thromb Haemost* **81**, 229–233. Case series describing the successful use of a continuous infusion of pasteurized factor VIII–vWf in 8 pregnant and nonpregnant patients. Use included bleeding prophylaxis in 2 women with severe vWD (type 3) during a vaginal delivery and a cesarean section. **III B**

5 Ljung R, Lindgren AC, Petrini P *et al.* (1994) Normal vaginal delivery is to be recommended for haemophilia carrier gravidae. *Acta Paediatr* **83**, 609–611. Retrospective analysis of 117 Swedish infants affected by hemophilia A or B. Vacuum extraction was associated with a high incidence (11 of 17) of subgaleal/cephalic hematoma or intracranial bleeding. Risk of serious hemorrhage following spontaneous vaginal delivery was low (8/87) and this mode of delivery is recommended. **III B**

31.6 Coagulation disorders: acquired

Philip Owen

Management option		Quality of evidence	Strength of recommendation	References
Disseminated intravascular coagulation (DIC)/massive hemorrhage (see also Section 31.9)	Interdisciplinary approach (obstetrics/ hematology)	IV	C	1,2
	Treat cause	IV	C	1,2
	Resuscitation volume replacement to maintain tissue perfusion	IV	C	1–3
	Replace fresh frozen plasma, cryoprecipitate and platelets on basis of laboratory results and clinical condition	IV	C	1–3
	Consider heparin in severe DIC due to amniotic fluid embolism	IV	C	1
Acquired inhibitors of coagulation	Interdisciplinary approach (obstetrics/ hematology)	IV	C	1
	Specific clotting factor concentrates (individualized management)	IV III	C B	1 4
	Immunosuppressive therapy	IV III	C B	1 4

References

1 Walker ID, Walker JJ, Colvin BT *et al.* (1994) Investigation and management of haemorrhagic disorders in pregnancy. *J Clin Pathol* **47**, 100–108. Review of inherited and acquired coagulation disorders in pregnancy. Recommendations for practice based upon literature review and the opinions of the authors. The method of literature review is not described. **IV C**

2 Giles AR (1994) Disseminated intravascular coagulation. In: Bloom AL, Forbes CD, Thomas DP, Taddenham EGD, eds. *Haemostasis and thrombosis*, 3rd edn, vol 2. Edinburgh: Churchill Livingstone, p. 969–986. Chapter in authoritative textbook describing the etiology, laboratory findings, clinical presentation and management of disseminated intravascular coagulation (DIC). No specific reference is made to the management of DIC complicating pregnancy and the puerperium. **IV C**

3 Blood Transfusion Task Force (1994) Conditional uses: fresh frozen plasma is only indicated in the presence of bleeding and disturbed coagulation. In: Wood K, ed. *Standard haematology practice* 2. Oxford: Blackwell Science, p. 231. Blood Transfusion Task Force recommendations on the use of fresh frozen plasma (FFP) and other blood concentrates. In the presence of massive transfusion, early laboratory assessment is required to determine the precise nature of any coagulation disorder. Prophylactic replacement with FFP or platelet concentrate is not recommended. **IV C**

4 Hauser I, Schneider B, Lechner K (1995) Post-partum factor VIII inhibitors: a review of the literature with special reference to the value of steroid and immunosuppressive treatment. *Thromb Haemost* **73**, 1–5. Literature review of the management of 51 cases developing factor VIII inhibitors post-delivery. Treatment included steroids, immunosuppressive agents, cytotoxic agents or no specific therapy. Immunosuppressive agents but not steroids may reduce the interval to complete remission in this condition. **III B**

31.7 Nonleukemic myeloproliferative disorders

Philip Owen

Management option		Quality of evidence	Strength of recommendation	References
Essential thrombo-cythemia	Conservative/observe only in most cases	III	B	1–4
	Consider low-dose aspirin	III	B	1,3,5,6
	?Hydroxyurea (avoid in first trimester)	IV	C	7
	More information needed about alpha interferon	III IV	B C	6 8–12
	Plateletpheresis gives only short-term benefit	III IV	B C	3 11
Polycythemia	?Venesection to keep hematocrit below 0.45	IV	C	13
	?Myelosuppressive therapy if associated thrombocytosis (and measures as under thrombocythemia, above)	IV	C	13
	Peripartum low-molecular-weight heparin prophylaxis	IV	C	13

References

1 Randi ML, Rossi C, Fabris F *et al.* (2000) Essential thrombocythemia in young adults: major thrombotic complications and complications during pregnancy – a follow-up study in 68 patients. *Clin Appl Thromb Hemost* **6**, 31–35. Prospective study of 68 consecutive young (< 40 years) men and women with essential thrombocythemia attending one center between 1980 and 1998. 16 pregnancies occurred in 13 women, with 13 pregnancies resulting in livebirths; 7 women received aspirin during pregnancy but no other treatment was given. **III B**

2 Beressi AH, Tefferi A, Silverstein MN *et al.* (1995) Outcome analysis of 34 pregnancies in women with essential thrombocythemia. *Arch Intern Med* **155**, 1217–1222. Well-described retrospective analysis of 31 pregnancies in 18 women with essential thrombocythemia referred to one specialist center. 17 (55%) resulted in live births and 14 (45%) in pregnancy losses. There was no correlation between pregnancy outcome and platelet count, treatment or history of disease complications. Interferon was not a treatment modality in this series. **III B**

3 Beard J, Hillmen P, Anderson CC *et al.* (1990) Primary thrombocythaemia in pregnancy. *Br J Haematol* **77**, 371–374. Retrospective analysis of 9 pregnancies in 6 women where essential thrombocythemia diagnosed before or during pregnancy. 8 pregnancies ended successfully with no major maternal morbidity. Treatments included aspirin, heparin and plateletpheresis. **III B**

4 Randi ML, Barbone E, Rossi C *et al.* (1994) Essential thrombocythemia and pregnancy: a report of six normal pregnancies in five untreated patients. *Obstet Gynecol* **83**, 915–917. Retrospective analysis of 6 pregnancies in 5 women with a prepregnancy diagnosis of essential thrombocythemia. No specific treatment was given. All pregnancies ended successfully with no maternal morbidity. **III B**

5 Pagliaro P, Arrigoni L, Muggiasca ML *et al.* (1996) Primary thrombocythemia and pregnancy: treatment and outcome in fifteen cases. *Am J Hematol* **53**, 6–10. Non-randomized retrospective study of 15 pregnancies in 9 women with essential thrombocythemia. Treatment included aspirin, heparin or no treatment. 9 pregnancies ended successfully. Treatment with aspirin and heparin was associated with a better fetal outcome than no treatment or treatment with aspirin alone. **III B**

6 Griesshammer M, Heimpl H, Pearson TC (1996) Essential thrombocythemia and pregnancy. *Leukemia Lymphoma* **22**, 57–63. Review of 106 pregnancies in 57 women with essential thrombocythemia. Live birth rate was 57% with first-trimester spontaneous loss the commonest unsuccessful outcome. There is no consensus on the optimal management of this condition in pregnancy. **III B**

7 Cinkotai KI, Wood P, Donnai P *et al.* (1994) Pregnancy after treatment with hydroxyurea in a patient with primary thrombocythaemia and a history of recurrent abortion. *J Clin Pathol* **47**, 769–770. Single case report of the successful use of hydroxyurea in treatment of prepregnancy essential thrombocythemia. Treatment was discontinued at 6 weeks gestation and no further specific treatment was required during the pregnancy. **IV C**

8 Williams JM, Schlesinger PE, Gray AG (1994) Successful treatment of essential thrombocythaemia and recurrent abortion with alpha interferon. *Br J Haematol* **88**, 647–648. Single case report of the successful use of preconceptual and gestational interferon in a case of essential thrombocythemia. **IV C**

9 Shpilberg O, Shimon I, Sofer O *et al.* (1996) Transient normal platelet counts and decreased requirement for interferon during pregnancy in essential thrombocythaemia. *Br J Haematol* **92**, 491–493. Report of two cases of pregnancy in women with essential thrombocythemia receiving prepregnancy interferon. Both women experienced a reduction in platelet counts to normal with consequent reduction in requirement for interferon. Both pregnancies ended successfully. **III B**

10 Pulik M, Lionnet F, Genet P *et al.* (1996) Platelet counts during pregnancy in essential thrombocythaemia treated with recombinant alpha-interferon. *Br J Haematol* **93**, 495. Single case report of prepregnancy-diagnosed essential thrombocythemia treated with interferon. The platelet count rose during pregnancy, requiring an increase in interferon. The pregnancy ended successfully. **III B**

11 Delage R, Demers C, Cantin G *et al.* (1996) Treatment of essential thrombocythemia during pregnancy with interferon-alpha. *Obstet Gynecol* **87**, 814–817. Single case report of the successful management of symptomatic essential thrombocythemia diagnosed in mid-trimester. Treatment involved interferon, aspirin and plateletpheresis. The pregnancy ended successfully. **III B**

12 Thornley S, Manoharan A (1994) Successful treatment of essential thrombocythemia with alpha interferon during pregnancy. *Eur J Haematol* **52**, 63–64. Single case report of the management of incidentally diagnosed essential thrombocythemia in the second half of pregnancy. Treatment was with aspirin and interferon with a successful outcome. **III B**

13 Ferguson JE II, Ueland K, Aronson WJ (1983) Polycythemia rubra vera and pregnancy. *Obstet Gynecol* **62**, 16s–20s. Report of the management of two consecutive pregnancies in one woman with polycythemia rubra vera. Both pregnancies ended successfully and uneventfully at term. No specific intervention was required during pregnancy and delivery. **IV C**

31.8 Hematological malignancies

Jane Gould

Hodgkin's disease

Management option		Quality of evidence	Strength of recommendation	References
Prepregnancy	Counsel about risks and prognosis	IIa	B	1
	Give contraceptive advice	III	B	2
Prenatal	Diagnosis by lymph node biopsy	–	✔	–
	Staging by clinical assessment and computed tomography/magnetic resonance imaging; counsel about prognosis and risks to fetus	IV	C	3
	Treatment – stage Ia/IIa ❑ Extra-abdominal: radiotherapy with shielding ❑ Intra-abdominal (depends on gestation and mother's wishes): – Deliver and radiotherapy – Continue pregnancy with chemotherapy and supportive care	 III Ib III Ib	 B A B A	 2,4 5 2,4 5
	Treatment – stage III/IV ❑ Chemotherapy with supportive care	 IIa	 B	 6
Postnatal	As for acute leukemia (see below)	–	✔	–

References

1 Lishner M, Zemlickis D, Degendorfer P *et al.* (1992) Maternal and foetal outcome following Hodgkin's Disease in pregnancy. *Br J Cancer* **65**, 114–117. Case-control study of 48 pregnant women with Hodgkin's disease. 20-year survival in Hodgkin's disease group was the same as their matched controls. **IIa B**

2 Jacobs C, Donaldson SS, Rosenberg SA *et al.* (1981) Management of the pregnant patient with Hodgkin's disease. *Ann Intern Med* **95**, 669–675. 15 patients with Hodgkin's disease were followed. 9 patients developed Hodgkin's disease during pregnancy, one relapsed during pregnancy and 5 became pregnant during treatment for Hodgkin's disease. Recommendations were for individualized treatment with the general principles of therapeutic abortion in the first trimester, monitoring of asymptomatic disease later in pregnancy, modified irradiation for supradiaphragmatic disease and single-agent chemotherapy for subdiaphragmatic and extranodal disease. **III B**

3 National Radiological Board (1993) Diagnostic medical procedures: advice and exposure to ionising radiation during pregnancy. *Doc NRPB (Oxon)* **4**, 1–14. Contents as stated in the title. Source and details of the information underlying the advice are not provided. **IV C**

4 Woo SY, Fuller LM, Cundiff JH *et al.* (1992) Radiotherapy during pregnancy for clinical stages IA–IIA Hodgkin's disease. *Int J Radiat Oncol Biol Phys* **23**, 407–412. Over a 34-year period 25/775 (3.2%) of women presenting to the MD Anderson had Hodgkin's disease. 6 out of 7 patients in the first trimester had abortions. 3 of the 8 women in the third trimester delivered. 16 remaining patients received supradiaphragmatic irradiation for stage IA (2 patients) and IIA (14 patients) – all delivered normal full-term infants. Emphasis was made on the necessity for shielding techniques. **III B**

5 Hoppe R, Coleman CN, Cox RS *et al.* (1982) The management of stage I–II Hodgkin's disease with irradiation alone or combined modality therapy: the Stanford experience. *Blood* **59**, 445–446. 230 patients with stage I–II Hodgkin's disease were treated between 1968 and 1978 with either irradiation alone or irradiation followed by adjuvant combination chemotherapy. There were no significant differences in survival or freedom from relapse at 10 years in the two groups. Radiation therapy alone is adequate for the treatment of stage I–II Hodgkin's disease. **Ib A**

6 Cullen MH, Stuart NS, Woodroffe C *et al.* (1994) ChlVPP/PABIOE and radiotherapy in advanced Hodgkin's disease. *J Clin Oncol* **12**, 779–787. A multicenter study with 216 patients treated with ChlVPP/PABIOE chemotherapy. ChlVPP/PABIOE chemotherapy has similar efficacy as MOPP/ABVD chemotherapy but with less toxicity (nausea and vomiting). The complete remission rate was 75% after chemotherapy, 85% with additional radiotherapy and the overall actuarial survival at 5 years was 78%. **IIa B**

Non-Hodgkin's lymphoma

Management option		Quality of evidence	Strength of recommendation	References
Prepregnancy	As for Hodgkin's disease	–	✔	–
Prenatal	Comments about staging and diagnosis are as for Hodgkin's disease	–	✔	–
	Treat as for nonpregnant patient. Options may vary from 'wait and watch' to aggressive combination chemotherapy with supportive care (termination or preterm delivery before chemotherapy are options)	Ib III	A C	1 2
	Counsel about prognosis and risk to fetus	III	C	2
Postnatal	As for acute leukemia (see below)	–	✔	–

References

1 Linch DC, Vaughan Hudson B, Hancock BW *et al.* (1996) A randomised comparison of a third generation regimen (PACEBOM) with a standard regimen (CHOP) in patients with histologically aggressive non-Hodgkin's lymphoma. A British National Lymphoma Investigation report. *Br J Cancer* **74**, 318–322. A randomized controlled trial of two different chemotherapy regimens for aggressive non-Hodgkin's lymphoma. 226 patients in the CHOP arm and 233 in the PACEBOM arm – no significant difference in the outcome of the two groups. **Ia A**

2 Aviles A, Diaz-Maqueo JC, Torras V *et al.* (1990) Non-Hodgkin's lymphomas and pregnancy: presentation of 16 cases. *Gynecol Oncol* **37**, 335–337. A report of 16 pregnant women treated with chemotherapy for non-Hodgkin's lymphoma (NHL). 8 were treated in the first trimester with no evidence of congenital malformations. 8 had enduring remissions and are considered cured. The article concluded that pregnancy was not a contraindication for treatment of NHL. **III C**

Acute leukemia

Management option		Quality of evidence	Strength of recommendation	References
Prepregnancy	Counsel about prognosis	–	✔	–
	Advise against conception until in remission and not on chemotherapy	IV III	C B	1,2 3
Prenatal	Start chemotherapy as for nonpregnant if diagnosed in pregnancy	IV	C	4,5
	Supportive therapy (blood, platelets, antibiotics, etc.)	–	✔	–
	Careful counseling, especially if treatment commenced in first trimester	IV	C	1,2
	Monitor fetal growth and health	IV	C	4
Labor and delivery	Expedite for normal obstetric indications	–	✔	–
	Ideally when mother in remission and fetus mature	–	✔	–
	Steroids if preterm delivery contemplated	–	✔	–
Postnatal	Contraceptive advice	III IV	B C	3,6 1,2,7
	Counseling about long-term prognosis	–	✔	–
	Avoid breastfeeding if on cytotoxic treatment	IV	C	8
	Examination and follow-up of newborn	–	✔	–

References

1 Kirshond B, Wasserstrum N, Willis R *et al.* (1988) Teratogenic effects of first trimester cyclophosphamide therapy. *Obstet Gynecol* **72**, 462–464. Case report of first-trimester cyclophosphamide therapy for a woman with systemic lupus erythematosus. The neonate had multiple anomalies thought to be secondary to the effects of cyclophosphamide. **IV C**

2 Powell HR, Ekert H (1971) Methotrexate induced congenital malformation. *Med J Aust* **2**, 1076–1077. Case report of methotrexate-induced congenital malformations primarily affecting the skull bones. The methotrexate was given for psoriasis in the first trimester of pregnancy. **IV C**

3 Selevan SG, Lindbohm ML, Hornung RW *et al.* (1985) Study of occupational exposure to antineoplastic drugs and fetal loss in nurses. *N Engl J Med* **313**, 1173–1178. Case-control study demonstrating a statistically significant association between fetal loss and occupational exposure to chemotherapy agents in the first trimester. Associations between fetal loss and the following drugs were suggested: cyclophosphamide, doxorubicin and vincristine. **III B**

4 Colbert N, Najman A, Gorin NC *et al.* (1980) Acute leukaemia during pregnancy: favourable course of pregnancy in two patients treated with cytosine arabinoside and anthracyclines. *Nouvelle Presse Med* **9**, 175–178. Case reports with chemotherapy beginning at 24 and 29 weeks respectively. Deliveries were at 36 and 33 weeks. Both children had a transient neutropenia aged 2 months but were well aged 13 months. **IV C**

5 Alegre A, Chunchurreta R, Rodriguez-Alarcon J *et al.* (1982) Successful pregnancy in acute promyelocytic leukemia. *Cancer* **49**, 152–153. Case report of daunorubicin being used to treat promyelocytic leukemia in the first trimester. **IV C**

6 Sanders JE, Buckner CD, Amos D *et al.* (1988) Ovarian function following marrow transplantation for aplastic anemia or leukemia. *J Clin Oncol* **6**, 813–818. Follow-up of ovarian function of 178 women aged 13–49 years following bone marrow transplantation. Multivariate analysis demonstrated that total body irradiation and greater patient age were significantly associated with a decreased probability of recovering normal ovarian function. **III B**

7 Milliken S, Powles R, Parikh P *et al.* (1990) Successful pregnancy following bone marrow transplantation for leukaemia. *Bone Marrow Transplant* **5**, 135–137. Case reports of three pregnancies in two women following allogeneic bone marrow transplantation for acute leukemia using a conditioning regimen of high-dose melphalan (but no total body irradiation). The pregnancies had normal outcomes. **IV C**

8 Committee on Drugs, American Academy of Pediatrics (1994) Transfer of drugs and other chemicals into breast milk. *Pediatrics* **93**, 137–150. Lists drugs and whether they are transferred into breast milk. Outlines possible effects on infant and lactation. Supports the avoidance of breastfeeding if on active cytotoxic treatment. Data obtained by a medical literature search but quality and strength of each individual recommendation not quoted. **IV C**

Chronic granulocytic leukemia

Management option		Quality of evidence	Strength of recommendation	References
Prepregnancy	Counsel about prognosis for pregnancy and in the long term	IV	C	1
	Give contraceptive advice	–	✔	–
Prenatal	Regular hematological monitoring	–	✔	–
	Consider leukapheresis	–	✔	–
	May try to control with busulfan, hydroxyurea or alpha interferon (avoid cytotoxics in the first trimester)	IV	C	2,3
	Manage accelerated phase and blast crisis as for nonpregnant patient and expedite delivery if possible (to allow possibility of bone marrow transplantation)	–	✔	–
Postnatal	As for acute leukemia	–	✔	–

References

1 Ozumba BC, Obi GO (1992) Successful pregnancy in a patient with chronic myeloid leukemia following therapy with cytotoxic drugs. *Int J Gynecol Obstet* **38**, 49–53. Case report. **IV C**

2 Jackson N, Shukri K, Ali K (1993) Hydroxyurea treatment for chronic myeloid leukaemia during pregnancy. *Br J Haematol* **85**, 203–204. Case report of a woman with chronic myeloid leukemia becoming pregnant while on hydroxyurea and being maintained on this treatment throughout pregnancy with no adverse events. **IV C**

3 Reichel RP, Linkesch W, Schetitska D (1992) Therapy with recombinant interferon alpha 2c during unexpected pregnancy in a patient with chronic myeloid leukaemia. *Br J Haematol* **82**, 472–473. Case report of a 29-year-old woman who became unexpectedly pregnant while on recombinant interferon-alpha 2c treatment for chronic phase myeloid leukemia. She presented at 20 weeks gestation. The treatment was initially stopped but was resumed after 3 weeks because of an increase in white cell count. No abnormalities of the placenta, fetus or baby were noted. **IV C**

31.9 Disseminated intravascular coagulation

Jane Gould

Management option	Quality of evidence	Strength of recommendation	References
Involve hematologist and support services (blood transfusion, etc.) early	–	✔	–
Treat/remove cause (e.g. empty uterus, antibiotics for sepsis)	–	✔	–
Hematological priorities are to replace blood constituents and coagulation factors	III	B	1
Heparin and antithrombolytic therapy have both been used in disseminated intravascular coagulation to break the cycle of consumptive coagulopathy. Neither has been subjected to controlled trials	IV	C	2

References

1 Maki M, Terao T, Ikenoue T *et al.* (1987) Clinical evaluation of antithrombin III concentrate (BI 6.013) for disseminated intravascular coagulation in obstetrics. Well-controlled multicenter trial. *Gynecol Obstet Invest* **23**, 230–240. Antithrombin III (AT III) is known to be the most important inhibitor of serine protease in the coagulation system. In the presence of heparin, AT III is converted from its progressive activity state to an immediate activity state. In disseminated intravascular coagulation (DIC) in the field of obstetrics, the treatment has to be initiated very early. Heparin treatment, on the other hand, is critical since postpartal or postoperative wound bleeding is frequently present. The authors established diagnostic criteria for the early diagnosis of DIC and investigated the clinical efficacy of a therapy with AT III in a well-controlled comparative study versus the injectable synthetic protease inhibitor FOY. The results of the trial showed that the AT III group (92%; $n = 24$) was significantly ($p < 0.001$) superior in clinical efficacy to the FOY group (60%; $n = 15$). No side effects whatsoever were observed after treatment with AT III concentrate (Behring Institute). From these results, it could be concluded that a single therapy with AT III concentrate can sufficiently control the symptoms of DIC in the field of obstetrics without the risk of increased bleeding. **III B**

2 Chung AF, Merkatz IR (1973) Survival following amniotic fluid embolism with early heparinization. *Obstet Gynecol* **42**, 809–881. Case report of heparinization in the management of a primigravida with an amniotic fluid embolus. **IV C**

Chapter 32

Respiratory disease

32.1 Breathlessness

Tracey Johnson

Management option	Quality of evidence	Strength of recommendation	References
Most breathlessness is due to physiological changes in pregnancy	III	B	1
Careful history and examination in all patients with this complaint	III	B	1
Investigate if pathological cause suggested from clinical features; tests might include: ❑ Oxygen saturation (± exercise; arterial blood gases and transfer factor in severe cases) ❑ Hemoglobin concentration ❑ Chest radiograph ❑ Ventilation–perfusion scan/magnetic resonance imaging/helical computed tomography ❑ Echocardiography	III	B	1

Reference

1 Milne J A, Howie AD, Pack AI (1978) Dyspnoea during normal pregnancy. *Br J Obstet Gynaecol* **85**, 260–263.

Observational study of 62 women assessed on eight occasions throughout a normal pregnancy. Complaint of dyspnea was more common as pregnancy advanced, with 76% complaining of this by 31 weeks gestation. After this time, few women noted any increase in symptoms. **III B**

32.2 Asthma

Tracey Johnson

Management option		Quality of evidence	Strength of recommendation	References
Prepregnancy	Adjust maintenance medication to optimize respiratory function	–	✔	–
	If possible, minimize precipitating factors by timing of pregnancy (seasonal) and avoidance of allergens	–	✔	–
	Advise early referral for prenatal care	–	✔	–
Prenatal	Adjust asthma medication as needed to control symptomatology	–	✔	–
	Inhalation rather than oral	III	B	1,2
	Regular assessment of peak flow	–	✔	–

Management option		Quality of evidence	Strength of recommendation	References
Prenatal (cont'd)	Use same drugs as outside pregnancy – steroids, beta-sympathomimetics, theophylline	IV III Ia IIa Ib	C B A B A	3 1,2,4,5 6–9 10 11
	If theophylline used, monitor blood levels, since blood volume expansion in pregnancy may mandate higher doses of the drugs	IV	C	12
	In the stable patient, antepartum nonstress testing is not necessary. If concerns over fetal wellbeing arise, begin antepartum testing in the late second or early third trimester	IV	C	1
	Seek anesthesiology consultation in preparation for delivery if general anesthesia anticipated	–	✔	–
Labor and delivery	Maintain adequate maternal oxygenation	IV	C	3
	Avoid prostaglandin $F_{2\alpha}$ and ergometrine	Ib	A	13
	Avoid general anesthesia if possible	–	✔	–
	Use parenteral steroids for patients on chronic oral therapy	–	✔	–
Postnatal	Physiotherapy to maintain adequate pulmonary toilet	–	✔	–
	Encourage respiratory therapy to minimize atelectasis	–	✔	–
	Restart maintenance drug therapy	–	✔	–
	Encourage breastfeeding	–	✔	–

References

1 Morrow Brown H, Storey G (1975) Treatment of allergy of the respiratory tract with beclomethasone dipropionate steroid aerosol. *Postgrad Med J* **51**, 59–94. Summary of one group's clinical experience with beclometasone dipropionate aerosol in control of allergic asthma and other respiratory allergy. In particular, the paper focuses on withdrawal of oral steroid therapy and replacement with inhaled steroid therapy for allergic asthma. They also assessed perennial allergic rhinitis and polyps and seasonal asthma and seasonal rhinitis. They showed that side effects were initial steroid withdrawal symptoms, which were controlled with modifying the oral steroid withdrawal regimen, and in those using beclometasone some cases of thrush were encountered. They also describe seven healthy babies being delivered with apparent side effects despite long-term treatment with inhaled beclometasone. **III B**

2 Stenius-Aarniala B, Hedman J, Teramo KA *et al.* (1996) Acute asthma during pregnancy. *Thorax* **51**, 411–414. Study following 504 pregnant asthmatics prospectively throughout pregnancy to try and assess the effect of an acute asthma attack on the course of pregnancy and delivery and the health of the newborn. Out of the 504 subjects 47 patients had an attack of asthma during pregnancy and their outcomes were compared with those of the 457 asthmatics with no recorded acute exacerbations and also with 237 healthy pregnant women. Of the 504 asthmatics 177 patients were not initially treated with inhaled corticosteroids and 17% of these had an acute attack of asthma during pregnancy compared with only 4% of the 257 patients who were on inhaled corticosteroids from the start of pregnancy. No differences were found between the groups with regard to birthweight, malformation, hypoglycemia or need for phototherapy. The authors concluded that inadequate inhaled anti-inflammatory treatment during pregnancy increases the risk of an acute attack of asthma but that if the attack was relatively mild and promptly treated it did not have any serious adverse effects on pregnancy outcome. **III B**

3 Clark SL (1993) Asthma in pregnancy. National Asthma Education Program Working Group on Asthma in Pregnancy. NIH, National Heart, Lung and Blood Institute. *Obstet Gynecol* **82**, 1033–1040. Summary of the

conference report issued by the working group on asthma in pregnancy from the National Institutes of Health, National Heart, Lung and Blood Institute. It reviews the pathogenesis of asthma and discusses the incidence. It highlights the fact that if maternal oxygen tension (P_{O_2}) falls below 60 mmHg this can result in a rapid and profound decrease in fetal oxygen saturation and fetal hypoxia and they recommend careful monitoring of fetal heart rate in the second or third trimester in the clinically unstable or hypoxic mother. The effects of asthma on pregnancy are discussed, in particular two large epidemiological studies that showed an increase in adverse perinatal outcome in women with asthma when compared to a controlled pregnant population. Both studies showed an increase in perinatal mortality rate and the other studies have reported an increased incidence of preterm delivery, low birthweight and preeclampsia in women with asthma. Treatment of asthma in pregnancy has been discussed and the group advocates objective measurement of lung volume or flow rates during pregnancy and in the case of severe asthma serial ultrasound evaluation of fetal growth. As far as drug therapy is concerned they recommend that the primary therapy of choice is inhaled anti-inflammatory agents such as cromolyn sodium or inhaled corticosteroids with the addition of oral corticosteroids when asthma escapes control. If asthma cannot be controlled long term on the maximum dose of bronchodilators and inhaled anti-inflammatories, long-term oral corticosteroids should be used but clinicians should be aware of the risks of long-term oral corticosteroid therapy. The paper then goes on to describe the management of acute severe asthma in pregnancy in a stepwise manner including oxygen, blood-gas analysis, pulmonary function tests and drug therapy with nebulizers or subcutaneous terbutaline. **IV C**

4 Schatz M, Patterson R, Zeitz S *et al.* (1975) Corticosteroid therapy for the pregnant asthmatic. *JAMA* **233**, 804–807. Descriptive study of 70 pregnancies and 55 asthmatic patients who received corticosteroids for management of their asthma during the course of their pregnancy. The study looks specifically at pregnancy outcome and there was only one spontaneous miscarriage in the series, all others being live births with no maternal, fetal or neonatal deaths. There was a slightly increased risk of prematurity but no other complications were encountered and the authors recommend the judicious use of corticosteroids during pregnancy for asthma control. **III B**

5 Bahna SL, Bjerkedal T (1972) The course and outcome of pregnancy in women with bronchial asthma. *Acta Allerg* **27**, 397–400. Retrospective study of pregnancy outcome in 381 asthmatics compared to a control group of 112530 pregnancies. Data were obtained from the Norwegian Medical Birth Registry. An increased incidence of pregnancy and labor complications, preterm delivery, low birthweight, hypoxia and neonatal death was described and the authors concluded that pregnant asthmatics and their newborns should be considered a high-risk population. **III B**

6 Manser R, Reid D, Abramson M (2000) Corticosteroids for acute severe asthma in hospitalised patients. In: *Cochrane database of systemic reviews*, issue 4. Oxford: Update Software. Meta-analysis of six trials comparing higher doses of systemic corticosteroids (oral, intravenous or intramuscular) with lower doses in the management of patients with acute severe asthma requiring hospital admission. No differences were identified among the different doses and the authors concluded that low doses of corticosteroids were adequate for initial management, with higher doses offering no therapeutic advantage. **Ia A**

7 Rowe BH, Spooner C, Ducharme FM *et al.* (2000) Early emergency department treatment of acute asthma with systemic corticosteroids. In: *Cochrane database of systemic reviews*, issue 4. Oxford: Update Software. Meta-analysis of 12 RCTs or quasi-RCTs including 863 patients, 435 who received systemic corticosteroids within 1 h of admission to the emergency department with acute asthma and 428 who received placebo. Use of corticosteroids significantly reduced the need for hospital admission, particularly in those with more severe asthma and those not currently receiving steroids. **Ia A**

8 Edmonds ML, Camargo CA, Pollack CV *et al.* (2000) Early use of inhaled corticosteroids in the emergency department treatment of acute asthma. In: *Cochrane database of systemic reviews*, issue 4. Oxford: Update Software. Meta-analysis of 6 (4 adult and 2 pediatric) RCTs or quasi-RCTs including 352 patients with acute asthma, 179 of whom received inhaled corticosteroids in the emergency department and 173 who were not treated with inhaled corticosteroids. Inhaled steroids reduced admission rates in patients who were not receiving concomitant systemic corticosteroids. **Ia A**

9 Adams NP, Bestall JB, Jones PW *et al.* (2000) Inhaled beclomethasone versus placebo for chronic asthma. In: *Cochrane database of systemic reviews*, issue 4. Oxford: Update Software. Meta-analysis of 52 trials including 3459 patients. The objectives were to compare inhaled beclometasone therapy to placebo in the control of chronic asthma, to assess the dose–response relationship and provide the best estimate of the efficacy of beclometasone as a benchmark for evaluation of newer asthma therapies. In non-oral-steroid-treated patients, beclometasone significantly improved pulmonary function test results and reduced rescue beta-2-agonist use compared to placebo. In oral-steroid-treated patients, beclometasone led to a significant reduction in oral prednisolone dose and increased the likelihood of discontinuing oral steroid therapy. There was little evidence for a dose–response effect. **Ia A**

10 Cydulka RK, Emerman CL, Schreiber D et al. (1999) Acute asthma among pregnant women presenting to the emergency department. *Am J Respir Crit Care Med* **160**, 887–892. Multicenter prospective cohort study comparing pregnant (51) versus nonpregnant (500) women presenting to the emergency department with acute asthma. The two groups were comparable in terms of asthma severity, but pregnant women were less likely to be treated with corticosteroids and less likely to be discharged home on corticosteroids if admitted. Pregnant women were more likely to report an ongoing exacerbation at a 2-week follow-up. The authors concluded that pregnant asthmatics were less likely to receive appropriate therapy than nonpregnant women. **IIa B**

11 Wendel PJ, Ramin SM, Barnett-Hamm C *et al.* (1996) Asthma treated in pregnancy: a randomized controlled study. *Am J Obstet Gynecol* **175**, 150–154. 84 pregnant women with 105 asthma exacerbations were studied. 65% required admission and were randomized to receive either intravenous aminophylline and inhaled beta-2-agonists or intravenous methylprednisolone and inhaled beta-2-agonists. At discharge they received either inhaled beta-2-agonists and corticosteroid taper plus inhaled beclometasone, or inhaled beta-2-agonists and corticosteroid taper alone. Intravenous aminophylline offered no therapeutic advantage and inhaled corticosteroids reduced the need for subsequent admissions. **Ib A**

12 Rubin PC (1986) Prescribing in pregnancy. *Br Med J* **293**, 1415–1417. Review article for practicing clinicians who prescribe drugs for women who are or may become pregnant, covering general principles for prescribing in pregnancy. The article briefly describes epidemiology of drug use during pregnancy and looks at the effect of pregnancy on those requirements, paying attention to increase in total body water, changes in serum proteins and an increase in liver metabolism and in particular points out that liver-enzyme-dependent clearance is twice the rate found in nonpregnant women. Renal drug clearance is covered, as is therapeutic drug monitoring during pregnancy, placental transfer of drugs and breastfeeding. The conclusion is that use of drugs during pregnancy and in the puerperium requires a fine balance that should be maintained taking into account both maternal and fetal welfare. **IV C**

13 Smith AP (1973) The effects of intravenous infusion of graded doses of prostaglandin F2 alpha and E2 on lung resistance in patients undergoing termination of pregnancy. *Clin Sci* **44**, 17–25. Randomized trial of 15 healthy women undergoing termination of pregnancy using intravenous prostaglandin E_2 in 7 cases and intravenous prostaglandin $F_{2\alpha}$ in 8 cases, where lung resistance was measured by the interrupter method. Both drugs led to an increase in lung resistance although no clinical problems were encountered and this was compared to lung resistance measured in 15 controls who did not have any intravenous prostaglandins. The author concluded that these drugs should be used with caution in women with lung problems and discusses the possible dangers of intravenous prostaglandin administration to patients with asthma and other lung disorders. **Ib A**

32.3 Sarcoid

Tracey Johnson

Management option		Quality of evidence	Strength of recommendation	References
Prepregnancy	Reassure patient of benign nature of sarcoidosis during pregnancy unless there is preexisting evidence of pulmonary fibrosis, hypoxemia or pulmonary hypertension	–	✔	–
	Baseline pulmonary function studies may assist in the evaluation of the patient's lung status prior to pregnancy	–	✔	–
Prenatal	Avoid multivitamins containing vitamin D	IV	C	1
	Watch for signs and symptoms of progressive pulmonary disease; institute steroid therapy with evidence of significant disease advancement	Ia	A	2
Labor and delivery	With substantial parenchymal disease avoid inhalation anesthesia	–	✔	–
	Recognize that high block conduction anesthesia may cause significant respiratory compromise	–	✔	–
	Obtain early anesthesiology consultation in patients with severe disease	–	✔	–
Postnatal	No specific disease-related needs	–	✔	–

References

1 James DG (1970) Sarcoidosis. *Disease-a-Month* **1**, 43. Review article that does not present original data. Calcium metabolism is discussed and the incidence of hypercalcemia and hypercalcuria in patients with sarcoid is highlighted. The author recommends that serum calcium is monitored throughout pregnancy as it may increase, particularly in those taking vitamin D supplements, as sarcoid patients are particularly susceptible to it. **IV C**

2 Paramothayan NS, Jones PW (2000) Corticosteroids for pulmonary sarcoidosis. In: *Cochrane database of systemic reviews*, issue 4. Oxford: Update Software. Meta-analysis of seven RCTs of the benefits of steroid therapy in the treatment of pulmonary sarcoid – five trials (516 patients) for oral steroids and two trials (66 patients) for inhaled steroids. Oral steroids improved chest X-ray appearances and the global score, symptoms and spirometry over 6–24 months but with little evidence of improved lung function. Oral steroids are indicated for stage 2 and 3 disease with moderate to severe or progressive symptoms or chest X-ray changes. Short-term (less than 6 months) courses of inhaled steroids may improve symptoms in those who mainly have cough. **Ia A**

32.4 Tuberculosis

Tracey Johnson

Management option		Quality of evidence	Strength of recommendation	References
Prepregnancy	It is best to establish this diagnosis, and treat the condition, prior to pregnancy. Therefore, screening of at-risk populations is advised	–	✓	–
	Counsel regarding the potential teratogenesis of streptomycin if being used (not standard therapy)	IV III	C B	1 2
Prenatal	Outside the first trimester, standard therapy (pyrazinamide, rifampin/rifampicin and isoniazid) for active tuberculosis should be employed. Pyrazinamide is usually reserved for severe illness	IV	C	1
	In the first trimester, one may withhold rifampin/rifampicin (and substitute with ethambutol) until later in pregnancy, and pyrazinamide should only be given with severe illness	IV	C	1
	Give pyridoxine when using isoniazid	III	B	3
Labor and delivery	No specific recommendations except that infection precautions are needed with active disease	–	✓	–
Postnatal	Only separate mother from baby if open	–	✓	–
	Administer isoniazid and BCG to neonate	–	✓	–
	Can breastfeed	–	✓	–
	Oral contraceptive efficacy impaired by drugs	–	✓	–

References

1 Snider DE, Layde PM, Johnson MW *et al.* (1980) Treatment of tuberculosis during pregnancy. *Am Rev Respir Dis* **122**, 65–79. Review article that does not present any original data but reviews the published observational data available on pregnancy outcome in women taking various combinations of four different antituberculous drugs: isoniazid, ethambutol, rifampin/rifampicin and streptomycin. They concluded that, with the exception of streptomycin-related ototoxicity, these drugs were safe to use in pregnancy, although the numbers were small with rifampicin, and that therapeutic abortion was not indicated because of teratogenic risk. **IV C**

2 Conway N, Birt BD (1965) Streptomycin in pregnancy: effect on the fetal ear. *Br Med J* **2**, 260–263. Study describing the results of audiograms and caloric tests carried out on 17 children whose mothers received streptomycin therapy for tuberculosis during pregnancy. Minor abnormalities of VIIIth nerve function were identified in 8, but no deafness was found in the speech frequencies. The authors concluded that further work was required to establish the risks to the fetus of streptomycin exposure *in utero*. **III B**

3 Atkins NA (1982) Maternal plasma concentration of pyridoxal phosphate during pregnancy: adequacy of vitamin B_6 supplementation during isoniazid therapy. *Am Rev Respir Dis* **126**, 714–716. Pyridoxal phosphate concentrations were measured serially throughout pregnancy in 12 women receiving isoniazid therapy for tuberculosis who were administered a prenatal vitamin supplement and 50mg of pyridoxine hydrochloride daily, to establish whether supplementation prevented vitamin B_6 deficiency. The author concluded that supplementation with 52–60mg of vitamin B_6 daily avoided deficiency. **III B**

32.5 Kyphoscoliosis

Tracey Johnson

Management option		Quality of evidence	Strength of recommendation	References
Prepregnancy	Counsel regarding risk for slight increase in pulmonary compromise as pregnancy advances, although not severe cardiopulmonary compromise. Previously reported high risks for fetal growth restriction and need for preterm delivery not confirmed by more recent data	B	III	1–3
	Assess pulmonary vital capacity if symptomatic	–	✔	–
Prenatal	Monitor respiratory function clinically and with oxygen saturation if symptomatic	B	III	1–3
	In unusual circumstance of severe cardiorespiratory compromise, begin prenatal surveillance for growth restriction and fetal wellbeing in early third trimester	–	✔	–
	May need early delivery for frank respiratory failure	–	✔	–
Labor and delivery	Supplementary oxygen if low oxygen saturation values	B	III	1–3
	Cesarean section if associated pelvic deformities but vaginal delivery possible with most cases; regional anesthesia possible in many cases	B	III	1–3
Postnatal	Physiotherapy especially if general anesthesia	–	✔	–

References

1 To WW, Wong MW (1996) Kyphoscoliosis complicating pregnancy. *Int J Gynaecol Obstet* **55**, 123–128. Observational study of 17 patients with 27 pregnancies complicated by kyphoscoliosis of varying etiology. 8 patients had previous spinal surgery. The vaginal delivery rate was high and none suffered cardiorespiratory embarrassment. There was no maternal or perinatal mortality. The authors concluded that the high risks previously reported are no longer valid. They speculate whether spinal surgery prior to pregnancy contributed to the improved outcome. **III B**

2 Siegler D, Zorab PA (1981) Pregnancy in thoracic scoliosis. *Br J Dis Chest* **75**, 367–370. Observational study of 118 pregnancies in 64 patients with thoracic scoliosis, two thirds of whom had curves in excess of 60°. Increased breathlessness was experienced in 17% of pregnancies but no serious cardiorespiratory problems were encountered. Spontaneous vaginal delivery was achieved in 65% and 17% had a cesarean section. **III B**

3 Orvomaa E, Hiilesmaa V, Poussa M *et al.* (1997) Pregnancy and delivery in patients operated by the Harrington method for idiopathic scoliosis. *Eur Spine J* **6**, 304–307. Observational study of 142 pregnancies in 146 patients after Harrington surgery for idiopathic scoliosis (1970–75). Pregnancy did not have a significant impact on spinal curvature. Cesarean section (23%) was significantly higher than in the background population (15%). Pregnancy and labor complication rates were no different from the background values. Backpain occurred in 40% but was only severe enough to require sick leave in 11%. **III B**

32.6 Cystic fibrosis (maternal)

Tracey Johnson

Management option		Quality of evidence	Strength of recommendation	References
Prepregnancy	Document baseline/prepregnancy respiratory function	III	B	1
	Counsel for maternal risks of respiratory failure and congestive cardiac failure, and preterm delivery if prepregnancy FEV_1 <60%	III	B	1
	Counsel for fetal risks of having cystic fibrosis or being a carrier. Gene testing of putative parents; in father, test will determine carrier status and in both parents it will examine the potential for informative prenatal diagnosis (genes for cystic fibrosis identifiable in about 99% of cases)	III	B	1
Prenatal	Monitor respiratory function	III	B	1
	Multidisciplinary management	III	B	1
	Vigilance for preterm delivery	III	B	1
Labor and delivery	Monitor respiratory function	III	B	1
	Supplemental oxygen if low oxygen saturation	III	B	1
Postnatal	Monitor respiratory function	III	B	1
	Breastfeeding is usually possible but avoid in nutritionally compromised patient	III	B	1

Reference

1 Edenborough FP, Stableforth DE, Webb AK *et al.* (1995) Outcome of pregnancy in women with cystic fibrosis. *Thorax* **50**, 170–174. Retrospective study of 22 pregnancies in 20 cystic fibrosis patients. 18 pregnancies were completed, producing healthy, non-cystic-fibrosis infants. Mothers lost 13% of FEV_1 and 11% of FVC during pregnancy, most of which was regained subsequently. Most mothers gained weight. Microbiological status remained unchanged. 6 infants were preterm and 2 were small-for-dates. 4 mothers died up to 3.2 years following delivery. Prepregnancy $\%FEV_1$ showed the best correlation with gestation, birth weight and maternal survival. **III B**

32.7 Pneumonia

Tracey Johnson

Management option		Quality of evidence	Strength of recommendation	References
Prepregnancy	None specifically related to pneumonia; in patients with underlying conditions, counsel regarding this possible complication	–	✔	–
	Influenza vaccine if second or third trimester during flu season	–	✔	–
	Pneumococcal vaccine if high-risk conditions, e.g. splenectomy	–	✔	–
Prenatal	Differentiate from other conditions, especially pulmonary embolus	–	✔	–

➡

Management option		Quality of evidence	Strength of recommendation	References
Prenatal (cont'd)	Use standard techniques for microbiological assessment	–	✔	–
	Do not avoid chest radiographs if pulmonary disease suspected	–	✔	–
	Begin appropriate antimicrobial therapy based on underlying conditions and presentation; avoid tetracycline therapy in pregnancy	–	✔	–
	Oxygen therapy if low oxygen saturation values	–	✔	–
Labor, delivery and postnatal	None specific	–	✔	–

Chapter 33

Hepatic and gastrointestinal disease

33.1 Obstetric cholestasis

Mike Maresh

Management option		Quality of evidence	Strength of recommendation	References
Prepregnancy	Not applicable, unless diagnosed in previous pregnancy	–	✔	–
	Counsel for 60–80% chance of recurrence	–	✔	–
	Biliary ultrasonography to detect stones or other disease	–	✔	–
Prenatal	Local antipruritic measures	–	✔	–
	Consider cholestyramine, ursodeoxycholic acid, steroids	Ib IV	A C	1,2 3
	Vitamin K supplements for mother	IV III	C B	3 4,5
	Monitor fetal wellbeing	–	✔	–
	Consider elective delivery at 37–38 weeks	–	✔	–
	Biliary tract ultrasonography to exclude other pathology	–	✔	–
Labor and delivery	Anticipate preterm labor	–	✔	–
	Increased risk of postpartum hemorrhage	–	✔	–
Postnatal	Monitor biochemical resolution	–	✔	–
	Vitamin K supplement for baby	–	✔	–
	Use oral contraceptives only with close clinical and biochemical monitoring	–	✔	–
	Consider liver biopsy if diagnosis is suspect or condition progressive	–	✔	–

References

1 Diaferia A, Nicastri PL, Tartagni M *et al.* (1996) Ursodeoxycholic acid therapy in pregnant women with cholestasis. *Int J Gynaecol Obstet* **52**, 133–140. Small controlled trial in which 16 women with intrahepatic cholestasis in the third trimester of pregnancy were randomized to ursodeoxycholic acid therapy or placebo. Active treatment was associated with a significant improvement in symptoms and a reduction in the level of bile acids and transaminases. **Ib A**

2 Riikonen S, Savonius H, Gylling H *et al.* (2000) Oral guar gum, a gel-forming dietary fiber, relieves pruritus in intrahepatic cholestasis of pregnancy. *Acta Obstet Gynecol Scand* **79**, 260–264. Controlled trial of 48 women with intrahepatic cholestasis were randomized to guar gum (a gel-forming fibre which increases fecal elimination of bile acids) or to placebo. Guar gum was associated with a reduction in pruritus and no increase in serum bile acids which did occur in controls. **Ib A**

3 Raine-Fenning N, Kilby M (1997) Obstetric cholestasis. *Fetal Matern Med Rev* **9**, 1–17. Detailed review including 150 references. It includes opinions on etiology and diagnosis. It reviews antenatal surveillance and the various treatments that have been studied. **IV C**

4 Fisk NM, Storey GNB (1998) Fetal outcome in obstetric cholestasis. *Br J Obstet Gynaecol* **95**, 1137–1143. Retrospective review of 83 pregnancies complicated by cholestasis. Antenatal cardiotocography and ultrasound assessment of amniotic fluid were not helpful in predicting fetal compromise. However, meconium did appear to be more predictive and the authors suggest that consideration should be given to amniocentesis to assess amniotic fluid. **III B**

5 Alsulyman OM, Ouzounian JG, Ames-Castro M *et al.* (1996) Intrahepatic cholestasis of pregnancy: perinatal outcome associated with expectant management *Am J Obstet Gynecol* **175**, 957–960. Study describing the outcome of 79 women with intrahepatic cholestasis having surveillance with antenatal cardiotocography and amniotic fluid assessments. They were compared with women who were having such surveillance because of a previous stillbirth. While the controls had more abnormal test results, those with cholestasis were associated with an increased incidence of meconium and two stillbirths. **III B**

33.2 Acute fatty liver of pregnancy

Mike Maresh

Management option		**Quality of evidence**	**Strength of recommendation**	**References**
Prepregnancy	None, except discussion of recurrence risks (see Postnatal)	–	✔	–
Prenatal	Establish diagnosis, resuscitate	–	✔	–
	Intensive care	–	✔	–
	Supportive therapy (see labor/delivery)	–	✔	–
	Plan delivery	–	✔	–
Labor and delivery	Maternal resuscitation by correction of: ❑ Hypoglycemia ❑ Fluid balance ❑ Coagulopathy	–	✔	–
	Treatment of liver failure	–	✔	–
	Intensive fetal monitoring	–	✔	–
	Urgent delivery when maternal condition is stabilized, vaginal delivery preferable for mother	–	✔	–
	Meticulous hemostasis including adequate wound drainage	–	✔	–
Postnatal	Continue intensive-care management	–	✔	–
	Watch for wound hematoma formation and sepsis, postpartum hemorrhage	–	✔	–
	Recurrence risk is difficult to estimate, perhaps as high as 10–20%	–	✔	–
	Support contraceptive measures	–	✔	–

33.3 Hyperemesis gravidarum

Mike Maresh

Management option		**Quality of evidence**	**Strength of recommendation**	**References**
Prepregnancy	Discuss recurrence risk	–	✔	–

➡

Management option		Quality of evidence	Strength of recommendation	References
Prenatal	Remember alternative diagnoses	–	✔	–
	Intravenous fluid and electrolyte therapy	–	✔	–
	Dietitian	–	✔	–
	Antiemetic regimen	Ia Ib	A A	1 2
	Nutrient and vitamin supplementation	–	✔	–
	Anti-gastroesophageal-reflux measures	–	✔	–
	Psychological and social support	–	✔	–
	Consider steroids	Ib	A	3,4
Postnatal	Review nutritional status	–	✔	–
	Discuss contraception	–	✔	–

References

1 Jewell D, Young G (2000) Interventions for nausea and vomiting in early pregnancy. In: *Cochrane database of systematic reviews*, issue 4. Oxford: Update Software. Systematic review that concludes that antiemetic drugs do reduce the frequency of nausea in early pregnancy. It also notes that pyridoxine (vitamin B_6) appears to be effective in reducing the severity of nausea. It does not review recent trials of steroid therapy. **Ia A**

2 Sullivan CA, Johnson CA, Roach H (1996) A pilot study of intravenous ondansetron for hyperemesis gravidarum. *Am J Obstet Gynecol* **174**, 1565–1568. RCT in 30 women with hyperemesis were randomized to intravenous ondansetron or intravenous promethazine. The newer and more expensive drug ondansetron appeared to offer no advantage over a conventional antiemetic. **Ib A**

3 Safari HR, Fassett MJ, Souter IC *et al.* (1998) The efficacy of methylprednisolone in the treatment of hyperemesis gravidarum: a randomized, doubled-blind, controlled study. *Am J Obstet Gynecol* **179**, 921–924. RCT of 40 women with severe hyperemesis randomized to promethazine or methylprednisolone. Almost all women in both groups responded initially by stopping vomiting. However, despite continuation of therapy for 2 weeks, significantly more women were readmitted within 2 weeks in the promethazine group. **Ib A**

4 Nelson-Piercy C, Fayers P, de Swiet M (2001) Randomized, double-blind placebo-controlled trial of corticosteroids for the treatment of hyperemesis gravidarum. *Br J Obstet Gynaecol* **108**, 9–15. RCT in 25 women with severe hyperemesis were randomized to prednisolone or placebo. Steroid therapy was associated with a significantly improved sense of wellbeing, appetite and weight gain. The improvement in nausea and vomiting with steroids was not significant nor was the reduced dependence on intravenous fluids. **Ib A**

33.4 The liver in severe preeclampsia

Mike Maresh

Management option		Quality of evidence	Strength of recommendation	References
Prepregnancy	None, other than counseling about a 10–30% recurrence risk of preeclampsia	–	✔	–
Prenatal	Control of hypertension	Ia	A	1–3
	Correct coagulation disturbance	–	✔	–
	Consider anticonvulsant prophylaxis	Ia	A	4

Management option		Quality of evidence	Strength of recommendation	References
Prenatal (cont'd)	Close fetal monitoring	–	✔	–
	Watch for fall in hemoglobin from hemolysis	–	✔	–
	Fluid and electrolyte management	–	✔	–
	Initiate delivery	–	✔	–
Postnatal	Anticipate delayed postnatal recovery	–	✔	–
	Continue monitoring platelets and renal function	–	✔	–
	Monitor for hemolysis	–	✔	–
	Control severe hypertension	Ia	A	1–4
See also Section 26.2.				

References

1 Abalos E, Duley L, Steyn DW *et al.* (2001) Antihypertensive drug therapy for mild to moderate hypertension during pregnancy (Cochrane Review). In: *The Cochrane library*, issue 2. Oxford: Update Software. Systematic review of randomized trials evaluating any hypertensive drug treatment for mild to moderate hypertension during pregnancy. 40 studies were included, involving 3797 women. 24 studies (2815 women) compared an antihypertensive drug with placebo or no drug. Antihypertensive drug treatment resulted in a halving of the risk of developing severe hypertension but little evidence of a difference in the incidence of preeclampsia (RR 0.99, 95% CI 0.84–1.18). There were no clear effects of treatment on the risk of preeclampsia, fetal or neonatal death, preterm birth or small-for-gestational-age babies. In trials comparing one antihypertensive drug with another, there were no clear differences between any of these drugs in the risk of developing severe hypertension and proteinuria/preeclampsia. Other antihypertensive agents appeared better than methyldopa for reducing the risk of the baby dying (14 trials, 1010 subjects, RR 0.49 (95% CI 0.24–0.99). **Ia A**

2 Magee LA, Duley L (2001) Oral beta-blockers for mild to moderate hypertension during pregnancy (Cochrane Review). In: *The Cochrane library*, issue 2. Oxford: Update Software. Systematic review of 27 randomized trials comparing beta-blockers with placebo/no therapy or other antihypertensive agents for women with mild–moderate pregnancy hypertension (i.e. blood pressure < 170mmHg systolic or 110mmHg diastolic). Oral beta-blockers decreased the risk of severe hypertension (14 trials, 1516 women, RR 0.37, 95% CI 0.26–0.53) and the need for additional antihypertensive drugs. Insufficient data prevented firm conclusions about the effect on perinatal mortality or preterm delivery. Beta-blockers appeared to be associated with an increase in small-for-gestational-age infants (RR 1.34, 95% CI 1.01–1.79). In 11 trials (787 women) comparing beta-blockers with methyldopa, there was no evidence of any differences between the drugs in efficacy or safety (either maternal or fetal). **Ia A**

3 Duley L, Henderson-Smart DJ (2001) Drugs for rapid treatment of very high blood pressure during pregnancy (Cochrane Review). In: *The Cochrane library*, issue 2. Oxford: Update Software. Systematic review of 14 randomized trials of intravenous drugs for severe hypertension in pregnancy. Ketanserin was found to be less effective than hydralazine in reducing blood pressure. Diazoxide was associated with profound hypotension, requiring treatment. Otherwise, there was no evidence that any one of the other antihypertensive agents was better than another. **Ia A**

4 Duley L, Gulmezoglu AM, Henderson-Smart DJ (2001) Anticonvulsants for women with pre-eclampsia (Cochrane Review). In: *The Cochrane Library*, issue 2. Oxford: Update Software. Systematic review of nine randomized trials of anticonvulsant usage in women with preeclampsia. In trials comparing magnesium sulfate with placebo/no anticonvulsant the relative risk (RR) of eclampsia was 0.33 (95% CI 0.11–1.02). Magnesium sulfate was better than phenytoin at reducing the risk of eclampsia (RR 0.05, 95% CI 0.00–0.84). Studies comparing magnesium sulfate and diazepam were too small for any reliable conclusions. Overall, there was not enough evidence to establish the benefits and hazards of anticonvulsants for women with preeclampsia but magnesium sulfate appeared to be the best choice. **Ia A**

33.5 Peptic ulceration in pregnancy

Mike Maresh

Management option		Quality of evidence	Strength of recommendation	References
Prepregnancy	Advise against agents that may exacerbate peptic ulcer disease (e.g. alcohol, smoking)	–	✔	–
	Anticipate improvement in clinical symptoms with pregnancy	–	✔	–
Prenatal	Adequate endoscopic investigation	–	✔	–
	Antacids or histamine-receptor blockers	–	✔	–
	Consider anti-*Helicobacter* treatment with positive diagnosis and if other therapy has been ineffective	–	✔	–
	Avoid oral steroids	–	✔	–
Postnatal	Repeat endoscopy if indicated by initial findings	–	✔	–

33.6 Celiac disease in pregnancy

Mike Maresh

Management option		Quality of evidence	Strength of recommendation	References
Prepregnancy	Preconception counseling and dietary control	IIa IIb	B B	1 2
	Folic acid supplementation	–	✔	–
Prenatal	Careful dietary surveillance by dietitian	–	✔	–
	Folic acid supplementation	–	✔	–
	Monitor nutritional status	–	✔	–
	Replace vitamins, minerals as indicated	–	✔	–
	Give iron	–	✔	–
	Screen for fetal abnormality, especially neural tube defect	–	✔	–
	Monitor fetal growth and wellbeing	IIa IIb	B B	1 2
Postnatal	Monitor nutritional and vitamin adequacy, particularly with lactation	–	✔	–
	Contraceptive advice and caution with oral preparations if disease active	–	✔	–

References

1 Sher KS, Mayberry JT (1996) Female fertility, obstetric and gynaecological history in coeliac disease: a case control study. *Acta Paediatr Suppl* **412**, 76–77. This is a case-controlled study of women with celiac disease. Prior to diagnosis women with celiac disease had more difficulty in conceiving and a higher risk of miscarriage than controls

but this difference was not present once diagnosed and treated. In addition, there was a trend towards more stillbirths in those with celiac disease. **IIa B**

2 Norgard, B, Fonager K, Sorensen HT *et al.* (1999) Birth outcomes of women with celiac disease: a nationwide historical cohort study. *Am J Gastroenterol* **94**, 2435–2440. Comparative study of 211 babies born to 127 mothers with celiac disease and 1260 control cases. Those women not on treatment (diet) had significantly lower newborn birthweights than the control group (after adjustment for confounders). In those on diet, the mean birthweight in the celiac cases was higher than the control group. The untreated group had a significantly increased risk of growth restriction. None of the babies in the treated group had growth restriction. **IIb B**

33.7 Inflammatory bowel disease in pregnancy

Mike Maresh

Management option		Quality of evidence	Strength of recommendation	References
Prepregnancy	Preconception counseling and control	–	✔	–
	Consider modification of drug therapy; steroids do not reduce the risk of relapse	Ia	A	1–3
	Ensure folate supplementation (5 mg daily)	–	✔	–
Prenatal	Continue appropriate drug therapy prenatally	Ia	A	1–3
	Attention to nutrition, iron and folate supplementation	–	✔	–
	Monitor fetal growth	–	✔	–
Labor and delivery	If abdominal delivery needed, anticipate peritoneal adhesions or anticipate difficulties from perineal scarring with vaginal delivery	–	✔	–
	Scrupulous attention to wound repair (abdominal and perineal) with Crohn's disease	–	✔	–
Postnatal	If severe diarrhea and malabsorption present, consider alternatives to oral contraceptives	–	✔	–

References

1 Steinhart A, Ewe K, Griffiths AM *et al.* (2000) Corticosteroids for maintaining remission of Crohn's disease. In: *Cochrane database of systematic reviews*, issue 3. Oxford: Update Software. Systematic review of the value of using corticosteroid therapy to maintain clinical remission in Crohn's disease. Three controlled trials were identified and in none of these did corticosteroids reduce the risk of relapse. However, whether any subgroups are more likely to benefit is yet to be established. **Ia A**

2 Pearson DC, May GR, Fick G *et al.* (2000) Azathioprine for maintaining remission of Crohn's disease. In: *Cochrane database of systematic reviews*, issue 4. Oxford: Update Software. Systematic review of the use of azathioprine to maintain remission in Crohn's disease. Analysis of five suitable studies, all conducted in the 1970s, showed that it was more effective than placebo in preventing remissions and also had a steroid-sparing effect. **Ia A**

3 Sutherland L, Roth D, Beck P *et al.* (2000) Oral 5-aminosalicylic acid for maintaining remission in ulcerative colitis. In: *Cochrane database of systematic reviews*, issue 4. Oxford: Update Software. Systematic review concluding that sulfasalazine is superior to the newer release formulations of 5-aminosalicylic acid to maintain remission in ulcerative colitis. Both were superior to placebo. The side effect profiles were similar. **Ia A**

Chapter 34

Neuromuscular disease

34.1 Seizures

Karen Brackley

Preeclampsia/eclampsia

Management option		Quality of evidence	Strength of recommendation	References
Prenatal, labor and delivery, postnatal	First aid measures: ❑ Avoid injury ❑ Semiprone position ❑ Maintain airway ❑ Administer oxygen ❑ Monitor maternal and fetal condition	Ia Ib IIa	A A B	1 2 3
	Control and prevent recurrence of seizures. Magnesium is the drug of choice (although some would use a short-acting benzodiazepine for immediate fit control, followed by magnesium for prophylaxis)	IV Ib Ia Ib	C A A A	4 5 6–8 9
	Treat hypertension	IV Ia	C A	4 1
	Avoid fluid overload	–	✔	–
	Check renal, liver and coagulation status	–	✔	–
	Deliver when stable	–	✔	–

References

1 Magee LA, Ornstein MP, von Dadelszen P (1999) Management of hypertension in pregnancy. *Br Med J* **318**, 1332–1336. Systematic review of the literature from 1966–97 with subsequent meta-analysis. Randomized controlled trials were identified that assessed the effectiveness of drug and nondrug therapies in chronic and pregnancy-induced hypertension to improve maternal and perinatal outcomes. As expected, antihypertensive treatment in mild–moderate hypertension reduces the incidence of severe hypertension and the need for additional hypertensives. The presence of proteinuria at delivery in pregnancy-induced hypertension is significantly reduced but there is no clear effect on other maternal or perinatal outcomes. The choice of antihypertensive drug does not matter, except that parenteral hydralazine in severe hypertension is associated with more maternal hypotension, cesarean sections and lowered Apgar scores. Women with early, severe preeclampsia have better perinatal outcomes if they are managed 'expectantly' but data are insufficient to estimate risks to the mother. The commentary criticizes the review for not providing guidance on when to implement antihypertensive drugs. The need for continued fetal surveillance following institution of antihypertensive treatment is stressed and 'expectant' management should be limited to experienced clinicians in tertiary referral units. **Ia A**

2 Phippard AF, Fischer WE, Horvath JS *et al.* (1991) Early blood pressure control improves pregnancy outcome in primigravid women with mild hypertension. *Med J Aust* **154**. 378–382. Small randomized, placebo-controlled trial that recruited primigravid women between 28 and 34 weeks gestation with effectively normal blood pressures (≥130/75 or 'more than 1 SD above the gestational mean'). Antihypertensive treatment with oral clonidine and hydralazine resulted in more subjects (22/25) reaching 38 weeks compared to controls (17/27) as a result of fewer third-trimester complications, including severe hypertension or preeclampsia and intrauterine growth restriction. The study had insufficient power to assess more important endpoints, including significant maternal and neonatal morbidity, and specifically was of poor quality and not relevant to seizures. **Ib A**

3 Fenakel K, Fenakel G, Appelman Z *et al.* (1991) Nifedipine in the treatment of severe preeclampsia. *Obstet Gynecol* **77**, 331–337. Quasi-randomized, controlled trial using week of the month as allocation method. 49 women

of mixed parity with severe preeclampsia, based primarily on blood pressure criteria, were recruited. 60% had superimposed preeclampsia. More consistent and prolonged control of hypertension occurred with nifedipine compared to hydralazine. Hydralazine was associated with more diagnoses of acute fetal distress (41% compared to 4%) but this was not reflected in significantly increased cesarean section rates. There were no significant differences in major neonatal outcomes in the nifedipine group. **IIb B**

4 Rey E, LeLorier J, Burgess E *et al.* (1997) Report of the Canadian Hypertension Society Consensus Conference: 3. Pharmacological treatment of hypertensive disorders in pregnancy. *Can Med Assoc J* **157**, 1245–1254. Members of the panel from the Canadian Hypertension Society performed a systematic review of the literature published from 1962 to September 1996 and produced evidence-based guidelines on the treatment of hypertension in pregnancy. Severe hypertension of 170/110mmHg should be urgently treated with either hydralazine, labetalol or nifedipine to prevent maternal intracerebral hemorrhage. The report highlights the limited evidence available to determine the benefits of treatment at lower blood pressure readings but suggests threshold levels in certain groups of patients. Antihypertensive treatment prevents severe hypertension but does not reduce the risk of developing proteinuric hypertension, intrauterine growth restriction or preterm delivery. Methyldopa is recommended as first-line therapy in nonsevere hypertension because of its safety record. Magnesium sulfate is recommended for the prevention and treatment of eclamptic seizures. **IV C**

5 Lucas MJ, Leveno KJ, Cunningham FG (1995) A comparison of magnesium sulfate with phenytoin for the prevention of eclampsia. *N Engl J Med* **333**, 201–205. RCT comparing magnesium sulfate with phenytoin as prophylaxis against eclamptic seizures in women with hypertension in the peripartum period. Eclampsia developed in 10/1089 women who received phenytoin prophylaxis whereas none of the 1049 women treated with magnesium sulfate had convulsions ($p = 0.004$). There were no significant differences in maternal or infant outcomes. This was a relatively low-risk study population with most of the subjects having mild to moderate hypertension without proteinuria. **Ib A**

6 Duley L, Henderson-Smart D (2000) Magnesium sulphate versus diazepam for eclampsia. In: *Cochrane database of systematic reviews*, issue 2. Oxford: Update Software. Systematic review of the literature comparing the effectiveness of magnesium sulfate (intravenous or intramuscular) and diazepam in women with eclampsia. Five trials of mostly good quality, involving 1236 subjects, were included in the meta-analysis. Magnesium sulfate was associated with a substantial reduction in the recurrence of convulsions (RR = 0.45, CI 0.35–0.58) when compared to diazepam. Maternal mortality was reduced, but with borderline significance (RR = 0.60, CI 0.36–1.00), and there were no differences in other measures of maternal morbidity. The only differences in neonatal outcome, when reported, were a reduction in low Apgar – less than 7 – at 5min and reduced length of stay on the neonatal unit with magnesium sulfate. **Ia A**

7 Duley L, Henderson-Smart D (2000) Magnesium sulphate versus phenytoin for eclampsia. In: *Cochrane database of systematic reviews*, issue 2. Oxford: Update Software. Systematic review of the literature comparing magnesium sulfate (intravenous or intramuscular) with phenytoin in the treatment of women with eclampsia. Four trials of good quality involving 823 women were included in the meta-analysis. Magnesium sulfate was associated with a substantial reduction in the recurrence of convulsions (RR = 0.30, CI 0.20–0.46). There was a trend to a reduction in maternal mortality and a significantly lower risk of pneumonia, ventilation and intensive care admission. Magnesium sulfate was also beneficial to the neonate with fewer admissions to the special-care baby unit (SCBU) and fewer babies who died or were in SCBU for more than 7 days (RR = 0.77, CI 0.63–0.95). **Ia A**

8 Duley L, Gulmezoglu AM, Henderson-Smart DG *et al.* (2000) Anticonvulsants for women with pre-eclampsia. In: *Cochrane database of systematic reviews*, issue 2. Oxford: Update Software. Systematic review of the literature comparing the effects of anticonvulsants with placebo or no anticonvulsant therapy and comparing different anticonvulsants in preeclampsia. In four trials comparing anticonvulsant therapy to none, involving over 1200 women, magnesium sulfate appeared to reduce the risk of eclampsia (RR = 0.33, CI 0.11–1.02) but the confidence intervals are wide. Magnesium sulfate was associated with a lower risk of eclampsia compared to phenytoin. There are few data concerning other clinically important maternal or neonatal outcomes. Overall, there is not enough evidence to establish whether anticonvulsant therapy in preeclampsia is beneficial or not and the MAGPIE trial is awaited. If an anticonvulsant is to be used, magnesium sulfate is the preferred agent. **Ia A**

9 Coetzee EJ, Dommisse J, Anthony J (1998) A randomised controlled trial of intravenous magnesium sulphate versus placebo in the management of women with severe pre-eclampsia. *Br J Obstet Gynaecol* **105**, 300–303. RCT involving women with severe preeclampsia requiring delivery who were all managed in a tertiary referral obstetric unit. All women initially received clonazepam and were given dihydralazine for severe hypertension if required. Significantly fewer women developed eclampsia on magnesium sulfate (1/345, 0.3%) compared to the placebo group (11/340, 3.2%), with a relative risk of 0.09 (CI 0.01–0.69). Using a regimen of 1g/h, there was only one adverse effect due to overdosage. The study was discontinued before the originally planned sample size of 1980 subjects was attained. The results of the larger MAGPIE trial are awaited. **Ib A**

Epilepsy

Management option		Quality of evidence	Strength of recommendation	References
Prepregnancy	Regular check of clinical control and serum anticonvulsant levels	IV	C	1
	Adjust anticonvulsant dose to control seizures with serum levels as a guide; avoid toxic doses	IV	C	1
	Folate supplementation	IV	C	2
Status epilepticus	First aid measures (see Preeclampsia/ Eclampsia, above)	–	✓	–
	Investigate and treat simultaneously	IV	C	1
	Control convulsions: ❑ Anticonvulsant drugs (intravenous benzodiazepine as boluses plus either i.v. phenytoin or i.v. magnesium if eclampsia is the cause) ❑ Ventilate while maintaining anticonvulsants if anticonvulsants alone fail to control seizures	Ia Ib –	A A ✓	3 4 –
	Avoid hypertension	–	✓	–
	Search for causes	IV	C	1
Prenatal	Regular check of clinical control and serum anticonvulsant levels	–	✓	–
	Adjust anticonvulsant dose to control seizures with serum levels as a guide; avoid toxic doses	IV	C	1
	Detailed fetal anomaly scan at 20 weeks	IV	C	2
	Short-acting benzodiazepine acutely if seizures recur	–	✓	–
	(Some advocate maternal administration of vitamin K over last 4 weeks)	–	✓	–
Labor and delivery	Continue anticonvulsant medication	–	✓	–
Postnatal	Examine newborn to confirm normality	–	✓	–
	Vitamin K to newborn	–	✓	–
	Monitor seizure control and serum levels; dose adjustment may be necessary	–	✓	–

References

1 Crawford P, Appleton R, Betts T *et al*. (1999) Best practice guidelines for the management of women with epilepsy. The Women with Epilepsy Guidelines Development Group. *Seizure* **8**, 201–217. A systematic review of the literature 1966–98 was performed and evidence-based UK clinical guidelines were produced. Preconception counseling should be offered to all females of childbearing potential. Changes to antiepileptic medication should be completed before conception and a single agent is preferred. The patient's seizures should be monitored in pregnancy and adjustments in dose made accordingly. The value of routinely measuring levels is uncertain, although a baseline preconception level may be helpful. Delivery should take place in an obstetric unit with facilities for maternal and neonatal resuscitation. The development of seizures during pregnancy warrants the same investigations as in the nongravid patient, including magnetic resonance imaging. **IV C**

2 Delgado-Escueta AV, Janz D (1992) Consensus guidelines: preconception counseling, management and care

of the pregnant woman with epilepsy. *Neurology* **42**, 149–160. Multinational workshop–symposium in 1990 produced these clinical guidelines concerning the use of antiepileptic drugs in pregnancy. Antiepileptic drugs are associated with a two- to threefold increased risk of congenital anomalies. Preconception counseling is advised and a detailed ultrasound scan should be offered. It is not known which antiepileptic drug is the least teratogenic. Folic acid supplements are recommended. If treatment is needed, monotherapy is preferred at the lowest effective dose. This group did recommend monitoring unbound or free plasma levels regularly. **IV C**

3. Duley L, Gulmezoglu AM, Henderson-Smart DG *et al.* (2000) Anticonvulsants for women with pre-eclampsia. In: *Cochrane database of systematic reviews*, issue 2. Oxford: Update Software. Systematic review of the literature comparing the effects of anticonvulsants with placebo or no anticonvulsant therapy and comparing different anticonvulsants in preeclampsia. In four trials comparing anticonvulsant therapy to none, involving over 1200 women, magnesium sulfate appeared to reduce the risk of eclampsia (RR = 0.33, CI 0.11–1.02) but the confidence intervals are wide. Magnesium sulfate was associated with a lower risk of eclampsia compared to phenytoin. There are few data concerning other clinically important maternal or neonatal outcomes. Overall, there is not enough evidence to establish whether anticonvulsant therapy in preeclampsia is beneficial or not and the MAGPIE trial is awaited. If an anticonvulsant is to be used, magnesium sulfate is the preferred agent. **Ia A**
4. Treiman DM, Meyers PD, Walton NY *et al.* (1998) A comparison of four treatments for generalized convulsive status epilepticus. *N Engl J Med* **339**, 792–798. Randomized, double-blind, multicenter trial of four intravenous regimens for the initial treatment of generalized convulsive status epilepticus. 570 patients were involved and pregnant women were excluded. Intention-to-treat analysis showed no differences in the success rates of lorazepam, phenobarbital, phenytoin or diazepam for overt or subtle status epilepticus. In 384 patients with confirmed overt status epilepticus, lorazepam had a higher success rate than phenytoin alone. There were no differences in recurrence rates or adverse effects. Belknap noted that accurate diagnosis and rapid treatment were more important than initial choice of anticonvulsant. Even the best treatments in this study were effective for only two thirds of patients with overt and one quarter of patients with subtle status epilepticus. **Ib A** (not pregnancy)

34.2 Cerebrovascular disease

Karen Brackley

Management option		Quality of evidence	Strength of recommendation	References
Ischemic stroke (arterial) and transient ischemic attacks	General supportive measures including seizure control (see Section 34.1)	–	✔	–
	Search for cause/associated factors and treat for thrombolic/embolic conditions	III	B	1
	Consider anticoagulation with heparin if no evidence of hemorrhage on computed tomography (CT) scan	–	✔	–
	Indications for surgery are as for nonpregnant patients	–	✔	–
Cerebral venous thrombosis	Control seizures	III	B	2,3
	Ensure adequate hydration	III	B	2
	One randomized case-controlled study suggests anticoagulation beneficial	Ib	A	4
	No experience in pregnancy with thrombolytic therapy	III	B	5
Intracerebral hemorrhage	**Diagnosis** (following high index of clinical suspicion) by, in order: ❑ CT scan ❑ Lumbar puncture ❑ Cerebral angiography (and/or magnetic resonance imaging)	IV	C	6

Management option		Quality of evidence	Strength of recommendation	References
Intracerebral hemorrhage (cont'd)	**Management – prenatal:**			
	❑ Interdisciplinary care with neurosurgeons	–	✔	–
	❑ In general, normal neurosurgical principles of management apply in pregnancy, although care needed intraoperatively with:			
	– Hypotension	IV	C	7
	– Hypothermia	IV	C	8
	– Anticonvulsants, high-dose steroids,	IV	C	9
	mannitol and nimodipine (safe in	Ib	A	10
	limited pregnancy experience) are used depending on clinical picture/problems	Ia	A	11
	Caution with epsilon aminocaproic acid (EACA)	III	B	12
	Management – labor/delivery:			
	❑ Regional analgesics preferable to narcotics and general anesthetics	–	✔	–
	❑ No evidence to support blanket policy of elective cesarean section, but most advocate: – Minimize pushing in second stage – Cesarean section for normal obstetric reasons – Consider life-support machine and care in patient with brain death to gain fetal maturity	IV	C	6,13

References

1 Kittner SJ, Stern BJ, Feeser BR *et al.* (1997) Pregnancy and the risk of stroke. *N Engl J Med* **335**, 768–774. The incidence of stroke in women of child-bearing age and the risk related to pregnancy was determined in this retrospective study involving 46 hospitals in two separate 12-month periods. For cerebral infarction, the risk adjusted for age and race was increased in the postpartum period (RR = 8.7, CI 4.6–16.7) but not during pregnancy. For intracerebral hemorrhage, the relative risk was 2.5 (CI 1.0–6.4) during pregnancy but 28.3 (CI 13.0–61.4) postnatally. **III B**

2 Srinivasan K, Natarajan M (1983) Cerebral venous and arterial thrombosis in pregnancy and puerperium: a study of 135 patients. *Angiology* **34**, 731–746. Study from India describing the presentation and management of 129 women with cerebral venous thrombosis and 6 with arterial thrombosis in the early puerperium over an 8-year period. Subjects with venous occlusions were more likely to present with impaired consciousness and convulsions compared to subjects with arterial occlusions, in whom there was a dense hemiparesis without signs of raised intracranial pressure. Investigations involved lumbar puncture, electroencephalograms and angiography rather than computed tomography or magnetic resonance imaging. Treatment options included anticonvulsants, antibiotics, mannitol or furosemide for cerebral edema and aspirin. Anticoagulants were used in particular circumstances and adequate therapy appeared to reduce mortality. 80 patients with venous thrombosis recovered without neurological disability but 35 patients died. Survival after arterial thrombosis was good (5 out of 6) but the neurological deficit tended to persist. **III B**

3 Bousser MG, Chiras J, Bories, J *et al.* (1985) Cerebral venous thrombosis – a review of 38 cases. *Stroke* **16**, 199–213. Retrospective French study describing 38 cases of angiographically proven cerebral venous thrombosis (CVT) over an 8-year period, of which only 2 were pregnancy-related. Electroencephalogram abnormalities were absent in 27% of cases and a normal dynamic isotope scan did not preclude sinus thrombosis. Cerebrospinal fluid was abnormal in 84% of cases with increased intracranial pressure, raised protein and the presence of red blood cells. The authors agree that computed tomography (CT) may reveal pathognomonic images of CVT but recommend angiography to exclude the diagnosis if these are absent. Anticonvulsants should be prescribed for seizures and antibiotics in the presence of infection. The management of raised intracranial pressure is controversial but dexamethasone is recommended initially. None of the 23 heparin-treated patients died and 19 made a complete recovery, suggesting that anticoagulants are not harmful. The authors recommend the use of heparin in patients who deteriorate despite symptomatic treatment, even if a hemorrhagic infarct is seen on CT scan. **III B**

4 Einhaupl KM, Villringer A, Meister W *et al.* (1991) Heparin treatment in sinus venous thrombosis. *Lancet*

338, 597–600. Report of a small, randomized, blinded trial involving 20 patients with cerebral venous thrombosis (CVT) comparing outcome following adjusted-dose intravenous heparin therapy to placebo. Heparin therapy appeared beneficial after 3 days and up to 3 months later. Importantly, heparin did not appear to promote intracranial hemorrhage in CVT. However, more subjects in the control group received corticosteroids, which may have adversely affected outcome and confounded the results. A further retrospective study of 102 patients with CVT suggested that mortality in patients with intracranial hemorrhage receiving heparin was lower than in patients receiving no heparin (15% vs 69%). The authors conclude that intracranial hemorrhage is not a contraindication for heparin treatment in CVT. **Ib A** (underpowered)

5 Horowitz M, Purdy P, Unwin H *et al.* (1995) Treatment of dural sinus thrombosis using selective catheterisation and urokinase. *Ann Neurol* **38**, 58–67. Paper describing the direct instillation of urokinase, a fibrinolytic agent, into the cerebral dural sinuses via a femoral catheter to hasten clot dissolution. 11 out of 12 patients had significant radiographic improvement or complete resolution of the thrombus associated with rapid neurological improvement. None of the cases were associated with pregnancy. The therapy appeared safe even in individuals with hemorrhagic or nonhemorrhagic venous infarcts. The authors recommend treating patients early and preferably within 72 hours. The indications for this intervention rather than expectant management or systemic heparinization are not yet established. **III B**

6 Tuttleman RM, Gleicher N (1981) Central nervous system hemorrhage complicating pregnancy. *Obstet Gynecol* **58**, 651–656. Presentation and management of three cases of intracerebral hemorrhage in the third trimester of pregnancy reported with a review of the literature. It is important to determine the underlying pathology using lumbar puncture, appropriate neuroimaging and cerebral angiography. A hypertensive disorder of pregnancy should be excluded. Vaginal delivery should be considered when feasible as cesarean section has not been shown to offer significant advantage, although an elective cesarean section may be appropriate in cases of untreated arteriovenous malformations. Epidural and outlet forceps are advised. **IV C**

7 Rigg D, McDonogh A (1981) Use of sodium nitroprusside in deliberate hypotension during pregnancy. *Br J Anaesth* **53**, 985–987. Paper describing the use of intravenous sodium nitroprusside to produce hypotension and facilitate surgery for ruptured cerebral aneurysms in two pregnant patients at 20 weeks gestation. There were no apparent adverse effects on the babies. The authors comment that concerns regarding cyanide toxicity in the fetus arise from animal experiments only. **IV C**

8 Stange K, Halldin M (1983) Hypothermia in pregnancy. *Anaesthesiology* **58**, 460–461. Hypothermia is used in neurosurgery to reduce metabolic rate and postoperative cerebral edema. This case report describes the use of hypothermia to 28°C during resection of an intracranial neurinoma in a 21-weeks-pregnant woman. The fetal heart rate slowed during cooling and increased during warming in parallel with the maternal heart rate. A healthy child was later delivered at term with normal progress to 1 year of age. **IV C**

9 Fisherman RA (1982) Steroids in the treatment of brain edema. *N Engl J Med* **306**, 359. Commentary addressing the use of steroids in the management of cerebral edema. The different pathophysiological mechanisms are outlined and the need for more controlled clinical trials is emphasized. The author criticizes the practice of automatically treating all causes of cerebral edema with high-dose steroids. The main indication should be vasogenic edema associated with mass lesions, including intracerebral hematomas. Confirmatory imaging with computed tomography is therefore important. **IV C**

10 Allen GS, Ahn HS, Preziosi TJ *et al.* (1983) Cerebral arterial spasm – a controlled trial of nimodipine in patients with subarachnoid hemorrhage. *N Engl J Med* **308**, 619–624. Randomized, double-blind placebo-controlled trial involving 121 patients presenting within 96 hours of a subarachnoid hemorrhage secondary to an aneurysm. The role of oral treatment with nimodipine, a calcium-channel antagonist, for 21 days in reducing neurological deficit due to arterial spasm was investigated. Pregnancy status is not given. Nimodipine was superior to placebo (1/56 compared to 8/60 patients) in reducing the occurrence of severe neurologic deficit (including death) from vasospasm ($p = 0.03$). There was no apparent increase in adverse effects including rebleeding with nimodipine. **Ib A**

11 Feigin VL, Rinkel GJ, Algra A *et al.* (2000) Calcium antagonists for aneurysmal subarachnoid haemorrhage. In: *Cochrane database of systematic reviews*, issue 2. Oxford: Update Software. Systematic review of the literature to compare the use of any calcium antagonist with control within 10 days of aneurysmal subarachnoid hemorrhage. 11 randomized trials involving 2804 patients (1376 treated and 1428 controls) were included in the meta-analysis. Overall, calcium antagonists significantly reduced the risk of poor outcome after subarachnoid hemorrhage (RR = 0.82, CI 0.72–0.93), ischemic neurological deficits (RR = 0.67, CI 0.59–0.76) and computed-tomography-documented cerebral infarction (RR = 0.80, CI 0.71–0.89). 20 patients needed to be treated to prevent one single poor outcome. The results depend mainly on the trials with oral nimodipine and the evidence for nicardipine and AT877 is inconclusive. The risk of death was not significantly reduced (RR = 0.94, CI 0.80–1.10). **Ia A**

12 Sengupta RP, So SC, Villarejo-Ortega FJ (1976) Use of epsilon aminocaproic acid (EACA) in the preoperative management of ruptured intracranial aneurysms. *J Neurosurgery* **44**, 479–484. Retrospective study describing the authors' clinical experience with epsilon aminocaproic acid (EACA), an antifibrinolytic agent, in the preoperative management of 66 patients with subarachnoid hemorrhage secondary to ruptured aneurysms. The incidence of rebleeding in this EACA group was compared to a group of 76 unmatched controls managed conservatively with bed rest and sedation. The authors suggest that EACA is beneficial as none of the treated patients rebled compared to 17 (22%) of controls. However, this conclusion is unreliable as the control group included more seriously ill patients than the EACA group. Because of the occurrence of two fatal thrombotic complications with EACA, the use of this therapy in pregnancy must be viewed with extreme caution. **III C**

13 Hunt HB, Schifrin BS, Suzuki K (1974) Ruptured berry aneurysms and pregnancy. *Obstet Gynecol* **43**, 827–837. The obstetric management of three women who had previously experienced ruptured berry aneurysms is described, followed by a comprehensive review of the literature. In a total of 20 cases of aneurysms rupturing before pregnancy, maternal outcome was reported as normal with no rebleeding. In over half of the aneurysms that ruptured during pregnancy or the puerperium (71 out of 127), the event occurred in the third trimester. The mortality rate for rupture in pregnancy was 22%. Elective cesarean section is not supported unless there is an obstetric reason. Continuous maternal and fetal monitoring is recommended in labor. The authors do not agree that the second stage of labor needs to be shortened but advise regional anesthesia. **IV C**

34.3 Headache

Diana Dunlop

Management option		Quality of evidence	Strength of recommendation	References
General	Indications for further investigation:			
	❑ Focal/abnormal neurological signs	–	✔	–
	❑ Impaired intellect	–	✔	–
	❑ Worsening and/or intractable pain	–	✔	–
	❑ Pain that disturbs sleep	–	✔	–
Migraine	Avoid precipitating factors	–	✔	–
	Nonpharmacological measures:			
	❑ Bed rest	–	✔	–
	❑ Avoidance of light	–	✔	–
	❑ Coping mechanisms	III	B	1
	❑ Ice	–	✔	–
	❑ Massage	–	✔	–
	❑ Sleep	–	✔	–
	Analgesics:			
	❑ Simple agents, e.g. paracetamol (acetaminophen)	–	✔	–
	❑ Short course of nonsteroidal anti-inflammatory drugs in first two trimesters but not third	IV	C	2
	❑ Narcotics, e.g. meperidine, morphine, for severe cases	IV	C	2
	❑ Short course of adjuvant gluco-corticoids for refractory cases (avoid benzodiazepines, ergot preparations and sumatriptan)	IV	C	2
	Prophylaxis:			
	❑ Propranolol (trial excluded pregnant women)	Ib	A	3
	❑ Tricyclic antidepressants	IV	C	2
	Antiemetics:			
	❑ Phenothiazines (trial excluded pregnant women)	Ib	A	4
Tension headaches	Reassurance, bed rest	–	✔	–
	Simple analgesia	III	B	5
Spinal headache	No evidence that injection of physiological saline at time of dural tap/puncture is of benefit	–	✔	–
	Analgesia	–	✔	–

Management option		Quality of evidence	Strength of recommendation	References
Spinal headache (cont'd)	Lying flat (trial may not be relevant to modern obstetric anesthetic practice)	Ib	A	6
	Autologous blood patch if analgesia and lying flat fail to work after 24 h	Ib	A	7
Benign intracranial hypertension	Exclude other causes of raised intracranial pressure	–	✔	–
	Monitor visual function	–	✔	–
	Avoid excess weight gain	IV	C	8,9
	If evidence of visual function deterioration consider: ❑ Acetazolamide ❑ Serial lumbar puncture	IV	C	8,9
	If these conservative measures fail (extrapolated from management in nonpregnant subjects): ❑ Shunting ❑ Optic nerve sheath fenestration if vision is still threatened	–	✔	–

References

1 Scharff L, Marcus DA, Turk DC (1996) Maintenance of effects in the non-medical treatment of headaches during pregnancy. *Headache* **36**, 285–290. This paper is not directly concerned with the treatment of headache during pregnancy. It looked at women up to 1 year after delivery, showing that the improvement in headaches that they obtained from relaxation training and biofeedback was maintained after pregnancy. **III B**

2 Silberstein SD (1993) Headaches and women: treatment of the pregnant and lactating migraineur. *Headache* **33**, 533–540. Review article. It emphasizes the importance of conservative management during pregnancy in order to reduce exposure of the fetus to drugs. Treatment should begin with rest, reassurance and ice packs. If these fail paracetamol (acetaminophen) should be used, followed by codeine and, if pain is still not controlled, then narcotics should be added. Aspirin, benzodiazepine and ergot-containing preparations should be avoided. Prophylaxis should only be considered in very severe cases and if propranolol is used the possible risks of intrauterine growth restriction should be discussed. **IV C**

3 Hesse J, Mogelvang B, Simonsen H (1994) Acupuncture versus metoprolol in migraine prophylaxis: a randomized trial of trigger point inactivation. *J Intern Med* **235**, 451–456. Randomized group-comparative study, showing that acupuncture and metoprolol were equipotent in reducing the frequency and duration of migraine attacks. Metoprolol was better at reducing the severity of attacks but had more side-effects. Pregnant women were excluded from the study. **Ib A**

4 Coppola M, Yealy DM, Leibold RA (1995) Randomized, placebo-controlled evaluation of prochlorperazine versus metoclopramide for emergency department treatment of migraine headache. *Ann Emerg Med* **26**, 541–546. Prospective, randomized, double-blind, placebo-controlled trial comparing prochlorperazine, metoclopramide and placebo in the treatment of migraine headache and associated nausea. Prochlorperazine performed better than either metoclopramide or placebo. However, pregnant subjects were excluded. **Ib A**

5 Maggioni F, Alessi C, Maggino T *et al.* (1997) Headache during pregnancy. *Cephalalgia* **17**, 765–769. In general the frequency of headaches declined during pregnancy and all responded to simple analgesia. **III B**

6 Thornberry EA, Thomas TA (1988) Posture and post-spinal headache. A controlled trial in 80 obstetric patients. *Br J Anaesth* **60**, 195–197. Lying flat provided symptomatic relief to patients with headaches following spinal anesthesia. However this paper is now out of date, as much finer needles with a 'pencil-point' end are now used for obstetric spinal anesthesia. These newer needles part rather than break the dural fibers and are associated with less headache. The relevance of early studies to current practice is therefore extremely questionable. **Ib A**

7 Seebacher J, Ribeiro V, Le Guillou JL *et al.* (1989) Epidural blood patch in the treatment of post-dural puncture headache: a double blind study. *Headache* **29**, 630–632. Small study with 6 patients in the treatment arm (of whom 5 benefited from blood patch) and 6 in the placebo arm (none of whom had symptom improvement). Again, the technique used in the original spinal anesthesia was not described and may well be outdated. **Ib A**

8 Weisberg LA (1975) Benign intracranial hypertension. *Medicine* **54**, 197–207. A review of 120 adults with benign intracranial hypertension, of whom 2 were pregnant. The patients were treated between 1964 and 1973; thus newer treatments such as optic nerve sheath fenestration are not even mentioned. The relevance to modern obstetrics of this paper is therefore questionable. **IV C**

9 Kassam SH, Hadi HA, Fadel HE *et al.* (1983) Benign intracranial hypertension in pregnancy: current diagnostic and therapeutic approach. *Obstet Gynaecol Surv* **38**, 314–321. Four case histories are presented with a review of the literature including the use of serial lumbar puncture, acetazolamide. Useful and less out of date than the first reference. **IV C**

34.4 Mononeuropathies

David Churchill

Management option		Quality of evidence	Strength of recommendation	References
Facial nerve palsy (Bell's palsy)	High-dose steroids, especially if severe and early presentation, though may not be as effective in pregnancy	III	B	1
	Protect eye on affected side	–	✔	–
Carpal tunnel syndrome	Explanation and reassurance	III	B	2,3
	Wrist exercises during the day, elevation at night	III	B	2–4
	Wrist splinting	III	B	2–4
	Diuretics if severe	III	B	4
	Decompression if severe and all else fails	III	B	4
	Local steroid injection for relief of symptoms (Note: reference not specific for pregnancy)	Ia III	A B	5 4
Lateral femoral cutaneous neuropathy (meralgia paresthetica)	Explanation and reassurance	IV	C	6,7
	Relief with certain positions, especially when sitting	IV	C	6,7
	Rarely anticonvulsants or antidepressants required	–	✔	–
Lumbar disc disease	Conservative approach (bed rest, firm supporting mattress)	III	B	8,9
	Surgery reserved for cases refractory to conservative measures persisting after pregnancy	III	B	9

References

1 Falco NA, Eriksson E (1989) Idiopathic facial palsy in pregnancy and the puerperium. *Surg Gynecol Obstet* **169**, 337–340. Systematic retrospective study of Bell's palsy in the pregnant population attending the Brigham and Women's Hospital between 1982 and 1987. The incidence of facial nerve palsy was calculated at 41/100000 deliveries, i.e. 1/2600 births. The majority occur in the third trimester. A variety of management policies were employed from expectant to systemic corticosteroids. The paper concluded that steroid therapy did not influence recovery of sufferers in pregnancy. **III B**

2 Ekman-Ordeberg G, Salgeback S, Ordeberg G (1987) Carpal tunnel syndrome in pregnancy. A prospective study. *Acta Obstet Gynecol Scand* **66**, 233–235. Prospective study of 56 women with carpal tunnel syndrome in pregnancy. The majority, 46/56, had symptomatic relief from using night-time wrist splints. Of the 10 who found no benefit from splinting, 3 had successful operative treatment and 7 continued with conservative treatment as they were close to term. **III B**

3 Stolp-Smith KA, Pascoe MK, Ogburn PL *et al.* (1998) Carpal tunnel syndrome in pregnancy: frequency, severity, and prognosis. *Arch Phys Med Rehabil* **79**, 1285–1287. Retrospective case review of pregnant women with carpal tunnel syndrome (CTS) $n = 87$ between 1987 and 1992. This paper is affected by ascertainment bias. Many of the cases of CTS in pregnancy are not recorded unless they had severe symptoms. The authors state that CTS in pregnancy usually responds to conservative measures. Surgical intervention is only occasionally needed. **III B**

4 Wand JS (1990) Carpal tunnel syndrome in pregnancy and lactation. *J Hand Surg* **15B**, 93–94. Epidemiological study of carpal tunnel syndrome (CTS) in pregnancy and lactation. Patients were recruited through an advert in a magazine and therefore the study was open to selection bias. Symptomatic relief was obtained by wearing a wrist splint in 85% of cases. Complete resolution 1 month following delivery occurred in all cases. Diuretics used in the puerperium benefited 82% of women but provided only temporary relief. Local steroid injections provided significant and lasting benefit in 62% of patients. CTS is often bilateral and more severe in the dominant hand. **III B**

5 Marshall S, Tardiff G, Ashworth N (2000) Local corticosteroid injection for carpal tunnel syndrome. In: *The Cochrane library*, issue 4. Oxford Update Software. Meta-analysis of local corticosteroid injection for carpal tunnel syndrome in the general population. Four randomized controlled trials were identified but two were excluded because of methodological difficulties. The methodological quality of the two remaining trials was judged to be good. However there were methodological differences in the treatments given. Both studies showed significant benefit from local steroid injection for 1 month following treatment, despite differences in populations and settings. **Ia A**

6 Pearson MG (1957) Meralgia paraesthetica. With reference to its occurrence in pregnancy. *J Obstet Gynaecol Br Empire* **64**, 427–430. Report of three pregnancies complicated by meralgia paresthetica. For mild cases, patients need reassurance. For severe cases, surgical freeing of the trapped nerve is suggested as a possible course of action. **IV C**

7 Peterson PH (1952) Meralgia paresthetica related to pregnancy. *Am J Obstet Gynecol* **64**, 690–691. Case report of meralgia paresthetica in pregnancy. Reassurance and general supportive measures were advocated as the management policy. **IV C**

8 Fast A, Shapiro D, Ducommun EJ *et al.* (1987) Low back pain in pregnancy. *Spine* **12**, 368–371. Cross sectional epidemiological study of backpain in pregnancy. Patients were interviewed 24–36 hours after labor. The percentage of those suffering from back pain was higher in Caucasians than in any other ethnic group. The onset of back pain occurred mainly from the fifth to seventh month of pregnancy. There was no relation between maternal age or weight gain in pregnancy, nor the baby's weight or the number of prior pregnancies, and back pain. The pain was aggravated by activity and relieved most often by rest and simple analgesics. **III B**

9 LaBan MM, Perrin JC, Latimer FR (1982) Pregnancy and the herniated lumbar disc. *Arch Phys Med Rehabil* **64**, 319–321. Case series ($n = 5$) of patients with lumbosacral and radicular leg pain. All patients were delivered by cesarean section and the disc prolapse was confirmed after delivery by myelography. All patients were treated by laminectomy and their symptoms resolved. The mechanical and postural stresses of pregnancy were identified as predisposing factors for disc herniation. **III B**

34.5 Polyneuropathies

David Churchill

Management option		Quality of evidence	Strength of recommendation	References
Acute inflammatory demyelinating polyneuropathy	Monitor respiratory function; ventilation may be necessary	–	✔	–
	Nursing and physiotherapy care	–	✔	–
	Prophylactic heparin	–	✔	–
	Therapy options: ❑ Plasmapheresis ❑ Intravenous immunoglobulin	Ib	A	1
Chronic inflammatory demyelinating polyneuropathy	Management similar to Guillain-Barré syndrome	IV III	C B	2 3
	Treatment with: ❑ Corticosteroids ❑ Plasmapheresis ❑ Intravenous immunoglobulin ❑ Interferon	IV	C	2,4

References

1 Van der Meche FG, Schmitz PI (1992) A randomized trial comparing intravenous immune globulin and plasma exchange in Guillain–Barré syndrome. *N Engl J Med* **326**, 1123–1129. RCT of plasma exchange versus immune globulin administration for Guillain–Barré syndrome (GBS). Nonpregnant patients with GBS were entered into the trial. There were more complications in the group receiving plasma exchange as well as more withdrawals from treatment. Analysis was carried out on an intention-to-treat basis. There was a significant functional improvement in the primary outcomes measure in patients receiving immunoglobulin. The results showed a similar benefit from immunoglobulin for secondary measures. There were significantly more complications in the plasma exchange group. It was concluded that immunoglobulin is both practical and safe when used as a treatment for GBS and appears superior to plasma exchange. **Ib A**

2 Dyck PJ, Phineas J, Pollard J (1993) Chronic inflammatory demyelinating polyradiculoneuropathy. In: Dyck PJ, Thomas P, Griffin JW *et al.* (eds) *Peripheral neuropathy*, 3rd edn. Philadelphia, PA: WB Saunders, pp. 1498–1517. Review chapter on treatment for chronic inflammatory demyelinating polyradiculoneuropathy (CIDP). The authors did not specifically deal with pregnancy. They reviewed all forms of treatment for CIDP and recommended the use of plasma exchange and steroid therapy. They did not advocate the use of immunoglobulin. **IV C**

3 McCombe PA, Pollard JD, McLeod JG (1987) Chronic inflammatory demyelinating polyradiculoneuropathy associated with pregnancy. *Ann Neurol* **21**, 102–104. Case series of 9 women who had a total of 30 pregnancies while they were suffering from chronic inflammatory demyelinating polyradiculoneuropathy (CIDP). There were more relapses of CIDP in pregnancy, especially in the third trimester and postpartum period. The relapses also tended to be more severe. Specifically the treatment of these patients was not approached in this paper. **III B**

4 Mancuso A, Ardita FV, Leonardi J *et al.* (1998) Interferon alpha-2a therapy and pregnancy. Report of a case of chronic inflammatory demyelinating polyneuropathy. *Acta Obstet Gynecol Scand* **77**, 869–872. Case report of a pregnancy complicated by chronic inflammatory demyelinating polyneuropathy and treated throughout with interferon-alpha. The pregnancy was complicated by fetal growth restriction but was otherwise successful in terms of outcome maternal and fetal outcome. **IV C**

34.6 Myotonic dystrophy

Mike Lumb

Management option		Quality of evidence	Strength of recommendation	References
Prepregnancy	Assess cardiorespiratory status; optimize treatment	III	B	1
	Genetic counseling	III	B	2
Prenatal	Monitor cardiorespiratory status	IV	C	3
	Discuss prenatal diagnosis	III	B	1,4,5
	Vigilance for hydramnios	III	B	1
	If hydramnios, vigilance for preterm labor	III	B	1
Labor and delivery	Augmentation with oxytocin if dystocia in first stage	III	B	1,6
	May need assisted second stage if significant weakness	III	B	1
	Active management of third stage	IV	C	7
	Regional analgesic preferable to narcotics and/or general anesthetic	III	B	1,6
	Pediatrician to be present for delivery	III	B	6
Postnatal	Careful neuromuscular examination and follow-up of newborn	III	B	1,6

Comments

Myotonic dystrophy is a rare condition where opportunities do not exist to carry out large comparative studies or RCTs. Extrapolation from nonpregnant patients has been used to support suggestions for anesthetic management. In many cases the recommendations are not based on the cases described but stem from earlier work quoted as references in the original papers.

References

1 Jaffe R, Mock M, Abramowicz J *et al.* (1986) Myotonic dystrophy and pregnancy: a review. *Obstet Gynecol Surv* **41**, 272–278. Review article and descriptive study of 20 women known to have myotonic dystrophy at the start of pregnancy, with the addition of a further case report. Prenatal diagnosis, problems of polyhydramnios and labor are discussed, together with the avoidance of general anesthesia and the need for neonatal follow-up are discussed. No management recommendations are supported by the data presented. **III B**

2 Norman AM, Floyd JL, Meredith AL *et al.* (1989) Presymptomatic detection and prenatal diagnosis of myotonic dystrophy by means of linked DNA markers. *J Med Genet* **26**, 750–754. Series of genetic studies in 99 families. Genetic counseling and presymptomatic detection in families is illustrated with examples. Prenatal diagnosis was performed in 10 cases, allowing the possibility of terminating a pregnancy with an affected fetus. No recommendations for any of the management options in the original text are supported by this paper. **III B**

3 Boyle R (1999) Antenatal and preoperative genetic and clinical assessment in myotonic dystrophy. *Anaesth Intens Care* **27**, 301–306. Case report of a patient with myotonic dystrophy undergoing cesarean section under spinal anesthesia. Cardiorespiratory assessment prior to delivery is discussed from an anesthetic perspective. A preference for regional blockade and precautions with general anesthesia are described. **IV C**

4 Erikson A, Forsberg H, Drugge U *et al.* (1995) Outcome of pregnancy in women with myotonic dystrophy and analysis of CTG gene expansion. *Acta Paediatr* **84**, 416–418. Review of 60 pregnancies in 32 women with myotonic dystrophy. If a previous child has severe congenital myotonic dystrophy, the other children would be similarly affected. The authors recommend that prenatal diagnosis should be offered to women with myotonic dystrophy, especially if they have previously given birth to a child with the congenital form. **III B**

5 Hojo K, Yamagata H, Moji H *et al.* (1995) Congenital myotonic dystrophy: molecular diagnosis and clinical study. *Am J Perinatol* **12**, 195–200. Case study of three pregnancies where the mothers had myotonic dystrophy and the children had the congenital form of myotonic dystrophy. Family members and the children were genotyped by Southern blot and polymerase chain reaction. Disease severity in the neonate did not correlate with gene expansion (number of trinucleotide repeats) but DNA analysis is a useful tool for prenatal diagnosis. **III B**

6 Shore RN, MacLachlan TB (1971) Pregnancy with myotonic dystrophy: course, complications and management. *Obstet Gynecol* **38**, 448–454. Review article of 8 pregnancies, including 6 previously published case reports and 2 further cases. In addition, *in-vitro* studies of myometrial contractility in one affected (but nonpregnant) and 'several hundred' unaffected patients are described, together with a study of serum muscle enzymes after delivery in normal and affected patients. Recommendations on the use of oxytocin in the first stage, avoidance of general anesthesia and pediatric assessment are based on the references quoted, not on the cases described. **III B**

7 Atlas I, Smolin A (1999) Combined maternal and congenital myotonic dystrophy managed by a multidisciplinary team. *Eur J Obstet Gynecol Reprod Biol* **87**, 175–178. Case report of a single pregnancy where congenital myotonic dystrophy was diagnosed by amniocentesis at 17 weeks but the patient elected to continue the pregnancy. Recommendations on the significance of polyhydramnios, oxytocin augmentation, need for assisted delivery, active management of the third stage and preference for regional block over general anesthesia are repeated from the listed references. **IV C**

34.7 Multiple sclerosis

Mike Lumb

Management option		Quality of evidence	Strength of recommendation	References
Prepregnancy	Counsel about risks to mother and baby	III	B	1,2
	Consider reducing therapy if disease in remission	–	✔	–
Prenatal	Monitor for relapse or worsening of disease activity (including use of magnetic resonance imaging)	IV	C	3

Management option		Quality of evidence	Strength of recommendation	References
Prenatal (cont'd)	If necessary increase therapy (NB. Lack of information on drugs in pregnancy)	III	B	1
	Maintain physical exercises, etc.	–	✔	–
Labor and delivery	'Stress dose' steroids for labor/delivery if patient on corticosteroids prenatally	IV	C	4
	Assisted second stage may be necessary	IV	C	4
	No data to suggest that spinal, epidural or general anesthetic is contraindicated	IV III	C B	5 6
Postnatal	Breast-feeding is acceptable	III IV	B C	6,7 4
	Vigilance for relapse	III	B	2

Comments

The combination of multiple sclerosis and pregnancy is uncommon and no RCTs were found. Many of the authors have addressed the issue of whether relapse rates and the course of the disease are influenced by pregnancy. These data are subject to bias in most cases because they rely on recollections by patients rather than data gathered prospectively on relapses. Further selection bias is present where patients are recruited on a clinic or hospital rather than population basis. Deliberate avoidance of pregnancy by some women with MS may confound conclusions about the natural history of the disease. Some authors do not differentiate between patients with the relapsing and progressive forms of multiple sclerosis. In many cases the recommendations for management are not based on the cases described but stem from earlier work quoted as references in the original papers.

References

1 Damek DM, Shuster EA (1997) Pregnancy and multiple sclerosis. *Mayo Clin Proc* **72**, 977–989. Systematic review of studies of multiple sclerosis (MS) and pregnancy. The frequency of attacks tends to decrease during pregnancy and increase postpartum. Immunological mechanisms in MS, safety of the drugs used in MS and the effects of oral contraceptives in MS are discussed. **III B**

2 Stenager E, Stenager EN, Jensen K (1994) Effect of pregnancy on the prognosis for multiple sclerosis. A 5-year follow-up. *Acta Neurol Scand* **90**, 305–308. Small prospective study of women with multiple sclerosis aged 25–45 at 5-year follow up from diagnosis. Only six had a relapsing/remitting course. It is not possible to determine the length of follow-up postpartum. The authors suggest discussing the situation with the couple antenatally and expecting exacerbations postnatally. **III B**

3 Van Walderveen MAA, Tas MW, Barkhof F *et al.* (1994) Magnetic resonance evaluation of disease activity during pregnancy in multiple sclerosis. *Neurology* **44**, 327–329. Case reports of two patients with multiple sclerosis in whom sequential magnetic resonance (MR) scans before, during and after pregnancy were used to visualize acute lesions in the brain. The number of these fell in the second half of pregnancy, with an increase in disease activity after delivery. No recommendations about the clinical monitoring of disease are made, but the paper supports the use of MR as a research tool to identify active lesions. **IV C**

4 Davis RK, Maslow AS (1992) Multiple sclerosis in pregnancy: a review. *Obstet Gynecol Surv* **47**, 290–296. Single case report of a patient with multiple sclerosis presenting in pregnancy. It includes a review of the epidemiology, pathophysiology, diagnosis, clinical care and treatment from the references listed in the paper, but no recommendations are based on the case report. **IV C**

5 Warren TM, Data S, Ostheimer GW (1982) Lumbar epidural anesthesia in a patient with multiple sclerosis. *Anesth Analg* **61**, 1022–1023. Case report of a single patient with multiple sclerosis who had two pregnancies and had epidurals for both deliveries. She experienced temporary areas of numbness that persisted for several weeks after delivery. Postulated mechanisms for neurotoxic effects of anesthetic agents on demyelinated neurons are offered to suggest that the epidurals caused disease exacerbation. **IV C**

6 Confavreux C, Hutchinson M, Hours MM *et al.* (1998) Rate of pregnancy-related relapse in multiple sclerosis. *N Engl J Med* **339**, 285–291. Prospective study of 254 women with multiple sclerosis during 269 pregnancies in 12 European centers. The frequency of relapses decreased during pregnancy, especially the third trimester, and increased

in the first 3 months post-partum, compared with the rate in the year before the pregnancy. Epidural analgesia and breastfeeding did not increase the risk of relapse post-partum. **III B**

7 Nelson LM and the Multiple Sclerosis Study Group (1988) Risk of multiple sclerosis exacerbation during pregnancy and breast feeding. *JAMA* **259**, 3441–3443. Retrospective study of 435 women with multiple sclerosis in whom 191 pregnancies had occurred during a nonprogressive phase of disease. The relapse data were collected by interview of patients and are liable to bias, while there appeared to be no matching of controls with subjects. The patients studied had been recruited for two other unrelated studies. The exacerbation rate at 3 months post-partum was 34% compared with 10% during the 9 months of pregnancy. Breastfeeding did not appear to affect the risk of exacerbation. **III B**

34.8 Cerebral tumors

Andrew Dawson

Primary tumors

Management option		Quality of evidence	Strength of recommendation	References
Prepregnancy	Tumors are best treated before commencing pregnancy	III	B	1,2
Prenatal	Management depends on: ❑ Tumor type and whether benign or malignant ❑ Its natural history ❑ Gestation ❑ Patient's wishes	III	B	1,2
	Most tumors are treated by surgery	III	B	1,2
	Adjuvant chemotherapy can be given after the first trimester	III	B	1,2
	Radiation is best delayed until after delivery	III	B	1,2
	High-dose steroids may be necessary with cerebral edema	III	B	1,2
Labor and delivery	Insufficient data to determine whether assisted second stage is of benefit	–	✔	–

References

1 Roelvink NC, Kamphorst W, van Alphen HA, Rao BR (1987) Pregnancy-related primary brain and spinal tumors. *Arch Neurol* **44**, 209–215. Review of 223 cases of primary brain or spinal tumor in 86 reports. The number of these cancers occurring in pregnancy, as with other cancers, was less than expected from age-matched women. The relative frequency of primary brain tumors is not influenced by pregnancy. **III B**

2 Burger PC, Green SB (1987) Patient age, histologic features, and length of survival in patients with glioblastoma multiforme. *Cancer* **59**, 1617–1625. Pathoclinical correlation study of 71 patients with glioblastoma multiforme. Despite wide variation in histologic features, patient age remained a significant factor in survival. Patients were of both sexes, with no consideration of pregnancy status as a factor. **III B**

Secondary/metastatic tumors

Management option	Quality of evidence	Strength of recommendation	References
Management depends on: ❑ Primary ❑ Site ❑ Its effects	III	B	1

Reference

1 Weed JC Jr, Woodward KT, Hammond CB (1982) Choriocarcinoma metastatic to the brain: therapy and prognosis. *Semin Oncol* **9**, 208–212. Case review of 23 patients with cerebral metastatic trophoblastic neoplasia identified retrospectively out of more than 400 women treated over an 11-year period with gestational trophoblastic neoplasia. A survival of 10/23 (43%) was less than that in a previous report, 7/14 (50%). Survival seemed to be related to the number of brain metastases, and optimal treatment constituted whole-brain radiation coincident with triple-agent therapy. **III B**

Prolactinoma

Management option		Quality of evidence	Strength of recommendation	References
Prenatal	Clinical surveillance (headaches and visual disturbance) for recurrence or expansion in pregnancy	III	B	1,2
	Some screen visual fields through pregnancy	–	✔	–
	Bromocriptine with tumor enlargement (confirmed with computed tomography and/or magnetic resonance imaging)	III	B	1–4
	Bromocriptine appears to be safe during pregnancy	III	B	1–3
	Hypophysectomy (radiotherapy rarely needed for failed medical management)	III	B	3

References

1 De Wit W, Coelingh Bennink HJ, Gerards LJ (1984) Prophylactic bromocriptine treatment during pregnancy in women with macroprolactinomas: report of 13 pregnancies. *Br J Obstet Gynaecol* **91** 1059–1069. Report of experience of 10 women treated with bromocriptine during 13 pregnancies. Bromocriptine does not appear to be teratogenic and does not interfere with the normal development of pregnancy. There is limited long-term follow-up information but some women may experience pituitary enlargement in late pregnancy if the drug is stopped. Women whose bromocriptine is stopped for pregnancy should be closely monitored for disease progression. **III B**

2 Hammond CB, Haney AF, Land MR *et al.* (1983) The outcome of pregnancy in patients with treated and untreated prolactin-secreting pituitary tumors. *Am J Obstet Gynecol* **147**, 148–157. Observational review of 92 patients, all with prolactinomas diagnosed by hyperprolactinemia and radiologically. There were three groups: women who became pregnant after transsphenoidal microsurgery, women who still had elevated prolactin levels after resection, and women who conceived after bromocriptine alone. Only two patients, in the latter group, developed signs of expanding tumor size in pregnancy. **III B**

3 Samaan NA, Schultz PN, Leavens TA *et al.* (1986) Pregnancy after treatment in patients with prolactinoma: operation versus bromocriptine. *Am J Obstet Gynecol* **155**, 1300–1305. In this observational study of 190 women, 88 were treated by microsurgery and 102 with bromocriptine. Fertility rates are described; higher prolactin levels after pregnancy were similar irrespective of the method of treatment. One patient treated by microsurgery required bromocriptine for advancing radiologic changes. **III B**

4 Kulkarni MV, Lee KF, McArdle CB *et al.* (1988) 1.5-T MR imaging of pituitary microadenomas: technical considerations and CT correlation. *Am J Neuroradiol* **9**, 5–11. Prospective evaluation with 1.5-T magnetic resonance (MR) compared with computed tomography (CT) imaging in 37 patients with suspected pituitary tumors. In 8 patients with surgically proved microadenomas, MR had a sensitivity of 83% and CT a sensitivity of 42%. For MR scanning the T1-weighted inversion recovery images were clearest in most cases. Other pulse sequences performed better in some circumstances. **III B**

34.9 Movement disorders

Andrew Dawson

Management option		Quality of evidence	Strength of recommendation	References
Chorea gravidarum	Management depends on cause	IV	C	1
	Treatment only given if: ❑ Dehydration ❑ Malnutrition ❑ Insomnia ❑ Violence ❑ Risk of maternal injury	IV	C	1
	Short-term, low-dose haloperidol commonly used	IV	C	1
Wilson's disease	Penicillamine is the treatment of choice, but lowest dose that gives disease control should be used (risk of fetal defects)	III IV	B C	2,3 4–6
Restless leg syndrome	Supportive treatment: ❑ Reassurance ❑ Massage, exercises and physiotherapy ❑ Walking	III	B	7
	Opiates for severe cases	III	B	7
Parkinson's disease	Levodopa/carbidopa is probably safe for the fetus (limited human data)	-	✔	-
	Bromocriptine is often added to this with severe cases	III	B	8
	Amantadine, selegiline and pergolide have limited published data	-	✔	-

References

1 Rogers JD, Fahn S (1994) Movement disorders and pregnancy. *Adv Neurol* **64**, 163–178. Detailed review of several movement disorders in pregnancy (49 references). Chorea gravidarum refers only to pregnancy, not to specific etiology. Patients with Wilson's disease have low serum ceruloplasmin levels. In pregnancy levels rise from increased mobilization of copper, especially in the second trimester. False-negative results for Wilson's disease may be obtained if ceruloplasmin levels are relied upon for diagnosis in pregnant women. **IV C**

2 Walsche JM (1977) Pregnancy in Wilson's disease. *Q J Med* **46**, 73–83. Study of the course of 15 pregnancies in 10 mothers with Wilson's disease. 9 mothers were taking D-penicillamine at the time of conception. Wilson's disease did not appear to alter the course of pregnancy in 8. The remaining woman may have been insufficiently 'de-coppered' because of constraints on treatment. Mothers taking D-penicillamine are advised to have vitamin B_6 supplements. **III B**

3 Scheinberg IH, Sternlieb I (1975) Pregnancy in penicillamine-treated patients with Wilson's disease. *N Engl J Med* **293**, 1300–1302. Review of 18 personal and published cases of Wilson's disease treated with D-penicillamine. None of these women suffered from exacerbation of their Wilson's disease during pregnancy. Recommendation for continuation of D-penicillamine during pregnancy, with reduction of dosage in late pregnancy 6 weeks before delivery if cesarean section is planned. **III B**

4 Dreifliss FE, McKinney WM (1966) Wilson's disease (hepatolenticular degeneration) and pregnancy. *JAMA* **195**, 960–962. Early single case report of successful pregnancy punctuating Wilson's disease. The patient was treated with dimercaprol. **IV C**

5 Biller J, Swiontoniowski M, Brazis PW (1985) Successful pregnancy in Wilson's disease: a case report and review of the literature. *Eur Neurol* **24**, 306–309. Single case report with publication review (12 references). Review contains some alternative therapies to D-penicillamine, including zinc. **IV C**

6 Mjolnerod OK, Dommerud SA, Rasmussen K, Gjeruldsen ST (1971) Congenital connective tissue defect probably due to D-penicillamine treatment in pregnancy. *Lancet* **1**, 673–675. Single case report of adverse outcome

of using D-penicillamine in pregnancy. The defect was a generalized connective tissue disorder with some features similar to Ehlers–Danlos syndrome. The mother had been taking D-penicillamine for severe cystinuria. **IV C**

7 Goodman JD, Brodie C, Ayida GA (1988) Restless leg syndrome in pregnancy. *Br Med J* **297**, 1101–1102. An assessment of the prevalence of this syndrome amongst 500 antenatal mothers attending a hospital clinic. 19% had the syndrome, although only 7/500 women had severe symptoms. The syndrome is not well known. It subsides after delivery. **III B**

8 Turkalj I, Braun P, Krupp P (1982) Surveillance of bromocriptine in pregnancy. *JAMA* **247**, 1589–1591. Report of outcome of pregnancy in 1410 pregnancies in 1335 women taking bromocriptine primarily in the early weeks of pregnancy. Not specifically focused on Parkinson's disease. The incidence rate of pregnancy losses was similar to normal populations. **III B**

34.10 Cerebral abscess

Andrew Dawson

Management option	Quality of evidence	Strength of recommendation	References
Aggressive intravenous antibiotics (broad-spectrum)	III	B	1
Find and treat source of infection	III	B	1
Surgical drainage for the few cases that fail to respond to the antibiotics	III	B	1

References

1 Aboukasm AG, Levine SR, Donaldson JO (1996) Pregnancy-related cerebral abscess. *Neurologist* **2**, 73–76. Two case reports of cerebral abscess during pregnancy and review of nine other pregnancy-related published cases suitable for analysis, published over 70 years. Pregnancy-related brain abscesses do not necessarily present with focal features. Mortality may be lower in noneclamptic patients. **III B**

Chapter 35

Renal disease

35.1 Chronic renal insufficiency

David Williams

Management option		Quality of evidence	Strength of recommendation	References
Prepregnancy	Pregnancy is not detrimental to long-term renal function in women who have chronic renal disease and *normal* renal function	III	B	1
	Conversely, most women (about 65%) with a serum creatinine above 2 mg/dl (177 µmol/l) will have an irreversible decline in renal function during pregnancy; a third of these women will rapidly decline to end-stage renal failure	III	B	2
	Low prepregnancy glomerular filtration rate (< 50 ml/min), hypertension and proteinuria each have an independent and additively negative effect on perinatal outcome and long-term maternal renal function	IIa III	B B	3 4,5
Prenatal	Frequent monitoring of: ❑ Blood pressure ❑ Renal function (serum urea and creatinine) ❑ Bacteriuria ❑ Fetal growth and health	–	✔	–
	Strict control of blood pressure (aim to keep below 140/85 mmHg)	III	B	6,7
	Consider low-dose aspirin	Ib	A	8
	Renal biopsy is indicated in the rare event that a steroid-responsive renal condition needs to be excluded before viability of the fetus	–	✔	–
Labor and delivery	Indications for delivery (similar to preeclampsia): ❑ Uncontrollable hypertension ❑ Deteriorating renal function ❑ Superimposed severe preeclampsia with either: – Mature gestation – Imminent eclampsia – Rapidly rising liver transaminases – Disseminated intravascular coagulation – Acute fetal compromise	–	✔	–
	Strive to control blood pressure perinatally	–	✔	–
Postnatal	Control of blood pressure (aim to keep below 140/85 mmHg)	–	✔	–
	Re-establish maintenance therapy	–	✔	–

References

1 Jungers P, Houillier P, Forget D *et al.* (1995) Influence of pregnancy on the course of primary glomerulonephritis. *Lancet* **346**, 1122–1124. Retrospective study examining the rate of progression to end-stage renal failure (ESRF) in 360 women with primary glomerulonephritis and initially normal renal function. After up to 30 years of follow-up, it found that those who had been pregnant did not progress to ESRF any quicker than matched controls who had never been pregnant. However, hypertension and the type of glomerulonephritis were influential on progression to ESRF. **III B**

2 Jones DC, Hayslett JP (1996) Outcome of pregnancy in women with moderate or severe renal insufficiency. *N Engl J Med* **335**, 226–232. Multicenter study documenting the outcome and types of complications affecting 67 pregnant women (82 pregnancies) with moderate to severe renal impairment. Women with the most severe preconceptional renal impairment had the worst perinatal outcome and were more likely to have long-term irreversible renal damage, especially with a preconception serum creatinine above 2 mg/dl (177 μmol/l). **III B**

3 Holley JL, Bernardini J, Quadri KH *et al.* (1996) Pregnancy outcomes in a prospective matched control study of pregnancy and renal disease. *Clin Nephrol* **45**, 77–82. Prospective, matched controlled study comparing the pregnancy outcome of 43 pregnancies in women with chronic renal disease with 43 controls (women with nonrenal medical problems). 42% of renal and nonrenal cases were diabetic. Adverse pregnancy outcome was worse in those with renal disease and was even worse in those who had hypertension (in any trimester) or proteinuria and in those with the worst renal impairment. The combination of hypertension and diabetic nephropathy was associated with a particularly poor pregnancy outcome. **IIa B**

4 Abe S (1991) An overview of pregnancy in women with underlying renal disease. *Am J Kidney Dis* **17**, 112–115. Retrospective report and overview of 240 pregnancies in 166 women (delivering between 1970 and 1988). Women with hypertension and a preconception glomerular filtration rate (GFR) of less than 70 ml/min had the worst perinatal outcome. Women without hypertension and a GFR above 70 ml/min had well-preserved long-term renal function. If GFR was below 50 ml/min with coexisting hypertension, then long-term maternal renal function was less likely to be preserved. Histological type of renal disease was less influential on pregnancy outcome than GFR and blood pressure. **III B**

5 Hemmelder MH, de Zeeuw D, Fidler V *et al.* (1995) Proteinuria: a risk factor for pregnancy related renal function decline in primary glomerular disease? *Am J Kidney Dis* **26**, 187–192. This retrospective study followed up 19 women who had had 30 pregnancies for 11 years. 10 of 30 pregnancies had an accelerated decline in renal function. These women had considerably higher preconception proteinuria than the 20 pregnancies not complicated by a postpregnancy accelerated decline in renal function. Surprisingly, such a relationship was not seen with renal function, blood pressure or histological diagnosis. **III B**

6 Jungers P, Chauveau D, Choukroun G *et al.* (1997) Pregnancy in women with impaired renal function. *Clin Nephrol* **47**, 281–288. Follow-up of 43 pregnancies complicated by moderate to severe renal impairment. Women who were hypertensive at conception or in early pregnancy had a fetal loss rate 10.6 times higher than those who had normal blood pressure either spontaneously or on therapy. Fetal loss or accelerated decline in renal function is more likely in those with a creatinine clearance lower than 25–30 ml/min. **III B**

7 Hou SH, Grossman SD, Madias NE (1985) Pregnancy in women with renal disease and moderate renal insufficiency. *Am J Med* **8**, 185–194. Report on the outcome of 25 pregnancies in 23 women who began pregnancy with moderate renal insufficiency (serum creatinine >1.4 mg/dl, 124 μmol/l). 14 pregnancies were complicated by the onset of worsening of hypertension. In 9 women the diastolic rose above 110 mmHg, necessitating delivery. Those with the worst renal function at conception were most likely to have an accelerated decline in renal function in relation to pregnancy. **III B**

8 CLASP (Collaborative Low-dose Aspirin Study in Pregnancy) Collaborative Group (1994) CLASP: a randomised trial of low dose aspirin for the prevention and treatment of pre-eclampsia among 9364 pregnant women. *Lancet* **343**, 619–629. Multicenter, randomized, placebo-controlled trial of aspirin 60 mg as prevention or treatment of preeclampsia. Prophylactic aspirin did not significantly reduce the risk of preeclampsia in a low-risk population, but may reduce the risk of early onset preeclampsia. Women with renal disease are at risk of early-onset preeclampsia and have a vulnerable glomerular capillary circulation. Therefore, aspirin (75 mg) is recommended to pregnant women with renal impairment to prevent early-onset preeclampsia and protect renal function. **Ib A**

35.2 Chronic hemodialysis

David Williams

Management option		Quality of evidence	Strength of recommendation	References
Prepregnancy	Fertility is reduced on dialysis but pregnancy is still possible	III	B	1–4
	Counsel about risks of pregnancy on dialysis (pregnancy is more likely to be successful after transplantation)	III	B	1–4
Prenatal	Careful attention to fluid balance	III	B	1–4
	Improved outcome with daily dialysis	III	B	1–4
	Improved outcome with better nutrition	III	B	1–4
	Most hemodialysis units offer regular human immunodeficiency virus and hepatitis screening	III	B	1–4
	Frequent monitoring of: ❑ Blood pressure ❑ Renal function (aim to keep predialysis urea below 15 mmol/l). ❑ Electrolyte balance (adjust conductivity to approximately 135) ❑ Bacteriuria (if still passing urine) ❑ Hemoglobin (likely to need more erythropoietin) ❑ Fetal growth and health (intrauterine growth restriction more likely)	III	B	1–4
	Strict control of hypertension	III	B	1–4
	Anemia should normally respond to more erythropoietin and iron	III	B	1–4
	Recommend low-dose aspirin and heparinizing the dialysis line as usual	III	B	1–4
	Daily dialysis should avoid sudden shifts in fluid and electrolytes	III	B	1–4
Labor and delivery	Indications for delivery are similar to those for chronic renal failure	–	✔	–
	Control blood pressure	–	✔	–
Postnatal	Review frequency of dialysis	–	✔	–

References

1 Bagon JA, Vernaeve H, De Muylder X *et al.* (1998) Pregnancy and dialysis. *Am J Kidney Dis* **31**, 756–765. Retrospective review of pregnancy on dialysis that went beyond the first trimester, including 5 cases from the reporting unit and 15 cases from the Belgian national register. 14 out of 15 required an increase in erythropoietin dose. Overall a successful pregnancy was achieved in 50% of cases in women on established hemodialysis and 80% who needed to start dialysis during the pregnancy. All pregnancies ended preterm with low-birthweight babies. Birthweight correlated with dialysis hours. 66% of women had a cesarean section. **III B**

2 Okundaye I, Abrinko P, Hou S (1998) Registry of pregnancy in dialysis patients. *Am J Kidney Dis* **31**, 766–773. Findings of a USA registry (National Transplantation Pregnancy Registry) that contains responses from 930 dialysis units. Over a 4-year period 2.4% of hemodialysis patients and 1.1% of peritoneal dialysis patients became pregnant. Among 182 women who conceived on dialysis, the infant survival rate was 40.2%. 57 women started dialysis having conceived and had 73.6% infant survival. Infant survival improved with more than 20 hours dialysis per week. 79% of women

had hypertension, 32 with a blood pressure above 170/110 mmHg. Only 5.9% had a hematocrit over 30. 77% of those not taking erythropoietin had blood transfusions. The mean gestational age at birth was 32.4 weeks. 84% of infants born to mothers who conceived on dialysis were premature, leading to a high frequency of long-term medical problems. **III B**

3 Hou S (1999) Pregnancy in chronic renal insufficiency and end-stage renal disease. *Am J Kidney Dis* **33**, 235–252. Review by an experienced clinician in renal disease during pregnancy focusing on dialysis and pregnancy. The author reviews the findings of the National Pregnancy Dialysis Registry (NPDR) and her own clinical experience to recommend management of pregnancies in women on dialysis. Limited data from the NPDR suggest best perinatal outcome with at least 20 hours dialysis per week. Nutritional advice suggests increasing protein and other minerals. Increased dialysis will clear increased urea. Increasing erythropoietin prevents blood transfusions. Preventing line-clotting with heparin remains important and safe in pregnancy. **III B**

4 Giatras I, Levy DP, Malone FD *et al.* (1998) Pregnancy during dialysis: case report and management guidelines. *Nephrol Dialysis Transplant* **13**, 3266–3272. Case report and review of 120 published cases of pregnancy on dialysis. Several management guidelines are recommended from reviewing observations of successful and unsuccessful pregnancy outcomes. These include aiming for maximum blood urea of 50 mg/dl (17 mmol/l); increasing to daily dialysis if necessary; adjusting dialysate to increase potassium concentration, decrease bicarbonate and adjust calcium according to maternal serum levels; monitoring the fetal heart towards the end of dialysis after 26 weeks; and being aware of the need to increase erythropoietin. **III B**

35.3 Renal transplantation

David Williams

Management option		Quality of evidence	Strength of recommendation	References
Prepregnancy	As fertility returns quickly after successful transplantation, ensure adequate contraception until ready to conceive	–	✔	–
	Avoid combined oral contraceptives	–	✔	–
	Barrier methods or, for selected women, a progesterone-secreting intrauterine contraceptive device	–	✔	–
	Counsel mothers of an increased risk of preterm delivery, intrauterine growth restriction (IUGR), low birthweight	III	B	1
	Counsel mothers regarding risk of pregnancy to long-term renal function	III	B	2,3
	Guidelines for suitability for pregnancy: ❑ Wait 1–2 years after transplantation before becoming pregnant ❑ Stable renal function with plasma creatinine below 2 mg/dl (170 µmol/l) ❑ Stable immune suppression levels ❑ Absent or controlled hypertension ❑ Sterile urine ❑ Good general health	III	B	2
Prenatal	Increased frequency of hospital attendance	–	✔	–
	Frequent monitoring of: ❑ Blood pressure ❑ Renal function ❑ Bacteriuria ❑ Liver function ❑ Hemoglobin, white cell count and platelet count ❑ Fetal growth and health	–	✔	–

Management option		Quality of evidence	Strength of recommendation	References
Prenatal (cont'd)	Maintain immunosuppressive therapy at prepregnancy levels	III	B	4
	Prednisolone/prednisone, azathioprine, cyclosporin and tacrolimus appear to be safe in pregnancy (?risk of IUGR with latter two)	III	B	5
	May require or need more erythropoietin	–	✔	–
	If rejection suspected, consider renal biopsy before aggressive antirejection therapy	–	✔	–
Labor and delivery	Steroid augmentation	–	✔	–
	Transplanted pelvic kidney rarely obstructs vaginal delivery, but cesarean section more likely, especially if pelvic osteodystrophy	–	✔	–
	Give peripartum antibiotics for instrumental delivery (amoxicillin and gentamicin)	–	✔	–
Postnatal	Contraception – as before pregnancy	–	✔	–
	No evidence that drugs in breast milk are detrimental	–	✔	–

References

1 Willis FR, Findlay CA, Gorrie MJ *et al.* (2000) Children of renal transplant recipient mothers. *J Paediatr Child Health* **36**, 230–235. Cross-sectional prevalence survey followed up 48 children born to 34 women transplanted at a single center between 1971 and 1992. There was an increased risk of preterm delivery (27/48 , 56%) and low birthweight (<2500g or <10th centile; 21/48, 44%). However, long-term development at median age 5.2 years was normal in 47/48 (98%). **III B**

2 Crowe AV, Rustom R, Gradden C *et al.* (1999) Pregnancy does not adversely affect renal transplant function. *Q J Med* **92**, 631–635. Follow-up of 33 pregnancies in 29 patients with reasonable renal function at conception (serum creatinine < 150μmol/l), proteinuria below 1g/d, no evidence of allograft rejection, controlled blood pressure and stable immunosuppression. All women with a serum creatinine above 200μmol/l were back on dialysis within 2 years of delivery. This study did not compare the outcome of women who had similar levels of impaired renal function but who had not been pregnant. **III B**

3 Sturgiss SN, Davison JM (1995) Effect of pregnancy on the long-term function of renal allografts: an update. *Am J Kidney Dis* **26**, 54–56. Study of renal transplant function in 17 women who became pregnant 15 years earlier, compared with 17 women who did not conceive. This concluded that there was no detrimental effect of pregnancy on long-term renal function. However, it must be noted that other studies have shown a detrimental effect of pregnancy, especially when renal function is impaired or if there is hypertension, heavy proteinuria or urinary infection. **III B**

4 Armenti VT, Radomski JS, Moritz MJ *et al.* (2000) Report from the National Transplantation Pregnancy Registry (NTPR): outcomes of pregnancy after transplantation. *Clin Transpl* 2000: 123–134. Update of a USA registry, including 200 transplant center reports on issues relating to organ transplants in pregnancy. Experience of the safety of newer immunosuppressive agents is reported. **III B**

5 Kainz A, Harabacz I, Cowlrick IS *et al.* (2000) Review of the course and outcome of 100 pregnancies in 84 women treated with tacrolimus. *Transplantation* **70**, 1718–1721. Retrospective analysis of published information between 1992 and 1998 found 100 pregnancies in 84 mothers who had taken tacrolimus throughout pregnancy. 66 were liver transplants, 27% renal transplants. The most common complications were graft rejection, preeclampsia, renal impairment and infection. All rejection episodes were successfully treated. There were 68/100 live births (24 terminations – 12 spontaneous and 12 induced). Mean gestation was 35 weeks. There were 4 neonatal malformations but no consistency of abnormality. It was concluded that complications were similar to those seen in other transplant patients on more established immunosuppressants. **III B**

35.4 Acute renal failure

David Williams

Management option		Quality of evidence	Strength of recommendation	References
Determine cause	Prerenal failure (following severe hypotension) ❑ Hemorrhage; antepartum or postpartum ❑ Miscarriage ❑ Hyperemesis gravidarum ❑ Septicemic shock (often with coagulopathy) ❑ Amniotic fluid embolus (usually with coagulopathy) If hypotension is severe and prolonged, acute tubular necrosis may follow	–	✔	–
	Intrinsic renal failure ❑ Acute tubular necrosis ❑ Preeclampsia ❑ Hemolytic uremic syndrome ❑ Pyelonephritis ❑ Acute glomerulonephritis ❑ Drug reaction ❑ Acute fatty liver of pregnancy	–	✔	–
	Postrenal failure (urinary tract obstruction) ❑ Calculus, clot or renal papilla in ureter ❑ Damage to ureters ❑ Pelvic hematoma ❑ Uterine obstruction of ureters	–	✔	–
Monitor	❑ State of hydration ❑ Fluid balance (fluid in and urine out) ❑ Renal function ❑ Blood pressure ❑ Urinalysis ❑ Urine microscopy ❑ Urine culture ❑ Renal ultrasound ❑ Coagulation ❑ Maternal oxygen saturation ❑ Central venous pressure when clinical monitoring difficult ❑ Fetal growth and health (if prenatal)	III	B	1–3
Treatment	❑ Fluid/blood replacement for hypovolemia ❑ Control hypertension ❑ Empty uterus with septic abortion and late pregnancy causes ❑ Antibiotics for infective causes ❑ Surgery or endoscopic correction of obstructive causes ❑ Dialysis for severe cases	III	B	1–3

References

1 Sibai BM, Villar MA, Mabie BC *et al.* (1990) Acute renal failure in hypertensive disorders in pregnancy. Pregnancy outcome and remote prognosis in thirty-one consecutive cases. *Am J Obstet Gynecol* **162**, 777–783. 18 pregnancies were complicated by preeclampsia, all of whom had acute tubular necrosis (9 needed dialysis, 2 maternal deaths). 13 women had chronic hypertension or acute on chronic renal disease (5 needed dialysis, one maternal death). Abruptio placentae and hemorrhage complicated almost all cases. Long-term renal prognosis was very good for women with preeclampsia and very poor for those with preexisting renal disease. **III B**

2 Nzerue CM, Hewan-Lowe K, Nwawka C (1998) Acute renal failure in pregnancy: a review of clinical outcomes at an inner-city hospital from 1986–1996. *J Natl Med Assoc* **90**, 486–490. Retrospective study of acute renal failure in pregnancy, in an inner-city hospital. The incidence (2/10000 pregnancies), maternal mortality (15.7%) and maternal and fetal morbidity were all high in this inner-city population. The authors suggest that improved antenatal care in this deprived population would improve these poor outcomes. **III B**

3 Stratta P, Besso L, Canavese C *et al.* (1996) Is pregnancy-related acute renal failure a disappearing clinical entity? *Renal Failure* **18**, 574–584. Retrospective analysis of pregnancy-related acute renal failure (ARF) assessed by nephrologists from 1958–94. The incidence of pregnancy-related ARF among all cases of ARF fell from 43% in 1956–67 to 0.5% in 1988–94. The worst maternal and renal prognosis was in women who had preeclampsia complicated by abruptio placentae and hemorrhage. Timely delivery and resuscitation with carefully monitored fluid replacement were critical to improved maternal and renal outcome. **III B**

35.5 Nephrolithiasis

David Williams

Management option		Quality of evidence	Strength of recommendation	References
Prepregnancy	In known 'stone formers', complete metabolic, hormonal and infectious evaluation for underlying etiologies, based on stone composition	–	✔	–
	Control underlying condition and eliminate existing stones	–	✔	–
	Counsel patients that complications from renal stones are no more likely during pregnancy than in the nongravid state	–	✔	–
Prenatal	Renal colic usually presents acutely: if suggestive symptoms check urinalysis, midstream specimen of urine, full blood count, urea and electrolytes and renal ultrasound	III	B	1,2
	If ultrasound nondiagnostic, proceed with intravenous urogram, limiting number of films and using modified pelvic shielding	III	B	1
	Most pregnant women will respond to conservative measures (hydration and analgesia)	III	B	1
	Treat associated urinary tract infections with antibiotics	III	B	1,2
	Try to avoid thiazides, xanthine oxidase inhibitors or penicillamine	–	✔	–
	With intractable pain, persistent infection, obstruction of a solitary kidney, recurrent preterm labor or evidence of deteriorating renal function, proceed with more invasive interventional strategies: ❑ Cystoscopy, stone removal, stent insertion/replacement ❑ Percutaneous or open nephrostomy ❑ Ureteric laser lithotripsy appears to be safe in pregnancy ❑ Extracorporeal shockwave lithotripsy should be avoided	III	B	1,3,4

➡

➡

Management option		Quality of evidence	Strength of recommendation	References
Postnatal	Delay complete diagnostic evaluation until at least 3 months post-partum (to allow resolution of gestational renal tract changes)	–	✔	–
	Reinstitute prepregnancy pharmacological agents as indicated	–	✔	–

References

1 Butler EL, Cox SM, Eberts EG *et al.* (2000) Symptomatic nephrolithiasis complicating pregnancy. *Obstet Gynecol* **96**, 753–756. Retrospective evaluation of perinatal outcome and management of nephrolithiasis in pregnancy between 1986 and 1999. 57 women had 73 admissions for symptomatic nephrolithiasis (1/3300 deliveries). Only 20% of women were known to have renal calculi before pregnancy. Renal calculi were visualized in 60% (21/35) of ultrasound examinations and 57% (4/7) who had a plain abdominal X-ray. However, renal stones were identified in 93% (13/14) of women who had single-shot intravenous pyelography as an initial diagnostic test. Conservative management improved symptoms in 75% (43/57) but 10 women needed ureteric stents, 3 needed percutaneous nephrostomy tubes and 2 underwent ureteral laser lithotripsy. **III B**

2 Coe FL, Parks JH, Lindheimer MD (1978) Nephrolithiasis during pregnancy. *N Engl J Med* **298**, 324–326. Retrospective series of 90 pregnancies in 78 women with renal stones, concluding that stone disease has no adverse effect on pregnancy, except an increased frequency of urinary tract infection (UTI). UTIs associated with renal stones should be treated for longer than isolated UTIs and followed up with antibiotic prophylaxis. **III B**

3 Asgari MA, Safarinejad MR, Hasseini SY et al. (1999) Extracorporeal shock wave lithotripsy of renal calculi during pregnancy. *Br J Urol* **84**, 615–617. Survey of 824 women found 6 who had inadvertently had extracorporeal shock wave lithotripsy (ESWL) during early pregnancy. All 6 went on to have healthy babies. This paper does not advocate the safety of ESWL in pregnancy but suggests that its inadvertent use in early pregnancy is not a cause for concern. **III B**

4 Carringer M, Swartz R, Johansson JE (1996) Management of ureteric calculi during pregnancy by ureteroscopy and laser lithotripsy. *Br J Urol* **77**, 17–20. Small case series of 4 women during 5 pregnancies reported that stones between 5 and 16 mm in diameter can be safely treated during pregnancy by ureteroscopy and laser lithotripsy. 2/5 cases were treated under topical anesthesia and fluoroscopy was not needed for any case. **III B**

Chapter 36

Autoimmune disease

36.1 Systemic lupus erythematosus

Janet Ashworth

Management option		Quality of evidence	Strength of recommendation	References
Prepregnancy	Establish good control of systemic lupus erythematosus (SLE)	–	✔	–
	Discontinue azathioprine, methotrexate and cyclophosphamide if possible (Reference is rat study)	(Ib) III	(A) B	1 2
	Laboratory assessment for anemia, thrombocytopenia, renal disease, antibodies (antiphospholipid, anti-Ro/SSA, anti-La/SSB)	–	✔	–
	Counsel patient regarding risks (exacerbations, primary idiopathic hypertension (PIH), fetal/neonatal)	–	✔	–
Prenatal	Multidisciplinary care	–	✔	–
	Dating scan	–	✔	–
	Frequent antenatal checks: 2-weekly in the first and second trimester, weekly in third	–	✔	–
	Vigilance for SLE flare, PIH, intrauterine growth restriction	–	✔	–
	Renal disease: 24 h urine every month	–	✔	–
	Drugs: ❑ Glucocorticoids are safe but there appears to be an increased risk of orofacial clefts when used in the first trimester ❑ Azathioprine if steroids are ineffective ❑ Methotrexate/cyclophosphamide as third choice ❑ Avoid antimalarials ❑ Avoid full-dose nonsteroidal anti-inflammatories	 III IV IV III IIb	 B C C B B	 3–5 6,7 6,7 8,9 10–12
	Serial biometry, Doppler studies and amniotic fluid volume	–	✔	–
	Begin prenatal testing at 30–32 weeks gestation (earlier in patients with worsening disease, evidence of fetal compromise or a history of poor pregnancy outcome)	III	B	13
	Consider low-dose aspirin	Ia	A	14

➡

Management option		Quality of evidence	Strength of recommendation	References
Labor/delivery	Deliver no later than at term	–	✔	–
	Continuous fetal heart rate monitoring	–	✔	–
	Extra steroids for those on steroid treatment	–	✔	–
Postnatal	Beware SLE exacerbation	–	✔	–
	Restart maintenance therapy	–	✔	–
	Check neonate for SLE manifestations	–	✔	–

References

1 Scott JR (1977) Fetal growth retardation associated with maternal administration of immunosuppressive drugs. *Am J Obstet Gynecol* **128**, 668–676. RCT on rats, studying effects of azathioprine and cyclophosphamide on pregnancy. Azathioprine was commonly embryocidal, although it did not inhibit implantation, and cyclophosphamide caused fetal loss in a dose-dependent manner. Both drugs were associated with fetal growth restriction. **Ib A**

2 Cote CJ, Meuwissen HJ, Pickering RJ (1974) Effects on the neonate of prednisone and azathioprine administered to the mother during pregnancy. *J Pediatr* **85**, 324–328. Case report of immunological changes (initial lymphopenia followed by chronic cytomegalovirus infection) in an infant exposed to azathioprine and prednisolone in pregnancy. Literature review of 21 case reports of similar *in-utero* exposure with 5 cases of lymphopenia. No documentation of baseline differences in study populations. **III B**

3 Bongiovanni AM, McPadden AJ (1960) Steroids during pregnancy and possible fetal consequences. *Fertil Steril* **11**, 181–186. Literature review of neonatal outcome from 260 pregnancies treated with reproductive or adrenal corticosteroids. No evidence of significant congenital abnormalities compared to animal studies of these drugs. Two incidences of cleft palate and one of transient neonatal adrenocortical failure. **III B**

4 Carmichael SL, Shaw GM (1999) Maternal corticosteroid use and risk of selected congenital anomalies. *Am J Med Genet* **86**, 242–244. Retrospective case-control study on the association of corticosteroid use in women 1 month before and 3 months after conception with selected congenital abnormalities (orofacial clefts (n = 662), conotruncal heart defects (n = 207), neural tube defects (n = 265) and limb reduction defects (n = 165)). Corticosteroid use was found to be associated with an increased risk for an isolated cleft lip (OR 4.3, 95% CI 1.1–17.2) and isolated cleft palate (OR 5.3, 95% CI 1.1–26.5). There was no increased risk for the other anomalies studied. **III B**

5 Rodriguez-Pinilla E, Martinez-Frias ML (1998) Corticosteroids during pregnancy and oral clefts: a case-control study. *Teratology* **58**, 2–5. Retrospective case-control study on the relationship of corticosteroid use during the first trimester of pregnancy and a nonsyndromic oral cleft in 1184 liveborns. Logistic regression analysis controlled for potential confounder factors shows a significantly increased risk of cleft lip (with or without cleft palate) when using corticosteroids during the first trimester (OR 6.55, 95% CI 1.4–29.8). **III B**

6 Connell W, Miller A (1999) Treating inflammatory bowel disease during pregnancy: risks and safety of drug therapy. *Drug Saf* **21**, 311–323. Review on the safety of drug therapy for inflammatory bowel disease during pregnancy. Current available information is largely derived from animal studies and clinical experience among patients with inflammatory bowel disease, autoimmune disorders and organ transplants. The review states that there is no causal relationship between exposure to sulfasalazine or other 5-aminosalicylic acid drugs and congenital malformations and that they may be used during pregnancy and lactation. Corticosteroids carry a very small risk to the developing fetus. Azathioprine is not teratogenic but impairs fetal immunity, may cause growth retardation and premature labor has been described. Preliminary data indicate no significant fetal toxicity following first trimester exposure to mercaptopurine. Cyclosporin is not teratogenic, but may be associated with growth retardation and prematurity. Methotrexate is an abortifacient and causes congenital malformations. Short courses of metronidazole or ciprofloxacin are safe; data on prolonged exposure are missing. **IV C**

7 Ostensen M (1992) Treatment with immunosuppressive and disease modifying drugs during pregnancy and lactation. *Am J Reprod Immunol* **28**, 148–152. Review of the literature on harmful effects of drugs used for autoimmune diseases. The author finds it appropriate not to use gold, penicillamine and chloroquine in pregnancy as long as their teratogenic effects are still disputed. Hydroxychloroquine, cyclosporin, azathioprine and sulfasalazine have been used in pregnancy without increasing the rate of congenital abnormalities. The latter may cause fetal growth retardation. Cyclophosphamide, chlorambucil and methotrexate are possibly teratogenic when given during early pregnancy but may be less harmful in late pregnancy. Because of insufficient data, breastfeeding is not recommended in patients on antimalarials, penicillamine, cyclosporin A and cytostatic drugs. Intramuscular gold and sulfasalazine seem to impose no major risk on the nursing infant. **IV C**

8 Hart C, Naughton RF (1964) The ototoxicity of chloroquine phosphate. *Arch Otolaryngol* **80**, 407–412. Case report of seven consecutive pregnancies in one mother with systemic lupus erythematosus (SLE). Those pregnancies where no treatment was given for SLE resulted in term deliveries of healthy infants. Two pregnancies where chloroquine phosphate was taken throughout resulted in infants with neurological problems (deafness, pyramidal signs, ataxia and learning difficulties). **III B**

9 Parke A (1988) Antimalarial drugs and pregnancy. *Am J Med* **85**, 30–33. Retrospective study of 14 pregnancies in 8 patients taking chloroquine or hydroxychloroquine for systemic lupus erythematosus throughout pregnancy. There were 6 live births, none with any congenital abnormalities. **III B**

10 Rumack CM, Guggenheim MA, Rumack BH *et al.* (1981) Neonatal intracranial hemorrhage and maternal use of aspirin. *Obstet Gynecol* **58**, 52S–56S. Prospective cohort study of 108 neonates born at or before 34 weeks gestation, or with birthweight no more than 1.5 kg, examining the effect of maternal aspirin ingestion in the last week of pregnancy on the incidence of intracranial hemorrhage. 17 infants had been exposed to aspirin and were compared with 20 exposed to acetaminophen/paracetamol and 71 with no drug exposure *in utero*. There was a significant increase in incidence of intracranial hemorrhage on computed tomography scan in the infants exposed to aspirin (71%) compared to both control groups (50% and 44% respectively). **IIb B**

11 Moise KJ, Huhta JC, Sharif DS *et al.* (1988) Indomethacin in the treatment of premature labor. Effects on the fetal ductus arteriosus. *N Engl J Med* **319**, 327–331. Prospective study of serial fetal echocardiography looking for premature closure of the ductus arteriosus in 14 cases of premature labor at 26–31 weeks being treated with indometacin. Half showed ductal constriction, unrelated to gestation or dose regimen, which resolved within 24 hours of stopping the drug, and none of the infants showed persistent fetal circulation postnatally. There was no control group. **IIb B**

12 Hickok DE, Hollenbach KA, Reilley SF *et al.* (1989) The association between decreased amniotic fluid volume and treatment with nonsteroidal anti-inflammatory agents for preterm labor. *Am J Obstet Gynecol* **160**, 1525–1531. Retrospective case review comparing reduction in amniotic fluid volumes in 17 women on nonsteroidal anti-inflammatory drugs (NSAIDs) and 10 on other tocolytic drugs for premature labor. Many of the liquor volume estimates were purely descriptive. The study reported a significant reduction in amniotic fluid volume in those taking NSAIDs ($p < 0.001$). **IIb B**

13 Druzin ML, Lockshin M, Edersheim TG *et al.* (1987) Second-trimester fetal monitoring and preterm delivery in pregnancies with systemic lupus erythematosus and/or circulating anticoagulant. *Am J Obstet Gynecol* **157**, 1503–1510. Prospective trial of nonstress-test CTG monitoring and measurement of anticardiolipin antibody titers in 8 patients with systemic lupus erythematosus (SLE) and 6 uncomplicated pregnancies. CTGs were performed serially from 19–26 weeks, followed up with contraction CTG testing or biophysical profiles if the CTG was not normal. All patients with active SLE had CTG abnormalities, 3 resulting in fetal demise without intervention and the 2 patients with inactive SLE and those with uncomplicated pregnancies all had normal CTGs. The study concluded that, while high anticardiolipin antibody titers and CTG were both good predictors of pregnancy outcome, only the CTG was helpful in determining optimal timing of delivery. **III B**

14 Imperiale TF, Petrulis AS (1991) A meta-analysis of low-dose aspirin for the prevention of pregnancy-induced hypertensive disease. *JAMA* **266**, 260–264. Meta-analysis of six controlled trials (five with randomization) of low-dose aspirin to prevent pregnancy-induced hypertension and severe low birthweight and to reduce cesarean section rate. In the 394 pregnancies studied, aspirin resulted in a significant reduction in relative risk of developing pregnancy-induced hypertension (RR 0.35, 95% CI 0.22–0.55, number needed to treat 4.4). No differentiation was made between nonproteinuric hypertension and preeclampsia, having a severe low-birthweight infant (RR 0.56, 95% CI 0.36–0.88) and requiring cesarean section (RR 0.34, 95% CI 0.25–0.48 but included all indications for cesarean section). There was no effect on perinatal mortality rate and no adverse effects of aspirin were reported. **Ia A**

36.2 Antiphospholipid syndrome

Janet Ashworth

Management option		Quality of evidence	Strength of recommendation	References
Prepregnancy	Counseling regarding risks	–	✔	–
	Check for: ❑ Anemia ❑ Thrombocytopenia ❑ Renal compromise	III	B	1
	Thromboprophylaxis for all?	III	B	1

➡

Management option		Quality of evidence	Strength of recommendation	References
Prenatal	Joint obstetrician and physician surveillance	–	✔	–
	Low-dose aspirin and subcutaneous heparin	III Ib	B A	2–5 6–9
	Increased frequency of attendance	III	B	2,10
	Surveillance of fetal growth and health	III	B	2,10
	Screen for preeclampsia	III	B	2

References

1 Munoz-Rodriguez FJ, Font J, Cervera R *et al.* (1999) Clinical study and follow-up of 100 patients with the antiphospholipid syndrome. *Semin Arthritis Rheum* **29**, 182–190. A retrospective study of 100 patients (86% female and 14% male; mean age, 36 years) with antiphospholipid syndrome (APS). 62% had primary APS and 38% had APS associated with systemic lupus erythematosus (SLE). During a median length of follow-up of 49 months, 53% had thromboses, 52% had thrombocytopenia and 60% of the women had pregnancy losses. APS patients with SLE had a higher prevalence of hemolytic anemia, thrombocytopenia, antinuclear antibodies and low complement levels. Thrombosis was recurrent in 53%. Recurrences were observed in 19% when treated with long-term oral anticoagulation, in 42% when treated prophylactically with aspirin and in 91% when anticoagulant/antiaggregant treatment was discontinued ($p = 0.0007$). Prophylactic treatment during pregnancy (usually with aspirin) increased the live birth rate from 38% to 72% ($p = 0.0002$). It was concluded that long-term oral anticoagulation appears to be the best prophylactic for recurrences. **III B**

2 Branch DW, Silver RM, Blackwell JL *et al.* (1992) Outcome of treated pregnancies in women with antiphospholipid syndrome: an update of the Utah experience. *Obstet Gynecol* **80**, 614–620. Retrospective case review of 82 consecutive pregnancies in women with antiphospholipid syndrome with varying treatment combinations, including prednisolone, aspirin, heparin and immunoglobulin infusion. Outcomes were similar in all treatment groups, with 73% live births, 60% intrauterine growth restriction, 50% preeclampsia or fetal distress, 37% delivering preterm and 5% postnatal thromboembolism. Number of previous pregnancy failures was the only significant predictor of adverse pregnancy outcome ($p = 0.02$). **III B**

3 Rosove MH, Tabsh K, Wasserstrum N *et al.* (1990) Heparin therapy for pregnant women with lupus anticoagulant or anticardiolipin antibodies. *Obstet Gynecol* **75**, 630–634. Prospective study of 15 pregnant women with antiphospholipid syndrome and poor obstetric histories treated with subcutaneous heparin from 10 weeks gestation. 14 had live births, with no cases of fetal growth restriction or maternal complications from the disease or the treatment. There was an increased rate of premature delivery and cesarean section. **III B**

4 Many A, Pauzner R, Carp H *et al.* (1992) Treatment of patients with antiphospholipid antibodies during pregnancy. *Am J Rep Immunol* **28**, 216–218. Retrospective study on the outcome of various treatment modalities using no medication (102 pregnancies) or corticosteroids, antiplatelet drugs and anticoagulant drugs alone or in combination (total154 pregnancies) in 31 women. Treatment increased live birth rate from 7% to 69%, some of these successes occurring in women with previous failed pregnancies on steroid and aspirin therapy. The authors conclude that therapy during pregnancy in these patients should be individualized according to their obstetric and medical history. **III B**

5 Branch DW, Silver RM, Blackwell JL *et al.* (1992) Outcome of treated pregnancies in women with well-characterized antiphospholipid syndrome. *Obstet Gynecol* **80**, 614–620. Retrospective comparison of 82 pregnancies in women with antiphospholipid syndrome on various treatment regimens (prednisone + aspirin/heparin + aspirin/prednisone, heparin + aspirin/immunoglobulin infusion), finding a neonatal survival rate of 73% with no differences between the treatment groups. There was a 37% preterm delivery rate and high incidences of preeclampsia and intrauterine growth restriction, with several postnatal thromboses occurring in spite of treatment. **III B**

6 Lockshin MD, Druzin ML, Oamar T (1989) Prednisone does not prevent recurrent fetal death in women with antiphospholipid antibody. *Am J Obstet Gynecol* **160**, 439–443. Prospective controlled study of the effects of aspirin, prednisone (prednisolone), both drugs or no treatment on pregnancy outcome in 32 women with antiphospholipid syndrome. A significantly worse outcome was reported in the 11 women treated with just prednisone, with some (not significant) protective effect of aspirin, but the numbers in each treatment arm were small and varying doses of prednisone were used in different individuals. **Ib A**

7 Cowchock FS, Reece EA, Balaban D et al. (1992) Repeated fetal losses associated with antiphospholipid antibodies: a collaborative randomized trial comparing prednisone with low-dose heparin treatment. *Am J Obstet Gynecol* **166**, 1318–1323. Multicenter, randomized trial, the controls consisting of those refusing or

unsuitable for randomization. 20 women with antiphospholipid syndrome were randomized to receive aspirin with low-dose heparin or prednisone (prednisolone) during pregnancy. Both groups had a 75% live birth rate but those treated with prednisone had a significantly higher rate of preterm delivery and of maternal morbidity. **Ib A**

8 Kutteh WH (1996) Antiphospholipid antibody-associated recurrent pregnancy loss: treatment with heparin and low-dose aspirin is superior to low-dose aspirin alone. *Am J Obstet Gynecol* **174**, 1584–1589. Prospective single-center trial, in which 50 women with antiphospholipid syndrome were randomized to treatment with aspirin alone or with heparin. The addition of heparin increased the live birth rate from 44% to 80%, with no difference in rates of preterm delivery, cesarean section or other complications. **Ib A**

9 Rai R, Cohen H, Dave M *et al.* (1997) Randomised controlled trial of aspirin and aspirin plus heparin in pregnant women with recurrent miscarriage associated with phospholipid antibodies (or antiphospholipid antibodies). *Br Med J* **314**, 253–257. Single-center RCT in which 90 pregnant women with antiphospholipid syndrome and recurrent miscarriage were randomized to aspirin alone or aspirin plus heparin therapy. The addition of heparin significantly increased the live birth rate, from 42% to 71%, with 90% of losses occurring in the first trimester, such that, for those pregnancies still viable at 13 weeks, no further differences were demonstrated between the two treatment groups. The only noted side-effect was a decrease in mean lumbar spine bone density of 5.4% in the group treated with aspirin and heparin. **Ib A**

10 Trudinger BH, Stewart GJ, Cook CM *et al.* (1988) Monitoring lupus anticoagulant-positive pregnancies with umbilical artery flow velocity waveforms. *Obstet Gynecol* **72**, 215–218. Observational study of umbilical artery Doppler waveform changes from 24 weeks gestation in six pregnancies of women with antiphospholipid syndrome on no therapy. All were delivered alive by cesarean section in the third trimester, four following abnormal Doppler studies and two for other obstetric indications. **III B**

36.3 Rheumatoid arthritis

Janet Ashworth

Management option		Quality of evidence	Strength of recommendation	References
Prepregnancy	Counseling regarding risks	III	B	1
	Review of therapy to improve disease control	–	✔	–
	Reduce dosage to lowest levels achieving therapeutic effect	–	✔	–
	Avoid known teratogens	IV	C	2
Prenatal	Regular review (joint obstetrician and physician surveillance)	–	✔	–
	Rest (general and local)	–	✔	–
	Physiotherapy	–	✔	–
	Drugs:			
	❑ Avoid full-dose aspirin and nonsteroidal anti-inflammatories if possible (or use minimum doses to control inflammation)	IV	C	3
	❑ Steroids for worsening disease (study not in pregnancy)	Ib	A	4
	❑ Avoid methotrexate in the first trimester	IV	C	2
	❑ D-penicillamine contraindicated	IV	C	2
Labor and delivery	Individualize care according to physical abilities	–	✔	–

References

1 Skomsvoll JF, Ostensen M, Irgens LM *et al.* (2000) Pregnancy complications and delivery practice in women with connective tissue disease and inflammatory rheumatic disease in Norway. *Acta Obstet Gynecol Scand* **79**, 490–495. Retrospective 28-year study comparing complications in pregnancies of women with connective tissue diseases and inflammatory arthritis with the rest of the population, using data from the national registry. Rheumatoid arthritis (documented in 0.43% of the pregnant population) was associated with an increased risk of developing

preeclampsia (OR 1.28, 95% CI 1.05–1.56), having labor induced and being delivered by cesarean section (OR 1.27, 95% CI 1.14–1.41). **III B**

2 Ostensen M (1992) Treatment with immunosuppressive and disease modifying drugs during pregnancy and lactation. *Am J Reprod Immunol* **28**, 148–152. Review of the literature on harmful effects of drugs used for autoimmune diseases. The author finds it appropriate not to use gold, penicillamine and chloroquine in pregnancy as long as their teratogenic effects are still disputed. Hydroxychloroquine, cyclosporin, azathioprine and sulfasalazine have been used in pregnancy without increasing the rate of congenital abnormalities. The latter may cause fetal growth retardation. Cyclophosphamide, chlorambucil and methotrexate are possibly teratogenic when given during early pregnancy but may be less harmful in late pregnancy. Because of insufficient data, breastfeeding is not recommended in patients on antimalarials, penicillamine, cyclosporin A and cytostatic drugs. Intramuscular gold and sulfasalazine seem to impose no major risk on the nursing infant. **IV C**

3 Briggs GG, Freeman RK, Yaffe SJ (1994) *Drugs in pregnancy and lactation*, 4th edn. Baltimore, MD: Williams & Wilkins. Adverse effects of nonsteroidal anti-inflammatory drugs in pregnancy include impaired hemostasis, prolonged gestation and premature closure of the ductus arteriosus. **IV C**

4 Kirwan JR (1995) The effect of glucocorticoids on joint destruction in rheumatoid arthritis. The Arthritis and Rheumatism Council Low-Dose Glucocorticoid Study Group. *N Engl J Med* **333**, 142–146. Multicenter RCT comparing oral prednisone (prednisolone) with placebo in 128 adults of both sexes. Prednisone therapy resulted in a significant reduction in hand joint destruction. Not studied in pregnancy. **Ib A**

36.4 Systemic sclerosis

Janet Ashworth

Management option		Quality of evidence	Strength of recommendation	References
Prepregnancy	Counseling regarding risks	IIa	B	1
	Review of therapy to improve disease control	III	B	2
	Assess cardiopulmonary and renal function (advise against conception if compromised?)	III	B	2
Prenatal	Joint obstetrician and physician surveillance	III	B	2
	Frequent visits	III IV	B C	2 3
	Monitor cardiopulmonary and renal function (consider termination of pregnancy if severe compromise)	IV	C	3
	Drugs: ❑ Anti-inflammatory for moderate joint problems ❑ Vasodilators for pulmonary problems ❑ Steroids for worsening disease	 – – –	 ✔ ✔ ✔	 – – –
	Vigilance for preeclampsia	IV	C	3
	Use of angiotensin-converting-enzyme inhibitors a dilemma if hypertension present	III	B	2
	Check fetal growth and health	IIa	B	1
Labor and delivery	Intensive/high-dependency care may be necessary	–	✔	–
	Special precautions to ensure wound healing if cesarean section	–	✔	–
Postnatal	Initial care in intensive/high dependency care setting	–	✔	–
	Review dosage of drugs	–	✔	–

References

1 Steen VD (1997) Scleroderma and pregnancy. *Rheum Dis Clin North Am* **23**, 133–147. A review on pregnancy in systemic sclerosis. The author states that, although pregnancy may be uneventful, complications do occur and antenatal evaluations, discussion of potential problems and participation in a high-risk obstetric monitoring program is crucial to optimize the best outcome. In diffuse scleroderma there is a greater risk for developing serious cardiopulmonary and renal problems early in the disease; pregnancy should be delayed until the disease stabilizes. The increased risk of premature and small infants may be reduced with intensive obstetric care. Renal crisis in scleroderma is the only truly unique aspect of these pregnancies, which, unlike blood pressure elevation in nonscleroderma pregnancies, must be treated aggressively with angiotensin-converting-enzyme inhibitors. Other pregnancy problems may not be unique to scleroderma but, because it is a chronic illness, any complication carries higher risks for both mother and child. Careful planning, close monitoring and aggressive management should allow women with scleroderma to have a high likelihood of a successful pregnancy. **IV C**

2 Steen VD (1999) Pregnancy in women with systemic sclerosis. *Obstet Gynecol* **94**, 15–20. 59 women with systemic sclerosis were observed prospectively over 91 pregnancies during 10 years. Miscarriage rates increased only in those with long-standing diffuse scleroderma; 29% ended in premature delivery and there was one neonatal death. Symptoms improved during pregnancy (particularly Raynaud's) except for reflux and 3 women with renal crises (all had early diffuse scleroderma), and postnatally some of those with diffuse scleroderma suffered increased skin thickening. It was advised that women with early diffuse scleroderma delay pregnancy until disease is stabilized. 5 babies were born without problems to mothers on angiotensin-converting-enzyme inhibitors. **III B**

3 Steen VD, Medsger TA (1999) Fertility and pregnancy outcome in women with systemic sclerosis. *Arthritis Rheum* **42**, 763–768. Retrospective case-control study on fetal morbidity and mortality in 214 women with systemic sclerosis (SSc), 167 women with rheumatoid arthritis (RA) and 105 healthy controls. There were no significant differences in miscarriage rate, premature births, small full-term births, or neonatal deaths between the three groups. Women with SSc were more likely than those without SSc to have adverse outcomes, particularly premature births (also seen in RA women) and small full-term infants. The authors conclude that women with SSc have acceptable pregnancy outcomes compared with the other groups studied. Further, they state that there are no excessive maternal or fetal pregnancy risks for women with SSc and that a well-timed pregnancy with careful obstetric monitoring will increase the likelihood of a successful outcome. **IIa B**

36.5 Myasthenia gravis

Janet Ashworth

Management option		Quality of evidence	Strength of recommendation	References
Prepregnancy	Counseling regarding risks	III	B	1, 2
	Review of therapy	IV	C	3
	Consider thymectomy	IV	C	3
Prenatal	Joint obstetrician and physician surveillance	III	B	1
	Continue preexisting drugs: ❑ Anticholinesterase ❑ Steroids ❑ Azathioprine	III	B	2
	Plasmapheresis for drug-resistant cases	III	B	2
	Fetal surveillance, especially activity (?biophysical profile score)	–	✔	–
	Avoid/minimize physical/emotional stress	IV	C	4
Labor and delivery	Minimize stress	IV	C	4
	Continue anticholinesterase drugs (parenteral)	IV	C	5
	Steroid cover if on steroids	–	✔	–

Management option		Quality of evidence	Strength of recommendation	References
Labor and delivery (cont'd)	Regional analgesia preferable to narcotics for pain relief and general anesthesia	III	B	6
	Experienced anesthetists if general anesthesia (advisable to consult in prenatal period)	IV	C	5
	Assisted second stage more likely	III	B	6
	Avoid magnesium sulfate (and other contra-indicated drugs) in patients with preeclampsia	IV	C	7,8
Postnatal	Special care and surveillance of newborn; may need short-term anticholinesterases	III	B	2
	Review dosage of drugs	III	B	2

References

1 Michell PJ, Bebbington M (1992) Myasthenia gravis in pregnancy. *Obstet Gynecol* **80**, 178–181. Retrospective case note review of 9 pregnancies complicated by myasthenia gravis. 4 women experienced antenatal exacerbations (the most severe being in a thymectomized patient) but there were no specific problems during labor or postnatally. One of the 11 babies had neonatal myasthenia gravis. There were no predictive factors for risk in pregnancy and a joint approach to care by obstetrician, neurologist and pediatrician was advocated. **III B**

2 Batocchi AP, Majolini L, Evoli A *et al.* (1999) Course and treatment of myasthenia gravis during pregnancy. *Neurology* **52**, 447–452. Descriptive study of 47 women with myasthenia gravis in 64 pregnancies. 17% relapsed, 39% improved, 4% had symptoms unchanged and 19% had deteriorating symptoms on treatment, while 28% deteriorated postnatally, although none had any long-term deterioration in their disease and its course in pregnancy was unpredictable. 43% of babies had anti-acetylcholine-receptor antibodies, and 9% developed neonatal myasthenia gravis. Immunosuppression, plasmapheresis and intravenous immunoglobulin therapy were all used without ill-effect. **III B**

3 Spring PJ, Spies JM (2001) Myasthenia gravis: options and timing of immunomodulatory treatment. *BioDrugs* **15**, 173–183. A review on the current options for treatment of myasthenia gravis: acute and long-term immunotherapies, acetylcholinesterase inhibitors and thymectomy. The many factors that influence the timing of initiation of immunomodulatory therapy such as stage and severity of the disease and patient factors, such as age, pregnancy and intercurrent illness, are considered. In general, acetylcholinesterase inhibitors alone are used only in mild ocular disease and immunomodulatory therapy in the majority of other patients (corticosteroids initially, followed by azathioprine). In refractory cases, the available options include immunosuppressants such as cyclosporin, mycophenolate mofetil and cyclophosphamide. Plasmapheresis and intravenous immunoglobulin are reserved for acute exacerbations, myasthenic crisis and perioperatively. The role of thymectomy in improving long-term outcome in nonthymomatous myasthenia gravis remains controversial. **IV C**

4 Bedlack RS, Sanders DB (2000) How to handle myasthenic crisis. Essential steps in patient care. *Postgrad Med* **107**, 211–214. A review on the management of myasthenic crises in patients with myasthenia gravis. It is stated that myasthenic crisis may be caused by infections, aspiration, physical and emotional stress, and changes in medication. Although no single factor determines the need for respiratory support, all patients with questionable respiratory status should be admitted to the intensive care unit. **IV C**

5 Rolbin WH, Levinson G, Shnider SM *et al.* (1978) Anesthetic considerations for myasthenia gravis and pregnancy. *Anesth Analg* **57**, 441–447. Review of anesthetic considerations in pregnant women with myasthenia gravis. Three cases are presented. It is stated that regional anesthesia is preferred for vaginal delivery and that anticholinesterase therapy should be maintained during labor, preferably by parenteral administration. **IV C**

6 Thoulon JM, Galopin G, Seffert P *et al.* (1978) Myasthenia and pregnancy. *Gynecol Obstet Biol Reprod* **7**, 1395–1403. Case review of 19 women with myasthenia gravis in 24 pregnancies over a period of 25 years. The severity of the disease was found to be variably affected by pregnancy. Worsening happens especially in the first trimester of the pregnancy. Labor can be normal but the second stage often has to be aided because of the patient's muscle tiredness. During labor and particularly in the second stage an acute crisis may occur, with difficulty in breathing. Resuscitation and aided ventilation maybe required. For this it is necessary to have an experienced anesthetist present. **III B**

7 Cohen BA, London RS, Goldstein PJ *et al.* (1976) Myasthenia gravis and preeclampsia. *Obstet Gynecol* **48**, 35S–37S. A case presentation of a patient with myasthenia gravis and preeclampsia with recommendations for

management. The authors conclude that magnesium is a contraindicated pharmacological agent in a myasthenic patient. **IV C**

8 Bashuk RG, Krendel DA (1990) Myasthenia gravis presenting as weakness after magnesium administration. *Muscle Nerve* **13**, 708–712. A case presentation of a pregnant patient with no prior history of neuromuscular disease who was diagnosed to have myasthenia gravis after becoming virtually quadriplegic after parenteral magnesium administration for preeclampsia with therapeutic serum magnesium levels. **IV C**

Chapter 37

Orthopedic, back and joint problems

37.1 General evaluation of back and pelvic pain

Aneesa Lala

Management option	Quality of evidence	Strength of recommendation	References
Consider extraskeletal etiologies for backache (e.g. obstetrical complications and urological disorders)	IV	C	1
Atypical presentations, or pain refractory to the usual care, may indicate more significant, although rare, pathology (e.g. disc herniation, infection, tumor)	IV	C	2,3
Differentiation of similar symptoms from direct fetal pressure on nerve roots (e.g. paresthesias in the distribution of the ilioinguinal and iliofemoral nerves and even quadriceps weakness and 'giving-way') is necessary	–	✔	–
Routine examination includes inspection of the patient while she is standing, then while forward bending, followed by palpation about the spine, paraspinal area and sacrum	–	✔	–
Radiographic evaluation, although undesirable during pregnancy, may be warranted if insidious etiologies for pain are suspected	IV	C	2
Magnetic resonance imaging may be particularly helpful in the diagnosis of tumor and infection	–	✔	–
Mass lesions compressing nerve roots, such as disc herniations, can be initially evaluated with electromyographic and nerve conduction studies	–	✔	–

References

1 Perkins J, Hammer RL, Loubert PV (1998) Identification and management of pregnancy-related low back pain. *J Nurse Midwifery* **43**, 331–340. Overview of recent research on pregnancy-related back pain. Two common back pain types are described and basic management techniques for women and primary caregivers are given. **IV C**

2 Ashkan K, Casey AT, Powell M *et al.* (1998) Back pain during pregnancy and after childbirth: an unusual cause not to miss. *J R Soc Med* **91**, 88–90. Case report of one antenatal and one postnatal patient presented with back pain, bilateral sciatica, motor weakness and sphincter involvement. Magnetic resonance imaging showed that both had a central disc prolapse L5–S1. Both required surgery. **IV C**

3 Magnusdottir R, Franklin J, Gestsson J (1996) Septic symphysial disruption presenting as severe symphysiolysis in pregnancy. *Acta Obstet Gynecol Scand* **75**, 681–682. Case report. **IV C**

37.2 Management of back and pelvic pain during pregnancy

Aneesa Lala

Management option	Quality of evidence	Strength of recommendation	References
Daily low back exercises and development of abdominal tone with standing, lateral bending and rotational trunk exercises	IV III	C B	1 2
The pelvic tilt exercise anecdotally provides marked relief of low back pain	IV III	C B	1 2
Simple measures taught in back-care programs, such as placing one foot on a foot stool when standing for a prolonged period, can give some relief	IV III	C B	1 2
For mild to moderate pain, general comfort measures (rest, activity modification) and physical therapy (massage and pelvic and low back exercises), as well as general back care, are helpful	IV III	C B	1 2
For night pain, the use of a 'maternity cushion' may give relief	Ib	A	3
Elastic compression stockings worn throughout the day may, by limiting lower extremity edema, diminish the fluid shifts and venous engorgement that occur at night	–	✔	–
Analgesic options are limited, and nonsteroidal anti-inflammatory drugs should be specifically avoided because of concern for potential adverse fetal effects	–	✔	–
Persistent pain not responsive to rest, including discogenic pain, may benefit from lumbar epidural steroids	–	✔	–
Transcutaneous electrical nerve stimulation may be helpful	–	✔	–
Muscle weakness is concerning, but only acute loss of bowel and bladder function or acute paralysis would indicate a need for decompressive surgery during pregnancy	IV	C	4
Mobilization techniques applied to the sacroiliac area have been reported to provide relief, commonly permanent, in some women	IV III	C B	1 2,5
Treatment with a trochanteric belt provides relief, particularly for women with posterior pelvic pain	IV III	C B	1,6 5
Sacroiliac injection with corticosteroids and local anesthetic may be indicated in severe cases	–	✔	–

References

1 Perkins J, Hammer RL, Loubert PV (1998) Identification and management of pregnancy-related low back pain. *J Nurse Midwifery* **43**, 331–340. Overview of recent research on pregnancy-related back pain. Two common back pain types are described and basic management techniques for women and primary caregivers are given. **IV C**

2 McIntyre IN, Broadhurst NA (1996) Effective treatment of low back pain in pregnancy. *Aust Fam Physician* **25**, S65–S67. Study of 20 patients treated with mobilizing techniques and home exercises. 15 had no pain and the remainder had a 50% improvement in their pain. Low back pain can be significantly improved with mobilization. **III B**

3 Young G, Jewell D (2000) Interventions for preventing and treating backache in pregnancy. In: *Cochrane Database of Systematic Reviews*, issue 2. Oxford: Update Software. 109 patient crossover trial. Comparison of Ozzlo pillow (special-shaped pillow to fit under women's abdomen) with a standard pillow. Women experience less back pain with the Ozzlo pillow (OR 0.32, 95%CI 0.18–0.58). **Ib A**

4 Ashkan K, Casey AT, Powell M *et al.* (1998) Back pain during pregnancy and after childbirth: an unusual cause not to miss. *J R Soc Med* **91**, 88–90. Case report of one antenatal and one postnatal patient presented with back pain, bilateral sciatica, motor weakness and sphincter involvement. Magnetic resonance imaging showed that both had a central disc prolapse L5–S1. Both required surgery. **IV C**

5 Berg G, Hammar M, Moller-Nielsen J *et al.* (1988) Low back pain during pregnancy. *Obstet Gynecol* **71**, 71–75. Questionnaire study. 862 women filled in a questionnaire in a Swedish antenatal clinic. 49% reported some form of low back pain. 79 were unable to continue work because of it. Most common etiology for severe low back pain was dysfunction of sacroiliac joints (51 women). 36 of these benefited from a trochanteric belt. **III B**

6 Ostgaard HC (1996) Assessment and treatment of low back pain in pregnant and working women. *Semin Perinatol* **20**, 61–69. Review. Defines backpain, suggests a method for classification and provides a model for treating pregnant women with these pain types. **IV C**

37.3 Scoliosis

Aneesa Lala

Management option		Quality of evidence	Strength of recommendation	References
Prepregnancy and prenatal	Curvature does not usually worsen	–	✔	–
	Compromise of respiratory function may occur in some (see Section 32.5)	–	✔	–
Labor and delivery	Regional analgesia may not be possible	–	✔	–
	Positioning for delivery may have to be individualized	–	✔	–
	For respiratory compromise see Section 32.5	–	✔	–

37.4 Pelvic arthropathy

Aneesa Lala

Management option	Quality of evidence	Strength of recommendation	References
Rest, with or without a pelvic band or girdle	–	✔	–
Analgesia and anti-inflammatory drugs	III	B	1
If this fails, consider injection of steroids and local anesthetic	III	B	1

Reference

1 Schwartz Z, Katz Z, Lancet M (1985) Management of puerperal separation of the symphysis pubis. *Int J Gynaecol Obstet* **23**, 125–128. Observational study of 13 postpartum patients with symphysiolysis treated by intrasymphysial injection of a combination of hydrocortisone, chymotrypsin and lidocaine. The injection was given once a day and the full treatment consisted of between three and seven injections according to the severity of the symptoms. No other medication was given. Immediate relief was obtained in all cases after the first injection and all symptoms disappeared after the completion of treatment. The average time of hospitalization was 9.8 days. No complications were seen as a result of the treatment and the patients resumed their normal activities after being discharged from hospital. In comparison with other modes of treatment, the intrasymphysial injection of the drug combination shortened the time of morbidity and effected complete recovery. **III B**

37.5 Rupture of the pubic symphysis

Aneesa Lala

Management option	Quality of evidence	Strength of recommendation	References
Treatment is generally nonsurgical, and complete recovery is to be expected	–	✔	–
Treat with steroids and anti-inflammatory drugs	IV	C	1
Treatment may begin with tight pelvic binding and rest in the lateral decubitus position	–	✔	–
Symptoms may last as little as 2 days, typically 8 weeks or reportedly up to 8 months	–	✔	–
For inadequate reduction, recurrent diastasis or persistent symptoms, external skeletal fixation is the treatment of choice to maintain stability while the ligaments heal	–	✔	–
Internal fixation by plate and screws or metallic cerclage wire is only considered in extreme cases	–	✔	–

Reference

1 Gonik B, Stringer A (1985) Post-partum osteitis pubis. *South Med J* **78**, 213–214. Case report, in which the patient presented 2 weeks postnatally with a rapid progression to inability to walk. X-rays showed typical appearance. Treatment was with strict bed rest and oral steroids. The prognosis for recovery is good. **IV C**

37.5 Hip problems

Aneesa Lala

Management option		Quality of evidence	Strength of recommendation	References
Transient osteoporosis	Conservation approach: limit weight-bearing, encourage movement, analgesia	IV	C	1
Avascular necrosis	As for transient osteoporosis (?separate entity)	–	✔	–
Hip arthroplasty	Usually no significant problem encountered nor special management required	–	✔	–

Reference

1 Bruinsam BJ, LaBan MM (1990) The ghost joint: transient osteoporosis of the hip. *Arch Phys Med Rehab* **71**, 295–298. Case report of three women in the third trimester experienced progressive hip pain upon weight-bearing, alleviated by rest and with minor limitations in range of movement. X-rays demonstrated varying degrees of osteopenia. Treatment is conservative and the condition is self-limiting. **IV C**

Chapter 38

Thromboembolic disease

38.1 Thromboembolic disease

Roy Farquharson

Treatment of established thromboembolism in pregnancy

Management option		Quality of evidence	Strength of recommendation	References
Initial management	Intravenous unfractionated heparin (UFH), 5000 IU loading dose then continuous 1000–2000 IU/h with daily surveillance for 1 week	Ib	A	1–3
	or Low-molecular-weight heparin (LMWH; e.g. Dalteparin 5000 IU three times daily subcutaneously) may be better alternative	Ib Ia	A A	4 5
	Control – double activated partial thromboplastin time (aPTT; UFH) or peak heparin level (anti-Xa) above 0.2 units/ml (LMWH)	Ib	A	3
Prenatal maintenance	UFH (10 000 IU s.c. twice daily) or LMWH (e.g. Dalteparin 5000 IU three times daily)	Ia	A	5
	Control – prolongation of APTT (1.5–2.5× control) for UFH; peak anti-Xa above 0.2 units/ml for LMWH	Ib IV	C A	3 6
Labor and delivery	Prophylaxis dose on day prior to induction, e.g. Dalteparin 5000 IU or UFH 7500 IU, both twice daily	III	B	7
	No further self-injection during labor	III	B	7
	Epidural block and instrumental delivery are not contraindicated if clotting normal	IV	C	8
Postnatal	Continue LMWH or UFH for 6 weeks	Ib IV	A C	3 9
	or At least 3 months anticoagulant treatment from thrombotic event	III IV	B C	7 9
	Checking maternal bone density is controversial	–	✔	–
	Repeat platelet count	–	✔	–
	Graduated elastic compression stockings worn for 2 years	Ib	A	10
	Breastfeeding is not contraindicated	III	B	11

References

1 Barritt DV, Jordan SC (1960) Anticoagulant drugs in the treatment of pulmonary embolism: a controlled trial. *Lancet* **1**, 1309–1312. RCT in nonpregnant patients with suspected pulmonary embolism, showing that treatment with anticoagulants (intravenous heparin and oral anticoagulants) reduced the risk of further thromboembolism compared to no treatment. **Ib A**

2 Brandjes DP, Heijboer H, Buller HR *et al.* (1992) Acenocoumarol and heparin compared with acenocoumarol alone in the initial treatment of proximal vein thrombosis. *N Engl J Med* **327**, 1485–1489. A double-blind trial of intravenous heparin plus oral anticoagulants versus oral anticoagulants alone in proven, proximal thrombosis showed inclusion of heparin reduced frequency of asymptomatic extension of deep venous thrombosis or pulmonary thromboembolism. **Ib A**

3 Hyers TM, Hull RD, Weg JG (1995) Antithrombotic therapy for venous thromboembolic disease. *Chest* **108**, 335–351. Two RCTs of unfractionated heparin in acute deep venous thrombosis showed that failure to achieve the appropriate therapeutic range of activated partial thromboplastin time was associated with a 10–15-fold increase in risk of recurrent venous thromboembolism. **Ib A**

4 Levine M, Gent M, Hirsh J *et al.* (1996) A comparison of low molecular weight heparin administered primarily at home with unfractionated heparin administered in hospital for proximal deep vein thrombosis. *N Engl J Med* **334**, 677–688. First paper to deal effectively with low-molecular-weight heparin (LMWH) efficacy, comparing low-cost domiciliary treatment versus hospitalized care. Showed clear benefit in favor of LMWH over unfractionated heparin and better compliance with patient-administered LMWH, and demonstrated full recovery and lower risk of embolism and clot propagation with LMWH. Findings applicable to pregnant population but untested as yet. **Ib A**

5 Gould MK, Dembitzer AD, Doyle RL *et al.* (1999) Low molecular weight heparins compared with unfractionated heparin for treatment of acute DVT. *Ann Intern Med* **130**, 800–809. Meta-analysis of all RCTs indicate that low-molecular-weight heparins and warfarin are more effective and are associated with fewer hemorrhagic complications and lower mortality than unfractionated heparin in the initial treatment of deep venous thrombosis. **Ia A**

6 Monreal M (2000) Long-term treatment of venous thromboembolism with low molecular weight heparin. *Curr Opin Pulm Med* **6**, 326–329. Women with antenatal venous thromboembolism can be managed with adjusted dose regimen of subcutaneous low-molecular-weight or unfractionated heparin for remainder of pregnancy but heparin handling altered in favor of heparin resistance so increased doses are required with advancing pregnancy. **IV C**

7 Toglia MR, Weg JG (1996) Venous thromboembolism during pregnancy. *N Engl J Med* **335**, 108–114. Good review and analysis of quality observational studies on antepartum and intrapartum use of heparin. **III B**

8 Checketts MR, Wildsmith JA (1999) Central nerve block and thromboprophylaxis – is there a problem? *Br J Anaesth* **82**, 164–167. The use of epidural block is not contraindicated as long as surveillance of clotting parameters is constantly maintained. **IV C**

9 Ginsberg JS, Greer I, Hirsh J (2001) Use of antithrombotic agents during pregnancy. *Chest* **119**(1 suppl), 122S–131S. Opinion on recommendation for 3 months' use of anticoagulant therapy since thrombotic event or use for at least 6 weeks postpartum. **IV C**

10 Brandjes DP, Buller HR, Heijboer H *et al.* (1997) Randomised trial of effect of compression stockings in patients with proximal venous thrombosis. *Lancet* **349**, 759–762. RCT showing a reduction in postthrombotic syndrome from 23% to 11% over a 2-year period of use. **Ib A**

11 Orme ML, Lewis PJ, de Swiet M *et al.* (1977) May mothers given warfarin breast-feed their infants? *Br Med J* **1**, 1564–1565. First paper to measure warfarin levels in breast milk and provide reassurance that breastfeeding is safe for infant. **III B**

Thromboembolism prophylaxis

Management option		Quality of evidence	Strength of recommendation	References
Low-risk patients (one previous episode, no thrombophilia, no family history)	Aspirin 75 mg from booking – watch for gastrointestinal side effects	Ia	A	1,2
	Start low-molecular-weight heparin (LMWH; e.g. Dalteparin 5000 IU s.c. daily) or unfractionated heparin (UFH) 7500 IU s.c. twice daily after delivery	Ia	A	3
	Continue LMWH or UFH for 6 weeks postnatally or convert to oral warfarin after 1 week of heparin	–	✔	–
	Breastfeeding is not contraindicated	–	✔	–

Management option		Quality of evidence	Strength of recommendation	References
High-risk patients (one previous episode and thrombophilia or family history)	Start LMWH, e.g. Dalteparin 5000 IU s.c. daily, increasing to twice daily after 20 weeks gestation or UFH 10 000 IU s.c. twice daily from booking	Ia	A	3
	Continue LMWH or UFH 7500 IU s.c. twice daily or LMWH in labor	–	✔	–
	Continue UFH or LMWH for 1 week	–	✔	–
	Then UFH, LMWH or warfarin for 5 weeks	–	✔	–
	Breastfeeding is not contraindicated	–	✔	–
Thrombo-prophylaxis for cesarean section	**Low risk:** early mobilization and hydration	IV	C	4
	Medium risk: s.c. heparin or stockings	Ia IV	A C	1 4
	High risk: heparin and stockings	Ia IV	A C	1 4

References

1 Amarigiri SV, Lees TA (2000) Elastic compression stockings for prevention of deep venous thrombosis. In: *Cochrane database of systematic reviews*, issue 4. Oxford: Update Software. 16 RCTs were identified. Graduated compression stockings (GCS) were applied on the day before surgery or on the day of surgery. They were worn until discharge or until the patients were fully mobile. In the majority of the included studies, deep venous thrombosis (DVT) was identified by radioactive iodine-125 uptake test. Nine RCTs were identified that tested the efficacy of GCS alone. In the treatment group of 624 patients, 81 developed DVT (13%) in comparison to the control group of 581 patients, where 154 (27%) had DVT (Peto's OR 0.34, 95% CI 0.25–0.46), favoring treatment with GCS. Seven RCTs were identified that tested GCS on a background of another prophylactic method. In the treatment group of 501 patients, 10 (2%) developed DVT whereas, in the control group of 505 patients, 74 (15%) developed DVT (OR 0.24, 95% CI 0.15–0.37). **Ia A**

2 Derry S, Loke YK (2000) Risk of gastrointestinal haemorrhage with long term use of aspirin: meta-analysis. *Br Med J* **321**, 1183–1188. Long-term use of low-dose aspirin carries an increased risk of gastrointestinal hemorrhage, occurring in approximately 2.3% of users from a meta-analysis of 24 RCTs. **Ia A**

3 Van den Belt AGM, Prins MH, Lensing AW *et al.* (2000) Fixed dose subcutaneous low molecular weight heparins versus adjusted dose unfractionated heparin for venous thromboembolism. In: *Cochrane database of systematic reviews*, issue 4. Oxford: Update Software. Meta-analysis of 14 studies showing that low-molecular-weight heparin is at least as effective as unfractionated heparin in preventing recurrent venous thromboembolism and significantly reduces risk of hemorrhage during initial treatment and overall mortality at end of follow-up. **Ia A**

4 Royal College of Obstetricians and Gynaecologists (1995) *Report of the RCOG working party on prophylaxis against thromboembolism in gynaecology and obstetrics*. London: RCOG. Consensus review and report. **IV C**

Chapter 39

Dermatological problems

39.1 Preexisting skin disorders

Fiona Fairlie

Infections

See Chapter 24.

Collagen vascular disease

Management option		Quality of evidence	Strength of recommendation	References
Systemic lupus erythematosus	Maternal skin and joint exacerbations respond to prednisolone (prednisone)	–	✔	–
	Fetal/neonatal lupus erythematosus: ❑ Skin biopsy if diagnosis uncertain ❑ Screen fetus/newborn for heart block (see Section 17.1 for management) ❑ Document maternal and neonatal anti-Ro, anti-La and anti-RNP status ❑ Electrocardiogram, liver function, platelets in newborn ❑ Topical steroids, protect from ultraviolet light	–	✔	–
Dermato-myositis/ polymyositis	**First attack in pregnancy:** ❑ Poor prognosis ❑ Prednisolone (prednisone; methotrexate as second line) ❑ Vigilance for intrauterine growth restriction and preterm labor ❑ Consider assisted vaginal delivery	–	✔	–
	Pre-existing disease: ❑ Prednisolone (prednisone) for exacerbation	–	✔	–
Systemic sclerosis	See Section 36.4			
Pseudo-xanthoma elasticum	Cervical suture if recurrent miscarriage	–	✔	–
	Monitor blood pressure and prompt treatment of hypertension	–	✔	–
	Monitor fetal growth and health	–	✔	–
See also Chapter 36.				

Tumors

Management option		Quality of evidence	Strength of recommendation	References
Malignant melanoma	Prompt excision	Ib IV	A C	1 2
Other tumors	Monitor blood pressure in patients with neurofibromatosis	–	✔	–

References

1 Crosby T, Manson D, Crosby D (2000) Malignant melanoma: non-metastatic. *Clin Evidence* **4**, 985–992. Narrow primary excision is as effective as wide excision with respect to overall survival and reduces the need for skin grafts. **Ib A**

2 Squatrito RC, Harlow SP (1998) Melanoma complicating pregnancy. *Obstet Gynecol Clin North Am* **25**, 407–416. Surgical treatment during pregnancy should be prompt. There is insufficient evidence to advocate the use of adjuvant therapy during pregnancy. **IV C**

Metabolic diseases

Management option		Quality of evidence	Strength of recommendation	References
Porphyria	Vigilance for recurrence/exacerbation	–	✔	–
	Consider venesection	–	✔	–
	Avoid chloroquine in first trimester	–	✔	–
	Avoid precipitating drugs	–	✔	–
Acrodermatitis enteropathica	Zinc supplementation	–	✔	–
	Careful screening for fetal normality	–	✔	–

Other skin diseases

Management option		Quality of evidence	Strength of recommendation	References
Generalized pustular psoriasis	Monitor maternal cardiac and renal function	–	✔	–
	Monitor fetal growth and health	–	✔	–
	High-dose corticosteroids	–	✔	–
	Methotrexate and cyclosporin A are second-line drugs	–	✔	–
	Vigilance for intrauterine growth restriction	–	✔	–
	Monitor maternal blood pressure, renal, cardiac and pulmonary function	–	✔	–
Pemphigus	Control maternal lesions with steroids	–	✔	–
	Monitor fetal growth and health	–	✔	–
	Examine newborn for lesions	–	✔	–

Connective tissue disorders

Management option		Quality of evidence	Strength of recommendation	References
Ehlers–Danlos syndrome	Prepregnancy counsel against conception	–	✔	–
	Vigilance for postpartum hemorrhage, wound dehiscence, rupture of viscera	–	✔	–
	Intravenous access and crossmatch blood for delivery	–	✔	–
	Avoid excessive trauma at operative delivery	–	✔	–
	Nonabsorbable sutures for cesarean section	–	✔	–
	Consider termination of pregnancy if no response to therapy	–	✔	–
Eczema	Emollients, soap substitutes, 1% hydrocortisone cream	Ia Ib	A A	1,2 3
Epidermolysis bullosa	Offer fetal skin biopsy for severe hereditary forms	–	✔	–
	Avoid skin trauma/irritation	–	✔	–

References

1 Kramer MS (2002) Maternal antigen avoidance during lactation for preventing atopic disease in infants of women at high risk. In: *Cochrane Database of Systematic Reviews*, issue 1. Oxford: Update Software. This review includes three trials involving 209 women. Although the combination data suggest that antigen avoidance diet in high-risk women during lactation may reduce the risk of atopic eczema, the trials have methodological shortcomings. The reviewers advise caution in applying the results. **Ia A**

2 Kramer MS (2002) Maternal antigen avoidance during pregnancy for preventing atopic disease in infants of women at high risk. In: *Cochrane Database of Systematic Reviews*, issue 1. Oxford: Update Software. Three trials involving 504 women are included in this review. The reviewers conclude that an antigen avoidance diet for high-risk women is unlikely to reduce their risk of giving birth to an atopic child. Such a diet could have an adverse effect of maternal and/or fetal nutrition. **Ia A**

3 Kramer MS (2002) Maternal antigen avoidance during lactation for preventing atopic eczema in infants. In: *Cochrane Database of Systematic Reviews*, issue 1. Oxford: Update Software. This review includes only one small trial, which reported a nonsignificant reduction in eczema severity associated with maternal antigen avoidance. The result should be interpreted with caution. **Ib A**

39.2 Pruritus in pregnancy

Fiona Fairlie

Management option		Quality of evidence	Strength of recommendation	References
Establish the diagnosis	Consider: ❑ Specific disorders and systemic diseases with skin involvement (see above) ❑ Other systemic diseases with pruritus (lymphoma, liver, thyroid) ❑ If rash present, consider pregnancy-specific dermatoses (see below) ❑ Pruritus gravidarum/obstetric cholestasis	–	✔	–

➡

Management option		Quality of evidence	Strength of recommendation	References
Management	Depends on cause – for **pruritus gravidarum/obstetric cholestasis:**			
	❑ Monitor fetal growth and health	III	B	1,2
		IIb	B	3
	❑ Delivery is the definitive treatment (induction of labor at 37–38 weeks)	–	✓	–
	❑ Monitor fetal health in labor	–	✓	–
	❑ Maternal treatment:			
	❑ – Cholestyramine (+ vitamin K)	–	✓	–
	❑ – Adenosyl-L-methionine	Ib	A	4,5
	❑ – Dexamethasone	III	B	6
	❑ – Ursodeoxycholic acid	Ib	A	5,7–9

References

1 Alsulyman OM, Ouzounian JG, Ames-Castro M, Goodwin TM (1996) Intrahepatic cholestasis of pregnancy: perinatal outcome associated with expectant management. *Am J Obstet Gynecol* **175**, 957–960. Perinatal outcome of 79 pregnancies with a clinical diagnosis of intrahepatic cholestasis of pregnancy was compared with 79 controls with a history of stillbirth – both groups underwent the same antepartum testing schemes. Two stillbirths occurred in the cholestasis group within 5 days of normal antepartum testing. Conclusion: conventional fetal surveillance may not predict adverse fetal outcome in intrahepatic cholestasis of pregnancy. **III B**

2 Fisk NM, Storey GNB (1988) Fetal outcome in obstetric cholestasis. *Br J Obstet Gynaecol* **95**, 1137–1143. Describes the outcome of 83 pregnancies complicated by obstetric cholestasis between 1975 and 1984. Management was at the discretion of the individual obstetrician but antenatal fetal monitoring and induction of labor were increasingly employed during the study period. The authors concluded that intensive fetal surveillance and induction of labor at term may reduce stillbirth rates in obstetric cholestasis. **III B**

3 Rioseco AJ, Ivankovic MB, Manzur A *et al.* (1994) Intrahepatic cholestasis of pregnancy: a retrospective case control study of perinatal outcome. *Am J Obstet Gynecol* **170**, 890–895. 320 women with cholestasis of pregnancy diagnosed by clinical criteria were compared to a control group comprising women who delivered immediately after a case of cholestasis. The cholestasis group was subject to daily fetal movement counts, weekly fetal heart rate recordings from 34 weeks and delivery at 38 weeks. Perinatal outcome in the cholestasis group was equal to that of the control group and better than previously reported for cholestasis of pregnancy. IIb B

4 Ribalta J, Reyes H, Gonzalez MC *et al.* (1991) *S*-Adenosyl-L-methionine in the treatment of patients with obstetric cholestasis of pregnancy: a randomized, double-blind, placebo-controlled study with negative results. *Hepatology* **13**, 1084–1089. Randomized double-blind placebo-controlled study. 18 women with pruritus, raised levels of bile acids and liver function tests were randomized to receive either intravenous *S*-adenosyl-L-methionine 800 mg or intravenous placebo daily for 20 days. No difference was observed during treatment between the two groups with respect to severity of pruritus or biochemical parameters. **Ib A**

5 Nicastri PL, Diaferia A, Tartagni M *et al.* (1998) A randomised placebo-controlled trial of ursodeoxycholic acid and *S*-adenosylmethionine in the treatment of intrahepatic cholestasis of pregnancy. *Br J Obstet Gynaecol* **105**, 1205–1207. 32 women with obstetric cholestasis were randomized into four groups receiving either ursodeoxycholic acid or *S*-adenosylmethionine, or a combination of both drugs, or placebo. Pruritus and biochemical abnormalities improved in all groups. A combination of ursodeoxycholic acid and *S*-adenosylmethionine was more effective than placebo or either drug alone. **Ib A**

6 Hirvioja ML, Timala R, Vuori J (1992) The treatment of obstetric cholestasis of pregnancy by dexamethasone. *Br J Obstet Gynaecol* **99**, 109–111. Observational study of 10 women diagnosed with intrahepatic cholestasis of pregnancy between 28 and 37 weeks. Daily treatment with 12 mg oral dexamethasone for 7 days was associated with disappearance or lessening of itching in all women and a fall in total bile acid levels. The authors concluded that a more extensive placebo-controlled study was required to confirm or refute this observation. **III B**

7 Floreani A, Paternoster D, Melis A *et al.* (1996) *S*-Adenosylmethionine versus ursodeoxycholic acid in the treatment of obstetric cholestasis of pregnancy: preliminary results in a controlled trial. *Eur J Obstet Gynaecol Reprod Biol* **67**, 109–113. 20 women with intrahepatic cholestasis were randomized to receive either *S*-adenosylmethionine (1000 mg daily intramuscularly) or ursodeoxycholic acid (450 mg daily) for at least 15 days before delivery. Ursodeoxycholic acid was more effective than *S*-adenosylmethionine in controlling pruritus and reducing bile acid levels. **Ib A**

8 Palma J, Reyes H, Ribalta J *et al.* (1997) Ursodeoxycholic acid in the treatment of cholestasis of pregnancy: a randomized, double-blind study controlled with placebo. *J Hepatol* **27**, 1022–1028. 15 women with pruritus,

abnormal levels of bile salts and aminotransferases presenting before 33 weeks gestation were randomized to receive either oral ursodeoxycholic acid 1 mg daily or placebo. Treatment with ursodeoxycholic acid was associated with a significant improvement in pruritus, serum bilirubin and aminotransferase levels compared with placebo. All women who received ursodeoxycholic acid delivered a healthy baby near term. In the placebo group there were 5 deliveries before 36 weeks, including one stillbirth. **Ib A**

9 Diaferia A, Nicastri PL, Tartagni M et al. (1996) Ursodeoxycholic acid therapy in pregnant women with cholestasis. *Int J Gynaecol Obstet* **52**, 133–140. 16 women with obstetric cholestasis were randomized to receive either ursodeoxycholic acid 600 mg daily (8 women) or placebo (8 women) for 20 days. The group receiving ursodeoxycholic acid showed a significant improvement in pruritus and biochemical parameters compared with the placebo group. **Ib A**

39.3 Rashes in pregnancy

Fiona Fairlie

Management option		**Quality of evidence**	**Strength of recommendation**	**References**
Establish the cause	Two possibilities: ❑ Preexisting skin conditions (see above) ❑ Dermatoses of pregnancy (DOP)	 – –	 ✔ ✔	 – –
DOP 1: Polymorphic eruption of pregnancy	Consider skin biopsy (if atypical or severe)	IV	C	1
	Explanation and reassurance	–	✔	–
	If treatment is required: ❑ Oral antihistamine (e.g. chlorpheniramine) ❑ Topical corticosteroids (moderate potency) ❑ Oral prednisolone (prednisone)	 Ib – III	 A ✔ B	 2 – 3
DOP 2: Pruritic folliculitis of pregnancy	Consider skin biopsy (if severe)	IV	C	1
	Explanation and reassurance	–	✔	–
	If treatment is required, topical 10% benzoyl peroxide or 1% hydrocortisone	–	✔	–
DOP 3: Prurigo of pregnancy	Explanation and reassurance	–	✔	–
	If treatment is required: ❑ Topical corticosteroids (moderate potency) ❑ Oral antihistamines	 – Ib	 ✔ A	 – 2
DOP 4: Pemphigoid gestationis	Skin biopsy if doubt about diagnosis	IV	C	1
	Oral antihistamines	–	✔	–
	Topical corticosteroids (moderate potency)	–	✔	–
	If severe/resistant form, oral prednisolone	–	✔	–
	Plasmapheresis if prednisolone fails	IV	C	4
	Monitor fetal growth and health (risk uncertain)	–	✔	–
DOP 5: Impetigo herpetiformis	Try high-dose oral prednisolone	–	✔	–
	Monitor maternal cardiac and renal function	–	✔	–
	Delivery is usually curative (with dexamethasone/betamethasone if preterm)	–	✔	–

References

1. Saurat J-H (1989) Immunofluorescence biopsy of pruritic urticarial papules and plaques of pregnancy. *J Am Acad Dermatol* **20**, 711. A letter supporting immunofluorescence biopsy for all cases of clinically typical pruritic urticarial papules and plaques of pregnancy with the purpose of confirming diagnosis and excluding other skin conditions. In the author's experience of more than 100 such cases, biopsy had revealed 2 women with herpes gestationis. **IV C**
2. Young GL, Jewell D (2002) Antihistamines versus aspirin for itching in late pregnancy. In: *Cochrane Database of Systematic Reviews*, issue 1. Oxford: Update Software. Only one trial involving 36 women is included in this review. Aspirin (600 mg four times daily) was compared with chlorpenamine (chlorpheniramine; 4 mg three times daily) for treating itching in late pregnancy. Aspirin was more effective in the absence of a skin rash but chlorphenamine (chlorpheniramine) was more effective if a rash was present. **Ib A**
3. Lawley TJ, Hertz KC, Wade TR *et al.* (1979) Pruritic urticarial papules and plaques of pregnancy. *JAMA* **241**, 1696–1699. Describes 7 cases of pruritic urticarial papules and plaques of pregnancy, 5 treated with steroid cream and 2 with oral prednisolone (prednisone). Treatment was associated with symptomatic relief in 5 cases. **III B**
4. Van de Wiel A, Hart HC, Flinterman J *et al.* (1980) Plasma exchange in herpes gestationis. *Br Med J* **281**, 1041–1042. Case report of a woman with histologically proven herpes gestationis from 20 weeks gestation unresponsive to antihistamines and pyridoxine. Authors withheld steroids because of pregnancy and hypertension but observed a rapid response to plasma exchange. **IV C**

Chapter 40

Benign gynecological disease

40.1 Subfertility

Ian Mahady and Farah Siddiqui

Management option		Quality of evidence	Strength of recommendation	References
Prepregnancy	Check for underlying medical disease (e.g. hypertension, diabetes, renal disease, chlamydial infection)	–	✔	–
	Commence folic acid	III	B	1
	Ensure rubella-immune	III	B	2,3
	Protocols to avoid hyperstimulation and multiple pregnancy	III	B	4
	Counsel about risks of aneuploidy with older mothers	–	✔	–
	Couples where the male partner has obstructive azoospermia should be screened for cystic fibrosis carrier status; males should also be screened for Y chromosome deletions	III	B	5
Prenatal	Check viability and number of intrauterine pregnancies	III	B	6
	Diagnose ectopic pregnancy early	–	✔	–
	Check progesterone levels until 12 weeks in those requiring clomiphene citrate or gonadotropin therapy	–	✔	–
	Screen for hypertension and gestational diabetes in women with polycystic ovary syndrome	IIb	B	7
	Check fetal growth and normality in *in-vitro*-fertilization pregnancies	–	✔	–
	Multiple pregnancies, see Chapter 45			
	Reassurance	IIb	B	8
Labor and delivery	Continuous fetal heart rate monitoring for psychological reasons	IIb	B	8
Postnatal	Contraception not usually an issue	–	✔	–
	Avoid intrauterine contraceptive devices with history of tubal disease	–	✔	–
	Avoid progestogens with a history of ovulatory disorders	–	✔	–

References

1 Whiteman D, Murphy M, Hey K *et al.* (2000) Reproductive factors, subfertility, and risk of neural tube defects: a case-control study based on the Oxford Record Linkage Study Register. *Am J Epidemiol* **152**, 823–828. This retrospective case-controlled study examined 694 women diagnosed with a neural tube defect in Oxfordshire or West Berkshire, UK. No evidence was found that the risk of neural-tube-defect (NTD)-affected pregnancies was increased by either subfertility or its treatment. After adjustment, NTD-affected pregnancies were associated with female offspring, multiple and higher numbers of pregnancies. The findings from this large, population-based study found no increased risk of NTD associated with exposure to fertility treatments but reported associations with various pregnancy outcomes. **III B**

2 Gyorkos TW, Tannenbaum TN, Abrahamowicz M *et al.* (1998) Evaluation of rubella screening in pregnant women. *Can Med Assoc J* **159**, 1091–1097. This was a cross-sectional study performed in 16 randomly selected hospitals in Quebec. The aim of the study was to assess the effectiveness of the prenatal rubella screening program. 2551 patients were selected randomly. The results showed that the overall screening rate was 94%. The larger hospitals had a higher screening rate than the smaller hospitals. **III B**

3 McElhaney RD Jr, Ringer M, DeHart DJ, Vasilenko P (1999) Rubella immunity in a cohort of pregnant women. *Infect Control Hosp Epidemiol* **20**, 64–66. Prospective cohort study of 350 pregnant women in Michigan, USA. The study reported that 15.1% of these women were not immune to rubella and that vaccination opportunities were missed. **III B**

4 Evans MI, Littman L, St Louis L *et al.* (1995) Evolving patterns of iatrogenic multifetal pregnancy generation: implications for aggressiveness of infertility treatments. *Am J Obstet Gynecol* **172**, 1750–1755. The methods of infertility treatment, number of fetuses and outcomes of 220 patients referred for multifetal pregnancy reduction were compared. Clomiphene, human menopausal gonadotropin and ovulation stimulation with urofollitropin were compared against gamete intrafallopian transfer, zygote intrafallopian transfer and *in-vitro* fertilization (assisted reproductive techniques). The proportion of multifetal pregnancies generated by assisted reproductive techniques has steadily risen from 26% to nearly half in the last 2 years. However, the number and proportion of quintuplet and greater pregnancies from assisted reproductive techniques have steadily fallen, while for ovulation stimulation the proportion has remained about one third. **III B**

5 Oliva R, Margarit E, Ballesca JL *et al.* (1998) Prevalence of Y chromosome microdeletions in oligospermic and azoospermic candidates for intracytoplasmic sperm injection. *Fertil Steril* **70**, 506–510. Prospective clinical study of patients recruited from the male infertility clinic. 186 men who were seen at an infertility clinic and who were referred to a genetic counseling service for genetic assessment before intracytoplasmic sperm injection; 50 of the men had azoospermia. The results demonstrated that 5.4% of the patients had Yq microdeletions. The number of microdeletions was much higher in azoospermic patients (8/50, 16%) than in oligospermic patients (2/136, 1.5%). Two of the azoospermic patients with Yq microdeletions also had sex chromosome aneuploidy mosaicism. No microdeletions were detected in 100 consecutively seen fathers who were included as controls. **III B**

6 Dunn A, Macfarlane A (1996) Recent trends in the incidence of multiple births and associated mortality in England and Wales. *Arch Dis Child Fetal Neonat Ed* **75**, F10–F19. This retrospective study reviewed the trends in multiple births and associated mortality in England and Wales since 1975, the extent of any association between multiple birth rates and assisted conception and drugs used for subfertility. The proportion of pregnancies that resulted in registered multiple births increased from a low of 9.9/1000 in 1975 to 13.6/1000 in 1994. The rise in the rate of triplet and other higher-order births was much steeper than that for all multiple births, increasing from 0.13 sets of triplets per 1000 maternities in 1975 to 0.41 in 1994. Prescriptions dispensed for selected drugs that may be used for the medical management of subfertility and assisted conception became more common over this period. **III B**

7 Wortsman J, de Angeles S, Futterweit W *et al.* (1991) Gestational diabetes and neonatal macrosomia in the polycystic ovary syndrome. *J Reprod Med* **36**, 659–661. Observational study of the incidence of gestational diabetes in 53 patients with polycystic ovary syndrome (PCOS) in comparison with over 2000 controls. The incidence of gestational diabetes in the PCOS patients was 7.5%, similar to the 6.6% frequency of gestational diabetes in the controls. The overall incidence of neonatal macrosomia (birthweight greater than 4000 g) was 7% (4 of 57) among infants born to PCOS women. That was similar to the 12.4% incidence of neonatal macrosomia among infants born to women with normal glucose tolerance and to the 14.5% incidence among infants born to women with gestational diabetes. Preexisting PCOS does not appear to increase the risk of developing gestational diabetes or neonatal macrosomia. **IIb B**

8 Black BP, Holditch-Davies D, Sandelowski M et al. (1995) Comparison of pregnancy symptoms of infertile and fertile couples. *J Perinat Neonat Nurs* **9**, 1–9. This study was undertaken to describe the most common symptoms experienced during pregnancy by couples with a history of infertility and to compare them with symptoms of expectant couples without a history of reproductive problems. The 10 most frequent symptoms reported and their rank order were very similar for the women from both groups. Men from the two groups frequently reported similar symptoms but differed on their rank order. This research provides evidence that in terms of pregnancy symptoms infertile and fertile couples are more alike than they are different. **IIb B**

40.2 Ovarian cysts

Ian Mahady and Farah Siddiqui

Management option		Quality of evidence	Strength of recommendation	References
Prepregnancy	Termination is rarely indicated	–	✔	–
	Treat symptomatic cysts, those that are sonolucent or echogenic cysts 8 cm or more in diameter	III	B	1
Prenatal	Treat ovarian hyperstimulation symptomatically; do not aspirate cysts but pleuro- or paracentesis for effusions/ascites may be necessary	–	✔	–
	Functional corpus luteum cysts regress by 16 cm	III	B	2
	Remove symptomatic cysts acutely	–	✔	–
	Laparotomy (not laparoscopy) to examine cysts 8 cm in diameter or more. Leave cysts due to endometriosis and tuberculosis; remove others. Ideal time for surgery is 18–20 weeks	III	B	3–5
	Progesterone support if corpus luteum cyst is removed before 10 weeks	III	B	6,7
	Tocolysis to cover operation and postoperative period	–	✔	–
	Avoid cyst aspiration (risk of missing malignancy)	III	B	8
Labor and delivery	For cysts impacted in pouch of Douglas perform lower segment cesarian section and ovarian cystectomy rather than cyst aspiration	–	✔	–

References

1 Kobayashi H, Yoshida A, Kobayashi M *et al.* (1997) Changes in size of the functional cyst on ultrasonography during early pregnancy. *Am J Perinatol* **14**, 1–4. Retrospective cohort study of 58 pregnant patients based in Japan. Of the 58 cases, 7 cases of functional cysts over 6cm in diameter and 5 cases after 15 weeks were observed. Percentage changes in cyst size per week of gestation were calculated and measured at weekly intervals. The results showed that the maximum cyst size is reached at about 7 weeks, with gradual diminution thereafter, and that the sonolucent ovarian cyst may be followed as a functional cyst, even if it is large or persists after 14 weeks. **III B**

2 Hill LM, Connors-Beaty DJ, Nowak A *et al.* (1998) The role of ultrasonography in the detection and management of adnexal masses during the second and third trimesters of pregnancy. *Am J Obstet Gynecol* **179**, 703–707. Prospective cohort study consisted of 7996 pregnant women between 13.0 and 42.8 weeks gestation. A total of 328 women in the study group (4.1%) had 335 ultrasonographically detectable adnexal masses; 309 of the masses were unilocular or had a single, thin septation and 26 were architecturally complex. Of the ovarian cysts 252 of 309 (81.6%) had a mean diameter of less than 3.0 cm; 60% of the 252 patients in this subgroup had serial ultrasonographic examinations; 43 of the unilocular cysts resolved and 17 have persisted for up to 2 years. There is a statistically significant trend toward decreasing frequency of ovarian cysts with increasing gestational age (χ^2 for linear trend; $p < 0.00001$). 18 of the 7996 had an exploratory laparotomy (one operation per 444 deliveries) during pregnancy or in the postpartum period. Pathologically confirmed lesions included 8 benign cystic teratomas, 3 mucinous cyst adenomas, 2 paratubal cysts, 2 corpus lutea, one serous cystadenoma, one follicular cyst, one endometrioma and one ovarian fibroma. **III B**

3 Yuen PM, Chang AMZ (1997) Laparoscopic management of adnexal mass during pregnancy. *Acta Obstet Gynecol Scand* **76**, 173–176. This is an observational study of six cases of pregnant women with asymptomatic adnexal masses detected by ultrasound carried out for gestational assessment. The masses were removed by laparoscopic

surgery at 13–15 weeks gestation. The size of the mass was not defined. Cystectomy or oophorectomy was performed using the bag retrieval technique. Median operating time was 37.5 min. No complications were reported and all patients were discharged on the second day. All pregnancies progressed to normal vaginal delivery. **III B**

4 Lachman E, Schienfeld A, Voss E *et al.* (1999) Pregnancy and laparoscopic surgery. *J Am Assoc Gynecol Laparosc* **6**, 347–351. Review of 518 reports in the literature of laparoscopic surgery in pregnancy. The most common procedure was a cholecystectomy (45%), followed by adnexal surgery (34%), appendectomy (15%) and other operations (6%). 33% were performed in the first trimester, 56% in the second and 11% in the third trimester. This review concludes that laparoscopy in pregnancy appears to be safe when performed by an experienced practitioner. **III B**

5 Mettler, L (2001) The cystic adnexal mass: patient selection, surgical techniques and long-term follow-up. *Curr Opin Obstet Gynecol* **13**, 389–397. Retrospective study of 641 patients treated surgically for an adnexal mass. Of 641 ovarian tumors, 76.9% (493) were treated by primary laparoscopy and 21.5% (138) by primary laparotomy. The criteria for laparotomy were either a high suspicion of malignancy or tumor size greater than 10 cm. Data were also reviewed concerning pregnant women who required surgery at the hospital (n = 26) and their fetal outcome. Although an adverse fetal outcome was suspected, 24 of the 26 patients delivered between 37 and 40 weeks gestation. One perinatal death and one abortion occurred. **III B**

6 Usui R, Minakami H, Kosuge S *et al.* (2000) Retrospective survey of clinical, pathologic, and prognostic features of adnexal masses operated on during pregnancy. *J Obstet Gynaecol Res* **26**, 89–93. Retrospective study of 69 patients with adnexal masses managed surgically during pregnancy. The pathologic features of the 69 lesions were as follows: 33 mature cystic teratomas, 13 functional cysts, 8 mucinous cystadenomas, 6 endometriotic cysts, 4 paraovarian cysts, 3 serous cystadenomas and 2 malignant neoplasms. 7 (12%) gave birth before 37 weeks of gestation, while 2 (3.3%) experienced spontaneous abortions. There were 3 perinatal deaths among the 60 infants. The results suggest that an adnexal mass might be associated with an adverse fetal outcome. Surgical intervention before 24 weeks of gestation might not *per se* have been related to the adverse outcomes. **III B**

7 Perkins KY, Johnson JL, Kay HH (1997) Simple ovarian cysts. Clinical features on a first-trimester ultrasound scan. *J Reprod Med* **42**, 440–444. Prospective study of 1001 pregnant patients scanned in the first trimester. Relationships were determined between the presence of a cyst and first-trimester pregnancy outcomes, including progression beyond the first trimester, blighted ovum, ectopic pregnancy and fetal demise. A simple ovarian cyst was observed in 29% of patients. Cysts were seen less often after 8 weeks gestation, and there was an equal distribution between those on the right and those on the left side of the pelvis. Cyst diameters did not vary with gestational age and most mean diameters were within a range of 1–3 cm. The absence of a cyst was more often associated with a blighted ovum on follow-up ultrasound scan (RR 2.8) but its presence or absence did not correlate with failure to progress beyond the first trimester, ectopic pregnancy or intrauterine fetal demise. The presence of simple ovarian cysts in the first trimester, which may represent corpus luteal cysts, appears to support early pregnancy development due to its association with a lower incidence of blighted ova. **III B**

8 Caspi B, Ben-Arie A, Appelman Z *et al.* (2000) Aspiration of simple pelvic cysts during pregnancy. *Gynecol Obstet Invest* **49**, 102–105. Study of 10 cases of simple ovarian cysts treated with sonographically guided cyst aspiration. 5 of the women did not require further treatment; the remaining patients required later definitive surgery. **III B**

40.3 Fibroids

Ian Mahady and Farah Siddiqui

Management option		Quality of evidence	Strength of recommendation	References
Prepregnancy	Remove endometrial/submucous fibroid polyps hysteroscopically	III	B	1–3
	Consider myomectomy for other fibroids if symptomatic and only after careful counseling	IIa (Ia	B A	4 1, p. 312)
Prenatal	Red degeneration: bed rest, analgesics, local heat/ice	III	B	5
	Removal of a pedunculated serosal fibroid producing severe symptoms should be rare	–	✔	–
	Ligate and avulse cervical fibroid polyps	–	✔	–

Management option		Quality of evidence	Strength of recommendation	References
Prenatal (cont'd)	Consider elective lower segment cesarian section (LSCS) if: ❑ Lower segment/cervical fibroids causing unstable lie or failure of engagement of fetal head ❑ Previous myomectomy for intramural fibroids	III	B	6
Labor and delivery	LSCS if fibroid leads to obstructed labor	III	B	7
	Vigilance for postpartum hemorrhage	–	✔	–
	Do not remove fibroids at LSCS	–	✔	–
	If delivery is by cesarean section only consider classical/upper segment approach if access through lower segment with 2–3 cm of normal tissue is not possible	III	B	6,8,9
Postnatal	Analgesia if excessive pain (?GnRH analog in extreme cases)	–	✔	–
See also Section 43.4.				

References

1 Narayan R, Rajat, Goswamy K (1994) Treatment of submucous fibroids, and outcome of assisted conception. *J Am Assoc Gynecol Laparosc* **1**, 307–311. This study of 100 women took place at an infertility clinic in London, UK and investigates the effect of hysteroscopic resection and goserelin in the treatment of submucous fibroids and their significance in assisted conception. Patients with history of subfertility and previous failed attempts at assisted conception were examined by transvaginal sonography before further attempts at assisted conception. Those diagnosed as having submucous fibroids were treated with goserelin injections, hysteroscopic resection or a combination of both. Saline sonohysterography was performed whenever the submucous nature of the fibroid was unclear. All patients underwent assisted conception within 3 months unless they conceived spontaneously in the interim. Their results concluded that submucous fibroids are a significant cause of subfertility. A combination of goserelin injections and hysteroscopic resection significantly improves pregnancy rates without increasing the miscarriage rate. **III B**

2 Rossetti A, Sizzi O, Soranna L *et al.* (2001) Fertility outcome: long-term results after laparoscopic myomectomy. *Gynecol Endocrinol* **15**, 129–134. Observational study of 29 women who had a laparoscopic myomectomy for symptomatic myomas measuring 5.4 ± 3.6 cm were studied. The overall rate of intrauterine pregnancy was 65.5% (19 pregnancies; 2 patients had 2 pregnancies each). Out of 9 patients with other infertility factors associated with uterine myomas, 3 (33.3%) became pregnant; out of 10 infertile patients with no other associated infertility factors, 7 (70%) became pregnant; out of 10 patients to whom myomectomy was performed for the rapid growth of the tumor or for myoma encroaching on the cavity, 9 (90%) had a pregnancy. 9 patients (73.4%) had a cesarean section (one twice), 4 (26.6%) had spontaneous vaginal delivery, one patient had a serious placental failure at the 28th week and 4 patients (19%) miscarried. Out of 21 pregnancies, the viable term delivery rate was 57.14%. No uterine ruptures were observed. The pregnancy rate after laparoscopic myomectomy was similar to that reported in other studies after laparotomic myomectomy. **III B**

3 Benson CB, Chow JS, Chang-Lee W *et al.* (2001) Outcome of pregnancies in women with uterine leiomyomas identified by sonography in the first trimester. *J Clin Ultrasound* **29**, 261–264. Prospective study of 143 women identified as having uterine fibroids on their first-trimester scan were studied. The pregnancy loss rates and modes of delivery in these cases were compared to a maternal-age-matched and gestational-age-matched control group (the control group comprised 715 patients) of women who had normal uteruses and first-trimester pregnancies with documented fetal heartbeats. The rate of spontaneous pregnancy loss in women with fibroids was almost twice the rate in women with normal uteruses (14.0% versus 7.6%; $p < 0.05$), and the loss rate was higher in women with multiple fibroids than in women with a single leiomyoma (23.6% vs 8.0%, $p < 0.05$). The loss rate was not significantly associated with fibroid size or location. The rate of cesarean-section delivery was higher in patients with fibroids than in patients with normal uteruses (38% vs 28%, $p < 0.05$). **III B**

4 Roberts WE, Fulp KS, Morrison JC *et al.* (1999) The impact of leiomyomas on pregnancy. *Aust N Z J Obstet Gynaecol* **39**, 43–47. Retrospective case-control investigation of 51 pregnant patients who were diagnosed by ultrasound with uterine fibroids compared to 102 randomly selected control patients. Women with uterine myomas were older

($p = 0.001$) and more likely to be African-American ($p = 0.001$) and to undergo cesarean delivery ($p = 0.03$) than controls. However, when women who underwent abdominal delivery for previous myomectomy ($n = 5$) were excluded, there was no significant difference in the incidence of cesarean delivery. Overall, there was no difference in the incidence of obstetric complications between groups even when the data were stratified for large and/or multiple leiomyomas. **IIa B**

5 Koike T, Minakami H, Kosuge S *et al.* (1999) Uterine leiomyoma in pregnancy: its influence on obstetric performance. *J Obstet Gynaecol Res* **25**, 309–313. Retrospective study of 102 women found to have uterine fibroids during the first half of the pregnancy. The medical notes were reviewed during the 7-year study period. The results showed that bleeding in early pregnancy occurred in 16% of the women. Pain localized to the fibroid requiring analgesia occurred in 28%. Tocolytic treatment was required in 25% of the pregnancies and preterm labor in 12%. 39% of the pregnancies resulted in a cesarian section. The study showed that, if the size of the fibroid was greater than 6cm, the preterm labor rate was 24%; 59% had bleeding greater than 500ml at delivery and 51% had a cesarian section. **III B**

6 Seinera P, Farina C, Todros T (2000) Laparoscopic myomectomy and subsequent pregnancy: results in 54 patients. *Hum Reprod* **15**, 1993–1996. Study examining the risk of uterine rupture following a laparoscopic myomectomy. 54 patients were studied prospectively during subsequent pregnancies. A total of 202 patients underwent laparoscopic myomectomy. A total of 65 pregnancies occurred in 54 patients who became pregnant following surgery. No cases of uterine rupture occurred. 4 multiple pregnancies occurred. 8 pregnancies resulted in a first-trimester miscarriage and another in an interstitial pregnancy requiring laparotomic removal of the cornual gestational sac. Of the remaining 56 pregnancies, 51 (91%) were uneventful. In 2 cases a cerclage was performed at 16 weeks. 2 pregnancies ended in preterm labor (26–36 weeks). Cesarean section was performed in 45 cases (54/57, 80%). **III B**

7 Sherer DM, Schwartz BM, Mahon TR (1999) Intrapartum ultrasonographic depiction of fetal malpositioning and mild parietal bone compression in association with large lower segment uterine leiomyoma. *J Matern Fetal Med* **8**, 28–31. This study used transabdominal ultrasound scanning on a small cohort of women with large lower segment uterine fibroids, to examine the extent of deflexion or extension of the fetal head at the level of the cervical spine during the first stage of labor. This is a review article discussing pregnancy in women with fibroids. Diagnosis and complications are considered in detail. The authors recommend that pregnant women with fibroids should receive counseling regarding the 18% risk of spontaneous abortion, 10–15% incidence of painful myomata, 20–30% incidence of preterm delivery, theoretical risk of fetal malformation and 7–15% incidence of fetal growth retardation. In patients with large lower-segment uterine fibroids exhibiting poor progress of labor, mild compression of the distal parietal fetal bone was demonstrated and considered consistent with compression by the fibroid. Following abdominal delivery, because of arrest of descent, significant deflexion of the fetal head (not suspected by intrapartum cervical examination) and mild parietal bone depression, consistent with the ultrasonographic examination, were noted. **III B**

8 Seago DP, Roberts WE, Johnson VK *et al.* (1999) Planned cesarean hysterectomy: A preferred alternative to separate operations. *Am J Obstet Gynecol* **180**, 1385–1393. Retrospective case-controlled study undertaken over 10 years at the University of Mississippi Medical Center, USA. 100 pregnant women who underwent planned cesarean hysterectomy were compared with 37 patients who underwent cesarean delivery followed by a hysterectomy performed within 6 months. The women undergoing planned cesarean hysterectomy did not have any demonstrable increase in intraoperative or postoperative complications compared to the cesarean delivery plus later hysterectomy group. Primarily as a result of significantly reduced hospital stay and shorter total operative time, there was a significant financial advantage associated with a single planned cesarean hysterectomy with respect to separate operations. **III B**

9 Coronado GD, Marshall LM, Schwartz SM (2000) Complications in pregnancy, labor, and delivery with uterine leiomyomas: a population-based study. *Obstet Gynecol* **95**, 764–769. Retrospective descriptive study of 2065 women correlated the presence of uterine fibroids with characteristics of pregnancy, labor and neonatal outcome recorded on birth certificates. From the remaining records, a comparison group of women without uterine leiomyomas diagnoses were selected at random and frequency-matched by birth year to women with leiomyomas. An association was detected between uterine leiomyomas and abruptio placentae (OR 3. 87, 95% CI 1.63–9.17), first-trimester bleeding (OR 1.82, 95% CI 1.05–3.20), dysfunctional labor (OR 1.85, 95% CI 1.26–2.72), and breech presentation (OR 3.98, 95% CI 3.07–5.16). The risk of cesarean was also higher among women with uterine leiomyomas (OR 6. 39, 95% CI 5.46–7.50) but a portion of the excess risk might have been due to biased detection of leiomyomas at cesarean delivery. **III B**

40.4 Prolapse

Ian Mahady and Farah Siddiqui

Management option		Quality of evidence	Strength of recommendation	References
Prepregnancy	Conservative management if possible until family complete	–	✔	–
Prenatal	Screen for urinary infection	–	✔	–

➡

Management option		Quality of evidence	Strength of recommendation	References
Prenatal (cont'd)	Physiotherapy and/or supportive pessaries if troublesome	–	✔	–
	Avoid corrective surgery during pregnancy	–	✔	–
Labor and delivery	Elective lower segment cesarian section if previous successful prolapse surgery	–	✔	–
Postnatal	Physiotherapy and exercises	–	✔	–
	Review 3–6 months after delivery for definitive long-term management plan	–	✔	–

40.5 Other gynecological diseases and problems

Ian Mahady and Farah Siddiqui

Management option		Quality of evidence	Strength of recommendation	References
Congenital anatomical defects	Evaluate prenatally and plan delivery	III IV	B C	1,2 3
	Divide vaginal septa	III IV	B C	1,2 3
Cervical stenosis	Evaluate prenatally and plan delivery	–	✔	–
	Vigilance for dystocia in labor and need for lower segment cesarian section	–	✔	–
Endometrial resection	Counseling and vigilance for higher risk of miscarriage, preterm delivery, intrauterine growth restriction and fetal death	IV	C	4–6
Previous third-degree repair	Evaluate prenatally and plan delivery, possibly as elective lower segment cesarian section (LSCS)	–	✔	–
Vulval varicosities	Avoid injection with sclerosants	–	✔	–
	Symptomatic treatment prenatally (bed rest, support)	–	✔	–
	Avoid trauma during delivery	–	✔	–
Female circumcision	Evaluate prenatally and plan delivery	III IV	B C	7–9 10
	Options: ❑ Prenatal surgical correction ❑ Early anterior and posterior episiotomies (cross-match blood) ❑ Elective LSCS	III IV	B C	7–9 10

References

1 Heinonen PK (1997) Unicornuate uterus and rudimentary horn. *Fertil Steril* **68**, 224–230. Retrospective study of 42 women who had a unicornuate uterus with or without rudimentary horn. The rudimentary horn was removed in 21 cases. A right unicornuate uterus with noncommunicating rudimentary horn was the most common type of

uterine anomaly. 34 women produced 93 pregnancies; ectopic pregnancy (rudimentary horn, tubal) occurred in 20 of these cases (22%). The pregnant uterine horn ruptured in 3 of 7 cases. The fetal survival rate was 61%, prematurity 17%, fetal growth retardation 5%, and the spontaneous intrauterine abortion rate was 16%. Pregnancy-induced hypertension (PIH) was more common in women lacking a kidney than in those with two kidneys. The prognosis of intrauterine pregnancy is not impaired in the unicornuate uterus although prematurity threatens. Unilateral renal agenesis is associated with PIH. **III B**

2 Malik E, Berg C, Sterzik K *et al.* (2000) Reproductive outcome of 32 patients with primary or secondary infertility and uterine pathology. *Arch Gynecol Obstet* **264**, 24–26. Retrospective study performed in Lubeck, Germany of 102 patients who had a laparoscopy and a hysteroscopy during investigations for primary or secondary infertility. 32 of the 102 patients had uterine pathology. 7 of them had septate uteri, 8 had uterine synechiae, another 6 had uterine fibroids, 4 had a bicornuate uterus, while the remaining 7 had either a combination of all or other uterine anomalies. After surgical treatment of these conditions, 10 women conceived and 5 pregnancies, including one twin pregnancy, resulted in term deliveries. **III B**

3 Matts SJ, Clark TJ, Khan KS *et al.* (2000) Surgical correction of congenital uterine anomalies. *Hosp Med* **61**, 246–249. Review article. Congenital uterine abnormalities have been associated with poor reproductive outcome. Anatomical correction using open or endoscopic surgery has been recommended to improve these. **IV C**

4 Hill DJ, Maher PJ (1992) Pregnancy following endometrial resection. *Gynaecol Endosc* **1**, 47–49. Single case report of pregnancy in a 35-year-old following endometrial resection with cutting loop and roller ball ablation. Post-operation, the patient still menstruated. Pregnancy, diagnosed 4 months post-operation, was uncomplicated and delivery was by elective cesarean section at 39 weeks because of three previous sections. The baby was in good condition at delivery and birth weight was normal. Histology of the placenta was normal. Filshie clips were applied to fallopian tubes at cesarean section. **IV C**

5 Hopkisson JF, Kennedy SH, Ellis JD (1994) Caesarean hysterectomy for intrauterine death after failed endometrial resection. *Br J Obstet Gynaecol* **101**, 810–811. Single case report of pregnancy 2 years after day case transcervical resection of endometrium (TCRE) for failed medical treatment of dysfunctional uterine bleeding in a patient with two previous cesarean sections. Pregnancy was uncomplicated until intrauterine death (IUD) occurred at 31 weeks gestation. Following failed induction of labor using prostaglandins and oxytocin, cesarean hysterectomy was carried out electively. Autopsy revealed no cause for the IUD. No placental pathology was found and no placenta accreta. The authors recommend sterilization at time of TCRE. **IV C**

6 Wood C, Rogers P (1993) A pregnancy after planned partial endometrial resection. *Aust N Z J Obstet Gynaecol* **33**, 316–318. Single case report of pregnancy after planned partial endometrial resection following multiple myomectomies for fibroids. Endometrium around and above the tubal ostia was left *in situ*. The pregnancy was complicated by spontaneous rupture of membranes at 22 weeks gestation, treated by bed rest. Spontaneous preterm labor occurred at 28 weeks and emergency cesarean section was carried out. There was partial placenta accreta. The baby died at 32 h post-delivery from pulmonary hypoplasia, bacterial septicemia, hypotension and persistent fetal circulation. **IV C**

7 McCaffrey M, Jankowska A, Gordon H (1995) Management of female genital mutilation: the Northwick Park Hospital experience. *Br J Obstet Gynaecol* **102**, 787–790. Observational study of 50 consecutive women attending an African Well Woman Clinic at Northwick Park Hospital, in whom antenatal deinfibulation was carried out. The series consisted of 13 nonpregnant, 14 primigravid and 23 multiparous women. The mean age at infibulation was 6.7 years. 13 (93%) of the primigravidae proceeded to spontaneous vaginal delivery with one cesarean section carried out for obstetric complications unrelated to infibulation. 14 (61%) of the multiparae had vaginal delivery, 3(13%) had instrumental delivery and 6 (25.1%) had a cesarean section. Reinfibulation post-delivery was not advised. **III B**

8 Haque MF, Brody BA (2000) The prevalence of female genital operations in the Houston metropolitan area. *Texas Med* **96**, 62–65. Study exploring the prevalence of female genital operations (FGOs), also known as female circumcision, among women in the Houston metropolitan area. The medical ramifications of the procedure and the specific type of procedure undergone were examined as well as the nationality and religious background of these women and their views regarding their experience. 30% of physicians reported treating patients with FGOs at some time in their practice. **III B**

9 Adinma JI (1997) Current status of female circumcision among Nigerian Igbos. *West Afr J Med* **16**, 227–231. The incidence of circumcision in 256 pregnant Nigerian Igbo women was 124 (48.4%). This incidence increased with increasing social class. Simple excision was the commonest type of circumcision, 122 (98.4%). The genital introitus was mildly scarred in 48 (38.7%) respondents, moderately scarred in 47 (37.9%) and severely scarred in 29 (23.4%). 94 (36.7%) of the respondents were not aware of their circumcision status, while 91 (96.8%) of the circumcised women had it performed during infancy. The incidence of episiotomy during delivery was similar for both circumcised (47, 18.4%) and uncircumcised (46, 18.0%) respondents ($p = 0.05$). Of the 118 female offspring of the respondents, 109 (92.4%) were not circumcised while 9 (7.6%) were. **III B**

10 Eke N, Nkanginieme KE (1999) Female genital mutilation: a global bug that should not cross the millennium bridge. *World J Surg* **23**,1082–1087. Review article studying the indications for the practice of female circumcision. The practice is only outlawed in the UK, Sweden and Belgium. Early complications include hemorrhage, urinary tract infection, septicemia and tetanus. Late complications include infertility, apareunia, clitoral neuromas, and vesicovaginal fistula. **IV C**

Chapter 41

Malignant disease (nonhematological)

41.1 Cervical cancer

John Williams and Farah Siddiqui

Management option		Quality of evidence	Strength of recommendation	References
Diagnosis	Physical examination and cervical smear at first prenatal visit in high-risk women and those without smear in previous 3 years	III	B	1
	Colposcopy and directed biopsies for suspicious lesions	III	B	2
	Cone biopsy when microinvasion suspected on directed biopsies; loop excision may be associated with increased preterm births	III IIb	B B	3,4 5
Treatment	**Cervical intraepithelial neoplasia:** ❑ Follow-up with colposcopy during pregnancy	IIb III	B B	5 4
	Microinvasive cancer: ❑ After careful maternal counseling consider delaying definitive therapy until fetal maturity reached (enhance with steroids) and delivery completed	III	B	6
	Invasive cancer – use same therapy guidelines as for nonpregnant patient: ❑ Before 20 weeks: consider termination and immediate therapy ❑ After 20 weeks: consider awaiting fetal maturity (enhance with steroids), then deliver and implement therapy postnatally	–	✔	–
	❑ Elective cesarean hysterectomy can be considered with early-stage disease ❑ Careful patient counseling required with either presentation	III	B	7

References

1 Coppola A, Sorosky J, Casper R *et al.* (1997) The clinical course of cervical carcinoma in situ diagnosed during pregnancy. *Gynecol Oncol* **67**, 162–165. Retrospective review of all women evaluated at the University of Iowa Colposcopy Clinic diagnosed with squamous cell cervical carcinoma-*in-situ* (CIS) during pregnancy. 34 pregnant women were studied. 20 (80%) had persistent disease, 2 (8%) had either missed disease or progressive disease postpartum and 3 (12%) resolved without treatment at postpartum evaluation. No statistical significance was found between route of delivery and persistence ($p = 0.34$). There is a high persistence rate of CIS complicating pregnancy. Given the relatively high rate of underestimation of disease severity by both cytology and colposcopic impression, the use of routine biopsy at the time of colposcopy is recommended. Invasive disease may be encountered on postpartum evaluation.
III B

2 De Sutter P, Coibion M, Vosse M *et al.* (1998) A multicentre study comparing cervicography and cytology in the detection of cervical intraepithelial neoplasia. *Br J Obstet Gynaecol* **105**, 613–620. Prospective comparative multicenter study, in three Belgian hospitals. Cervical cytology and cervicography were performed on 5724 women. Overall detection of cervical intraepithelial neoplasia (CIN) is improved but this is mainly due to the detection of more low-grade lesions. The lower sensitivity and specificity in high-grade lesions compared with cervical cytology is the

main limitation of cervicography in screening for CIN. An important finding was that the performance of cervicography was highly dependent on the assessor's experience. **III B**

3 Robinson WR, Webb S, Tirpack J *et al.* (1997) Management of cervical intraepithelial neoplasia during pregnancy with LOOP excision. *Gynecol Oncol* **64**, 153–155. The purpose of this prospective cohort study of 20 women is to determine the efficacy of LOOP excision performed during pregnancy (between 8–34 weeks gestation). 14 of 20 (70%) had dysplastic changes in the LOOP specimen. 8 of 14 (57%) had involved margins. 9 of 19 (47%) had residual dysplasia 3 months postpartum, including 3 patients whose initial LOOP specimens were negative for dysplasia. Significant morbidity included 3 preterm births, 2 patients who required blood transfusion following LOOP, and one unexplained intrauterine fetal demise. The gestational age range of those patients who had significant morbidity was 27–34 weeks. **III B**

4 Ueki M, Ueda M, Kumagai K *et al.* (1995) Cervical cytology and conservative management of cervical neoplasias during pregnancy. *Int J Gynecol Pathol* **14**, 63–69. This prospective cohort study was set in Japan. To elucidate the clinical significance of cervical cytology during pregnancy, 7725 pregnant women were examined. Abnormal cytological findings were recorded in 65 cases (0.8%). Colposcopically directed punch biopsies revealed cervical dysplasia and carcinoma in 27 cases (0.35%). Cytological findings of the patients with cervical neoplasia during pregnancy agreed well (76%) with their histological findings. Colposcopically, the squamocolumnar junction was visible in many cases and white epithelium was most commonly observed during pregnancy. Pre- and postpartum follow-up study revealed that progression from dysplasia was seen only in 2 (10%) of 20 cases. **III B**

5 Baldauf JJ, Dreyfus M, Ritter J *et al.* (1995) Colposcopy and directed biopsy reliability during pregnancy: a cohort study. *Eur J Obstet Gynecol Reprod Biol* **62**, 31–36. Prospective cohort study of 117 pregnant women and 234 control nonpregnant women undergoing colposcopy, based in France. Findings showed that the reliability of cytology, colposcopy and directed biopsy was not related to pregnancy. These data show that the physiological changes that occur in pregnancy do not significantly alter the reliability of colposcopy and directed biopsy if the colposcopist is aware of the peculiar difficulties and does not overreact to the accentuated patterns that may occur during pregnancy. **IIb B**

6 Duggan B, Muderspach LI, Roman LD *et al.* (1993) Cervical cancer in pregnancy: reporting on planned delay in therapy. *Obstet Gynecol* **82**, 598–602. Retrospective cohort study of 27 pregnant patients with invasive cervical cancer, Los Angeles. Most patients had stage I lesions. 8 patients with stage Ia or Ib cervical cancer postponed therapy to optimize fetal outcome, with a mean diagnosis-to-treatment interval of 144 days (range 53–212). 19 patients elected immediate treatment, with a mean diagnosis-to-treatment interval of 17 days (range 2–42). Fetal outcome was uniformly good for the delayed-treatment group. 9 fetal deaths and 2 neonatal deaths occurred in the immediate-treatment group. All patients who delayed therapy were free of disease after a median follow-up of 23 months. The delay of therapy to achieve fetal maturity appears to be a reasonable option for patients with stage I cervical cancer complicating pregnancy. **III B**

7 Hoffman MS, Roberts WS, Fiorica JV *et al.* (1993) Elective cesarean hysterectomy for treatment of cervical neoplasia. An update. *J Reprod Med* **38**, 186–188. 37 patients underwent elective cesarean hysterectomy for early cervical neoplasia. 34 patients had cervical intraepithelial neoplasia III and 3 patients had stage IA-1 squamous-cell carcinoma of the cervix. 28 were primary cesarean sections; 9 had obstetric indications. The mean operative time was 128 min; mean estimated blood loss was 1400 ml. One patient experienced an intraoperative hemorrhage (3500 ml). There were no other recognized intraoperative complications. Four significant postoperative complications included a vaginal cuff abscess, a wound dehiscence and pelvic abscess, one patient with febrile morbidity and an ileus and ligation with partial transection of a ureter. Patients were discharged on a mean of postoperative day 5.7. **III B**

41.2 Ovarian cancer

John Williams and Farah Siddiqui

Management option		Quality of evidence	Strength of recommendation	References
Diagnosis	Often as chance finding during an obstetric ultrasound examination	IV	C	1
	CA-125 levels are unhelpful, as they can be raised in normal pregnancy	IV	C	2
	Magnetic resonance imaging helpful	III	B	3
Treatment	Surgical exploration ideally performed in second trimester	III	B	4,5

Management option		Quality of evidence	Strength of recommendation	References
Treatment (cont'd)	Pregnancy preservation and conservative surgery with unilateral salpingo-oophor-ectomy and staging biopsies are possible in most early stage ovarian cancers (uncommon)	III	B	4,5
	Chemotherapy if needed, has risks (see Section 31.8)	III	B	4,5
	Salvage of the pregnancy may not be possible with advanced disease	III	B	4,5

References

1 Grendys EC Jr, Barnes WA (1995) Ovarian cancer in pregnancy. *Surg Clin North Am* **75**, 1–14. Review article. A pelvic mass in pregnancy is relatively common; the majority will resolve with observation into the second trimester. Masses persisting into the second trimester should be surgically evaluated, given the decreased risk to both mother and fetus at this time. For masses persisting into the third trimester, a 2–5% risk of malignancy is to be expected. Potentially life-saving therapy should not be withheld from patients because they are pregnant, especially considering that chemotherapy is apparently safe in the second and third trimesters. **IV C**

2 Meden H, Fattahi-Meibodi A (1998) CA-125 in benign gynecological conditions. *Int J Biol Markers* **13**, 231–237. Review article. The tumor marker CA-125 was initially thought to be specific for ovarian malignancies. Subsequently it was found to be raised in a variety of benign conditions, including pregnancy, endometriosis, hyperstimulation syndrome, ectopic pregnancy, fibroids, pelvic inflammatory disease, tuberculosis and cirrhosis of the liver. These results demonstrate that CA-125 is a marker of nonspecific peritoneal conditions. **IV C**

3 Kier R, McCarthy SM, Scoutt LM *et al.* (1990) Pelvic masses in pregnancy: MR imaging. *Radiology* **176**, 709–713. The value of magnetic resonance (MR) imaging was assessed for 17 pregnant patients with sonograms suggestive of a pelvic mass. The MR imaging improved lesion characterization in 47% (8/17) of cases. The origin of the pelvic mass was accurately determined on 100% (17/17) of the MR images versus 71% (12/17) of the sonograms. In 3 cases, the results of MR imaging led to cancellation of surgery, which would have proceeded on the basis of the sonographic results alone. MR imaging is a valuable complement to sonography for preoperative evaluation of pelvic masses in pregnant patients. **III B**

4 Ueda M, Ueki M (1996) Ovarian tumors associated with pregnancy. *Int J Gynaecol Obstet* **55**, 59–65. Among 106 cases undergoing ovarian surgery during pregnancy, 31 (29.2%), 70 (66%) and 5 (4.7%) were diagnosed as physiological, benign and malignant, respectively. The incidence of benign neoplastic tumor was 1/112 deliveries and that of malignant neoplastic tumor was 1/1684 deliveries. Dermoid cyst was the most common lesion found. Of the 70 benign tumors, 51 (72.9%) were greater than 8 cm in diameter and 55 (78.6%) were preoperatively diagnosed before the 10th gestational week; 44 (62.9%) were operated before the 15th gestational week. The spontaneous abortion rate in 80 cases followed up after surgery was only 10%, 61 patients (76.3%) progressing to full-term delivery. 5 malignant tumors included 3 epithelial carcinomas, one embryonal carcinoma and one dysgerminoma. Ovarian surgery in the first trimester for persistent or enlarging masses is important to obtain a final histological diagnosis and rule out malignancy. **III B**

5 Hess LW, Peaceman A, O'Brien WF *et al.* (1988) Adnexal mass occurring with intrauterine pregnancy: report of fifty-four patients requiring laparotomy for definitive management. *Am J Obstet Gynecol* **158**, 1029–1034. 54 cases in which surgical intervention during pregnancy was required for definitive therapy of adnexal masses were reviewed. The calculated incidence of adnexal masses that required surgical intervention during pregnancy in the primary population (patients who were not referred for evaluation of an already identified mass) was one case per 1300 live births. A malignant tumor was found in 5.9% of the pregnant patients who underwent exploratory celiotomy for therapy of an adnexal mass. Those pregnant women who underwent emergency laparotomy because of hemorrhage or torsion as a complication of an adnexal mass spontaneously aborted or underwent premature delivery more frequently than those patients who underwent elective laparotomy for removal of the mass ($p < 0.001$). **III B**

41.3 Other gynecological malignant disease

John Williams and Farah Siddiqui

Management option		Quality of evidence	Strength of recommendation	References
Vulval carcinoma	Rare; histological varieties most commonly encountered are invasive squamous-cell carcinomas and melanomas	IV	C	1,2
	Radical excision of the primary lesion and inguinal femoral node dissection is the treatment of choice for stage I and II squamous-cell cancer	IV	C	1,2
	Timing of treatment and mode of delivery are usually dependent on the time of diagnosis during pregnancy. It has been recommended to proceed with definitive surgical treatment at any time during pregnancy up to 36 weeks of gestation. Patients can be allowed to deliver vaginally provided the wounds have healed	IV	C	1,2
Endometrial carcinoma	There have been 12 cases of endometrial carcinomas reported during pregnancy. Surprisingly, 5 cases were associated with a viable fetus. The remaining cases were diagnosed at the time of dilatation and curettage performed for irregular bleeding	IV	C	3–5

References

1. Regan MA, Rosenzweig BA (1993) Vulvar carcinoma in pregnancy: a case report in literature review. *Am J Perinatol* **10**, 334–335. Single case report of invasive vulval carcinoma in pregnancy. Literature review. **IV C**
2. Monaghan JM, Lindegue G (1986) Vulvar carcinoma in pregnancy. Commentary. *Br J Obstet Gynaecol* **93**, 785–786. Editorial commentary. **IV C**
3. Carinelli SG, Cefis F, Merlo D (1987) Epithelial neoplasia of the endometrium in pregnancy. A case report. *Tumori* **73**, 175–180. Single case report. Focal atypical hyperplasia/adenocarcinoma-*in-situ* found T.O.P. 10 other cases from the literature reviewed, all adenocarcinoma. The authors advocate conservative treatment. **IV C**
4. Fine BA, Baker TR, Hempling RE *et al.* (1994) Pregnancy coexisting with serous papillary adenocarcinoma involving both uterus and ovary. *Gynecol Oncol* **53**, 369–372. Single case report. Pregnancy plus uterine adenocarcinoma. Viable preterm infant. Cisplatin therapy. **IV C**
5. Ojomo EO, Ezimokhai M, Reale FR *et al.* (1993) Recurrent postpartum hemorrhage caused by endometrial carcinoma co-existing with endometrioid carcinoma of the ovary in a full-term pregnancy. *Br J Obstet Gynaecol* **100**, 489–491. Single case report. Postpartum hemorrhage from carcinoma of the endometrium with endometrioid carcinoma of the ovary concurrently at term. **IV C**

41.4 Breast cancer

Paul Ayuk

Management option		Quality of evidence	Strength of recommendation	References
Diagnosis	Physiological changes of pregnancy reduce the sensitivity of physical examination and mammography	III	B	1

➡

Management option		Quality of evidence	Strength of recommendation	References
Diagnosis (cont'd)	Fine-needle aspiration of any suspicious lesion	III	B	2
	Open biopsy if the results of needle biopsy are equivocal	III	B	2
Treatment	Radical mastectomy is the preferred treatment for early cancers	III Ib	B A	3 4
	Adjuvant chemotherapy may be indicated for some patients with high-risk cancers. Both maternal benefits and potential risks to the fetus should be weighed carefully	III IV	B C	3 5
	If diagnosis is made late in pregnancy and chemotherapy or radiation treatment are indicated, consider delaying therapy until after delivery	IIb	B	6
	Routine therapeutic abortions are not indicated	III	B	3,7
	Termination of pregnancy may be considered in patients with advanced disease if chemotherapy and/or radiation treatment are indicated in early pregnancy	IIb	B	6
	Recommend delaying conception for 2–3 years after treatment	IIa	B	8,9

References

1 Liberman L, Giess CS, Dershaw DD *et al.* (1994) Imaging of pregnancy-associated breast cancer. *Radiology* **191**, 245–248. Retrospective analysis on the use of mammography prior to biopsy ($n = 21$) in diagnosing pregnancy-associated breast cancer in women with breast cancer diagnosed during pregnancy or within 1 year after pregnancy ($n = 85$). Mammographic findings were present in 18 of 23 cases of invasive carcinoma (78%). It is concluded that pregnancy-associated breast cancer is often advanced at diagnosis and that breast imaging studies usually demonstrate focal findings when clinically evident. **III B**

2 Carrillo JF, Mendivil MF, Dominguez JR *et al.* (1999) Accuracy of combined clinical findings and fine needle aspiration cytology for the diagnosis in palpable breast tumors. *Rev Invest Clin* **51**, 333–339. Prospective study on the accuracy of fine-needle aspiration in the investigation of breast lumps. A single aspirate was obtained from 213 patients who also underwent biopsy for histological examination. Fine-needle aspiration had a sensitivity of 93.2%, a specificity of 97.3% and a positive predictive value of 96.9% in the diagnosis of breast cancer. **III B**

3 King RM, Welch JS, Martin JK *et al.* (1985) Carcinoma of the breast associated with pregnancy. *Surg Gynecol Obstet* **160**, 228–232. This study describes the management of breast cancer diagnosed during pregnancy over a 30-year period. The data do not allow conclusions to be drawn on the most suitable therapeutic procedure (radical mastectomy/modified radical mastectomy ± adjuvant chemotherapy). Pregnancy interruption does not appear to influence 5-year survival. **III B**

4 Jacobson JA, Danforth DN, Cowan KH *et al.* (1995) Ten-year results of a comparison of conservation with mastectomy in the treatment of stage I and II breast cancer. *N Engl J Med* **332**, 907–911. RCT of 237 women with stage I or II breast cancer treated by modified radical mastectomy ($n = 116$) or lumpectomy, axillary dissection and radiotherapy ($n = 121$) and followed up for a median of 10.1 years. There was no significant difference in overall 10-year survival or disease-free survival in the two groups. Disease-free survival was assessed on the assumption that 'recurrence within the breast that was successfully treated by mastectomy was not considered a local or regional recurrence unless it was followed by a further local or regional event'. The figures suggest that initial local/regional recurrence occurred in 17% in the lumpectomy group and 9% in the mastectomy group. **Ib B**

5 Petrek JA (1994) Breast cancer and pregnancy. *J Natl Cancer Inst Monogr* **16**, 113–121. Review article, which does not present original data. The potential fetal complications of radiotherapy and chemotherapy are discussed. The review concludes that pregnant women present with more advanced disease, but, when matched stage-for-stage with nonpregnant controls, outcome is not significantly affected. **IV C**

6 Nettleton J, Long J, Kuban D et al. (1996) Breast cancer during pregnancy: quantifying the risk of treatment delay. *Obstet Gynecol* **87**, 414–418. This is a theoretical analysis using published data on the relationship between primary breast tumor size and the risk of positive axillary nodes to estimate the effect of delayed treatment for breast cancer in pregnancy on the risk of axillary metastasis and therefore survival. The model developed estimates the daily increase in risk of axillary metastasis due to delayed treatment at 0.028–0.057%. This risk should be considered, together with gestation age at diagnosis, in making decisions on the timing of treatment. **IIb B**

7 Clark RM, Chua T (1989) Breast cancer and pregnancy: the ultimate challenge. *Clin Oncol* **1**: 11–18. Observational study reporting outcome for breast cancer treatment in 154 women diagnosed during pregnancy, 96 women diagnosed within 12 months of delivery and 136 women who subsequently became pregnant. Women diagnosed with breast cancer during pregnancy had significantly poorer survival, as did those who had therapeutic abortions. The conclusions of this study are unreliable as no correction was made for stage of disease at diagnosis or histological type. **III B**

8 Kroman N, Jensen MB, Melbye M *et al.* (1997) Should women be advised against pregnancy after breast-cancer treatment? *Lancet* **350**, 319–322. Observational case-controlled study examining the effect of subsequent pregnancy on survival following treatment for breast cancer. 173 women treated for breast cancer who subsequently became pregnant were compared with 5552 women (aged < 45 years) without subsequent pregnancy. This well-designed study found that pregnancy after treatment for breast cancer did not significantly affect prognosis. **IIa B**

9 Dow KH, Harris JR, Roy C (1994) Pregnancy after breast-conserving surgery and radiation therapy for breast cancer. *J Natl Cancer Inst Monogr* **16**, 131–137. Observational case-controlled study comparing outcomes in 23 women with breast cancer managed by conservative surgery plus radiotherapy and who subsequently became pregnant with 23 matched controls without subsequent pregnancy. There was no significant difference in disease-free survival in the two groups. Subsequent pregnancy did not significantly affect prognosis following treatment for breast cancer. The number of cases is too small to allow firm conclusions. **IIa B**

41.5 Malignant melanoma

Paul Ayuk

Management option		Quality of evidence	Strength of recommendation	References
Diagnosis	Biopsy any suspicious lesion	III	B	1
Treatment	Surgery is the most effective cure for early-stage disease	IV III	C B	2 3,4
	Role of radiotherapy and chemotherapy uncertain	IV III	C B	2 5
	Routine therapeutic abortion not indicated	IV	C	6
	Recommend delaying conception for 2–3 years after treatment	IV IIb	C B	6 7

References

1 Hallock GG, Lutz DA (1998) Prospective study of the accuracy of the surgeon's diagnosis in 2000 excised skin tumors. *Plast Reconstr Surg* **101**, 1255–1261. Prospective study on the accuracy of clinical diagnosis in 2058 skin lesions with histological examination as the gold standard. 65% of all tumors were identified correctly preoperatively. Approximately 90% of all lesions were removed appropriately. It is concluded that any suspicious or equivocal lesion will require histological examination, as clinical diagnosis does not have 100% accuracy. **III B**

2 Squatrito RC, Harlow SP (1998) Melanoma complicating pregnancy. *Obstet Gynecol Clin North Am* **25**, 407–416. Review of the management of malignant melanoma in pregnancy. Suspected lesions should be investigated promptly and managed surgically during pregnancy. Although the results of published studies are conflicting, the authors conclude that pregnancy does not appear to affect prognosis. The role of adjuvant chemotherapy or immunotherapy in pregnancy remains uncertain. **IV C**

3 Slingluff CL, Reintgen DS, Vollmer RT *et al.* (1990) Malignant melanoma arising during pregnancy. A study of 100 patients. *Ann Surg* **211**, 552–557. Study describing the management of 100 patients with malignant melanoma during pregnancy and compares the outcome with 86 matched controls. Patients were treated by local excision with node dissection in 16 pregnant women and immunotherapy in 83 patients. Pregnancy did not affect overall survival. Disease-free survival was significantly reduced in the pregnant group with pregnancy being a significant prognostic factor. **III B**

4 MacKie RM, Bufalino R, Morabito A *et al.* (1991) Lack of effect of pregnancy on outcome of melanoma. For The World Health Organization Melanoma Programme. *Lancet* **337**, 653–655. This study compares tumor characteristics and outcome in women with stage I malignant melanoma treated before any pregnancy (n = 85), during pregnancy (n = 92), between pregnancies (n = 68) and after completing their family (n = 143). Women treated during pregnancy had tumors of significantly greater thickness. Pregnancy did not affect survival. **III B**

5 Hill GJ, Ruess R, Berris R *et al.* (1974) Chemotherapy of malignant melanoma with dimethyl triazeno imidazole carboxamide (DITC) and nitrosourea derivatives (BCNU, CCNU). *Ann Surg* **180**, 167–174. Paper describing clinical experience in the use of chemotherapy in the management of metastatic malignant melanoma in 80 patients, one of whom was pregnant. Patients were treated with dimethyl triazeno imidazole carboxamide (DTIC) and the nitrosoureas BCNU and CCNU with a 28% response rate. DTIC was the most effective drug. Other chemotherapeutic agents available at the time proved ineffective. **III B**

6 Kjems E, Krag C (1993) Melanoma and pregnancy. *Acta Oncol* **32**, 371–378. Review article outlining the presentation, management and prognosis of malignant melanoma in pregnancy. Pregnant women have thicker tumors at presentation but stage-for-stage have no significant difference in survival. The advice to avoid pregnancy for 3 years following diagnosis is based on the observation that 80–90% of recurrences appear during this period. There is no conclusive evidence that therapeutic abortion alters the prognosis. **IV C**

7 Reintgen DS, McCarty KS, Vollmer R *et al.* (1985) Malignant melanoma and pregnancy. *Cancer* **55**, 1340–1344. Observational case-controlled study examining outcome in 58 women with malignant melanoma diagnosed during pregnancy, 43 women who became pregnant within 5 years of diagnosis and matched controls. Pregnancy did not affect overall survival. Pregnancy at the time of diagnosis had an adverse effect on disease-free survival but this effect was not seen in women who became pregnant after treatment. **IIb B**

41.6 Colorectal carcinoma

Paul Ayuk

Management option		Quality of evidence	Strength of recommendation	References
Surgery is the mainstay of treatment. Management options include the following		–	✔	–
In early pregnancy	Pregnancy termination before definitive surgery	–	✔	–
	Hysterectomy may be indicated as part of surgical procedure for rectosigmoid tumors	IV	C	1,2
In late pregnancy	Elective delivery when fetus viable followed by definitive surgery; hysterectomy is determined by surgical access	IV	C	1–4
	Definitive surgery without disturbing uterus and contents	IV	C	2,3
	Oophorectomy for all low-lying tumors because of high metastasis rate	IV	C	1,3,4

References

1 Bernstein MA, Madoff RD, Caushaj PF *et al.* (1993) Colon and rectal cancer in pregnancy. *Dis Colon Rectum* **36**, 172–178. Paper reviewing the presentation and management options in women diagnosed with colorectal carcinoma in pregnancy. It recommends definitive surgical excision before 20 weeks gestation with hysterectomy if the uterus is invaded or access is required. Cesarean section should be performed only if there is a pelvic obstructing tumor, otherwise surgical excision should await uterine involution. The risk of ovarian metastases is high (~22%); therefore, bilateral oophorectomy is advised, although there is no evidence that this alters prognosis. Stage-for-stage, pregnancy does not affect prognosis. **IV C**

2 Nesbitt JC, Moise KJ, Sawyers JL (1985) Colorectal carcinoma in pregnancy. *Arch Surg* **120**, 636–640. Five cases of colorectal cancer in pregnancy are reported with a review of the literature and a proposed management strategy. Surgical resection may be undertaken up to 20 weeks gestation without disturbing the uterus. Hysterectomy should only be performed if the uterus is invaded or access is required. Bilateral oophorectomy is not recommended in the first half of pregnancy because of the risk of miscarriage. Tumors diagnosed after 20 weeks gestation should await fetal viability, vaginal delivery if possible and uterine involution prior to resection. **IV C**

3 Ringenberg QS, Doll DC (1989) Endocrine tumors and miscellaneous cancers in pregnancy. *Semin Oncol* **16**, 445–455. Review of the presentation and management of colorectal cancer in pregnancy. In the first/second trimester, surgical resection is recommended regardless of the fetus. Pelvic tumors may require delivery by cesarean section with simultaneous surgical resection. If vaginal delivery occurs, surgical resection should be delayed for a few days to reduce the risk of infection. Pregnancy does not affect prognosis. **IV C**

4 Heres P, Wiltink J, Cuesta MA *et al.* (1993) Colon carcinoma during pregnancy: a lethal coincidence. *Eur J Obstet Gynecol Reprod Biol* **48**, 149–152. Presentation of a single case of colorectal carcinoma in pregnancy with a review of the literature. Surgical resection was the initial treatment. Bilateral oophorectomy was subsequently required for metastatic disease. Chemotherapy was also employed. The risk of ovarian metastasis in colorectal cancer diagnosed during pregnancy is quoted at 25%. **IV C**

41.7 Thyroid cancer

Paul Ayuk

Management option		Quality of evidence	Strength of recommendation	References
Diagnosis	Fine-needle biopsy of thyroid nodule for diagnosis	III IV	B C	1,2 3
	Radioisotope scans are contraindicated in pregnancy	IV	C	3
Treatment	For patients with papillary or follicular carcinomas, surgical resection can be performed during pregnancy or deferred until after delivery	III	B	2,4
	Anaplastic carcinomas carry a very poor prognosis and should be treated immediately and aggressively. In addition to radical surgery, chemotherapy and/or radiation may be indicated in these cases	III	B	5,6

References

1 Vini L, Hyer S, Pratt B *et al.* (1999) Management of differentiated thyroid cancer diagnosed during pregnancy. *Eur J Endocrinol* **140**, 404–406. Case reports on nine women with differentiated thyroid cancer diagnosed during pregnancy and followed up for a median of 14 years. The diagnosis was made by fine-needle aspiration cytology in all patients. One patient had a subtotal thyroidectomy in the second trimester while the others were operated upon 3–10 months post-partum with good outcomes. Treatment of differentiated thyroid cancer diagnosed during pregnancy may safely be delayed until after delivery. **III B**

2 Choe W, McDougall IR (1994) Thyroid cancer in pregnant women: diagnostic and therapeutic management. *Thyroid* **4**, 433–435. Report of four cases of thyroid cancer diagnosed during pregnancy with a review of the literature on management strategies. The authors recommend fine-needle aspiration as the investigation of choice for thyroid nodules diagnosed in pregnancy. Thyroid cancer in early pregnancy should be managed by thyroidectomy with suppressive doses of thyroxine and assay of serum thyroglobulin to monitor therapy. Treatment for cancers diagnosed in late pregnancy can be deferred until after delivery. **III B**

3 Ringenberg QS, Doll DC (1989) Endocrine tumors and miscellaneous cancers in pregnancy. *Semin Oncol* **16**, 445–455. This review article describes the management of thyroid cancer in pregnancy. Diagnosis should be by fine-needle aspiration, which has a quoted accuracy of over 80%. Thyroid surgery should be deferred until the second or third trimester and suppressive doses of thyroxine should be used. There are no indications for therapeutic abortion and iodine-131 therapy is contraindicated during pregnancy. **IV C**

4 Moosa M, Mazzaferri EL (1997) Outcome of differentiated thyroid cancer diagnosed in pregnant women. *J Clin Endocrinol Metab* **82**, 2862–2866. Observational case-controlled study examining the presentation, management and outcome for differentiated thyroid cancer in 61 pregnant women and 528 matched controls. Malignant thyroid nodules tend to be asymptomatic in pregnancy but pregnancy did not affect the histological type, stage at diagnosis or prognosis. Patients were treated by thyroidectomy ± iodine-131 chemotherapy with suppressive doses of thyroxine. A mean delay in treatment of up to 16 months in the pregnant group did not significantly affect outcome. Thyroid surgery may safely be performed during pregnancy and treatment of differentiated thyroid cancer may safely be delayed until after delivery. **III B**

5 Kober F, Heiss A, Keminger K *et al.* (1990) Chemotherapy of highly malignant thyroid tumors. *Wien Klin Wochenschr* **102**, 274–276. Study describing a phase II trial of surgery plus chemotherapy in 15 patients with anaplastic thyroid carcinoma or thyroid sarcoma. 10 patients responded to chemotherapy, although the prognosis remained poor, with a median survival of 20.8 months in responders and 4.5 months in nonresponders. **III B**

6 Hadar T, Mor C, Shvero J *et al.* (1993) Anaplastic carcinoma of the thyroid. *Eur J Surg Oncol* **19**, 511–516. Study describing clinical experience in 48 cases of anaplastic carcinoma of the thyroid gland. Patients were treated by thyroidectomy (total or subtotal) ± radiotherapy or chemotherapy. The overall prognosis was poor, with a 2-year survival rate of 28%. **III B**

Chapter 42

Trauma

42.1 General management options

Michelle Mohajer

Management option		Quality of evidence	Strength of recommendation	References
Major trauma	Multidisciplinary approach	IV	C	1
	Increased risk of thromboembolism	III	B	2
	Consider low-molecular-weight heparins for prophylaxis	Ib	A	3
	Nasogastric tube placement for ruptures of the left diaphragm	IV	C	4
Diagnosis	X-rays	IV	C	5
	Peritoneal lavage	III IIb	B B	6,7 8
	Computed tomography scan	III	B	7
	Ultrasound	IIb III	B B	8 9,10
	Contrast imaging (duodenum, urinary tract)	IV	C	4,5

References

1 Dudley DJ, Cruikshank DP (1990) Trauma and acute surgical emergencies during pregnancy. *Semin Perinatol* **14**, 42–51. Review of the diagnosis and management of trauma and surgical emergencies in the pregnant patient. The anatomical and physiological changes associated with pregnancy may create difficulties and require close cooperation between the trauma surgeon, the anesthetist and the obstetrician to ensure the best outcome possible for mother and fetus. A wide range of areas is covered, including major trauma, (blunt and penetrating), burns, appendicitis, bowel obstruction, cholecystitis, pancreatitis, visceral rupture, pulmonary embolism and esophageal varices. **IV C**

2 Geerts WH, Code KI, Jay RM *et al.* (1994) A prospective study of venous TE after major trauma. *N Engl J Med* **331**, 1601–1606. Prospective cohort study of 716 patients admitted to a regional trauma unit who were investigated for deep-vein thrombosis by serial impedance. Venous thromboembolism was found in over half of the trauma cases by plethysmography and lower-extremity contrast venography. A multivariate analysis identified five independent risk factors for deep-vein thrombosis: older age (OR 1.05 per year of age, 95%CI 1.03–1.06), blood transfusion (OR 1.74, 95%CI 1.03–2.93), surgery (OR 2.30, 95%CI 1.08–4.89), fracture of the femur or tibia (OR 4.82, 95%CI 2.79–8.33) and spinal-cord injury (OR 8.59, 95%CI 2.92–25.28). **III B**

3 Geerts WH, Jay RM, Code KI *et al.* (1996) A comparison of low-dose heparin with low-molecular weight heparin as a prophylaxis against VTE after major trauma. *N Engl J Med* **335**, 701–707. Randomized double-blind clinical trial comparing the efficacy of heparin (5000 units) or enoxaparin (30 mg) every 12 h in 344 major trauma (no intracranial bleeding) patients in the prevention of deep-vein thrombosis as assessed by contrast venography performed on or before day 14. 60 patients given heparin (44%) and 40 patients given enoxaparin (31%) had deep-vein thrombosis ($p = 0.014$); 15% and 6% respectively had proximal-vein thrombosis ($p = 0.012$). It is concluded that low-molecular-weight heparin was more effective than low-dose heparin in preventing venous thromboembolism after major trauma. **Ib A**

4 McAnena OJ, Moore EE, Marx JA *et al.* (1990) Initial evaluation of the patient with blunt abdominal trauma. *Surg Clin North Am* **70**, 495–513. Review on the investigation of patients with blunt abdominal trauma. Important diagnostic tools include radiology, laboratory investigations, computed tomography scan, ultrasound, intravenous pyelogram and contrast duodenography. However, the cornerstone of management in these patients appears to be peritoneal lavage, for its diagnostic accuracy. Special reference is made to trauma in children, pregnancy and the elderly. **IV C**

5 Goldman SM, Wagner LK (1996) Radiological management of abdominal trauma in pregnancy. *AJR* **166**, 763–767. Review on the role of radiological investigations in the pregnant woman following abdominal trauma. It outlines the risk of radiation following investigations such as plain X-rays, abdominal computed tomography, angiography and contrast imaging but concludes that the benefit of these tests outweighs the potential harmful effects of radiation. **IV C**

6 Fischer RP, Beverlin BC, Engrav LH *et al.* (1978) Diagnostic peritoneal lavage. Fourteen years and 2,586 patients later. *Am J Surg* **36**, 701–704. Retrospective descriptive study on the results from diagnostic peritoneal lavage in blunt abdominal trauma over a 14-year period in 2586 patients. Peritoneal lavage was found to be 98.5% accurate, with a 0.2% false-positive rate and a 1.2% false-negative rate. **III B**

7 Esposito TJ, Gens DR, Smith LG *et al.* (1989) Evaluation of blunt abdominal trauma occurring during pregnancy. *J Trauma* **29**, 1628–1632. Review of the management of a series of 40 pregnant patients admitted to a trauma unit following blunt abdominal trauma. Management consisted of either diagnostic peritoneal lavage (32%), laparotomy and cesarean section (7%), computed tomography (CT) imaging of abdomen (7%) or clinical observation (55%). Peritoneal lavage had high diagnostic accuracy (92%) but could not assess intrauterine pathology. CT imaging was advantageous in this latter area. Clinical observation was felt to be safe – however, fetal mortality in the study was 100%. **III B**

8 Gruessner R, Mentges B, Duber C *et al.* (1989) Sonography versus peritoneal lavage in blunt abdominal trauma. *J Trauma* **29**, 242–244. Prospective study in which 71 trauma patients underwent ultrasound examination of the abdomen prior to peritoneal lavage. The results of both examinations were compared with the operative findings or clinical course. Peritoneal lavage was found to be significantly more accurate than ultrasound in diagnosing intraperitoneal injury. The authors concluded that the two examinations should be complementary. **IIb B**

9 Bode PJ, Niezen RA, van Vugt AB *et al.* (1993) Abdominal ultrasound as a reliable indicator for conclusive laparotomy in blunt abdominal trauma. *J Trauma* **34**, 27–31. Retrospective study reviewed 353 patients subjected to blunt abdominal trauma. Ultrasound of the abdomen was performed in all cases. Hemoperitoneum and intraperitoneal damage were correctly diagnosed in 99.4% of cases. Although other imaging modalities (computed tomography, angiography, magnetic resonance imaging) are accurate, they are time-consuming and costly. The authors argue that the ultrasound should be performed by an experienced individual, and hence that a radiologist should be part of the trauma team. **III B**

10 Rozycki GS, Ochsner MG, Jaffin JH *et al.* (1993) Prospective evaluation of surgeons' use of ultrasound in the evaluation of trauma patients. *J Trauma* **34**, 516–527. In this study, trauma specialists and surgical residents were trained in the use of ultrasound for the detection of free fluid in the abdomen and thorax. They evaluated their ability to accurately detect free fluid in a series of 476 trauma patients. Accurate detection was made in 79% of cases. The authors concluded that ultrasound is a rapid, safe test and that skills are easily learned. **III B**

42.2 Blunt trauma

Michelle Mohajer

Management option	Quality of evidence	Strength of recommendation	References
Increased risk of fetomaternal transfusion	IIa	B	1
Preterm labor, fetal distress and placental abruption occur more often but are rare in nonmajor trauma cases	III IIb	B B	2 3
Observation at least 4 h in nonmajor trauma	IIb	B	1,3
Assessment of the fetal condition: ❑ Fetal heart rate ❑ Kleihauer–Betke test ❑ Ultrasound	 IIa III III	 B B B	 1,3 2,4 4
Consider tocolysis	III	B	2,5
Aim to repair a ruptured uterus	IV	C	6

References

1 Pearlman MD, Tintinalli JE, Lorenz RP (1990) A prospective controlled study of outcome after trauma during pregnancy. *Am J Obstet Gynecol* **62**, 1502–1510. Study comparing the outcome of 85 pregnant women subjected to trauma with a matched control group. Fetomaternal transfusion occurred significantly more often following trauma and was more likely if the placenta was situated anteriorly. Continuous fetal heart rate monitoring was recommended for at least 4h following trauma to detect fetal compromise. **IIa B**

2 Dahmus MA, Sibai BM (1993) Blunt abdominal trauma: are there any predictive factors for abruptio placentae or maternal-fetal distress? *Am J Obstet Gynecol* **169**, 1054–1059. Retrospective study on outcome in a cohort of 233 pregnant women who had sustained nonmajor trauma. Preterm labor, fetal distress and placental abruption were all extremely rare (1%, 1.7% and 2.6% respectively). Coagulation studies and Kleihauer–Betke tests were not predictive of fetal or maternal morbidity. It was concluded that hospitalization for more than 4h is not indicated. **III B**

3 Goodwin TM, Breen MT (1990) Pregnancy outcome and fetomaternal hemorrhage after non catastrophic trauma. *Am J Obstet Gynecol* **162**, 665–671. Study prospectively evaluating the outcome of a group of 205 pregnant women subjected to nonmajor trauma against a group of matched controls. Trauma patients were managed by strict protocol. Pregnancy complications occurred in 8.8%. Preterm labor (10), placental abruption (5), fetal injury (1) and fetal death (1) occurred more often than in the control group. In the absence of contractions, uterine tenderness and bleeding, complications were rare (0.9%). Clinical signs were felt to be a good predictor of outcome. Lacking these, it was felt that observation beyond 2–3h was not indicated. **IIa B**

4 Lowery R, English TP, Wisner D *et al.* (1993) Evaluation of pregnant women after blunt injury. *J Trauma* **35**, 731–736. Retrospective review of 125 pregnant women who had sustained blunt trauma. It examines the usefulness of three diagnostic tests – fetal ultrasound, external fetal heart rate monitoring and Kleihauer–Betke test (K–B) – in detecting fetal complications. Fetal heart rate monitoring and fetal ultrasound were far more effective than K–B in detecting these complications. **III B**

5 Connolly A, Katz VL, Bash KL *et al.* (1997) Trauma and pregnancy. *Am J Perinatol* **14**, 331–336. Review of 476 pregnancies complicated by trauma (road traffic accidents, domestic abuse, falls, burns and animal bites). Regular uterine contractions occurred in 18%, preterm labor in 11.4%, preterm delivery in 25%, and placental abruptions in 1.58% of cases. Fetal heart rate monitoring was abnormal in 3% of cases. 14 perinatal deaths were related to trauma. Clinical signs and a positive Kleihauer–Betke test were not predictive of an adverse pregnancy outcome. The authors recommend continuous fetal heart rate monitoring for the first 4h. **III B**

6 Smith AJ, LeMire WA, Hurd WW *et al.* (1994) Repair of the traumatically ruptured gravid uterus. *J Reprod Med* **39**, 825–828. Two case reports are described in which major trauma resulted in ruptured uterus with fetal death. Both cases underwent uterine repair and successfully conceived and delivered healthy infants thereafter. The authors recommend hysterosalpingography prior to conception to examine the integrity of the initial surgical repair. **IV C**

42.3 Penetrating trauma

Diana Fothergill

Management option		Quality of evidence	Strength of recommendation	References
General management	Examine for entrance and exit wounds	–	✔	–
	Exploratory laparotomy	–	✔	–
	Midline vertical incision	–	✔	–
	Uterine evacuation is not mandatory	–	✔	–
	Cesarean hysterectomy if uncontrollable hemorrhage or extensive uterine damage	–	✔	–
Gunshot wounds	Flat plate and lateral radiograph if no exit wound visible	IV	C	1
	Surgical exploration if:			
	❏ Signs of intra-abdominal injury	III	B	2,3
	❏ Positive peritoneal lavage	III	B	4
	❏ Persistent unexplained shock	–	✔	–

Management option		Quality of evidence	Strength of recommendation	References
Gunshot wounds (cont'd)	Consider conservative management if:			
	❑ Hemodynamically stable mother	IV	C	1,5
	❑ Bullet entered below uterine fundus	III	B	3
	❑ Bullet can be localized to the uterus	III	B	3
	❑ Fetus is without injury or dead	III	B	3
	❑ Absence of maternal genitourinary or gastrointestinal injury	III	B	2,3
	Deliver fetus if:			
	❑ Evidence of fetal hemorrhage	IV	C	5
	❑ Uteroplacental insufficiency	IV	C	5
	❑ Infection	–	✔	–
Stab wounds	Determine peritoneal penetration – options:			
	❑ Probe wound	–	✔	–
	❑ Fistulogram	IV	C	6
	❑ Diagnostic peritoneal lavage	III	B	4,7
	Surgical exploration if:			
	❑ Peritoneal penetration	IV	C	6
	❑ Entry above the uterine fundus	–	✔	–
	❑ Hemodynamically unstable mother	IV	C	8
	❑ Fetal compromise at viable gestation	IV	C	6
	Consider conservative management if:			
	❑ No peritoneal penetration	IV	C	6
	❑ Entry below the uterine fundus	IV	C	6,8
	Delivery of the fetus: same as for gunshot wounds (above)	IV	C	6
	Uterine injury with lower abdominal stab wound – options:			
	❑ Observation	IV	C	6,8
	❑ Uterine repair with delivery	IV	C	6,8
	❑ Uterine repair and fetus remains *in utero*	IV	C	

References

1 Iliya FA, Hajj SN, Buchsbaum HJ (1980) Gunshot wounds of the pregnant uterus: Report of two cases. *J Trauma* **20**, 90–92. Description of two cases that demonstrate the protective shielding effect of the pregnant uterus, as the bullets came to rest within the uterus. Both women underwent laparotomy and cesarean section to deliver stillborn infants. The women survived but the authors questioned whether conservative treatment would have been more appropriate, as the cesarean section only added to morbidity. Based on these cases and a review of the literature they advise avoiding exploration if the fetus is dead, the entrance wound is below the fundus and the bullet shown on X-ray to be within the uterus. **IV C**

2 Muckart DJ, Abdool-Carrim AT, King B (1990) Selective conservative management of abdominal gunshot wounds: a prospective study. *Br J Surg* **77**, 652–655. Prospective study on the management of 111 patients with gunshot wounds of the abdomen. 89 patients (80%) had a laparotomy, of which 7 were negative. 22 (20%) were managed conservatively. Of these, 8 were considered to have peritoneal penetration. None required delayed laparotomy. 8 patients (7%) died; all were in the laparotomy group. The incidence of significant intra-abdominal injury if the peritoneal cavity had been penetrated was 89%. It was concluded that selective conservative management may be appropriate with gunshot wounds of the abdomen. **III B**

3 Awwad JT, Azar GB, Seoud MA *et al.* (1994) High-velocity penetrating wounds of the gravid uterus: review of 16 years of civil war. *Obstet Gynecol* **83**, 259–264 Retrospective study on 14 pregnant women with high-velocity abdominal penetrating trauma to the uterus. At surgical exploration, visceral injuries were present when the entrance of the missile was in either the upper abdomen or the back. They were absent in all 6 women with an anterior entry site below the uterine fundus. Half of these suffered a perinatal death due to maternal shock, uteroplacental or direct fetal injury. Delayed delivery after surgical exploration was successful in the 3 cases managed as such. Selective laparotomy may be considered in pregnant women with anterior penetrating abdominal trauma, depending on the location of the penetrating wound. **III B**

4 Esposito TJ, Jurkovich GJ, Rice CL *et al.* (1991) Trauma during pregnancy. A review of 79 cases. *Arch Surg* **126**, 1073–1078. Retrospective analysis of women admitted to a trauma center from 1980–89. The maternal mortality rate was 10%, which was similar to the nonpregnant population. The fetal loss rate was 34%. 21 women underwent peritoneal lavage: 9 in the first trimester, 9 in the second and 3 in the third. 7 of these were positive and there was one false negative. **IV C**

5 Franger AL, Buchsbaum HJ, Peaceman AM (1987) Abdominal gunshot wounds in pregnancy. *Am J Obstet Gynecol* **160**, 1124–1128. Report of 3 cases, 2 of which were deliberate attempts to end the pregnancy. In each of these cases the bullet passed through the uterus. One case, involving a 28-week fetus, resulted in delivery of a hypotensive but viable fetus with multiple fractures of the femur. An algorithm for management based on these cases and 7 other cases of self-inflicted injury advises conservative management if the fetus is either dead or not compromised and the entrance wound is below the fundus or the bullet is in the uterus. Laparotomy is advised if the entrance point is above the uterus or the bullet is not in the uterus. **IV C**

6 Sakala EP, Kort D (1988) Management of stab wounds to the pregnant uterus: a case report and a review of the literature. *Obstet Gynecol Surv* **43**, 319–324. Case report and review of a deliberate stabbing at 26 weeks as an abortifacient, and review of 18 published cases. In 14 cases where the uterus was perforated, only one fetus escaped injury; 7/14 died either *in utero* or in the neonatal period. All the mothers survived. Conservative management was advised if a fistulogram did not demonstrate entry into the peritoneal cavity. The authors consider that cesarean section is indicated when uterine size prevents adequate exploration or repair of visceral damage, if a viable fetus has identifiable distress, or when there is penetrating uterine injury of a live fetus at term. **IV C**

7 Alyono D, Perry JF (1981) Value of quantitative cell count and amylase activity of peritoneal lavage fluid. *J Trauma* **21**, 345–348. Retrospective analysis of 1588 patients who underwent diagnostic peritoneal lavage. When lavage fluid was not grossly bloody an aliquot was quantitated for red cell count, white cell count and amylase content. The test had a sensitivity of 94.3% and specificity of 99.8%. The false-positive rate was 0.1% and the false-negative 1.3%. In 8 patients the only abnormal finding was a raised white cell count; they all had bowel injuries. **III B**

8 Grubb DK (1992) Nonsurgical management of penetrating uterine trauma in pregnancy: a case report. *Am J Obstet Gynecol* **166**, 583–584. Case report of multiple abdominal stab wounds in a 30-week pregnancy managed conservatively. The woman was hemodynamically stable and the fetal heart satisfactory, one of the stab wounds was directly over the fetal head. Amniocentesis showed no evidence of infection, and the Kleihauer test was negative. Spontaneous labor occurred at 34 weeks; at delivery there was a small laceration over the parietal bone. **IV C**

42.4 Burns

Diana Fothergill

Management option		Quality of evidence	Strength of recommendation	References
Minor burns	Outpatient treatment if burn does not cover area of critical function and is not of cosmetic importance	–	✔	–
	Superficial burn:			
	❑ Analgesia	–	✔	–
	❑ Keep burned area clean and protected	–	✔	–
	Partial full-thickness burn:			
	❑ Clean, debride and irrigate	–	✔	–
	❑ Bacitracin ointment	–	✔	–
	❑ Non adherent dressing	–	✔	–
	❑ Adequate analgesia	–	✔	–
	❑ Reevaluate in 24 h	–	✔	–
Major burns	Fluid balance management:			
	❑ Adequate fluid administration (Parkland, Brooke or Evans formula)	Ib	A	1
	❑ Monitor urinary output to maintain 0.5 ml/kg/h	IV	C	2
	Examine entire body surface: assess depth of burn and surface area involved	IIa	B	3,4
	Arterial blood gas analysis and carbon monoxide level	IV	C	5

➡

Management option		Quality of evidence	Strength of recommendation	References
Major burns (cont'd)	Wound care: ❑ Sterile technique ❑ Topical antimicrobial agent ❑ Silver sulfadiazine relatively contraindicated in late pregnancy ❑ Surgery for debridement, prevention of cicatrization ❑ Cicatrized abdominal wounds may require release in pregnancy	 – IV IV IV IV	 ✔ C C C C	 – 6 6 6 7
Carbon monoxide poisoning	100% inspired oxygen by face mask if CO level above 10%	IIb	B	5,8
	Treat five times longer than required to lower maternal level below 5%	IIb	B	5
	Hyperbaric oxygen therapy if: ❑ Maternal CO level over 20% ❑ Neurological changes regardless of CO level ❑ Signs of fetal compromise	IV	C	9
Inhalation injury	Intubation if laryngeal edema develops	IV	C	8
	Warm humidified oxygen	IV	C	8
	Pulmonary toilet	IV	C	8
	Mechanical ventilation as indicated	IV	C	8
	Therapeutic bronchoscopy	IV	C	8
Labor and delivery	Cautious use of tocolysis if preterm labor	III	B	10
	Consider delivery of the fetus if: ❑ Significant medical complications in gravida with moderate to severe burns ❑ Gravely ill woman who develops complications ❑ Extensive burns at more than 32 weeks gestation ❑ More than 40–50% total body surface area burned	 IIb IIb IIb IIb	 B B B B	 3 3 3,4 3,4

References

1 Goodwin CW, Dorethy J, Lam V *et al.* (1983) Randomized trial of efficacy of crystalloid and colloid resuscitation on hemodynamic response and lung water following thermal injury. *Ann Surg* **197**, 520–531. RCT of the use of crystalloid or colloid fluid replacement in thermally injured patients. Measurement of lung water in 50 patients (25 in each therapeutic arm) showed a progressive increase in the colloid group; 5/25 had radiographic changes of pulmonary edema, compared with 1/25 in the crystalloid group. Colloid showed no other overall benefit. **Ib A**

2 Monafo WW (1996) Current concepts: initial management of burns. *N Engl J Med* **335**, 1581–1586. Review article covering the initial treatment of burn shock, inhalation injury and burn wound management. Crystalloid therapy is based on maintaining an hourly urine output of 0.5 ml/kg in the first 24 h. Inhalation injury remains a major cause of death and there are no randomized trials to advise best management. Topical antimicrobial agents are a mainstay of treatment; the three agents with proven efficacy are 11.1% mafenide acetate, 1% silver sulfadiazine and 0.5% silver nitrate. (None are regarded as safe in pregnancy; sulfadiazine may cause kernicterus if used near term.) **IV C**

3 Taylor JW, Plunkett GD, McManus WF *et al.* (1976) Thermal injury during pregnancy. *Obstet Gynecol* **47**, 434–438. Observational study of 19 pregnant women who sustained burn areas of 6–92% was found to be similar to that of 258 nonpregnant women of reproductive age who were treated in the same time period. 7 women died; they all sustained burns of more than 60%, and only one baby in this group survived. There was one stillbirth among the surviving women; this was associated with severe burn cellulitis. The authors recommend reserving obstetric intervention for very severely burned third-trimester patients who have become septic, hypotensive or hypoxic. **IIb B**

4 Akhtar MA, Mulawkar PM, Kulkarni HR *et al.* (1994) Burns in pregnancy: effect on maternal and fetal outcomes. *Burns* **20**, 351–355. A prospective case controlled study to identify risk factors for poor maternal and fetal outcome in 50 pregnant burned patients compared to 50 uncomplicated singleton pregnancies and 50 nonpregnant burned females. 64% had burns more than 60% of the total body surface area (TBSA) with 100% fetal and maternal mortality. There was 50% maternal and fetal loss in the 40–59% TBSA group. A fetal loss of 11.1% was found in the 20–39% TBSA group with no maternal loss. TBSA burned was the only variable found to be statistically significantly ($p < 0.0001$) that was responsible for the adverse fetal and maternal outcome. Pregnancy did not alter the maternal survival. Adequate shock management and early excision with grafting could reduce the mortality figures. **IIa B**

5 Longo LD (1997) The biological effects of carbon monoxide on the pregnant woman, fetus, and newborn infant. *Am J Obstet Gynecol* **129**, 69–97. Comprehensive review of the physiological and biological effects of carbon monoxide. Experimental work in animals has shown that CO uptake and elimination occur relatively more slowly in the fetus than in the mother. Mathematical modeling of the CO elimination curve in the fetus leads to the recommendation that a pregnant woman should receive 100% oxygen five times as long as is necessary to reduce her own carboxyhemoglobin concentration to less than 3–4%. **IV C**

6 Nguyen TT, Gilpin DA, Meyer NA *et al.* (1996) Current treatment of severely burned patients. *Ann Surg* **223**, 14–25. Review article summarizes current treatment. Burn shock is no longer the major cause of death as adequate fluid replacement is given according to the various formulae derived from retrospective analysis of patient data. The Parkland formula gives Ringer lactate 4 ml/kg/% burn surface area in the first 24 h. Sepsis remains a major challenge and is controlled by early excision of burn wounds and topical antimicrobials. Inhalational injury is treated by fluid resuscitation, humidified oxygen and occasional ventilatory support. Prophylactic antibiotics are of no proven benefit in reducing the mortality rate. **IV C**

7 Widgerow AD, Ford TD, Botha M *et al.* (1991) Burn contracture preventing uterine expansion. *Ann Plast Surg* **27**, 269–271. Report of two cases of surgical release of contractures at approximately 4 months, following burns sustained in childhood. Both pregnancies subsequently progressed normally and were delivered vaginally. **IV C**

8 Heimbach DM, Waeckerle JF (1988) Inhalation injuries. *Ann Emerg Med* **17**, 1316–1320. Review on inhalation injuries, which are stated to occur in approximately one-third of all major burns and to be the cause of death in a significant number of burns patients as a result of carbon monoxide poisoning, hypoxia and smoke inhalation. Thermal burns of the upper airway usually manifest within 48 h of injury. Diagnosis is by direct visualization of the upper airway. Treatment is with humidified oxygen, pulmonary toilet and bronchodilators and prophylactic endotracheal intubation as needed. Carbon monoxide poisoning is the most common cause of death in inhalation injury and is a result of combustion. Symptoms and signs correlate with blood levels and arterial blood gases determine the degree of intoxication. Treatment is based on the principle that carbon monoxide dissociation occurs much faster if the patient is placed on 100% oxygen. Smoke inhalation damages respiratory physiology, resulting in injury progressing from acute pulmonary insufficiency to pulmonary edema to bronchopneumonia, depending on the severity of exposure. Diagnosis is based on history, but clinical findings, arterial blood gases and fiberoptic bronchoscopy are helpful. **IV C**

9 VanHoesen KB, Camporesi EM, Moon RE *et al.* (1987) Should hyperbaric oxygen be used to treat the pregnant patient for acute carbon monoxide poisoning? A case report and literature review. *JAMA* **261**, 1039–1043. Case report of a maternal carboxyhemoglobin level of 42.7% at 37 weeks. On admission the fetal heart was abnormal with a tachycardia, decreased variability and late decelerations. Following administration of hyperbaric oxygen the CTG improved, after 90 min the maternal carboxyhemoglobin level was 2.4%. The baby was delivered several weeks later; there were no abnormal findings on fundoscopy. **IV C**

10 Matthews RN (1982) Obstetric implications of burns in pregnancy. *Br J Obstet Gynaecol* **89**, 603–609. Study of the outcomes in 50 pregnant women from local experience (16 women) and published cases. The author concludes that any woman in the second or third trimester who sustains more than 50% burns should be delivered, as there is no likelihood of improving fetal survival by delay and maternal outlook is poor. If the burn area is less than 40% then tocolysis may be appropriate. Vaginal delivery is possible even in the presence of perineal burns but there is no good evidence that cesarean section is harmful if obstetrically indicated – the wounds heal well and infection risk is not increased. **III B**

42.5 Electrical injury

Michelle Mohajer

Management option	Quality of evidence	Strength of recommendation	References
Fetal assessment	IV	C	1
Continued fetal surveillance for delayed effects	IV	C	2–4
Maternal injury may not correlate with fetal injury	IV	C	1,3

References

1 Fatovich DM (1993) Electric shock in pregnancy. *J Emerg Med* **11**, 175–177. Review of all case reports (15) in the English language literature of electric shock in pregnancy. Fetal mortality ($n = 11$) was 73% and there was only one normal pregnancy following electric shock. It was concluded that the fetus is much less resistant to electric shock than the mother and needs to be monitored carefully after such an event. **IV C**

2 Steer RG (1992) Delayed fetal death following electrical injury in the first trimester. *Aust N Z J Obstet Gynaecol* **32**, 377–378. Case report outlining the possibility of delayed fetal death following electrical shock in the first trimester. There is evidence in the literature that effects of electrical injury may be delayed as well as immediate. The authors also warn against the hazards of electrical fences in rural areas. **IV C**

3 Strong TH, Gocke SE, Levy AV *et al.* (1987) Electrical shock in pregnancy: a case. *J Emerg Med* **5**, 381–383. Case report of electrical shock in pregnancy and review of the literature. The authors suggest that the severity of the maternal injury does not correlate well with fetal injury and advise close fetal surveillance under such circumstances. **IV C**

4 Leiberman JR, Mazor M, Molcho J *et al.* (1986) Electrical accidents during pregnancy. *Obstet Gynecol* **67**, 861–863. Six case reports of electrical injury during pregnancy. Three cases resulted in stillbirth at varying intervals from the initial accident. The authors suggest close monitoring of the pregnancy following electrical injury and also that pregnant women should notify their doctor if they have sustained any minor electrical accident. **IV C**

42.6 Perimortem cesarean section

Michelle Mohajer

Management option	Quality of evidence	Strength of recommendation	References
Timing: at cardiopulmonary arrest, not sooner	IV	C	1
Consider performing the procedure to aid maternal resuscitation	IV	C	2
Initiate delivery within 4 min after arrest when resuscitation is unsuccessful	IV	C	1,3
Aim to deliver 5 min after arrest	IV	C	1,3
Continue cardiopulmonary resuscitation during delivery	IV	C	1
No need for sterility	IV	C	3
Quickest incision possible	IV	C	3
Consider low uterine incision	IV	C	3
Deliver if signs of fetal life and more than 4 min passed since maternal arrest	IV	C	1,3

References

1 Weber CE (1971) Postmortem cesarean section: review of the literature and case reports. *Am J Obstet Gynecol* **110**, 158–165. Review covering all aspects of perimortem cesarean section, from the historical aspects to the medicolegal perspective. It is clearly recommended as a management option in particular circumstances: where the pregnancy has exceeded 28 weeks gestation and when the fetus can be delivered within 15 minutes of maternal death. Additional recommendations were of continued maternal cardiopulmonary support and prompt neonatal resuscitation. **IV C**

2 Whitten M, Irvine LM (2000) Postmortem and perimortem caesarean section: what are the indications? *J R Soc Med* **93**, 6–9. Report considering the merits of perimortem cesarean section, particularly in the light of the Confidential Enquiry into Maternal Deaths. Although the total cases are few, the procedure should always be considered, not only for the life of the infant but also in the interests of resuscitation of the mother, which is facilitated by emptying the uterus. The report also claims that, with acute maternal shock, neurodevelopmental handicap is extremely rare as the fetus usually survives intact or perishes. **IV C**

3 Katz VL, Cefalo RC, McCune BK *et al.* (1986) Perimortem cesarean delivery. *Obstet Gynecol* **68**, 571–576. Review of the practice of perimortem cesarean section, in particular the changing pattern of maternal mortality, which obviously affects the situation. Prompt delivery is essential (within 4 min of death), otherwise serious neurodevelopmental problems may occur. The authors also review the medicolegal perspective, concluding that liability is virtually unknown. **IV C**

Chapter 43

Abdominal pain

Conditions dealt with elsewhere

- Miscarriage (see Section 7.1)
- Ectopic pregnancy (see Section 6.1)
- Placental abruption (see Section 46.1)
- Chorioamnionitis (see Section 24.12)
- Preterm labor (see Section 46.1)
- Inflammatory bowel disease (see Section 33.7)
- Peptic ulcer disease (see Section 33.5)
- Urinary tract (see Section 24.11,acute cystitis; acute pyelonephritis; Section 35.5, nephrolithiasis)
- Acute fatty liver of pregnancy (see Section 33.2)
- Severe preeclampsia–eclampsia (see Chapter 26)
- Sickle-cell crisis (see Section 31.1)
- Porphyria (see Section 39.1)
- Malaria (see Section 24.17)
- Tuberculosis (see Section 24.16)

43.1 Round ligament pain

Petra Deering

Management option	Quality of evidence	Strength of recommendation	References
Exclude pathological causes of pain	–	✔	–
Reassure	–	✔	–
Reduce physical activity	–	✔	–
Local heat	–	✔	–

43.2 Severe uterine torsion

Petra Deering

Management option	Quality of evidence	Strength of recommendation	References
Exclude pathological cause of pain	–	✔	–
Conservative ❑ Bed rest ❑ Analgesia ❑ Altering maternal position ❑ Screen for acute and chronic fetal hypoxia	–	✔	–
Surgical (diagnosed at laparotomy) ❑ Correct the torsion ❑ Delivery by cesarean section during laparotomy or later if preterm	IV	C	1

Reference

1 Gronkjaer Jensen J (1992) Uterine torsion in pregnancy. *Acta Obstet Gynecol Scand* **71**, 260–265. Review article of 212 reported cases of uterine torsion (defined as rotation of more than 45% around the long axis of the uterus). 6% occurred in the first, 26% in the second and 49% in the third trimester. The degree of torsion is most often 180°. The symptoms (pain, shock, intestinal complaints, urinary symptoms, bleeding, obstructed labor) are related to the degree of torsion and can be acute, subacute, chronic or intermittent. The maternal mortality is influenced by the degree of torsion: less than 90°, 2%; 90–180°, 7%; 180–360°, 36%, more than 360°, 67%. Since 1960 only one woman has died as a result of torsion. The propagated treatment for uterine torsion is laparotomy and detorsion of the uterus. If the fetus is viable, cesarean section is performed following detorsion of the uterus. **IV C**

43.3 Heartburn, excess vomiting and constipation

Petra Deering

Management option		Quality of evidence	Strength of recommendation	References
Heartburn	Reassure	–	✔	–
	Avoid bending	–	✔	–
	Avoid lying flat in bed (more pillows/raise head of bed)	–	✔	–
	Antacids	Ib	A	1,2
	H_2 antagonists if severe	Ia	A	3
Excess vomiting	Exclude pathological cause	–	✔	–
	Reassure	–	✔	–
	Dietary adjustment	–	✔	–
	Rectal antiemetics (?avoid first trimester)	–	✔	–
	Consider hospital admission (especially if dehydration/ketosis): ❑ Nil else as first measure ❑ Consider intravenous fluids and intravenous antiemetics if continued problem	–	✔	–
Constipation	Dietary adjustment, increase fiber	IIb	B	4
	Stop iron therapy unless absolutely indicated	–	✔	–
	Consider laxatives	III	B	5,6
	Consider suppositories/enema only if severe	–	✔	–

References

1 Shaw RW (1978) Randomized controlled trial of Syn-Ergel and an active placebo in the treatment of heartburn of pregnancy. *J Int Med Res* **6**, 147–151. RCT to study the efficacy of Syn-Ergel (aluminium/aluminum phosphate gel) versus an active placebo in the treatment of heartburn of pregnancy in 92 patients (third trimester; 7-day course). Syn-Ergel was significantly better ($p < 0.001$) in all groups of pretreatment pain severity in relieving the symptoms and had a longer duration of action than the active placebo. Complete relief of pain was achieved in 79.5% of Syn-Ergel treatments with a further 10% of treatments resulting in marked easing of discomfort at 1 h following administration. The corresponding figures for the active placebo were 56% and 20%. **Ib A**

2 Atlay RD, Weekes AR, Entwistle GD, Parkinson DJ (1978) Treating heartburn in pregnancy: comparison of acid and alkali mixtures. *Br Med J* **2**, 919–920. A randomized double-blind crossover trial performed in 41 pregnant women with heartburn to see whether acid and alkali treatment alleviated it. 51% of women found complete symptom

relief or alleviation with alkali, 68% with acid and 44% with placebo (alkali vs acid $p = 0.18$, alkali v placebo $p = 0.66$, acid v placebo $p = 0.045$). **Ib A**

3 Redstone HA, Barrowman N, Veldhuyzen Van Zanten SJ (2001) H2-receptor antagonists in the treatment of functional (non-ulcer) dyspepsia: a meta-analysis of randomised controlled clinical trials. *Aliment Pharmacol Ther* **15**, 1291–1299. 22 studies met the inclusion criteria, 15 of which reported the active drug superior to placebo. Many studies suffered from suboptimal study design. The OR in favor of active drug was 1.48 (95% CI 0.9–2.3) for global assessment of dyspepsia symptoms, 2.3 (95% CI, 1.6–3.3) for improvement of epigastric pain and 1.8 (95% CI, 1.2–2.8) for complete relief of epigastric pain. **Ia A**

4 Anderson AS, Whichelow MJ (1985) Constipation during pregnancy: dietary fiber intake and the effect of fiber supplementation. *Hum Nutr Appl Nutr* **39**, 202–207. 40 women complaining of constipation during the third trimester of pregnancy completed weighed diet records and bowel function charts over a 4-week period. After an initial 2 weeks of baseline observation the women were randomly allocated into three groups (A, B, C). Groups A and B were asked to take 10g dietary fiber supplements per day in the form of either a corn-based biscuit or wheat bran; group C carried on without further intervention. In the final 2 weeks, the mean increase in fiber intake for group A was 7.2 ± 1.0g ($p < 0.001$) and 9.1 ± 1.6g for group B ($p < 0.001$); group C showed a mean decrease of 3.5 ± 1.6g per day ($p < 0.005$). These changes were accompanied by an increase in the number of bowel movements (OR 0.18, 95% CI 0.05–0.67) and a change to a softer stool consistency in groups A and B, with no change in Group C. **IIb B**

5 Muller M, Jaquenoud E (1995) Treatment of constipation in pregnant women. A multicenter study in a gynaecological practice. *Schw Med Wochenschr* **125**, 1689–1693. In an open, baseline-controlled multicenter study, 62 pregnant women aged between 19–40 years were treated with lactulose for 4 weeks. The frequency of defecation was significantly increased after 1 week (median per week 4.0 vs 2.5 times, $p < 0.001$) and normalized after 2 weeks (6 stools per week). Also, the consistency of the stools was normalized during treatment. **III B**

6 Signorelli P, Croce P, Dede A (1996) [A clinical study of the use of a combination of glucomannan with lactulose in the constipation of pregnancy]. (In Italian). *Minerva Ginecol* **48**, 577–582. 50 pregnant women affected by constipation were treated with sachets containing a preparation of glucomannan (1.45g) and lactulose (4.2g) in a posology of two (one to four) sachets a day for 1–3 months. Treatment induced a return to normal frequency of weekly number of evacuations (4.9–5.8/week). **III B**

43.4 Uterine fibroids

Petra Deering

Management option		Quality of evidence	Strength of recommendation	References
Prepregnancy	The majority of women with fibroids will have no problems in conceiving or with pregnancy	Ia	A	1
	Myomectomy: only consider cautiously in cases with uterine cavity distortion and problems such as menorrhagia, recurrent miscarriage and/or infertility. Even then, only undertake after careful counseling	Ia III	A B	1 2
	Exclude other pathological causes of pain	–	✔	–
Prenatal	If asymptomatic, reassure	–	✔	–
	If associated with pain, exclude other diagnoses first	–	✔	–
	Red degeneration: ❑ Bed rest ❑ Analgesia ❑ ? Local ice packs	(III	B	5, p.289)
	Avoid surgery unless pedunculated	–	✔	–
	Review mode of delivery at 36–38 weeks (? malpresentation, possible dystocia)	–	✔	–

Management option		Quality of evidence	Strength of recommendation	References
Labor and delivery	If obstructed labor, cesarean section may be necessary (possibly via upper segment)	(III	B	7, p.289)
Postnatal	Analgesia for excess pain with involution	–	✔	–
See also Section 40.3.				

References

1 Pritts EA (2001) Fibroids and infertility: a systematic review of the evidence. *Obstet Gynecol Surv* **56**, 483–491. Systematic literature review was performed to determine whether fibroids are associated with decreased fertility rates and whether removal increases fertility rates. Meta-analysis was conducted when multiple studies addressed a single issue and were sufficiently homogenous. Data were analyzed for effect of any fibroid upon fertility, as well as specific fibroid location. Subgroup analysis failed to indicate any effect on fertility of fibroids that did not have a submucous component. Women with submucous myomas demonstrated lower pregnancy rates (RR 0.30, 95% CI 0.13–0.7) and implantation rates (RR 0.28, CI 0.10–0.72). Results of surgical intervention were similar. When all fibroid locations were considered together, myomectomy results were widely disparate. When considering women with submucous fibroids separately, pregnancy was increased after myomectomy compared with infertile controls (RR 1.72, 95% CI 1.13–2.58) and delivery rates were then equivalent to infertile women without fibroids (RR 0.98; 95% CI 0.45–2.41). The current data suggest that only those fibroids with a submucosal or an intracavitary component are associated with decreased reproductive outcomes and that hysteroscopic myomectomy may be of benefit. **Ia A**

2 Vercellini P, Zaina B, Yaylayan L *et al.* (1999) Hysteroscopic myomectomy: long-term effects on menstrual pattern and fertility. *Obstet Gynecol* **94**, 341–347. Observational study of 108 women who had first-line hysteroscopic resection of submucous pedunculated ($n = 54$), sessile ($n = 30$) or intramural ($n = 24$) fibroids at the First Department of Obstetrics and Gynecology of the University of Milan were studied to determine the effects of myomectomy on menorrhagia and infertility. Menorrhagia was the main indication for two thirds of the subjects. After a mean (± SD) follow-up of 41 ± 23 months there was a myoma recurrence in 27 subjects (12/54 with pedunculated lesions, 7/30 with sessile lesions and 8/24 with intramural lesions), with a corresponding overall 3-year cumulative myoma recurrence rate of 34%. 80% achieved long-term control of menorrhagia (more than 3 years; significant reduction in menstrual blood loss and increase in hemoglobin level; paired t test, $p < 0.01$). The 3-year cumulative probability of conception was 49% in women with pedunculated lesions ($n = 22$), 36% in those with sessile lesions ($n = 12$) and 33% in those with intramural lesions ($n = 6$). **III B**

43.5 Uterine rupture

Petra Deering

Management option		Quality of evidence	Strength of recommendation	References
Prepregnancy	Discuss sterilization in the patient with a history of uterine rupture	III	B	1,2
Prenatal	Careful counseling and vigilance in those with risk factors	–	✔	–
	Consider delivery by cesarean section if diagnosis is suspected	–	✔	–
Labor and delivery	In women at 'high risk' (uterine scar, high parity, prolonged oxytocic stimulation), vigilance for uterine rupture:	III IIb	B B	3 4
	❑ Continuous fetal heart rate monitoring	III	B	3,5
	❑ Regular vaginal examinations to ensure normal progress	–	✔	–
	❑ Regard any fresh bleeding seriously	III	B	3

Management option		Quality of evidence	Strength of recommendation	References
Labor and delivery (cont'd)	If diagnosis is suspected, proceed to laparotomy, delivery by cesarean section and repair uterus (hysterectomy may occasionally be necessary)	–	✔	–
	Correct blood loss	–	✔	–

References

1 O'Connor RA, Gaughen B (1989) Pregnancy following simple repair of the ruptured gravid uterus. *Br J Obstet Gynaecol* **96**, 942–944. Retrospective review of 67 cases of rupture of the gravid uterus. 34 of these ruptures were considered suitable for repair. In this study 18 pregnancies in 15 patients in whom a simple repair was performed were traced. 13 involved rupture of the lower uterine segment, 2 the upper uterine segment (one a previous classical scar, the other a small fundal rupture). 17 of the pregnancies had a successful outcome. 16 of these were delivered by elective lower segment cesarean section between 37 and 40 weeks gestation; the patient with a previously ruptured classical scar was delivered at 35 weeks by lower segment cesarean section. The one unsuccessful outcome occurred in a twin pregnancy, both fetuses were diagnosed as intrauterine deaths at 28 weeks. In young patients with uterine rupture and patients who have not completed their family, simple repair without tubal ligation should be considered, with elective delivery by lower segment cesarean section. **III B**

2 Aguero O, Kizer S (1968) Obstetric prognosis of the repair of uterine rupture. *Surg Gynecol Obstet* **124**, 528–530. Report of 66 subsequent pregnancies in 62 patients in whom a simple repair following uterine rupture was performed. 15 had spontaneous vaginal deliveries, 8 had a forceps delivery and 43 were delivered by cesarean section. 4 cases of recurrent rupture occurred, all in patients in whom vaginal delivery was allowed to take place. **III B**

3 Chen LH, Tan KH, Yeo GS (1995) A ten-year review of uterine rupture in modern obstetric practice. *Ann Acad Med Singapore* **24**, 830–835. Retrospective study of 26 proven cases of uterine rupture. Incidence of rupture was 1/6331 deliveries. The incidence of rupture in unscarred uteri was 1/27 433 cases, the incidence of scar dehiscence was 1/1183 lower segment cesarean sections (0.08%). Ratio of cases with scarred uteri against unscarred was 3:1. The commonest cause of rupture in the unscarred group was undiagnosed cephalopelvic disproportion (67%) half of which received oxytocin augmentation. The main clinical presentations were cardiotocogram abnormalities (25%) and bloodstained liquor (20%) in the scarred group, and postpartum hemorrhage (50%) and shock (33%) in the unscarred group. 95% of patients in the scarred group had a uterine repair, 67% in the unscarred group required a hysterectomy. There was one maternal death. Commonest cause for maternal morbidity was anemia. The average blood loss was significantly higher in the unscarred group – all patients required a blood transfusion versus 35% in the scarred group. Overall fetal loss was 7.4%. **III B**

4 Leung AS, Farmer RM, Leung EK *et al.* (1993) Risk factors associated with uterine rupture during trial of labor after cesarean delivery: a case-control study. *Am J Obstet Gynecol* **168**, 1358–1363. A case-control study of 70 patients with prior cesarean delivery with uterine rupture during trial of labor between January 1983 and June 1990 was conducted at the Women's Hospital of the Los Angeles County-University. Oxytocin was administered to 77% of patients in the case group and 56% of patients in control group (OR 2.7, 95% CI 1.2–6.0). Dysfunctional labor increased risk of rupture (OR 7.2, 95% CI 2.7–20.0). More specifically, arrest disorders (arrest of descent or of dilatation) were experienced by 84% of the case group and 28% of the control group. Risk of uterine rupture for women with two or three prior cesarean deliveries was increased (OR 2.6, 95% CI 1.1–6.4). Epidural anesthesia, macrosomia, history of successful vaginal delivery after cesarean section and history of cesarean delivery because of cephalopelvic disproportion were not associated with uterine rupture. **IIb B**

5 Ayres AW, Johnson TR, Hayashi R (2001) Characteristics of fetal heart rate tracings prior to uterine rupture. *Int J Gynaecol Obstet* **74**, 235–240. The cardiotocogram strips during the 2-hour period preceding uterine rupture of 11 patients who delivered at the University of Michigan Hospital from 1985–99 were reviewed. 8 fetal heart rate tracings were available. 87.5% revealed recurrent late decelerations and 50% terminal bradycardia. All 4 patients with fetal bradycardia were preceded by recurrent late decelerations. **III B**

43.6 Torsion of adnexa

Petra Deering

Management option		Quality of evidence	Strength of recommendation	References
Prenatal	Laparotomy: untwisting and then deciding on ovarian cystectomy versus oophorectomy depending on viability	–	✔	–
	? Intravenous tocolysis	–	✔	–
	If corpus luteum removed before 8 weeks, progesterone support up to 10 weeks	–	✔	–

43.7 Appendicitis

Petra Deering

Management option	Quality of evidence	Strength of recommendation	References
Diagnosis is not easy; risk to mother and fetus greatly increased with perforation	III	B	1
Laparotomy with right paramedian incision at site of maximal tenderness	–	✔	–
? Use of prophylactic tocolysis postoperatively for 2–3 days	III	B	1,2
Postoperative antibiotics	–	✔	–

References

1 Al-Mulhim AA (1996) Acute appendicitis in pregnancy. *Int Surg* **81**, 295–297. Retrospective study of 52 pregnant patients who underwent laparotomy for suspected acute appendicitis, revealing a histopathological diagnosis in 29 (56%) patients. The hospital incidence for acute appendicitis in pregnancy was 0.09% (1/1102 deliveries). Abdominal pain in the right lower quadrant was the most common presenting symptom. Abdominal tenderness and rebound tenderness were the most common physical signs, although the latter was less marked in late pregnancy. Preoperative white cell count (WBC) was of little diagnostic help; however the left shift in WBC differential signified infection, which was present in 72% of patients with acute appendicitis versus only 32% of women with normal appendix. Among the patients with proven appendicitis, 5 fetuses were lost (17%), 4 of them associated with perforated appendix with symptoms exceeding 24 h before operation. Maternal morbidity was limited in the current series to 5 cases of postoperative wound infection; 3 of these were associated with perforated appendix. Antibiotics were used in all cases of gangrenous or perforated appendix. The authors recommend the use of tocolytics when appendicitis is suspected. **III B**

2 To WW, Ngai CS, Ma HK (1995) Pregnancies complicated by acute appendicitis. *Aust N Z J Surg* **65**, 799–803. 38 obstetric cases who had an appendicectomy performed during pregnancy were reviewed. In 31 cases acute appendicitis was proven at laparotomy and by subsequent histopathology. The overall pregnancy loss rate among those with confirmed appendicitis, including miscarriages and neonatal death, was 16%. The major cause in the 3 cases of fetal loss beyond the first trimester in the series has been related to late second trimester miscarriage and premature labor, so the authors advise the use of prophylactic tocolytics. In total there were 4 cases of premature labor within 3–10 days of onset of symptoms at 26, 28, 34 and 36 weeks gestation. **III B**

43.8 Intestinal obstruction

Petra Deering

Management option	Quality of evidence	Strength of recommendation	References
Once diagnosis is made, conservative versus surgical approach is cause for debate:	IV	C	1
If surgical option chosen: ❑ Conservative (nasogastric suction, i.v. fluids) may be considered for a few hours if no strangulation/perforation ❑ Surgical approach (laparotomy and surgical correction of obstruction) always if strangulation/perforation, although some would advocate early surgery for all cases ❑ Obstetrician and surgeon operating together is advisable ❑ Adequate vertical incision ❑ Cesarean section may be necessary for adequate surgical field in late pregnancy	IV	C	1
Careful attention to fluid and electrolyte balance	–	✔	–
? Tocolysis for 2–3 days after surgery	–	✔	–
Perioperative antibiotics	–	✔	–

Reference

1 Connolly MM, Unti JA, Nora PF (1995) Bowel obstruction in pregnancy. *Surg Clin North Am* **75**, 101–113. Review article of all cases reported in the English literature from 1945–95. Adhesions are the leading cause of bowel obstruction in pregnancy (55%); intestinal volvulus is responsible for 25% of cases, assuming a far greater role in the pregnant woman (only 3–5% of nonpregnant cases of bowel obstruction are caused by volvulus). The mortality rate is much higher in pregnancy because of delay in diagnosis, in part related to initial avoidance of radiological studies and hesitancy to perform surgery on pregnant patients. A multidisciplinary approach incorporating both the surgeon and obstetrician is deemed mandatory. When fever, tachycardia, localized abdominal pain and leukocytosis are not present, conservative management may be attempted, otherwise gangrene must be suspected and immediate laparotomy should be performed. Failure of improvement within 48 h of tube decompression should also lead to laparotomy. Fluid resuscitation, correction of acid–base and electrolyte imbalances, gastrointestinal decompression and antibiotic prophylaxis are recommended as part of preoperative preparation. Maternal mortality over the past 30 years has decreased to 6%. Fetal mortality rates have remained constant at 20–26%. **IV C**

43.9 Cholecystitis

Petra Deering

Management option		Quality of evidence	Strength of recommendation	References
Prepregnancy	Consider cholecystectomy prior to conception with symptomatic gallstones	–	✔	–
Prenatal	Conservative approach first: ❑ Bed rest ❑ Analgesia/sedation ❑ Intravenous fluids ❑ Nasogastric suction ❑ Antibiotics (e.g. amoxicillin, cefradine or co-amoxiclav; chenodeoxycholic acid is contraindicated because of possible teratogenic effects) ❑ Dietary adjustment after attack has subsided (avoiding fatty foods, etc.)	III	B	1

➡

Management option		Quality of evidence	Strength of recommendation	References
Prenatal (cont'd)	Indications for cholecystectomy (preferably in second trimester): ❑ Recurrent cholecystitis attacks ❑ Jaundice ❑ Abnormal liver function ❑ Empyema of gall bladder ❑ Bile duct dilatation suggestive of obstruction ❑ Pancreatitis ❑ Laparotomy is also indicated if appendicitis cannot be excluded	III IV	B C	2 3

References

1 Landers D, Carmona R, Crombleholme W *et al.* (1987) Acute cholecystitis in pregnancy. *Obstet Gynecol* **69**, 131–133. 30 cases of acute cholecystitis in pregnancy were identified between 1972 and 1985. 25 were initially treated medically with bed rest, intravenous fluids, analgesics and intravenous ampicillin if febrile. 21 (84%) patients responded to conservative treatment and 4 were judged to need cholecystectomy during pregnancy. 3 patients underwent cholecystectomy at 16, 17 and 29 weeks gestation and delivered live infants at term. One patient underwent exploratory laparotomy complicated by *Salmonella* septicemia and went into preterm labor and delivery of a 1620g infant, who survived. Subsequent cholecystectomy confirmed the gallbladder as the source of the *Salmonella* sepsis. For 5 patients surgery was the primary mode of management, for unknown reasons. One patient underwent cholecystectomy at 9 weeks gestation and aborted postoperatively. A second patient at 16 weeks had no pregnancy-related complications, a patient at 30 weeks went into preterm labor postoperatively. A further 2 patients had elective terminations precholecystectomy in the first trimester. **III B**

2 Dixon NP, Faddis DM, Silberman H (1987) Aggressive management of cholecystitis during pregnancy. *Am J Surg* **154**, 292–294. Report of 44 patients with the diagnosis of biliary colic or cholecystitis. 26 patients were treated conservatively, of whom 56% had recurrent episodes of biliary colic during the course of pregnancy. Spontaneous miscarriage occurred in 3 patients (12%) at 7, 12, 14 weeks gestation after biliary symptoms, and termination of pregnancy was performed in 3 patients in the first trimester prior to undergoing elective cholecystectomy. 3 patients underwent cholecystectomy in the first trimester (unaware of pregnancy), of whom all opted for termination postoperatively. 14 patients underwent surgery in the second trimester with 11 babies born at term, one born following induction of labor for preeclampsia at 36 weeks and 2 lost to follow-up. One patient operated on at 28 weeks went into preterm labor postoperatively that was successfully arrested with magnesium sulfate. Surgery performed during the second trimester was associated with little maternal morbidity, no fetal loss and a substantial reduction in total hospital days. **III B**

3 Ghumman E, Barry M, Grace PA (1997) Management of gallstones in pregnancy. *Br J Surg* **84**,1646–1650. Review article of management of symptomatic cholelithiasis in pregnancy. Most clinicians recommend surgery in cases of repeated attacks of biliary colic, acute cholecystitis, obstructive jaundice, gallstone pancreatitis, peritonitis or uncertainty of diagnosis. The treatment of choice for uncomplicated cholecystitis is nonoperative, with elective cholecystectomy performed after delivery. Conservative treatment in particular is advocated for during the first and third trimester because of increased loss of pregnancy/induction of preterm labor. Surgery is performed best during the second trimester because organogenesis is complete, uterine size does not interfere with the operative field and the risk of spontaneous miscarriage is low. **IV C**

43.10 Acute pancreatitis

Petra Deering

Management option		Quality of evidence	Strength of recommendation	References
Prepregnancy	Discuss specific measures in women with risk factors: ❑ Cholecystectomy in women with known gallstones and previous attacks of cholecystitis or pancreatitis ❑ Various strategies in women with alcohol abuse ❑ Change treatment in women taking thiazide diuretics	–	✔	–
Prenatal	Prevention and treatment of shock with intravenous fluids and monitoring electrolyte, calcium and glucose concentrations	III	B	1
	Analgesia	–	✔	–
	Prophylactic antibiotics (such as amoxicillin, cefradine or co-amoxiclav)	III	B	1
	Suppression of pancreatic activity (no RCTs): ❑ Anticholinergic drugs ❑ Steroids ❑ Prostaglandins ❑ Glucagon ❑ Cimetidine ❑ Trypsin inhibitors	–	✔	–
	Use of nasogastric suction is questioned	–	✔	–
	Prompt recognition and treatment of surgical complications	–	✔	–
	Laparotomy, usually with cholecystectomy, if conservative measures fail	–	✔	–
	Cholecystectomy as an early option when pancreatitis occurs with gallstones in first or second trimester	–	✔	–
Postnatal	Cholecystectomy if pancreatitis with gallstones successfully treated conservatively in pregnancy	–	✔	–

Reference

1 Ramin KD, Ramin SM, Richey SD *et al.* (1995) Acute pancreatitis in pregnancy. *Am J Obstet Gynecol* **173**, 187–191. Review of 43 cases of acute pancreatitis in pregnancy. The incidence was 1/3333 pregnancies. Pancreatitis was associated with biliary disease in 68% and was more common with advanced pregnancy (19% first, 26% second, 53% third trimester). The women were seen in consultation by the surgical service. Management was based on resolution of symptoms and improvement of laboratory findings and included bowel rest, intravenous hydration, antibiotics and analgesics. Symptoms resolved over a mean of 5.5 days and the patients were hospitalized for a mean of 8.5 days (range 2–15 days). 8 women failed to respond to conservative treatment and underwent cholecystectomy. Perinatal outcomes were available for 39 women, of whom 74% were delivered of healthy term infants. There were 6 preterm deliveries associated with the acute episode of pancreatitis, from which 2 babies survived. **III B**

43.11 Abdominal pregnancy

Petra Deering

Management option		Quality of evidence	Strength of recommendation	References
With dead fetus	Delivery by laparotomy, possibly with a delay to reduce complication rates	IV	C	1
With a live fetus before 24 weeks	Delivery by laparotomy	–	✔	–
	Consider a conservative approach after careful counseling, possibly undertaken as inpatient	–	✔	–
With a live fetus after 24 weeks	Laparotomy and delivery if oligohydramnios and/or compressional deformities	–	✔	–
	Laparotomy and delivery: ❑ Ideally performed jointly with general/vascular surgeon ❑ Several units of blood available ❑ Midline vertical incision in abdomen ❑ Incision of sac away from placenta ❑ Avoid placental manipulation during delivery ❑ If blood supply to placenta can be secured, remove placenta completely ❑ If blood supply to placenta cannot be secured, ligate cord only (greater postoperative morbidity)	IV	C	1

Reference

1 Opare-Addo HS, Deganus S (2000) Advanced abdominal pregnancy: a study of 13 consecutive cases seen in 1993 and 1994 at Komfo Anokye Teaching Hospital, Kumasi, Ghana. *Afr J Reprod Health* **4**, 28–39. A total of 13 cases of advanced abdominal pregnancy were managed at the Komfo Anokye Teaching Hospital over a 2-year period. Only abdominal pregnancies with fetal weights greater than 500g (gestation 20 weeks or more) were included in this study. An incidence ratio of one advanced abdominal pregnancy to 1320 deliveries occurred during this period. The perinatal mortality rate and maternal case fatality rates were 69.6% and 15.3% respectively. In the case of a dead fetus it was found that delay of laparotomy reduced complication rates because of easy removal of the placenta (2/13). Hemorrhage following partial separation of the placenta and during hysterectomy to remove the attached placenta resulted in major hemorrhage and 2 maternal deaths; in one of the cases insufficient blood was available for transfusion. All the patients whose placenta remained *in situ* survived but the long-term morbidity was 100%. **IV C**

LATE PREGNANCY

Chapter 44

Bleeding in late pregnancy

44.1 Bleeding in late pregnancy

David Penman

Management option		Quality of evidence	Strength of recommendation	References
Prenatal	Identification of at-risk women and book for delivery in unit with facilities for blood transfusion and cesarean section:	III IIb	B B	1–3 4,5
	❑ Previous antepartum/postpartum hemorrhage	IIb	B	4
	❑ Proven placenta previa	III	B	3
	❑ Anemia at the onset of labor	–	✔	–
	❑ Previous cesarian section (risk of placenta previa)	IIb	B	4
	Initial assessment of severity of bleeding	III	B	3,6
	Severe and continuing:			
	❑ Resuscitate (intravenous access, blood and clotting factors)	III	B	3,7
	❑ A major obstetric hemorrhage protocol should be available	IV	C	8
	❑ Deliver/empty uterus (route depends on gestation, fetal condition, maternal condition and amount of blood loss, fetal presentation, whether patient is in labor)	IIa III	B B	9 7,10
	Mild/moderate and settling: establish cause and manage appropriately	–	✔	–
	Placental abruption:			
	❑ Serial fetal assessment	III	B	11,12
	❑ ? Elective delivery at term	III	B	13,14
	Placenta previa:			
	❑ Controversy whether to admit asymptomatic patient	III	B	15
	❑ Hospital admission (and readiness for blood transfusion and cesarian section) if symptomatic (though considerable variation in practice)	IIb III	B B	16 17
	Anti-D for rhesus-negative woman	IV	C	18
Labor and delivery	Cross-match with severe/active bleeding or placenta previa	III	B	3,7
Postnatal	Vigilance for postpartum hemorrhage	IV	C	19
	Anti-D for rhesus-negative woman if not already given	IV	C	18
	High dependency/intensive care may be necessary	III	B	1
	Treat anemia	–	✔	–

References

1 Silver R, Depp R, Sabbagha RE *et al.* (1984) Placenta previa: aggressive expectant management. *Am J Obstet Gynecol* **50**, 15–22. 95 consecutive cases of placenta previa managed at a major perinatal center between 1974 and 1980 are reported. A regime of aggressive expectant management was used, along with selective outpatient management. The perinatal mortality rate of 4.3% was considerably less than quoted in other studies. The paper comments that an overriding factor in their success was the immediate access to resources of a perinatal center, including 24-hour obstetric and anesthetic cover. **III B**

2 Abdella TN, Sibai BM, Hays JM *et al.* (1984) Relationship of hypertensive disease to abruptio placentae. *Obstet Gynecol* **63**, 365–370. Retrospective study of 265 cases of abruptio placentae conducted to examine the relationship between hypertension and abruptio placentae. The incidence of abruption was highest in eclampsia (23.6%), followed by chronic hypertension (10.0%) and preeclampsia (2.3%). Hypertensive disease affects both the incidence and outcome of abruptio placentae. **III B**

3 Golditch IA, Boyce NE (1970) Management of abruptio placentae. *JAMA* **212**, 288–293. Retrospective study of 130 cases of abruptio placentae among 26 743 deliveries. It is concluded that early recognition of high-risk patients, immediate hospitalization of all women with third-trimester bleeding, prompt resuscitation and early definitive diagnosis are the mainstay of good management. Mild cases, or cases of fetal demise, may be delivered vaginally. With moderate or severe cases, unless delivery is imminent, delivery should be by cesarean section after prompt resuscitation. **III B**

4 Lydon-Rochelle M, Holt VL, Easterling TR *et al.* (2001) First-birth cesarean and placental abruption or previa at second birth. *Obstet Gynecol* **97**, 765–769. Control cohort study of a second pregnancy population of 96 975 women on the incidence of placental abruption and placenta previa in those who were delivered by cesarean section in their first pregnancy. It was found that women with first birth by cesarean section had a significantly increased risk at second birth of abruptio placentae (OR 1.3, 95% CI 1.1–1.5) and placenta previa (OR 1.4, 95% CI 1.1–1.6) compared with women with prior vaginal deliveries. **IIa B**

5 Tan NH, Abuy M, Woo JL *et al.* (1995) The role of transvaginal sonography in the diagnosis of placenta praevia. *Aust N Z J Obstet Gynaecology* **35**, 42–45. Transvaginal (TV) sonography was performed in 70 women diagnosed to have placenta previa by transabdominal (TA) sonography. The diagnostic accuracy of the TV route was 92.8%, compared with 75.7% for the TA route. The results suggest that TV sonographic localization of the placenta is safe and superior to the TA route for type 1 and 2 placenta previa but no better for type 3 or 4. **IIb B**

6 Lunan CB (1973) The management of abruptio placentae. *Br J Obstet Gynaecol* **80**, 120–124. Retrospective review of 379 cases of abruptio placentae that occurred between 1966 to 1970 in a single maternity unit (out of a total of 29,456 deliveries). The retroplacental clot size at the time of delivery was used to divide the cases into three groups, mild (< 30 ml), moderate (30–150 ml) and severe (> 150 ml). The authors concluded that intensive fetal monitoring and a readiness to deliver by lower segment cesarean section, especially in babies judged to weigh more than 2000 g, would minimize the perinatal mortality rate. **III B**

7 Hurd WW, Miodovnik M, Hertzberg V *et al.* (1983) Selective management of abruptio placentae: a prospective study. *Obstet Gynecol* **61**, 467–473. Prospective study of 59 consecutive cases of abruptio placentae managed in a single institution over a 17-month period. Management included intravenous access, cross-matching, hematological and clotting studies and continuous fetal monitoring. There was a live fetus at the time of admission in 50 cases and the diagnosis of abruptio placentae was made antenatally in 31 (62%) of these cases. No fetus died *in utero* following the diagnosis of placental abruption using the suggested management regime. **III B**

8 Bonnar J (2000) Massive obstetric haemorrhage. *Baillière's Best Pract Res Clin Obstet Gynaecol* **14**, 1–18. Review on massive obstetric hemorrhage stating that a delay in the correction of hypovolemia, diagnosis, treatment of defective coagulation and surgical control of bleeding are the avoidable factors in maternal mortality. Guidelines on appropriate management incorporating all these are given. The importance of a multidisciplinary team approach in specific cases is underlined. **IV C**

9 Chan CC, To WW (1999) Antepartum hemorrhage of unknown origin – what is its clinical significance? *Acta Obstet Gynecol Scand* **78**, 186–190. Retrospective case control study on antepartum hemorrhage in 718 singleton pregnancies after 24 weeks. There was a significant increase in the incidence of preterm labor, induction of labor and cesarean section in the study group. Birthweights, major antepartum complications and neonatal complications did not differ between the groups. More infants in the study group had congenital abnormalities. It was concluded that, at term, induction of labor should depend only on other obstetric indications. **IIa B**

10 Knab DR (1978) Abruptio placentae: an assessment of the time and method of delivery. *Obstet Gynecol* **52**, 625–629. Literature review and an analysis of 388 cases of abruptio placentae. 75% of fetal deaths occurred more than 90 min after admission to hospital. The data suggest that rapid resuscitation and immediate delivery, generally by lower segment cesarean section, would reduce the perinatal mortality rate and that a prospective randomized study should be conducted. **III B**

11 Brenner WE, Edelman WE, Hendricks CH (1978) Characteristics of patients with placenta previa and results of 'expectant management'. *Am J Obstet Gynecol* **132**, 180–189. Retrospective study to determine the differences between pregnancies complicated by placenta previa and those without. Of a total of 31 070 consecutive deliveries at a single institution, 185 cases of placenta previa were identified. A higher proportion of these patients were multiparous, older, had had previous abortion and were carrying a male fetus or twins. Rates of prematurity, antepartum

and intrapartum fetal death, neonatal death, congenital abnormality and low Apgar scores were higher among the placenta previa group. **III B**

12 Rivera-Alsima ME, Saldana LR, Maklad N *et al.* (1983) The use of ultrasound in the expectant management of abruptio placentae. *Am J Obstet Gynecol* **146**, 924–927. Three case reports of the use of ultrasound in the management of patients with abruptio placentae are presented. The authors suggest that the use of ultrasound and nonstress testing in the expectant management of abruptio placentae could result in a decrease in maternal and perinatal mortality and morbidity. **IV C**

13 Sampson MB, Lastres O, Tomasi AM *et al.* (1984) Tocolysis with terbutaline sulfate in patients with placenta previa complicated by premature labor. *J Reprod Med* **29**, 248–250. Six patients with ultrasound confirmed total placenta previa between 24 and 36 weeks gestation with painful, regular uterine contractions of less than 10 min frequency and without significant vaginal bleeding were treated with terbutaline sulfate. The average prolongation of pregnancy was 3.5 weeks. There is no control group and, although the administration of the tocolytic appeared to be safe, this study does not demonstrate that it is of clinical advantage to mother or baby. **III B**

14 Willocks J (1971) Antepartum haemorrhage of uncertain origin. *J Obstet Gynaecol Br Commonw* **78**, 987–991. A retrospective review of 307 cases of antepartum hemorrhage of uncertain origin occurring in a 6-year period (1964–69). No fetal loss could have been avoided by routine induction of labor at 38 weeks. **III B**

15 Rosen DMB, Peek MJ (1984) Do women with placenta praevia without antepartum haemorrhage require hospitalisation? *Aust N Z J Obstet Gynaecol* **34**, 130–134. Retrospective study of 69 consecutive cases of patients diagnosed with placenta previa in the third trimester. The outcome of 15 cases who had no bleeding is compared to those who had one or more episodes of vaginal bleeding. The study concluded that outpatient management in patients with placenta previa and no bleeding may be safe and cost-effective, and warrants a randomized prospective study. **III B**

16 Cotton DB, Read JA, Paul RH *et al.* (1980) The conservative aggressive management of placenta previa. *Am J Obstet Gynecol* **137**, 687–695. Retrospective comparative study of cases of placenta previa managed in one hospital between 1969 and 1975–78. A reduction in the perinatal mortality in the later group was half that of the 1969 group. This difference was attributed to greater use of expectant management and aggressive use of antenatal transfusion. **IIb B**

17 D'Angelo LJ, Irwin LF (1984) Conservative management of placenta previa: a cost benefit analysis. *Am J Obstet Gynecol* **149**, 320–323. Retrospective study of 38 patients with placenta previa. Their management had been based on the policies of the attending obstetricians and two groups of patients were available for study according to whether they had been managed by an inpatient or outpatient expectant approach. Mean maternal hospital days and costs were significantly higher in the inpatient group but the overall costs for maternal–neonatal pairs were 69% higher in the outpatient group. **III B**

18 Consensus Conference (1998) Consensus Conference on Anti-D Prophylaxis. Edinburgh, United Kingdom, 8–9 April 1997. Papers and abstracts. *Br J Obstet Gynaecol* **105**(suppl 18), 1–44. UK consensus statement on the reduction of rhesus isoimmunization, listing evidence-based guidelines at various levels of evidence. **IV C**

19 Jouppila P (1995) Postpartum hemorrhage. *Curr Opin Obstet Gynecol* **7**, 446–450. An extensive review on postpartum hemorrhage stating causes (uterine atony, maternal soft-tissue trauma, retained placenta or its parts and obstetric coagulopathy), associated factors (advanced maternal age, prolonged labor, preeclampsia, obesity, multiple pregnancy, a birth weight of more than 4000 g, previous postpartum hemorrhage) and prophylaxis and treatment options. **IV C**

Chapter 45

Multiple pregnancy

45.1 Multiple pregnancy: general

Etelka Moll

Management option		Quality of evidence	Strength of recommendation	References
Prepregnancy	Counsel women undergoing assisted conception techniques about multiple pregnancy risks	III	B	1,2
	Pre- and periconceptual folate supplementation	Ia	A	3
Prenatal	Documentation at 10–14 weeks of chorionicity	III	B	4
	Routine anomaly ultrasound scan at 18–20 weeks	III	B	5
	Conjoined twins: ❑ Careful ultrasonographic evaluation of anatomy ❑ Interdisciplinary discussion of therapeutic options	III	B	6
	Iron and folate supplementation from the second trimester	IIb	B	7
	Increased surveillance if monochorionic	IIb	B	8
	Vigilance for the early symptoms of preterm labor; prompt self-referral if suspected	Ib	A	9
	Possible ultrasound assessment of cervical change and fetal fibronectin as preterm delivery screening	IIa	B	10
	Prenatal corticosteroids when considered at risk of preterm birth before 34 weeks	Ia	A	11
	No evidence that hospitalization to prevent preterm labor and delivery is effective	Ia	A	12
	No evidence that prophylactic cervical cerclage is effective to prevent preterm labor and delivery	Ia	A	13
	Screening for hypertension	IIa	B	14
	Conflicting evidence of value of screening for gestational diabetes	IIa	B	15,16
	Regular fetal ultrasound assessment of growth and umbilical artery Doppler	III	B	17
	Hospitalization at woman's request or if complications are detected	Ia	A	12

Management option		Quality of evidence	Strength of recommendation	References
Prenatal (cont'd)	Consider therapeutic amniocentesis (repeated if necessary) for extreme hydramnios and maternal distress	IIb	B	18
	Prenatal education of possible modes of delivery, analgesia and care in labor	IV	C	19
Labor and delivery	Hospital delivery	III	B	20
	Experienced obstetrician	III	B	20
	Await spontaneous labor if no complications	III	B	21
	Pediatrician, neonatal nurse and anesthetist to be available at delivery. One pediatrician per baby if preterm, operative delivery or fetal problems anticipated	–	✔	–
	Continuous monitoring of all fetuses during labor	III	B	20
	Intravenous access	–	✔	–
	Epidural analgesia recommended	III	B	20
	Aim for vaginal delivery unless leading twin nonlongitudinal lie. Some advocate elective cesarean if the first twin is not cephalic	III	B	21,22
	Vaginal delivery of the first twin, if appropriate	III	B	22
	Synthetic oxytocin infusion for uterine inertia, especially after first twin delivered	–	✔	–
	If second twin longitudinal lie, amniotomy and delivery	III	B	23
	If nonlongitudinal lie, convert to longitudinal lie by external version or, if this fails internal podalic version	III	B	23
	Prophylactic oxytocin infusion after delivery to reduce risk of postpartum hemorrhage	Ia	A	24
	Some do not advocate elective cesarean section for triplets and higher-order births	IIb	B	25
Postnatal	Extra support while in hospital to assist with care of babies	–	✔	–
	Offer longer inpatient stay	–	✔	–
	Arrange support at home	–	✔	–
	Adequate contraceptive advice	–	✔	–

References

1 Bollen N, Camus M, Staessen C *et al.* (1991) The incidence of multiple pregnancy after in vitro fertilization and embryo transfer, gamete or zygote intra fallopian transfer. *Fertil Steril* **55**, 314–318. Retrospective study during a 2-year period on the incidence of multiple pregnancy after 713 *in-vitro* fertilization–embryo transfers with three embryos, 190 gamete intrafallopian transfers with three oocytes and 161 zygote intrafallopian transfers with three zygotes. The rate of multiple pregnancy at 20 weeks was 32%, 16% and 27% respectively. **III B**

2 Northern Region Perinatal Mortality Survey Steering Group (1998) Time trends in twin perinatal mortality in northern England, 1982–94. *Twin Res* **1**, 189–195. A retrospective study on all twin perinatal deaths between 1982 and 1994 in the northern region of the NHS in England. Of the 10734 twin pregnancies, 421 resulted in 530 deaths. There was a significantly higher perinatal mortality rate in like-sexed twins compared to unlike-sexed twins. **III B**

3 Lumley J, Watson L, Watson M *et al.* (2000) Periconceptional supplementation with folate and/or multivitamins for preventing neural tube defects (Cochrane Review). In: *The Cochrane library*, issue 2. Oxford: Update Software. Meta-analysis of four randomized trials or quasi-randomized trials involving 6425 women comparing supplementation by multivitamins, folate and placebo for the prevention of neural tube defects. It was concluded that periconceptional folate supplementation reduced neural tube defects (OR 0.28, CI 0.15–0.53). **Ia A**

4 Sepulveda W, Sebire NJ, Hughes K *et al.* (1996) The lambda sign at 10–14 weeks of gestation as a predictor of chorionicity in twin pregnancies. *Ultrasound Obstet Gynecol* **7**, 421–423. Prospective study on the accuracy of chorionicity determination by ultrasound at 10–14 weeks in 81 monochorionic and 288 dichorionic twins. The outcome demonstrated a high reliability of ultrasound examination for the determination of chorionicity between 10 and 14 weeks gestation. **III B**

5 Edwards MS, Hirigoyen M, Burge PD *et al.* (1995) Predictive value of antepartum ultrasound examination for anomalies in twin gestations. *Ultrasound Obstet Gynecol* **6**, 43–49. Retrospective study on 245 twin pregnancies between 1988 and 1994 that were all screened by ultrasound for malformations. The overall prevalence of congenital malformations was 4.9%. The detection of each individual anomaly had a sensitivity of 82% and a specificity of 100%. The positive predictive value was 100% and the negative predictive value 98%. **III B**

6 Barth RA, Filly RA, Goldberg JD *et al.* (1990) Conjoined twins: prenatal diagnosis and assessment of associated malformations. *Radiology* **177**, 201–207. Retrospective study on 14 cases of conjoined twins. 9 cases (64%) had shared hearts with little chance on successful postnatal correction. Early determination of the degree of conjoining allows for the option of pregnancy termination prior to 24 weeks gestation and vaginal delivery. **III B**

7 Blickstein I, Goldschmidt R, Lurie S (1995) Hemoglobin levels during twin vs. singleton pregnancies. Parity makes the difference. *J Reprod Med* **40**, 47–50. Retrospective, case-control study of 200 consecutive twin and singleton gestation controls, matched for parity. There were no significant differences in third-trimester values between the groups. The statistically significant lower hemoglobin levels during the first and second trimester in twins versus singletons (11.8g/dl vs 12.2g/dl, $p = 0.015$ and 11.0g/dl vs 11.5g/dl, $p = 0.0001$, respectively) resulted from lower values in multiparous twins compared to their controls associated with multiparity. It was concluded that this subgroup of twin pregnancies may benefit from closer hematologic surveillance and iron supplementation. **IIb B**

8 Minakami H, Honma Y, Matsubara S *et al.* (1999) Effects of placental chorionicity on outcome in twin pregnancies. A cohort study. *J Reprod Med* **44**, 595–600. Cohort study on the effects of chorionicity in 44 monochorionic and 164 dichorionic twins at 1 year of corrected age and a retrospective review from less than 20 weeks gestational age. In conclusion, monochorionic twins had an increased risk of adverse outcomes (10% vs 3.7%, $p < 0.05$), which was mainly due to twin–twin transfusion syndrome. In both types a birthweight discordance of 25% or more was associated with an adverse outcome ($p < 0.01$). **IIb B**

9 Knuppel RA, Lake MF, Watson DL *et al.* (1990) Preventing preterm birth in twin gestation: home uterine activity monitoring and perinatal nursing support. *Obstet Gynecol* **76**, 24S–27S. Multicenter RCT of 45 twin pregnancies randomly assigned to daily home uterine activity monitoring (19) or counseling regarding the common signs and symptoms of preterm labor (45). 62 vs 74% developed preterm labor (not significant). The mean cervical dilatation at the first preterm labor episode was 1.6 vs 2.9cm ($p = 0.01$). In the home monitoring group there were fewer preterm births and fewer deliveries with failed tocolysis ($p = 0.03$). **Ib A**

10 Goldenberg RL, Iams JD, Miodovnik M *et al.* and the National Institute of Child Health and Human Development Maternal–Fetal Medicine Units Network (1996) The preterm prediction study: risk factors in twin gestations. *Am J Obstet Gynecol* **175**, 1047–1053. Prospective study on 147 twin gestations screened at 24 and 28 weeks gestation for different potential risk factors for spontaneous preterm birth. At 24 weeks cervical length of 25mm or less was the best predictor of preterm birth before 32, 35 and 37 weeks with an OR of 6.9 (CI 2.0–24.2), 3.2 (CI 1.3–7.9) and 3.2 (CI 1.1–7.7) respectively. Fetal fibronectin (at 28 weeks) was the only significant predictor of preterm birth at less than 32 weeks ($p = 0.047$). **III B**

11 Crowley P (2000) Prophylactic corticosteroids for preterm birth (Cochrane Review). In: *The Cochrane library*, issue 4. Oxford: Update Software. Meta-analysis of 18 randomized trials with data on over 3700 babies. Antenatal administration of 24mg betamethasone, 24mg dexamethasone or 2g hydrocortisone given to women with expected preterm birth significantly reduced mortality (OR 0.60, CI 0.48–0.75) and respiratory distress syndrome (OR 0.53, CI 0.44–0.63). **Ia A**

12 Crowther CA (2000) Hospitalisation and bed rest for multiple pregnancy (Cochrane Review). In: *The Cochrane library*, issue 4. Oxford: Update Software. Six RCTs involving over 600 women and 1400 babies. Rather than a reduction in preterm birth, an increase was seen in births at less than 34 weeks gestation (OR 1.84, CI 1.01–3.34). There were no differences in perinatal mortality or morbidity. There was a suggestion of improved fetal growth. **Ia A**

13 Grant A (1989) Cervical cerclage to prolong pregnancy. In: Chalmers I, Enkin M, Keirse MJNC (eds) *Effective care in pregnancy and childbirth*. Oxford: Oxford University Press, pp. 633–645. Meta-analysis of two RCTs showing an increase in gestational age at delivery with prophylactic cerclage in twin pregnancies at the cost of an increase in miscarriages resulting from the procedure. The routine use of prophylactic cerclage is not recommended in twin pregnancy. **Ia A**

14 Santema JG, Koppelaar I, Wallenburg H (1995) Hypertensive disorders in twin pregnancy. *Eur J Obstet Gynecol Reprod Biol* **58**, 9–13. Case-control study in which 187 twin pregnancies were matched with singleton pregnancies for maternal age, parity and gestational age at delivery. Pregnancy-induced hypertension occurred in 21% vs 13% ($p < 0.05$) of cases. This was due to a significant difference in pregnancy-induced hypertension in nulliparous women (15% vs 6%, $p < 0.05$). There was no difference in the incidence of preeclampsia (6% vs. 6.5%). **IIa B**

15 Henderson CE, Scarpelli S, LaRosa D *et al.* (1995) Assessing the risk of gestational diabetes in twin gestation. *J Natl Med Assoc* **87**, 757–758. Retrospective analysis of twin and singleton pregnancies matched for maternal age, weight, parity. A 1h oral glucose challenge test was used for screening of 9185 women. Gestational diabetes was diagnosed in 5.8% vs 5.4% (NS) cases. **IIa B**

16 Schwartz DB, Daoud Y, Zazula P *et al.* (1999) Gestational diabetes mellitus: metabolic and blood glucose parameters in singleton versus twin pregnancies. *Am J Obstet Gynecol* **181**, 912–914. Case-control study in which gestational diabetes was found to be increased in twins (7.7% vs. 4.1%, $p < 0.05$). Maternal weight at booking was significantly less in singletons and the 3h glucose tolerance test value was significantly higher in twins. Insulin requirements were not different. **IIa B**

17 Joern H, Rath W (2000) Correlation of Doppler velocimetry findings in twin pregnancies including course of pregnancy and fetal outcome. *Fetal Diagn Ther* **15**, 160–164. Retrospective study in which 206 twin pregnancies had an umbilical Doppler examination in a median of 9 days before delivery. In 32 cases with abnormal findings of at least one twin, intrauterine growth retardation and preeclampsia occurred five times more often, premature delivery rate was 3.4 times higher, the rate of small-for-gestational-age was 6.3 times higher and perinatal mortality was increased by 1.5 as compared to the normal Doppler group. The median birth weight and gestational age at birth were significantly lower in the abnormal Doppler group (1660g, 35 weeks vs 2460g, 37 weeks, $p < 0.001$). **III B**

18 Hecher K, Plath H, Bregenzer T *et al.* (1999) Endoscopic laser surgery versus serial amniocenteses in the treatment of severe twin–twin transfusion syndrome. *Am J Obstet Gynecol* **180**, 717–724. Retrospective comparative study of two centers with two different treatments of 116 cases of severe twin–twin transfusion syndrome (TTTS) between 17 and 25 weeks gestation. 73 were treated with laser coagulation, 43 with serial amniocenteses. Overall fetal survival was similar (61% vs 51%, $p = 0.239$) but at least one survivor occurred more often in the laser group (79% vs 60%, $p = 0.033$). Spontaneous intrauterine fetal death of both fetuses occurred in 3% vs 19% ($p = 0.003$) of cases respectively. There were significantly less abnormal ultrasonographic findings in the brain in the laser group (6% vs 18%, $p = 0.03$) and significantly higher birthweights in donor (1750g vs 1145g, $p = 0.034$) but not in recipient twins (2000g vs 1560g, $p = 0.076$). It was concluded that laser coagulation of placental vascular anastomoses offers a more effective alternative as treatment of TTTS. **IIb B**

19 Hofmeyr GJ, Drakeley AJ (1998) Delivery of twins. *Baillière's Clin Obstet Gynaecol* **12**, 91–108. Review on the delivery of twins. It is thought that particular attention needs to be paid to the emotional needs during labor, delivery and afterwards of the parents of the twins. The routine use of cesarean section is not supported by evidence of improved neonatal outcome. **IV C**

20 Osbourne GK, Patel NB (1985) An assessment of perinatal mortality in twin pregnancies in Dundee. *Acta Genet Med Gemellol (Roma)* **34**, 193–199. Retrospective study on all twins born in Dundee between 1956 and 1983 showing a fall in perinatal mortality rate from 116/1000 to 16/1000 births. It was concluded that factors such as early routine ultrasound scanning, tocolytic drugs, intrapartum fetal monitoring, epidural anesthesia and an increase in cesarean section rate from 2% to 39% may be a possible cause for this. **IV C**

21 Chasen ST, Madden A, Chervenak FA (1999) Cesarean delivery of twins and neonatal respiratory disorders. *Am J Obstet Gynecol* **181**, 1052–1056. Retrospective study comparing neonatal morbidity in twin pregnancies delivered by cesarean section at 36–38 weeks ($n = 79$) with vaginal delivery at 38–40 weeks ($n = 47$). Neonatal respiratory disorders were significantly more common in the first group ($p = 0.04$). **III B**

22 Morales WJ, O'Brien WF, Knuppel RA *et al.* (1989) The effect of mode of delivery on the risk of intraventricular hemorrhage in non-discordant twin gestations under 1500g. *Obstet Gynecol* **73**, 107–110. Retrospective study on neonatal morbidity of 59 vertex/vertex, 59 vertex/nonvertex and 38 twin-one-nonvertex presentation in nondiscordant twins weighing less than 1500g. In vertex-presenting twins there was a significant increase in respiratory distress syndrome when delivered by cesarean section (66% vs 54%, $p < 0.05$). Birthweight rather than mode of delivery (spontaneous or cesarean section) accounted for differences in neonatal outcome of nonvertex-presenting twins. **III B**

23 Kaplan B, Peled Y, Rabinerson D *et al.* (1995) Successful external version of B-twin after the birth of A-twin for vertex–non-vertex twins. *Eur J Obstet Gynecol Reprod Biol* **58**, 157–160. Retrospective study of 408 twin deliveries weighing more than 1500g at birth. External cephalic version of the second twin and subsequent vaginal delivery in vertex–nonvertex was successful in 75% of cases. Internal podalic version and assisted breech delivery was performed in 20 cases and the remaining two were delivered by cesarean section. Apgar scores were not significantly different among the various groups and no complications arose from external cephalic version performed on second nonvertex twins. **III B**

24 Prendiville WJ, Elbourne D, McDonald S *et al.* (2000) Active versus expectant management in the third stage of labour (Cochrane Review). In: *The Cochrane library*, issue 4. Oxford: Update Software. Meta-analysis consisting of four RCTs. Compared to expectant management, active management was associated with a reduced risk of maternal blood loss (weighted mean difference 79.33ml, 95% CI −94.29 to −64.37) and postpartum hemorrhage of more than 500ml (RR 0.38, 95% CI 0.32–0.46). It is concluded that routine active management of the third stage is superior to expectant management in terms of blood loss and postpartum hemorrhage. **Ia A**

25 Wildschut HI, van Roosmalen J, van Leeuwen E *et al.* (1995) Planned abdominal compared with planned vaginal birth in triplet pregnancies. *Br J Obstet Gynaecol* **102**, 292–296. Retrospective study, comparing 30 abdominal vs 39 vaginal deliveries in triplet pregnancies. Planned abdominal delivery was associated with a significantly higher perinatal mortality rate ($p = 0.02$), primarily due to respiratory distress syndrome, and a higher recorded neonatal complication rate ($p = 0.03$), especially sepsis, respiratory distress syndrome and necrotizing enterocolitis. **IIb B**

45.2 Multiple pregnancy: specific problems

Etelka Moll

Single fetal death

Management option		Quality of evidence	Strength of recommendation	References
Prenatal	Counseling and support for mother and family	–	✔	–
	Screening for maternal coagulopathy	IIa	B	1
	If dichorionic pregnancy, continue fetal surveillance in survivor	IIa	B	1
	If monochorionic pregnancy and early delivery not undertaken, fetal surveillance in surviving twin, although this may not accurately predict neurodevelopmental prognosis	IIa	B	1
	Role of high-resolution ultrasound of fetal brain in survivor is uncertain	III	B	2
Labor and delivery	Steroids if preterm delivery contemplated	Ia	A	3
	If dichorionic pregnancy, delay delivery until 37 weeks provided no maternal coagulopathy or fetal compromise in survivor	IIa	B	1
	If monochorionic pregnancy, options are early delivery vs delay until 37 weeks (if fetal surveillance is normal). Multicenter randomized trial is necessary as no clear evidence of which is better	IIa	B	1
Postnatal	Counseling and support for the mother and family	–	✔	–
	Pediatric assessment and neurodevelopmental follow-up and appropriate management depending on problems	III	B	4,5

References

1 Santema JG, Swaak AM, Wallenburg HC (1995) Expectant management of twin pregnancy with single fetal death. *Br J Obstet Gynaecol* **102**, 26–30. Case-controlled retrospective study on 29 twin pregnancies with a single fetal death after 20 weeks gestation matched for parity with 58 twin pregnancies without a fetal death. No differences were found in median gestational age at delivery (33 weeks vs 34 weeks) and median birthweight of liveborn infants (1880g vs 2160g). There were significantly more cases with pregnancy-induced hypertensive disorders in the study group. No maternal coagulopathy occurred in any of the 29 cases. **IIa B**

2 Levine D, Barnes PD, Madsen JR *et al.* (1999) Central nervous system abnormalities assessed with prenatal magnetic resonance imaging. *Obstet Gynecol* **94**, 1011–1019. Retrospective study on 90 fetuses comparing ultrasound with magnetic resonance imaging (MRI) findings. MRI led to changed diagnosis in 40% of 66 fetuses with abnormal confirmatory sonograms. When a central nervous system anomaly is detected by sonography or suspected on ultrasound, MRI findings may lead to altered diagnosis and patient counseling. **III B**

3 Crowley P (2000) Prophylactic corticosteroids for preterm birth (Cochrane Review). In: *The Cochrane library*, issue 4. Oxford: Update Software. Meta-analysis of 18 randomized trials with data on over 3700 babies. Antenatal administration of 24 mg betamethasone, 24 mg dexamethasone or 2 g hydrocortisone given to women with expected preterm birth significantly reduced mortality (OR 0.60, CI 0.48–0.75) and respiratory distress syndrome (OR 0.53, CI 0.44–0.63). **Ia A**

4 Rydhstrom H, Ingemarsson I (1993) Prognosis and long-term follow-up of a twin after antenatal death of the co-twin. *J Reprod Med* **38**, 142–146. Retrospective study of 206 twin pregnancies with the death of at least one twin. Perinatal mortality for a twin after the antenatal death of the co-twin was considerable. 50% of survivors died before 34 weeks gestation and 18.7% thereafter. At follow-up, 8 years or more after birth, 3 twins (4.6%) were handicapped. **III B**

5 Pharoah PO, Adi Y (2000) Consequences of in-utero death in a twin pregnancy. *Lancet* **355**, 1597–1602. Cohort study of 434 same-sex twin pairs with one fetal death. The liveborn co-twin of a fetus who died *in utero* was found to be at increased risk of cerebral impairment, the overall risk is 20% (95% CI 16–25%). **III B**

Twin reversed arterial perfusion sequence

Management option	Quality of evidence	Strength of recommendation	References
Control hydramnios with serial amniocenteses or indomethacin	IV	C	1
Fetal surveillance of 'pump' twin; intervention prematurely if compromise (see Section 46.1)	III	B	2,3
Role of umbilical occlusion or hysterotomy not yet established	III IV	B C	4 5
Mode of delivery depends on factors such as presentation and fetal health	III	B	2

References

1 Ash K, Harman CR, Gritter H (1990) TRAP sequence – successful outcome with indomethacin. *Obstet Gynecol* **76**, 960–962. Case of twin reversed arterial perfusion sequence (acardiac twin) complicated by hydramnios was managed by maternal administration of indomethacin. Successful outcome was achieved after 8.5 weeks of therapy with delivery of a normal liveborn infant at 34 weeks. **IV C**

2 Brassard M, Fouron JC, Leduc L *et al.* (1999) Prognostic markers in twin pregnancies with an acardiac fetus. *Obstet Gynecol* **94**, 409–414. Retrospective study of nine pregnancies with twin reversed arterial perfusion sequence. The PI of the acardiac umbilical artery was significantly lower than that of the normal twin (OR 0.71 compared with OR 1.04 for good outcome, $p < 0.05$). An elevated shortening fraction in the second trimester and a rapid growth rate of the mass were associated with a poor prognosis. **III B**

3 Moore TR, Gale S, Benirschke K (1990) Perinatal outcome of forty-nine pregnancies complicated by acardiac twinning. *Am J Obstet Gynecol* **163**, 907–912. Retrospective study on 49 acardiac twin pregnancies determining prognostic factors for the normal twin. Perinatal outcome was found to be strongly related to the weight ratio of the acardiac and pump twin. A ratio over 70% was related to an incidence of preterm delivery of 90%, 40% hydramnios, 30% heart failure compared to 75%, 30% and 10% retrospectively if lower than 70% (all $p < 0.05$). **III B**

4 Quintero RA, Romero R, Reich H *et al.* (1996) In utero percutaneous umbilical cord ligation in the management of complicated monochorionic multiple gestations. *Ultrasound Obstet Gynecol* **8**, 16–22. Retrospective analysis of 11 successful cases ($n = 13$) of percutaneous cord occlusion with a range in gestational age between 16 and 25 weeks (10 acardiacs, 2 twin–twin transfusion syndrome and one acranial twin). 7 of the 11 cases had living children. The incidence of premature rupture of the membranes was 30%. **III B**

5 Ginsberg NA, Applebaum M, Rabin SA *et al.* (1992) Term birth after midtrimester hysterotomy and selective delivery of an acardiac twin. *Am J Obstet Gynecol* **167**, 33–37. Case report on a hysterotomy and removal of an acardiac twin at 23 weeks gestation in which the normal twin was delivered at 37 weeks by cesarean section. **IV C**

Monoamniotic twins

Management option	Quality of evidence	Strength of recommendation	References
Surveillance of fetal health until term (see Section 10.1)	III	B	1,2
Delivery at term, or sooner if evidence of fetal compromise, but consider steroid administration	IIa III	B B	3 4
Vaginal delivery is not contraindicated provided continuous fetal heart rate monitoring of both twins and facilities for immediate cesarean section	IIa	B	3

References

1 Belfort MA, Moise KJ Jr, Kirshon B *et al.* (1993) The use of color flow Doppler ultrasonography to diagnose umbilical cord entanglement in monoamniotic twin gestations. *Am J Obstet Gynecol* **168**, 601–604. Report on three monoamniotic twins followed with color flow Doppler to identify umbilical cord entanglement. It was concluded that this method may provide a means of monitoring for evidence of cord compression. **III B**

2 Rodis JF, Vintzileos AM, Campbell WA *et al.* (1987) Antenatal diagnosis and management of monoamniotic twins. *Am J Obstet Gynecol* **157**, 1255–1257. Retrospective study on 13 monoamniotic twin pregnancies monitored with serial ultrasound scans and nonstress tests and a literature review. Comparison of these 13 cases with 77 cases without prenatal diagnosis from the literature showed a 71% reduction in relative risk of perinatal mortality. The average gestational age in the study group was 32.9 weeks. **III B**

3 Tessen JA, Zlatnik FJ (1991) Monoamniotic twins: a retrospective controlled study. *Obstet Gynecol* **77**, 832–834. Retrospective study comparing 20 monoamniotic twin pregnancies with 40 monochorionic, diamniotic controls regarding antepartum and intrapartum complications. More monoamniotic twins were more likely to die *in utero* and were delivered earlier, but not when only liveborns were considered. No fetal death occurred after 32 weeks, suggesting that preterm delivery may not be indicated in all cases. Labor and vaginal delivery were not associated with an increased risk of fetal death. **IIa B**

4 Carr SR, Aronson MP, Coustan DR *et al.* (1990) Survival rates of monoamniotic twins do not decrease after 30 weeks' gestation. *Am J Obstet Gynecol* **163**, 719–722. Retrospective study on 24 sets of monoamniotic twins. No further fetal deaths occurred in the 17 cases with at least one twin alive who reached 30 weeks gestation. **III B**

Twin–twin transfusion syndrome

Management option	Quality of evidence	Strength of recommendation	References
Serial therapeutic amniocentesis	IIb	B	1
Laser ablation	IIb	B	2
Amniotomy of dividing membrane	III	B	3
Selective feticide (see Section 9.5)	III	B	4
Fetal venesection and transfusion	–	✔	–
Therapeutic abortion	–	✔	–

References

1 Mari G, Detti L, Oz U *et al.* (2000) Long-term outcome in twin–twin transfusion syndrome treated with serial aggressive amnioreduction. *Am J Obstet Gynecol* **183**, 211–217. Retrospective study on 33 pregnancies with twin–twin transfusion syndrome who underwent one or more amnioreductions. If both twins were delivered alive after 27 weeks gestation without congenital malformations and survived the neonatal period, no major neurological handicaps developed. Hydrops of the recipient and absence of end-diastolic flow velocity waveforms of the umbilical artery in one of the twins were poor prognostic signs. **IIb B**

2 Hecher K, Plath H, Bregenzer T et al. (1999) Endoscopic laser surgery versus serial amniocenteses in the treatment of severe twin–twin transfusion syndrome. *Am J Obstet Gynecol* **180**, 717–724. Retrospective

comparative study of two centers with two different treatments of 116 cases of severe twin–twin transfusion syndrome (TTTS) between 17 and 25 weeks gestation. 73 were treated with laser coagulation, 43 with serial amniocenteses. Overall fetal survival was similar (61% vs 51%, $p = 0.239$) but at least one survivor occurred more often in the laser group: 79% vs 60% $p = 0.033$. Spontaneous intrauterine fetal death of both fetuses occurred in 3% vs 19% ($p = 0.003$) of cases. There were significantly fewer abnormal ultrasonographic findings in the brain in the laser group (6% vs.18%, $p = 0.03$) and significantly higher birthweights in donor (1750g vs1145 g, $p = 0.034$) but not in recipient twins (2000g vs 1560g $p = 0.076$). It was concluded that laser coagulation of placental vascular anastomoses offers the more effective alternative as treatment of TTTS. **IIb B**

3 Saade GR, Belfort MA, Berry DL *et al.* (1998) Amniotic septostomy for the treatment of twin oligohydramnios–polyhydramnios sequence. *Fetal Diagn Ther* **13**, 86–93. Retrospective study on 12 twin–twin transfusion syndrome cases treated with piercing of the intertwin membrane. The combined survival rate was 83.3% with a septostomy-to-delivery interval of between 0.6 and 13 weeks (mean 8.3 ± 4.8 weeks). **III B**

4 Quintero RA, Romero R, Reich H *et al.* (1996) In utero percutaneous umbilical cord ligation in the management of complicated monochorionic multiple gestations. *Ultrasound Obstet Gynecol* **8**, 16–22. Retrospective analysis of 11 successful cases ($n = 13$) of percutaneous cord occlusion with a range in gestational age between 16 and 25 weeks (10 acardiacs, 2 twin–twin transfusion syndrome and one acranial twin). 7 of the 11 cases had living children. The incidence of premature rupture of the membranes was 30%. **III B**

Congenital anomaly in one twin

Management option	Quality of evidence	Strength of recommendation	References
Continuation of pregnancy	–	✔	–
Termination of pregnancy	–	✔	–
Selective termination/feticide (see Section 8.5)	III	B	1

Reference

1 Quintero RA, Romero R, Reich H *et al.* (1996) In utero percutaneous umbilical cord ligation in the management of complicated monochorionic multiple gestations. *Ultrasound Obstet Gynecol* **8**, 16–22. Retrospective analysis of 11 successful cases ($n = 13$) of percutaneous cord occlusion with a range in gestational age between 16 and 25 weeks (10 acardiacs, 2 twin–twin transfusion syndrome and one acranial twin). 7 of the 11 cases had living children. The incidence of premature rupture of the membranes was 30%. **III B**

Chapter 46

Prematurity

46.1 Threatened and actual preterm labor

Rajesh Varma

Management option		Quality of evidence	Strength of recommendation	References
Prepregnancy	Establish possible risk factors – overall value limited	III	B	1
	Discuss value of preventative measures: patient education, cervical assessment, biochemical markers, ambulatory uterine activity monitoring, infection screening and nutrient supplementation	IV	C	2
	General non specific strategies:			
	❑ Stop smoking and substance abuse	III	B	3
	❑ Reduce heavy work load	IIb	B	4
Prenatal – possible strategies	Formal scoring system to assess risk – low predictive value	III	B	5
	Consider value of general preventative measures as described above	–	✔	–
	Cervical suture in women with clinical diagnosis of cervical incompetence – benefit in reducing preterm delivery	Ib	A	6
	Subclinical infection screening	IV	C	7
	Patient education about clinical features – may alert clinician but overall has poor predictive value	Ia	A	8
	Increased attendance and discussion for increased-risk women – helpful for decision on place, timing and mode of delivery	IV	C	9
Prenatal – strategies needing further evaluation	Monitoring uterine contractility – as yet no consistent evidence of any benefit	Ia	A	10
	Regular clinical cervical assessment – may be of some value	III	B	11
	Ultrasound assessment of cervical dilatation or length – poor predictive value	III	B	12
	Vaginal infection screening – may identify at-risk group for possible treatment and prevention	IV	C	13
	Fetal fibronectin screening at 24–28 weeks – good sensitivity and negative predictive value but poor positive predictive value	IIb	B	14
	Treatment of bacterial vaginosis with systemic metronidazole and erythromycin reduces preterm delivery	Ia	A	15

➡

Management option		Quality of evidence	Strength of recommendation	References
Labor and delivery	Transfer to tertiary-care hospital reduces preventable mortality	III	B	16
	Tocolysis for at least 48h if gestation less than 34 weeks to allow for transfer and/or steroids. Subsequent maintenance tocolytic therapy to prevent recurrence not recommended	Ia	A	17,18
	Antibiotics – of no benefit in labor with intact membranes and associated with increased perinatal morbidity	Ia	A	19
	Antibiotics for those with group B streptococcal colonization may be of some benefit	Ia	A	20
	Corticosteroids recommended	Ia	A	21
	If cephalic, aim for vaginal delivery – no clear evidence of benefit from cesarean delivery	Ia	A	22
	Continuous electronic fetal heart rate monitoring commonly used but unproven	-	✔	-
	Epidural analgesia commonly used but unproven	-	✔	-
	Antibiotics in established preterm labor, particularly for group B streptococcus, recommended	Ia	A	19
	Prophylactic outlet forceps do not improve neonatal outcome	III	B	23
	Prophylactic episiotomy does not improve neonatal outcome	III	B	23

References

1 Meis PJ, Goldenberg RL, Mercer BM *et al.* (1998) The preterm prediction study: risk factors for indicated preterm births. Maternal–Fetal Medicine Units Network of the National Institute of Child Health and Human Development. *Am J Obstet Gynecol* **178**, 562–567. Large comparative multicenter study evaluated women (n = 2929) at 24 weeks gestation between 1992 and 1994. The study identified a preterm delivery rate of 14.4%. Of these preterm births 28.4% (n = 120) were indicated preterm births. Reasons for preterm delivery included proteinuric hypertension, fetal distress, intrauterine growth restriction, abruption, fetal death or a combination of these. Risk factors common to all preterm births were lung disease, black ethnicity, employment and previous preterm birth. Risk factors unique to indicated rather than spontaneous preterm birth include müllerian duct abnormality, proteinuria at less than 24 weeks and chronic hypertension. Those unique to spontaneous preterm birth included poor socioeconomic status, vaginal bleeding, low body mass index, bacterial vaginosis, cervicovaginal fetal fibronectin and shortening of cervix. **III B**

2 Goldenberg RL, Rouse DJ (1998) Prevention of premature birth. *N Engl J Med* **339**, 313–320. Comprehensive and up-to-date review of strategies to reduce preterm delivery involving: prenatal care, patient education programs, cervical cerclage, maternal progesterone supplementation, smoking prevention, nutritional supplementation (e.g. zinc, calcium and other minerals), home uterine activity monitoring, tocolytics, bed rest/hydration and treating infection. **IV C**

3 Fox SH, Brown C, Koontz AM *et al.* (1990) Perceptions of risks of smoking and heavy drinking during pregnancy: 1985 NHIS findings. *Public Health Rep* **102**, 73–79. Questionnaire study, administered as part of the 1985 National Health Interview Survey, with nearly 20000 respondents aged 18–44 years. The study assessed the awareness of the risks of smoking and heavy drinking during pregnancy; smoking was perceived to pose less risk to pregnancy than heavy drinking. **III B**

4 Mozurkewich EL, Luke B, Avni M *et al.* (2000) Working conditions and adverse pregnancy outcome: a meta-analysis. *Obstet Gynecol* **95**, 623–635. Meta-analysis of 29 studies (mainly case-control, prospective cohort and cross-sectional) based on 160988 women. Physically demanding work was significantly associated with preterm birth. Preterm birth was also significantly associated with prolonged standing, shift and night work, and high cumulative work fatigue score. There was no association between long working hours and preterm birth. **IIb B**

5 Mercer BM, Goldenberg RL, Das A *et al.* (1996) Maternal–Fetal Medicine Units Network of the National Institute of Child Health and Human Development. The preterm prediction study: a clinical risk assessment system. *Am J Obstet Gynecol* **174**, 1885–1893. Large comparative multicenter study evaluated women (n = 2929) at 24 weeks gestation between 1992 and 1994. Multivariate regression analysis showed that a graded risk assessment (based upon a combination of medical history, socioeconomic, obstetric and cervical risk factors) was associated with the occurrence of spontaneous preterm delivery in nulliparous and multiparous women; the sensitivities were 24.2% and 18.2% and positive predictive values 28.6% and 33.3%, respectively for nulliparous and multiparous women. **III B**

6 MRC/RCOG Working Party on Cervical Cerclage (1993) Final report of the Medical Research Council/Royal College of Obstetricians and Gynaecologists multicentre randomised trial of cervical cerclage. *Br J Obstet Gynaecol* **100**, 516–523. Multicenter RCT (n = 647 cerclage, n = 645 no cerclage). All women had a history of early delivery or cervical surgery and their obstetrician was uncertain whether to advise cerclage or not. There were fewer deliveries before 33 weeks in the cerclage group (RR 0.75 95% CI 0.57–0.98; NNT 24, 95% CI 14–275). However, there was no statistically significant reduction in the rate of miscarriage, stillbirth or neonatal death. The use of cervical cerclage was associated with increased medical intervention and risk of puerperal pyrexia (RR 2.13 95% CI 1.06–4.15). **Ib A**

7 Gibbs RS, Romero R, Hillier SL *et al.* (1992) A review of premature birth and subclinical infection. *Am J Obstet Gynecol* **166**, 1515–1528. Review of the evidence linking subclinical infection and premature birth. Evidence of subclinical infection as a cause of preterm labor is raised by finding elevated maternal serum C-reactive protein and abnormal amniotic fluid organic acid levels in some patients in preterm labor. Biochemical mechanisms for preterm labor in the setting of infection are suggested by both *in-vitro* and *in-vivo* studies of prostaglandins and their metabolites, endotoxin and cytokines. Some, but by no means all, antibiotic trials conducted to date have reported decreases in prematurity. These results support the hypothesis that premature birth results in part from infection caused by genital tract bacteria. In the next few years, research efforts must be prioritized to determine the role of infection and the appropriate prevention of this cause of prematurity. **IV C**

8 Hueston WJ, Knox MA, Eilers G *et al.* (1995) The effectiveness of preterm-birth prevention educational programs for high-risk women: a meta-analysis. *Obstet Gynecol* **86**, 705–712. Meta-analysis of six RCTs (n = 3258 intervention group, n = 3187 control group) showed no beneficial effect of preterm-birth prevention educational programs (involving patient education with weekly cervical examination or patient education with home visitation) on neonatal survival, low birth weight rates and preterm delivery rates. However, these programs increase the risk (OR 1.7, 95% CI 1.41–2.08) of being diagnosed as having preterm labor during pregnancy. **Ia A**

9 Bowes WA (1992) Editorial. *Obstet Gynecol Surv* **47**, 474. Brief editorial highlighting the many unanswered questions regarding preterm labor and the management of those who go into labor very early. The author summarizes the consensus rather than evidence of the contribution of prenatal care in preterm birth management by suggesting that success is related to the continuity of care, time available for patients to talk about their problems, ready access to ancillary services when needed and a prenatal record that provides fail-safe reminders of critical procedures and screening tests. **IV C**

10 Colton T, Kayne HL, Zhang Y *et al.* (1995) A meta-analysis of home uterine activity monitoring. *Am J Obstet Gynecol* **173**, 1499–1505. Meta-analysis of six trials of home uterine activity monitoring (published 1987–1992). Overall, for all pregnancies, home uterine activity monitoring was associated with a statistically significant reduced risk (OR 0.48, p = 0.001) of preterm labor combined with cervical dilatation of more than 2cm, and a statistically significant increase of 86g in mean birthweight. The reduction in risk of preterm labor combined with cervical dilatation of more than 2cm was more pronounced in twin (OR 0.44) than singleton pregnancies (OR 0.76). There was no significant effect on infant referral to the intensive care unit. **Ia A**

11 Smeltzer J, Lewis J, van Dorsten P *et al.* (1992) Cervical dilation is the best predictor of risk for preterm birth. Society of Perinatal Obstetricians. *Am J Obstet Gynecol* **166**, S364 (abstract no. 318). Comparative prospective study (n = 981) evaluating risk factors for preterm delivery. Consecutive pregnancies (n = 981) were evaluated for general pregnancy risk factors (derived from social, medical and current pregnancy history) and prospectively assessed by weekly cervical examination from 25 to 37 weeks. A history of multiple pregnancy and progressive cervical dilation of the internal os were identified as statistically significant risk factors for preterm birth. **III B**

12 Vendittelli F, Volumenie J (2000) Transvaginal ultrasonography examination of the uterine cervix in hospitalized women undergoing preterm labour. *Eur J Obstet Gynecol Reprod Biol* **90**, 3–11. Qualitative analysis of nine studies (mainly nonexperimental descriptive type). Using a cervical length cutoff (18–30mm), the sensitivity for predicting preterm birth varied from 68% to 100% and the specificity ranged from 54% to 90%. **III B**

13 Goldenberg RL, Hauth JC, Andrews WW (2000) Intrauterine infection and preterm delivery. *N Engl J Med* **342**, 1500–1507. Comprehensive up-to-date review discussing epidemiology, timing of infection, bacterial vaginosis, mechanisms of preterm delivery due to infection, markers of infection and treatment of infection to prevent preterm delivery. **IV C**

14 Faron G, Boulvain M, Irion O *et al.* (1998) Prediction of preterm delivery by fetal fibronectin: a meta-analysis. *Obstet Gynecol* **92**, 153–158. Meta-analysis of 29 studies (mainly prospective cohort studies) showed that cervicovaginal fetal fibronectin (FFN) appears to be an effective predictor of preterm delivery in both low-risk women (OR 7.5, 95% CI 4.6–12.3) and high-risk women (OR 3.5, 95% CI 2.6–4.6). In high-risk women a negative FFN test was associated with a reduced risk of preterm delivery (OR 0.4, 95% CI 0.3–0.5). **IIb B**

15 Brocklehurst P, Hannah M, McDonald H (2001) Interventions for treating bacterial vaginosis in pregnancy (Cochrane Review). In: *The Cochrane library*, issue 1. Oxford: Update Software. Meta-analysis of five RCTs (n = 1504) comparing pregnancy outcomes in women infected with bacterial vaginosis and treated with one or more antibiotic regimens. Compared to placebo, antibiotic treatment caused a nonsignificant reduction in preterm delivery (<37 weeks) (RR 0.78, 95% CI 0.60–1.02), which became statistically significant in a subgroup analysis of women with a history of previous preterm birth (RR 0.37, 95% CI 0.23–0.60; NNT 4, 95% CI 3–8). **Ia A**

16 Powell SL, Holt VL, Hickok DE *et al.* (1995) Recent changes in delivery site of low-birth-weight infants in Washington: impact on birth weight-specific mortality. *Am J Obstet Gynecol* **173**, 1585–1592. Retrospective comparative study comparing birthweight-specific mortality rates, for tertiary and non-tertiary hospitals, for low-birthweight infants (500–2499 g) born in Washington between 1980 and 1991. Nontertiary delivery of infants under 2000 g was associated with higher preventable mortality than tertiary center delivery. Nontertiary hospital delivery of 2000–2499 g infants was associated with lower overall mortality, but higher-risk deliveries in this birthweight range tended to occur in tertiary hospitals. **III B**

17 Gyetvai K, Hannah ME, Hodnett ED *et al.* (1999) Tocolytics for preterm labor: a systematic review. *Obstet Gynecol* **94**, 869–877. Meta-analysis of 17 RCTs examining the effectiveness of any tocolytic (n = 1184 women) compared with placebo or no tocolytic (n = 1100 women) for preterm labor. Three trials included women with ruptured membranes. Tocolytics used in the intervention group included: isoxsuprine, ethanol, terbutaline, ritodrine (five trials), indomethacin, magnesium sulfate and atosiban. Beta-mimetics, indomethacin, atosiban and ethanol, but not magnesium sulfate, were associated with significant prolongation of pregnancy for women in threatened preterm labor. Tocolytics were not associated with significantly reduced rates of perinatal death, neonatal morbidity, low birthweight, or births before 30/32/37 weeks gestation. **Ia A**

18 Sanchez-Ramos L, Kaunitz AM, Gaudier FL *et al.* (1999) Efficacy of maintenance therapy after acute tocolysis: a meta-analysis. *Am J Obstet Gynecol* **181**, 484–490. Meta-analysis of 12 RCTs (n = 1590 patients: 855 maintenance tocolysis and 735 placebo or no treatment) assessing the efficacy of maintenance tocolytic therapy after successful short-term tocolysis in patients with an acute episode of preterm labor. Tocolytics used in the treatment of the acute preterm labor episode included magnesium sulfate (8 trials), ritodrine (1 trial), terbutaline (1 trial), ethanol (1 trial), and atosiban (1 trial). Tocolytics used in the maintenance therapy included terbutaline (7 trials), ritodrine (3 trials), sulindac (1 trial) and atosiban (1 trial). Maintenance tocolytic therapy did not reduce the incidence of recurrent preterm labor (RR 0.81, 95% CI 0.64–1.03), preterm delivery (RR 0.95 95% CI 0.77–1.17), or improve perinatal outcome (neonatal respiratory distress syndrome, perinatal deaths or differences in birthweight). The results of this meta-analysis do not support the use of maintenance tocolytic therapy after successful treatment of preterm labor. **Ia A**

19 King J, Flenady V (2001) Antibiotics for preterm labour with intact membranes (Cochrane Review). In: *The Cochrane library*, issue 1. Oxford: Update Software. Meta-analysis of 10 RCTs comparing antibiotic treatment (various regimens) with placebo or no treatment for women in preterm labor (between 20 and 36 weeks gestation) with intact membranes. Antibiotic use was associated with a statistically significant prolongation of pregnancy (5.4 days, 95% CI 0.9–9.8 days), and a statistically significant reduction in maternal infection (RR 0.59, 95% CI 0.36–0.97) and neonatal necrotizing enterocolitis (RR 0.33, 95% CI 0.13–0.88). No statistically significant effect was detected on neonatal sepsis (RR 0.67, 95% CI 0.42–1.07). However, an increase in perinatal mortality was observed in the group receiving antibiotics (RR 3.36, 95% CI 1.21–9.32), which included postnatal deaths due to complications of prematurity. This review fails to demonstrate a clear overall benefit from antibiotic treatment for preterm labor with intact membranes on neonatal outcomes and raises concerns about increased perinatal mortality for those who received antibiotics. **Ia A**

20 Smaill F (2001) Intrapartum antibiotics for Group B streptococcal colonisation (Cochrane Review). In: *The Cochrane library*, issue 1. Oxford: Update Software. Meta-analysis of five trials, although most studies had methodological flaws. Intrapartum antibiotic treatment of women colonized with group B streptococcus reduces the incidence of neonatal infection (RR 0.17, 95% CI 0.07–0.39) without a significant beneficial effect on neonatal mortality (RR 0.12, 95% CI 0.01–2.00). **Ia A**

21 Crowley P (2001) Prophylactic corticosteroids for preterm birth (Cochrane Review). In: *The Cochrane library*, issue 1. Oxford: Update Software. Meta-analysis of 18 RCTs involving over 3700 babies (1972–95) comparing corticosteroids (betamethasone, dexamethasone, hydrocortisone) with placebo or no treatment in women before anticipated preterm delivery (elective or after spontaneous onset of preterm labor). Corticosteroid treatment was associated with a significant reduction in mortality (RR 0.60, 95% CI 0.48–0.75), respiratory distress syndrome (RR 0.53, 95% CI 0.44–0.63) and intraventricular hemorrhage in preterm infants. **Ia A**

22 Grant A (2001) Elective versus selective caesarean section for delivery of the small baby. In *The Cochrane library*, issue 2. Oxford: Update Software. Meta-analysis of five trials of 105 women in which no significant differences were found between elective and selective cesarean delivery for any of the fetal, neonatal and maternal outcomes. **Ia A**

23 Bottoms S (1995) Delivery of the premature infant. *Clin Obstet Gynecol* **38**, 780–789. Review article suggesting that selective use of episiotomy may be beneficial but not based on any good-quality trials. The author also states that the suggestion that cesarean delivery before the onset of labor reduces intraventricular hemorrhage in very-low-birthweight (VLBW) infants has not been demonstrated clearly. A vertical uterine incision may be needed for cesarean delivery of VLBW infants. Cesarean delivery is often employed for VLBW infants in breech presentation or if either fetus in a twin gestation is not in vertex presentation, but is usually not needed for face or compound vertex presentations. **IV C**

46.2 Premature rupture of the membranes

Rajesh Varma

Management option		Quality of evidence	Strength of recommendation	References
Prepregnancy	Establish possible risk factors – overall value limited	III	B	1
	Stress value of preventative measures – patient education and smoking	III	B	2
Prenatal: prevention	Vaginal infection screening – may identify at-risk group for possible treatment and prevention	Ia	A	3
	Cervical assessment with fetal fibronectin in women with previous history of premature rupture of the membranes may be of benefit	III	B	4
Prenatal: confirm diagnosis	History and clinical examination	–	✔	–
	Alkaline pH, ferning, nitrazine test useful but some limitations at early gestation (?< 32 weeks)	–	✔	–
	Presence of fetal fibronectin may predict likelihood of ensuing preterm labor	III	B	4
Prenatal: treatment <31 weeks – no evidence of chorioamnionitis or fetal distress	Expectant management:			
	❑ Look for clinical evidence of chorioamnionitis (CA)	–	✔	–
	❑ One small RCT suggests that management at home is not associated with poorer outcome	Ia	B	5
	Active management is indicated where there is clinical CA, fetal distress or maternal hemorrhage	–	✔	–
	Where there is none of above gestation at which active management is initiated will depend on local survival rates	–	✔	–
	Look for evidence of subclinical infection:	–	✔	–
	❑ Elevated polymorphonuclear white cell count or serial rise indicates infection	Ib	A	6
	❑ Amniotic fluid gram stain, culture and white cells of some value	III	B	7
	❑ C reactive protein may be an early indicator of chorioamnionitis	III	B	7
	Oligohydramnios may be associated with increased risk of CA	III	B	8
	Nonstress test alone and biophysical profile are poor predictors of intrauterine infection	IIb	B	9

Management option		Quality of evidence	Strength of recommendation	References
Prenatal: treatment <31 weeks (cont'd)	Prophylactic antibiotics (particularly combination of erythromycin and amoxicillin) reduces neonatal morbidity	Ia Ib	A A	10 11,12
	Corticosteroid therapy reduces respiratory distress, intraventricular hemorrhage, necrotizing enterocolitis and neonatal death without increasing risk of infectious morbidity	Ia	A	13
	There is some evidence that concomitant use of glucocorticoids may reduce the beneficial effects of antibiotic therapy	Ia	A	14
	Long-term tocolysis has not been shown to be of any benefit in prolonging pregnancy	Ia	A	15
Prenatal treatment: 34–37 weeks	Common practice is to wait for 24–48h and then induce labor. This has been shown to improve spontaneous vaginal delivery rate and reduce maternal sepsis morbidity	Ib	A	16
Prenatal treatment: >37 weeks	Induction of labor is indicated as this reduces infectious maternal morbidity	Ia	A	17
Labor and delivery	Continue observing for evidence of infection	–	✔	–
	Treatment of confirmed or suspected group B streptococcus reduces maternal and neonatal infectious morbidity	Ia	A	18
	Amnioinfusion for oligohydramnios reduces intervention for fetal distress, cesarean section, acidotic delivery artery pH and hospital stay	Ia	A	19
	Insufficient evidence to promote cesarean delivery apart from for obstetric indications	Ia	A	20
	Ensure pediatrician present at delivery	–	✔	–
	Continue observing mother and neonate for infection post-partum	–	✔	–

References

1 Meis PJ, Goldenberg RL, Mercer BM *et al.* (1998) The preterm prediction study: risk factors for indicated preterm births. Maternal–Fetal Medicine Units Network of the National Institute of Child Health and Human Development. *Am J Obstet Gynecol* **178**, 562–567. Large comparative multicenter study evaluated women (*n* = 2929) at 24 weeks gestation between 1992 and 1994. The study identified a preterm delivery rate of 14.4%. Of these preterm births 28.4% (*n* = 120) were indicated preterm births. Reasons for preterm delivery included proteinuric hypertension, fetal distress, intrauterine growth restriction, abruption, fetal death or a combination of these. Risk factors common to all preterm births were lung disease, black ethnicity, employment and previous preterm birth. Risk factors unique to indicated rather than spontaneous preterm birth include müllerian duct abnormality, proteinuria at less than 24 weeks and chronic hypertension. Those unique to spontaneous preterm birth included poor socioeconomic status, vaginal bleeding, low body mass index, bacterial vaginosis, cervicovaginal fetal fibronectin and shortening of cervix. **III B**

2 Harger JH, Hsing AW, Tuomala RE et al. (1990) Risk factors for preterm premature rupture of fetal membranes: a multicenter case-control study. *Am J Obstet Gynecol* **163**, 130–137. Case-control study in six US tertiary perinatal centers. The study involved completion of a comprehensive questionnaire for 341 women with preterm premature rupture of membranes in singleton pregnancies from 20–36 weeks gestation and 253 control women matched for maternal age, gestational age, parity, clinic or private patient status and previous vaginal or cesarean delivery. Univariate analysis revealed 11 variables associated with a significantly ($p < 0.05$) increased risk of preterm PROM. After multiple logistic regression analysis, three variables remained in the model as independent risk factors: antepartum vaginal bleeding in more than one trimester (OR 7.4, 95% CI 2.2–25.6), current cigarette smoking (OR 2.1, 95% CI 1.4–3.1), and previous preterm delivery (OR 2.5, 95% CI 1.4–2.5). Cessation of cigarette smoking by pregnant women may reduce the risk of preterm PROM. **III B**

3 Brocklehurst P, Hannah M, McDonald H *et al.* (2001) Interventions for treating bacterial vaginosis in pregnancy (Cochrane Review). In: *The Cochrane library*, issue 1. Oxford: Update Software. Meta-analysis of five RCTs ($n = 1504$) comparing pregnancy outcomes in women infected with bacterial vaginosis and treated with one or more antibiotic regimens. Compared to placebo, antibiotic treatment caused a nonsignificant reduction in preterm delivery (<37 weeks) (RR 0.78, 95% CI 0.60–1.02), which became statistically significant in a subgroup analysis of women with a history of previous preterm birth (RR 0.37, 95% CI 0.23–0.60; NNT 4, 95% CI 3–8). **Ia A**

4 Mercer BM, Goldenberg RL, Meiss PJ *et al.* (2000) The Preterm Prediction Study: prediction of preterm premature rupture of membranes through clinical findings and ancillary testing. *Am J Obstet Gynecol* **183**, 738–745. A total of 2929 women were evaluated in 10 centers at 23–24 weeks gestation. Premature rupture of membranes (PROM) at less than 37 weeks gestation complicated 4.5% of pregnancies, accounting for 32.6% of preterm births. Univariate analysis revealed low body mass index, pulmonary disease, contractions within 2 weeks, short cervix (≤25 mm), positive results of fetal fibronectin screening, bacterial vaginosis, and a previous preterm birth caused by PROM (in multiparous women) to be significantly associated with preterm birth caused by PROM in the current gestation. Short cervix, previous preterm birth caused by PROM in multiparous women, and presence of fetal fibronectin were the strongest predictors for preterm birth caused by PROM at both less than 37 and less than 35 weeks gestation. Women with positive fetal fibronectin screening results and a short cervix had greater risks of preterm birth caused by PROM at both less than 37 weeks gestation (RR 4.9) and less than 35 weeks gestation (RR 13.5). Multiparous women with all three risk factors had a 31.3-fold increased risk of preterm birth caused by PROM at less than 35 weeks gestation. **III B**

5 Lewis DF, Adair CD, Weeks JW *et al.* (1999) A randomized clinical trial of daily non-stress testing versus biophysical profile in the management of preterm premature rupture of membranes. *Am J Obstet Gynecol* **181**, 1495–1499. In a RCT, 135 patients with preterm premature rupture of membranes (at 23–34 weeks of gestation) were assigned to either a daily nonstress test or a biophysical profile, after a 24 h observation period. Demographics, pregnancy characteristics and neonatal outcomes were similar. Neither the daily nonstress test nor the daily biophysical profile had good sensitivity for predicting infectious complications (39.1% and 25.0% respectively). **Ib A**

6 Carlan SJ, O'Brien WF, Parsons MT *et al.* (1993) Preterm premature rupture of membranes: a randomized study of home versus hospital management. *Obstet Gynecol* **81**, 61–64. RCT comparing pregnancy outcomes in a carefully selected group of women ($n = 67$) with preterm premature rupture of the membranes who were randomized by sealed envelope to home versus hospital expectant management. The groups were managed similarly with pelvic and bed rest. Management included recording of temperature and pulse every 6 h, daily charting of fetal movements, twice-weekly nonstress test and complete blood count, and weekly ultrasound and visual examination of the cervix. There was no significant difference in clinical characteristics or perinatal outcome between the groups. There was, however, a significant decrease in both days of maternal hospitalization and maternal hospital expenses in the home group. **Ib A**

7 Yoon BH, Jun JK, Park KH *et al.* (1996) Serum C-reactive protein, white blood cell count, and amniotic fluid white blood cell count in women with preterm premature rupture of membranes. *Obstet Gynecol* **88**, 1034–1040. Maternal C-reactive protein, white blood cell count (WBC) and amniocentesis were performed in 90 women with preterm premature rupture of membranes. Women with positive amniotic fluid (AF) culture and clinical chorioamnionitis had significantly higher median C-reactive protein, WBC, and AF WBC than did women without these conditions ($p < 0.05$), whereas women with histological chorioamnionitis and significant neonatal morbidity had higher median C-reactive protein and AF WBC, but not WBC, than those without the conditions ($p < 0.05$). An AF WBC of at least 20 cells/mm^3 had a greater sensitivity than C-reactive protein (cutoff 0.7 mg/dl) and WBC (cutoff 13 000 cells/mm^3) in the detection of positive AF culture and histologic chorioamnionitis. Logistic regression analysis indicated that, among AF WBC, C-reactive protein and WBC, AF WBC was the best predictor of positive AF culture (OR 24.2, 95% CI 6.0–97.5, $p < 0.001$), histological (OR 74.0, 95% CI 7.4–736.3, $p < 0.001$) and clinical chorioamnionitis (OR 8.9, 95% CI 0.9–85.6, $p = 0.057$) and neonatal morbidity (OR 4.3, 95% CI 1.1–16.6, $p < 0.05$). **III B**

8 Nowak M, Oszukowski P, Szpakowski M *et al.* (1998) Intrauterine infections. I. The role of C-reactive protein, white blood cell count and erythrocyte sedimentation rate in pregnant women in the detection of intrauterine infection after preliminary rupture of membranes. *Ginekol Pol* **69**, 615–622. A group of 80 patients with premature rupture of membranes before 35 weeks gestation were evaluated prospectively and managed expectantly. 59 (73.7%) patients had significant chorioamnionitis on histopathology and only 15 of them had clinical chorioamnionitis. Serum C-reactive protein (CRP) serial determinations (definition of abnormal tests: 1) >1.2 mg/dl; 2) >2.0 mg/dl; 3) >1.2 mg/dl and increasing in two consecutive days) were found to be the most reliable, with a sensitivity 1) 91.5%; 2) 85%; 3) 88%, specificity 57%; 76%; 86%, positive predictive value 86%; 90%; 94.5%, negative predictive value 70.5%; 64%; 72% and accuracy 82.5%; 82.5%; 87.5% respectively. The efficacy of white blood cell count (WBC; abnormal tests: >12 500/mm^3; >15 000/mm^3; >12 500/mm^3 and increasing in two consecutive days) and erythrocyte sedimentation rate (ESR; abnormal tests: >60 mm/h; >60 mm/h and increasing in two consecutive days)

serial evaluations was significantly lower. Moreover, in cases of chorioamnionitis CRP increased above the upper limit of normal 3 days earlier than WBC or ESR. CRP was found to be the most reliable indicator of histological chorioamnionitis and indicated the presence of intrauterine infection earlier than WBC or ESR. **III B**

9 Vermillion ST, Kooba AM, Soper DE *et al.* (2000) Amniotic fluid index values after preterm premature rupture of the membranes and subsequent perinatal infection. *Am J Obstet Gynecol* **183**, 271–276. Nonconcurrent prospective analysis of 225 singleton pregnancies complicated by preterm premature rupture of the membranes, with delivery between 24 and 32 weeks gestation. Patients were categorized into two groups on the basis of a 4-quadrant amniotic fluid index (AFI) of less than 5 cm (n = 131) or 5 cm or above (n = 94). Both groups were similar with respect to selected demographics, gestational age at rupture of the membranes, birthweight and maternal group B streptococcal colonization. Patients with an AFI below 5 cm demonstrated a shorter mean latency until delivery (5.5 ± 4.0 vs 14.1 ± 5.2 days (mean ± SD; p = 0.02)), greater frequency of amnioinfusion therapy (23.6% vs 5.3%, p < 0.001), and cesarean delivery for nonreassuring fetal testing (18.3% vs 4. 3%, p =001). Multiple logistic regression analysis showed that an AFI of less than 5 cm was the only significant risk factor independently associated with early-onset neonatal sepsis (p = 0.004) and chorioamnionitis (p = 0.024). **IIb B**

10 Kenyon S, Boulvain M (2001) Antibiotics for preterm premature rupture of membranes (Cochrane Review). In: *The Cochrane library*, issue 3. Oxford: Update Software. Meta-analysis of 12 RCTs (n = 1599 women) examining the use of antibiotics (various regimens) in women with preterm premature rupture of membranes. Compared to placebo, antibiotic treatment increased the latency period and reduced the risk of chorioamnionitis and neonatal infection; there was no statistically significant reduction in perinatal mortality or neonatal necrotizing enterocolitis. However, most of the trials did not include antenatal administration of corticosteroids, which may explain the lack of beneficial effect on neonatal mortality. **Ia A**

11 Mercer BM, Miodovnik M, Thurnau GR *et al.* (1997) Antibiotic therapy for reduction of infant morbidity after preterm premature rupture of the membranes. A randomized controlled trial. *JAMA* **278**, 989–995. Randomized, double-blind, placebo-controlled trial of 614 gravidas with preterm premature rupture of the membranes between 24 and 32 weeks gestation, treated with ampicillin (2 g every 6 h) and erythromycin (250 mg every 6 h) for 48 h followed by oral amoxicillin (250 mg every 8 h) and erythromycin base (333 mg every 8 h) for 5 days versus a matching placebo regimen. The primary outcome included pregnancies complicated by at least one of the following: fetal or infant death, respiratory distress, severe intraventricular hemorrhage, stage 2 or 3 necrotizing enterocolitis, sepsis within 72 h of birth. The primary outcome (44.1% vs 52.9%; p = 0.04), respiratory distress (40.5% vs 48.7%; p = 0.04), and necrotizing enterocolitis (2.3% vs 5.8%; p = 0.03) were less frequent with antibiotics. In the group-B-streptococcus (GBS)-negative cohort, the antibiotic group had less frequent primary outcome (44.5% vs 54.5%; p = 0.03), respiratory distress (40.8% vs 50.6%; p = 0.03), overall sepsis (8.4% vs 15.6%; p = 0.01), pneumonia (2.9% vs 7.0%; p = 0.04), and other morbidities. Among GBS-negative women, significant pregnancy prolongation was seen with antibiotics (p < 0.001). **Ib A**

12 Kenyon SL, Taylor DJ, Tarnow-Mordi W *et al.* (2001) Broad-spectrum antibiotics for preterm, prelabour rupture of fetal membranes: the ORACLE I randomised trial. ORACLE Collaborative Group. *Lancet* **357**, 979–988. In a randomized multicenter trial 4826 women with preterm premature rupture of the membranes were randomly assigned to 250 mg erythromycin (n = 1197), 325 mg co-amoxiclav (250 mg amoxicillin plus 125 mg clavulanic acid; n = 1212), both (n = 1192), or placebo (n = 1225) four times daily for 10 days or until delivery. The primary outcome measure was a composite of neonatal death, chronic lung disease or major cerebral abnormality on ultrasonography before discharge from hospital. Among the 2415 infants born to women allocated erythromycin only or placebo, fewer had the primary composite outcome in the erythromycin group (151/1190, 12.7% vs 186/1225, 15.2%, p = 0.08) than in the placebo group. Among the 2260 singletons in this comparison, significantly fewer had the composite primary outcome in the erythromycin group (125/1111, 11.2% vs 166/1149, 14.4%, p = 0.02). Co-amoxiclav only and co-amoxiclav plus erythromycin had no benefit over placebo with regard to this outcome in all infants or in singletons only. Use of erythromycin was also associated with prolongation of pregnancy, reductions in neonatal treatment with surfactant, decreases in oxygen dependence at 28 days of age and older, fewer major cerebral abnormalities on ultrasonography before discharge and fewer positive blood cultures. Although co-amoxiclav only and co-amoxiclav plus erythromycin were associated with prolongation of pregnancy, they were also associated with a significantly higher rate of neonatal necrotizing enterocolitis. **Ib A**

13 Harding JE, Pang J, Knight DB *et al.* (2001) Do antenatal corticosteroids help in the setting of preterm rupture of membranes? *Am J Obstet Gynecol* **184**, 131–139. Meta-analysis of 15 RCTs, involving over 1400 women with preterm premature rupture of the membranes, showing antenatal corticosteroid administration to reduce the risk of respiratory distress syndrome (RR 0.56, 95% CI 0.46–0.70), intraventricular hemorrhage (RR 0.47, 95% CI 0.31–0.70), necrotizing enterocolitis (RR 0.21, 95% CI 0.05–0.82), and neonatal death (not significant, RR 0.68, 95% CI 0.43–1.07). There is no statistically significant increased risk of infection in either mother or infant following corticosteroid administration. **Ia A**

14 Leitich H, Egarter C, Reisenberger K *et al.* (1998) Concomitant use of glucocorticoids: a comparison of two meta-analyses on antibiotic treatment in preterm premature rupture of the membranes. *Am J Obstet Gynecol* **178**, 899–908. A group receiving antibiotic treatment with concomitant glucocorticoids (five RCTs, n = 509) was compared against a group receiving antibiotic treatment without glucocorticoids (seven RCTs, n = 657). The beneficial effects of antibiotic treatment (reducing the incidence of chorioamnionitis, postpartum endometritis, neonatal sepsis and intraventricular hemorrhage) might be diminished when glucocorticoids are used concomitantly. **Ia A**

15 Gyetvai K, Hannah ME, Hodnett ED *et al.* (1999) Tocolytics for preterm labor: a systematic review. *Obstet Gynecol* **94**, 869–877. Meta-analysis of 17 RCTs examining the effectiveness of any tocolytic (n = 1184 women) compared with placebo or no tocolytic (n = 1100 women) for preterm labor. Three trials included women with ruptured membranes. Tocolytics used in the intervention group included: isoxsuprine, ethanol, terbutaline, ritodrine (five trials), indomethacin, magnesium sulfate and atosiban. Beta-mimetics, indomethacin, atosiban and ethanol, but not magnesium sulfate, were associated with significant prolongation of pregnancy for women in threatened preterm labor. Tocolytics were not associated with significantly reduced rates of perinatal death, neonatal morbidity, low birthweight, or births before 30/32/37 weeks gestation. **Ia A**

16 Ladfors L, Mattsson LA, Eriksson M *et al.* (1996) A randomised trial of two expectant managements of prelabour rupture of the membranes at 34 to 42 weeks. *Br J Obstet Gynaecol* **103**, 755–762. RCT comparing pregnancy outcome in women (n = 1385) with prelabor rupture of the membranes (between 34 and 42 weeks and without contractions 2h after admission), randomly allocated to early induction (the next morning) or late induction (2 days later). In nulliparous women, a higher rate of spontaneous deliveries occurred in the late induction group compared with the early induction group. The ventouse rate was significantly lower in the late-induction group. **Ib A**

17 Mozurkewich EL, Wolf FM (1997) Premature rupture of membranes at term: a meta-analysis of three management schemes. *Obstet Gynecol* **89**, 1035–1043. Meta-analysis of 23 studies (n = 7493 women) compared the pregnancy outcomes in women with premature rupture of membranes at term following immediate induction of labor with intravenous oxytocin, immediate induction with vaginal prostaglandin E_2 or conservative management (or delayed oxytocin induction). There were no differences in the rates of cesarean section or neonatal sepsis amongst the three management options. Vaginal prostaglandins resulted in more chorioamnionitis than immediate oxytocin induction but less chorioamnionitis than conservative management. Immediate oxytocin induction resulted in less chorioamnionitis (RR 0.67, 95% CI 0.52–0.85) and endometritis (RR 0.71, 95% CI 0.51–0.99) than conservative management. **Ia A**

18 Smaill F (2001) Intrapartum antibiotics for Group B streptococcal colonisation (Cochrane Review). In: *The Cochrane library*, issue 3. Oxford: Update Software. Meta-analysis of five trials, although most studies had methodological flaws. Intrapartum antibiotic treatment of women colonized with group B streptococcus reduces the incidence of neonatal infection (RR 0.17, 95% CI 0.07–0.39) without a significant beneficial effect on neonatal mortality (RR 0.12, 95% CI 0.01–2.00). **Ia A**

19 Hofmeyr GJ (2001) Amnioinfusion for umbilical cord compression in labour (Cochrane Review). In: *The Cochrane library*, issue 3. Oxford: Update Software. 12 studies were included in this review. Transcervical amnioinfusion for potential or suspected umbilical cord compression was associated with the following reductions: fetal heart rate decelerations (RR 0.54, 95% CI 0.43–0.68); cesarean section for suspected fetal distress (RR 0.35, 95% CI 0.24–0.52); neonatal hospital stay greater than 3 days (RR 0.40, 95% CI 0.26–0.62); maternal hospital stay greater than 3 days (RR 0.46, 95% CI 0.29–0.74). Transabdominal amnioinfusion showed similar results. Transcervical amnioinfusion to prevent infection in women with membranes ruptured for more than 6h was associated with a reduction in puerperal infection (RR 0.50, 95% CI 0.26–0.97). **Ia A**

20 Grant A, Penn ZJ, Steer PJ (1996) Elective or selective caesarean delivery of the small baby? A systematic review of the controlled trials. *Br J Obstet Gynaecol* **103**, 1197–1200. Meta-analysis of six trials (n = 122) showed that a policy of elective cesarean delivery for women in spontaneous preterm labor increases the risk of serious maternal morbidity (OR 6.2; 95% CI 1.3–30.1) without showing clear neonatal benefits. **Ia A**

LABOR AND DELIVERY

Chapter 47

Labor and delivery problems

47.1 Breech presentation

Ian Scudamore

Breech presentation at term

Management option		Quality of evidence	Strength of recommendation	References
Version in prenatal period	Evidence for reduced breech presentation at delivery and in cesarean section rate with external cephalic version (ECV) at term	Ia	A	1
	Tocolysis is associated with fewer ECV failures	Ia	A	2
	Fetal vibroacoustic stimulation in midline fetal position is associated with fewer ECV failures	Ia	A	2
	Need for fetal heart rate monitoring before and after ECV	III	B	3
	Apparent safety in women with a previous cesarean section	IIa	B	4
	No evidence to support postural management to encourage spontaneous version	Ia	A	5
Fetal assessment	Confirm diagnosis and determine placental site	-	✔	-
	Confirm normality as association of breech presentation with congenital anomaly	III	B	6
	Assess fetal attitude – hyperextension of fetal head is associated with spinal cord injury during vaginal delivery	III	B	7
Labor and delivery	Evidence that planned cesarean section for breech at term as preferred method of delivery significantly reduced perinatal mortality and morbidity	Ia	A	8

References

1 Hofmeyr GJ, Kulier R (2000) External cephalic version for breech presentation at term. In: *Cochrane database of systematic reviews*, issue 4. Oxford: Update Software. Six RCTs of external cephalic version (ECV) for breech presentation at term were reviewed. ECV was associated with fewer noncephalic births (RR 0.42, 95% CI 0.35–0.50) and cesarean section (RR 0.52, 95% CI 0.39–0.71) with no difference in perinatal mortality (RR 0.44, 95% CI 0.07–2.92). These data support the value of ECV in reducing the rate of breech birth and cesarean section but do not provide enough evidence to definitively assess any risks of ECV at term. **Ia A**

2 Hofmeyr GJ (2000) External cephalic version facilitation for breech presentation at term. In: *Cochrane database of systematic reviews*, issue 4. Oxford: Update Software. Review evaluating the evidence from six randomized and quasi-randomized trials of the value of tocolysis, fetal acoustic stimulation, epidural anesthesia and amnioinfusion in external cephalic version (ECV). Fewer failures at ECV were associated with both tocolysis (RR 0.77, 95% CI 0.64–0.92) and fetal acoustic stimulation (RR 0.17, 95% CI 0.05–0.60). No appropriate trials of epidural anesthesia or amnioinfusion were identified. **Ia A**

3 Hofmeyr GJ, Sonnendecker EWW (1983) Cardiotocographic changes after external cephalic version. *Br J Obstet Gynaecol* **90**, 914–918. The findings of cardiotocography before and after 53 consecutive attempts at external cephalic version (ECV) are reported with a transient fetal bradycardia occurring in 5 cases. No bradycardia persisted for more than 5 min and the proposed cause was relative fetal hypoxia caused by the uterine manipulation. The authors recommend that duration and force of manipulation should be limited and, despite not monitoring during the ECV, they suggest that the fetal heart should be continuously monitored and manipulation discontinued if bradycardia occurs. **III B**

4 Flamm BL, Fried MW, Lonky NM *et al.* (1991) External cephalic version after previous cesarean section. *Am J Obstet Gynecol* **165**, 370–372. As previous cesarean section is considered a contraindication to external cephalic version (ECV) the authors studied 56 patients with a previous cesarean section who underwent ECV for breech presentation at more than 36 weeks gestation. A control group of 56 consecutive attempts at ECV for breech presentation after 36 weeks on women with no previous history of cesarean section was identified for comparison. ECV was more successful in the study group (82% vs 61%), reflecting differences in parity. Fetal heart rate abnormalities during the ECV leading to cesarean section occurred in one patient in each group. There were no other major complications and no evidence of uterine rupture or scar complications in the study group. While the numbers were small, this study provides some evidence that a policy of previous cesarean section being an absolute contraindication to ECV is not justified. **IIa B**

5 Hofmeyr GJ, Kulier R (2000) Cephalic version by postural management for breech presentation. In: *Cochrane database of systematic reviews*, issue 4. Oxford: Update Software. Review including randomized and quasi-randomized trials comparing postural management by pelvic elevation for breech presentation with a control group. Five studies were included. Analysis of 392 pregnancies demonstrated no effect of postural management in facilitating cephalic birth. There is no evidence to support postural management of breech presentation. **Ia A**

6 Schutte MF, van Hemel OJ, van de Berg C *et al.* (1985) Perinatal mortality in breech presentations as compared to vertex presentations in singleton pregnancies: an analysis based upon 57819 computer-registered pregnancies in The Netherlands. *Eur J Obstet Gynecol Reprod Biol* **19**, 391–400. After 1982, 70% of Dutch hospitals participated in a nationwide collection of obstetric data. The authors of this paper used the database to study the perinatal outcome of breech presentation. They found that perinatal mortality was persistently higher in breech presentation than vertex and that this was the case even after allowing for a higher congenital anomaly rate and after correcting for birthweight and gestational age. They postulate that breech presentation may not be coincidental but a product of factors intrinsic to the fetus themselves associated with a poorer outcome. If so, they surmise, routine cesarean section would be unlikely to improve neonatal outcome. **III B**

7 Ballas S, Toaff R (1976) Hyperextension of the fetal head in breech presentation: radiological evaluation and significance. *Br J Obstet Gynaecol* **83**, 201–204. Case report and a review of published cases of hyperextension of the fetal head in breech presentation. Hyperextension of the fetal head (extension angle >90°) was present on radiographic assessment of the case reported and elective cesarean section was performed. The child was developing normally at age 30 months. 38 cases of hyperextension but with a measured angle of less than 90° were identified in the literature and 25 of these were delivered vaginally without any reported damage to the cervical cord. In contrast, of 20 babies reported to have an extension angle of more than 90°, 11 delivered vaginally and 8 sustained cervical cord lesions. The 9 babies delivered by cesarean section had no cervical damage. The authors suggest that hyperextension of the fetal head should be sought when considering a trial of vaginal delivery and that it is a contraindication to labor. **III B**

8 Hofmeyr GJ, Hannah ME (2001) Planned caesarean section for term breech delivery. In: *Cochrane database of systematic reviews*, issue 3. Oxford: Update Software. Review of RCTs shows that cesarean delivery occurred in 550/1227 (45%) of those women allocated to a vaginal delivery protocol. Planned cesarean section was associated with modestly increased maternal morbidity (RR 1.29, 95% CI 1.03–1.61). Perinatal and neonatal death (excluding fatal anomalies) were greatly reduced (RR 0.29, 95% CI 0.10–0.86). The reductions were similar for countries with low and high perinatal mortality rates. Perinatal/neonatal death or neonatal morbidity was also greatly reduced (RR 0.31, 95% CI 0.19–0.52). The difference was smaller for countries with a high national perinatal mortality rate. **Ia A**

Preterm breech presentation

Management option		Quality of evidence	Strength of recommendation	References
Prenatal	Evidence that external cephalic version is not useful in preterm breech presentation	Ia	A	1
Labor and delivery – general	Infant outcome worse with breech presentation than vertex	III	B	2,3
	Routine cesarean section would cause iatrogenic prematurity	Ib	A	4

➡

Management option		Quality of evidence	Strength of recommendation	References
Preterm breech presenting in labor	Confirm in labor, including vaginal examination	–	✔	–
	Confirm normality	–	✔	–
	Confirm type of breech	–	✔	–
	No strong evidence of benefit but probably cesarean section preferred, especially for 1000–1500 g baby	III	B	5–9
	For babies less than 1000 g no evidence of benefit from either mode of delivery	III	B	9,10

References

1 Hofmeyr GJ (2000) External cephalic version for breech presentation before term. In: *Cochrane database of systematic reviews*, issue 4. Oxford: Update Software. Review of three randomized or quasi-randomized trials containing a total of 889 women. External cephalic version (ECV) before term had no significant effect on noncephalic presentation, cesarean section, low Apgar scores or perinatal mortality. The evidence from these trials does not support a practice of ECV before term. **Ia A**

2 Gravenhorst JB, Schreuder AM, Veen S *et al.* (1993) Breech delivery in very preterm and very low birthweight infants in The Netherlands. *Br J Obstet Gynaecol* **100**, 411–415. Neonatal mortality and childhood handicap rates at age 2 and 5 of survivors were studied from a nationwide collaborative collection of perinatal and follow-up data relating to 899 preterm infants (< 32 weeks or < 1500 g) delivered in the Netherlands in 1983. Logistic regression analysis suggested a poorer outcome for breech than vertex presentation and a possible trend to better outcome for breech presentation delivered by cesarean section. The authors recognize potential selection bias in such an observational study and question the ethical justification of a policy of cesarean section for preterm breech. **III B**

3 Danielian PJ, Wang J, Hall MH (1996) Long term outcome by method of delivery of fetuses in breech presentation at term: population based follow up. *Br Med J* **312**, 1451–1453. Population-based retrospective review of long-term outcome of infants delivered in breech presentation according to intended mode of delivery. There were 1645 term breech deliveries over the study period, of whom 590 (35.9%) were delivered by cesarean section and 1055 (64.1%) were intended to have a vaginal delivery. 269 children (19.4%) were identified as having handicap or other health problems and seemed to have been proportionately delivered by elective cesarean section (100/269, 37.2%) or after intention to deliver vaginally (169/269, 62.8%). Also there was no apparent difference between the two groups in the distribution of severe handicap. Case review suggested that only one case was a severe handicap possibly attributable to vaginal delivery. The authors conclude that carefully selected and supervised trial of vaginal delivery is not associated with poor neonatal outcome and that routine cesarean section for breech presentation at term is not justified. They indicate the need for an appropriate randomized trial to establish the safest method of delivery for breech presentation at term. **III B**

4 Penn ZJ, Steer PJ, Grant A (1996) A multicentre randomised controlled trial comparing elective and selective caesarean section for the delivery of the preterm breech infant. *Br J Obstet Gynaecol* **103**, 684–689. Multicenter RCT of intention to deliver vaginally versus intention to deliver by cesarean section in preterm breech labor at gestational age 26–32 weeks. The trial was closed after 17 months as only 13 patients were recruited. One baby randomized to cesarean section at 26 weeks was not in labor and was delivered by cesarean section at 29 weeks in cephalic presentation. Two other babies randomized as breech presentations were cephalic at delivery. The study shows that a policy of elective cesarean section will lead to some babies being delivered unnecessarily early. Also, maternal morbidity was restricted to those women who had cesarean sections. The authors recognize the difficulties of conducting such a randomized trial and indicate that, until evidence from such study is available, individualized decisions will need to be made in consultation with the woman herself. **Ib A**

5 Goldenberg RL, Nelson KG (1977) The premature breech. *Am J Obstet Gynecol* **127**, 240–244. Retrospective review of 141 singleton breech deliveries of birthweight 500–2499 g. While the authors assert that prophylactic cesarean section is likely to benefit the preterm infant in breech presentation, the study is likely to have been heavily biased by obstetricians selectively avoiding cesarean section in situations of extreme prematurity and anticipating a poor neonatal outcome. It is not surprising that the outcomes for the babies of birthweight between 750 and 1500 g were better if delivered by cesarean section, as the use of cesarean section was highly selective. Method of delivery was associated with little difference in perinatal outcome in the babies of birthweight between 1500 and 2500 g, suggesting fundamentally different obstetric decision making and perhaps also different levels of success with neonatal care. The findings of the study justify further investigation but not definitive change in practice. **III B**

6 Weissman A, Blazer S, Zimmer EZ *et al.* (1988) Low birthweight breech infant: short-term and long-term outcome by method of delivery. *Am J Perinatol* **5**, 289–292. Retrospective case review of breech deliveries of infants weighing 500–1999g between 1980 and 1986. There was a recognized preference for cesarean section if the fetus was estimated to be over 1000g and for vaginal delivery if less than 1000g or the woman arrived in the delivery suite in advanced labor. In the group of babies of birthweight 1000–1999g there was a benefit in perinatal mortality associated with cesarean section (17/78, 21.8%) compared with vaginal delivery (12/27, 44.4%). There also appeared to be a benefit in longer-term function as the babies delivered vaginally were more likely to suffer from cerebral palsy, blindness, sensorineural deafness or developmental delay. The authors contend that their data support a policy of cesarean section in breech presentation of birthweight 1000–1999g. **III B**

7 Viegas OA, Ingemarsson I, Sim LP *et al.* (1985) Collaborative study on preterm breeches: vaginal delivery versus caesarean section. *Asia-Oceania J Obstet Gynaecol* **11**, 349–355. Uncontrolled review of perinatal outcome and infant development in 73 preterm deliveries (28–36 weeks). It attempts to identify outcome associations with mode of delivery and appears to have initially been an attempt at a randomized trial of cesarean section vs a trial of labor. Of 73 patients, only 23 agreed to randomization and the remaining 50 formed a descriptive study group; the two groups were combined for analysis. Vaginal delivery occurred in 41/73 (56%) and cesarean section in 32 (44%). Perinatal mortality was 7/41 (17%) and 2/32 (6%) respectively. No statistical analysis is presented. Review of a number of papers is presented. Despite the authors' acknowledgment that these studies are retrospective and exposed to potential bias, they use the accumulated data and their own limited data to argue a case for cesarean section as the preferred mode of delivery in the preterm breech. **III B**

8 Paul RH, Koh KS, Monfared AH *et al.* (1979) Obstetric factors influencing outcome in infants weighing from 1001 to 1500 grams. *Am J Obstet Gynecol* **133**, 503–508. Retrospective evaluation of obstetric factors that may have affected the neonatal outcome in 201 infants of birthweight 1001–1500g. 25 of the babies were breech presentation at birth. Neonatal death occurred in 1/15 delivered by cesarean section and in 4/10 delivered vaginally. These data are not considered specifically in the paper, which addresses factors generally applicable to prematurity rather than breech presentation. **III B**

9 Yu VYH, Bajuk B, Cutting D *et al.* (1984) Effect of mode of delivery on outcome of very-low-birthweight infants. *Br J Obstet Gynaecol* **91**, 633–639. Retrospective study reviewing the management and outcomes of 72 singleton breech infants in birthweight bands 501–1000g and 1001–1500g. The hospital survival of babies delivered by cesarean section in the 1001–1500g group was significantly higher than the vaginal delivery group (28/29, 94% vs 8/12, 67%). There were no differences in survival in the 501–1000g group. At 2-year follow-up the differences in normal survival were no longer present. The authors provide a useful review of the literature and recognize the deficiencies in retrospective studies preventing firm conclusions. They cautiously note that their results suggest a potential benefit of cesarean section for the breech presentation of birthweight 1001–1500g recommending prospective, randomized study. **III B**

10 Kitchen W, Ford GW, Doyle LW *et al.* (1985) Cesarean section or vaginal delivery at 24 to 28 weeks' gestation: comparison of survival and neonatal and two-year morbidity. *Obstet Gynecol* **66**, 149–157. Well-conducted retrospective study assessing the effect of mode of delivery on outcome of breech delivery between 24 and 28 weeks gestation. Stepwise multiple regression analysis was performed to allow for differences in gestation and 14 obstetric variables that could have influenced survival. From January 1977 to March 1982 172/326 (52.8%) babies appropriate for the study were delivered and survived their primary hospitalization. There was no policy favoring cesarean section and the cesarean section rate over the course of the study was 51/326 (15.6%). Initial analysis suggested a trend toward increased survival after delivery by cesarean section but this trend disappeared when survival was adjusted for other prognostic factors. The variables that were associated with improved survival included increasing gestational age ($p < 0.0001$), absence of maternal hypertension ($p = 0.007$), singleton pregnancy ($p = 0.007$) and antenatal steroid administration ($p = 0.018$). 2-year follow-up of 162/167 surviving infants demonstrated no association between mode of delivery and incidence of handicap. The authors contend that their analysis argues against the routine use of cesarean section in infants before 28 weeks gestation but that a randomized controlled trial would be required to provide a definitive answer with regard to the influence of mode of delivery on neonatal outcome. **III B**

47.2 Unstable lie

Sandra Newbold

Management option		Quality of evidence	Strength of recommendation	References
Prenatal	**Expectant management:** ❑ If noncephalic after 36 weeks – wait-and-see policy. Danger is that patient may be admitted with cord prolapse or in advanced labor with a malpresentation	–	✔	–

Management option		Quality of evidence	Strength of recommendation	References
Prenatal (cont'd)	**Expectant management (cont'd):**			
	❑ Advice to adopt knee–chest maneuver to promote cephalic version has not been shown to be of value and thus not recommended	Ia	A	1
	Active management:			
	❑ If noncephalic after 36 weeks, external cephalic version (ECV) should be attempted if no contraindications	Ia	A	2
	❑ Admit into hospital and assess daily *or* see from home every 2–3 days to ensure baby remaining cephalic and advise to come into hospital as soon as labor begins or membranes rupture	-	✓	-
	❑ Stabilizing induction between 38–39 weeks	III	B	3
	❑ Cesarean section if ECV fails or version contraindicated	Ia	A	4
Labor and delivery	Intrapartum management depends on the presentation in labor and these issues are discussed elsewhere in the relevant section	-	✓	-

References

1 Hofmeyr GJ, Kulier R (2001) Cephalic version by postural management for breech presentation. In: *The Cochrane Library*, Issue 2. Oxford: Update Software. Many postural techniques have been used to promote cephalic version. This review was to assess the effects of postural management of breech presentation on measures of pregnancy outcome. Five studies involving a total of 392 women were included. No effect of postural management on the rate of noncephalic births was detected, either for the subgroup in which no external cephalic version was attempted, or for the group overall (RR 0.95, 95% CI 0.81–1.11). No differences were detected for cesarean sections or Apgar scores below 7 at 1 min. There is therefore no evidence to support the use of postural management for breech presentation. The numbers of women studied to date remain relatively small. **Ia A**

2 Hofmeyr GJ, Kulier R (2001) External cephalic version for breech presentation at term (Cochrane Review). In: *The Cochrane library*, issue 2. Oxford: Update Software. The objective of this review was to assess the effects of external cephalic version at term on measures of pregnancy outcome. Six studies were included. External cephalic version at term was associated with a significant reduction in noncephalic births (RR 0.42, 95% CI 0.35–0.50) and cesarean section (RR 0.52, 95% CI 0.39–0.71). There was no significant effect on perinatal mortality (RR 0.44, 95% CI 0.07–2.92). Attempting cephalic version at term appears to reduce the chance of noncephalic births and cesarean section. There is not enough evidence to assess any risks of external cephalic version at term. **Ia A**

3 Edwards RL, Nicholson HO (1969) The management of the unstable lie in late pregnancy. *J Obstet Gynaecol Br Commonw* **76**, 713–718. Observational study of 254 cases of unstable lie at term managed over an 8-year period. Orthodox management occurred in 152 cases and was compared to a 'stabilizing induction' performed in 102 cases. In the orthodox management group cephalic vaginal delivery occurred in 73.5% of cases if spontaneous stabilization occurred before the onset of labor but only in 40.7% of cases if the lie remained unstable when either spontaneous labor or intervention (induction of labor or elective cesarean section) occurred. The rate of cephalic vaginal delivery was much higher (88.2%) after a stabilizing induction. **III B**

4 Hofmeyr GJ, Hannah ME (2001) Planned caesarean section for term breech delivery (Cochrane Review). In: *The Cochrane library*, issue 2. Oxford: Update Software. This review was to assess the effects of planned cesarean section for breech presentation on measures of pregnancy outcome. Randomized trials comparing planned cesarean section for breech presentation with planned vaginal delivery were identified. Cesarean delivery occurred in 550/1227 (45%) of those women allocated to a vaginal delivery protocol. Planned cesarean section was associated with modestly increased maternal morbidity (RR 1.29, 95% CI 1.03–1.61). Perinatal and neonatal death (excluding fatal anomalies) was greatly reduced (RR 0.29, 95% CI 0.10–0.86). The reductions were similar for countries with low and high perinatal mortality rates. Perinatal/neonatal death or neonatal morbidity was also greatly reduced (RR 0.31, 95% CI 0.19–0.52). The difference was smaller for countries with a high national perinatal mortality rate. Planned cesarean section greatly reduces both perinatal/neonatal mortality and neonatal morbidity, at the expense of somewhat increased maternal

morbidity. Cost, and future morbidity due to the cesarean section scar were not assessed. The option of external cephalic version is dealt with in separate reviews. The data from this review will help to inform individualized decision-making regarding breech delivery. **Ia A**

47.3 Prolonged pregnancy

Sandra Newbold

Management option		Quality of evidence	Strength of recommendation	References
Prenatal: general	Establish accurate gestational age as early as possible	III	B	1
	Menstrual dates overestimate gestation. Routine early scan of value in preventing induction for 'post dates'	Ia	A	2
	Breast stimulation does not reduce incidence of postterm pregnancy	Ia	A	2
	Sweeping membranes at term reduces chance of pregnancy going beyond 41 weeks	Ia	A	3
Prenatal: at 41 weeks	Reevaluate for possible risk factors	–	✔	–
	Routine induction of labor reduces perinatal mortality	Ia	A	2
	Active management:			
	❑ Cervical ripening reduces risk of failed induction	Ib	A	4
	❑ Labor induction does not increase rate of cesarean section or operative vaginal delivery if cervix made favorable first	Ia	A	2
	Expectant management:			
	❑ Routine fetal movement counts alone have not been shown to be of value in reducing perinatal deaths – but no specific data in postdate pregnancies	Ib	A	5
	❑ Maternal perception of sound-provoked fetal movements may be of value where facilities for frequent nonstress testing (NST) are not available	III	B	6
	❑ Serial NST twice weekly at least helpful in monitoring fetal wellbeing in postterm pregnancies	IIa	B	7
	❑ Fetal acoustic stimulation test may be of value in those with a nonreactive NST	Ia	B	8
	❑ Assessment of amniotic fluid index versus vertical pockets of amniotic fluid increases obstetric intervention	Ib	A	9
	❑ Biophysical profile twice weekly may be helpful for monitoring fetal wellbeing but is time-consuming	IIb	B	10
	❑ Combination of just amniotic fluid volume and fetal acoustic stimulation test may be acceptable	III	B	11
	❑ Umbilical artery Doppler has not been shown to be any better than NST	III	B	12
Labor and delivery	Manage as high-risk pregnancy	–	✔	–
	If umbilical cord compression from oligohydramnios – amnioinfusion is useful	Ia	A	13
	Be vigilant for shoulder dystocia	III	B	14

References

1 Gardosi J, Vanner T, Francis A (1997) Gestational age and induction of labour for prolonged pregnancy. *Br J Obstet Gynaecol* **104**, 792–797. Retrospective analysis of computerized obstetric records in which a record of both the last menstrual period and a dating ultrasound scan were found. Menstrual dates systematically overestimated gestational age when compared with scan dates. Analysis suggested that most pregnancies considered 'prolonged' according to menstrual dates are in fact misdated. Therefore most pregnancies induced for 'post-dates' are not postterm when assessed by ultrasound dates. **III B**

2 Crowley P (2000) Interventions for preventing, or improving the outcome of delivery at or beyond term. In: *Cochrane database of systematic reviews*, issue 4. Oxford: Update Software. Meta-analysis of 26 randomized or quasi-randomized trials of intervention involving the intention to induce labor at a specific gestational age. Findings: routine early pregnancy ultrasound scanning (four trials) reduced the incidence of postterm pregnancy (OR 0.68, 95% CI 0.57–0.82); breast and nipple stimulation at term (two trials) did not affect the incidence of postterm pregnancy (OR 0.53, 95% CI 0.28–0.96); routine induction of labor (19 trials) reduced perinatal mortality (OR 0.2, 95% CI 0.06–0.70) – this benefit is due to induction of labor after 41 weeks but about 500 inductions of labor may be necessary to prevent one perinatal death; routine induction of labor had no effect on cesarean section rates. **Ia A**

3 Boulvain M, Stan C, Irion O (2001) Membrane sweeping for induction of labour (Cochrane Review). In: *The Cochrane library*, issue 2. Oxford: Update Software. Meta-analysis of 17 randomized trials comparing membrane sweep with no treatment. Sweeping the membranes at term reduced the frequency of pregnancy continuing beyond 41 weeks (RR 0.62, 95% CI 0.49–0.79) and beyond 42 weeks (RR 0.28, 95% CI 0.15–0.50). To avoid one formal induction of labor, membrane sweep needs to be performed on 7 women. There was no evidence of a difference in maternal or neonatal infection. Discomfort during vaginal examination and other adverse effects (bleeding, irregular contraction, etc.) were more frequently reported by women allocated to sweeping. **Ia A**

4 Kemp B, Winkler M, Rath W (2000) Induction of labor by prostaglandin E_2 in relation to the Bishop score. *J Gynecol Obstet* **71**, 13–17. Prospective multicenter RCT, 470 patients with unfavorable Bishop scores (3–4) were randomized to receive prostaglandin vaginal gel (2 mg) or intracervical gel (0.5 mg). In patients with unfavorable Bishop scores the intravaginal application route resulted in a better cervical ripening, a shorter induction to delivery interval and a higher cumulative rate of deliveries during 24 h ($p = 0.01$). **Ib A**

5 Grant A, Elbourne D, Valentin L *et al.* (1989) Routine formal fetal movement counting and risk of antepartum late death in normally formed singletons. *Lancet* **1**, 345–349. Multicenter RCT with 'cluster' allocation. 31 993 women were asked to keep daily formal fetal movement records after trial entry at 28–32 weeks gestation. Pregnancy outcome of this 'counting' group was compared to that in 36 661 control pregnancies in which antenatal care was routine. The antepartum death rate for normally formed singletons was similar in the two groups. Most of the stillborn babies were dead before the mother received medical attention whether formal fetal movement counting was employed or not. Therefore, formal fetal movement counting was not found to be helpful. **Ib A**

6 Arulkumaran S, Anandakumar C, Wong YC *et al.* (1989) Evaluation of maternal perception of sound-provoked fetal movement as a test of antenatal fetal health. *Obstet Gynecol* **73**, 182–186. Observational study of maternal perception of sound-provoked fetal movement in 1097 high-risk pregnancies, all beyond 28 weeks. 92% of women felt fetal movements with the stimulus and all but 3 had a reactive nonstress test (NST). Of the 88 women who did not feel fetal movements with the stimulus 10 had a nonreactive NST; the outcome in 9 of these 10 suggested fetal compromise. Maternal perception of sound-provoked fetal movements correlated well with the result of the NST, with a sensitivity of 76.9%, a specificity of 92.8% and a negative predictive value of 99.7%. However, the positive predictive value was only 11.4%. **III B**

7 Almstrom H, Granstrom L, Ekman G (1995) Serial antenatal monitoring compared with labor induction in post-term pregnancies. *Acta Obstet Gynecol Scand* **74**, 599–603. Prospective controlled study, without randomization, comparing induction of labor at 42 weeks gestation (205 cases) with serial monitoring (cardiotocogram and amniotic fluid volume assessment on three occasions over one week) until spontaneous labor, or induction at 43 weeks (193 cases). The frequency of labor induction was lower in the conservatively managed group but the two groups did not differ in obstetric or perinatal outcome. **III B**

8 Smith CV, Phelan JP, Platt LD *et al.* (1986) Fetal acoustic stimulation testing. II: A randomized clinical comparison with the nonstress test. *Am J Obstet Gynecol* **155**, 567–568. RCT of antenatal testing with a nonstress test (NST) or fetal acoustic stimulation test (FAST-test) in 715 high-risk pregnancies between 28 and 44 weeks gestation (307 were post-dates). The incidence of a nonreactive antenatal test was significantly reduced when the FAST-test was used as compared to the NST alone (9% vs 14%, $p = 0.004$). A significant reduction in testing time was also observed. **Ib A**

9 Alfirevic Z, Luckas M, Walkinshaw SA *et al.* (1997) A randomised comparison between amniotic fluid index and maximum pool depth in the monitoring of post-term pregnancy. *Br J Obstet Gynaecol* **104**, 207–211. Prospective RCT in 500 women with singleton, uncomplicated pregnancies with gestational age of 290 days or more, in which fetal monitoring by either amniotic fluid index (AFI) and computerized cardiotocography, or maximum pool depth and computerized cardiotocography were compared. The number of abnormal AFIs was significantly higher than the number of abnormal maximum pool depths (10% vs 2.4%; OR 4.51, 95% CI 1.82–11.21; $p = 0.0008$), which resulted in more inductions for abnormal postterm monitoring in the amniotic fluid index group (14.8% vs 8.4%; OR

1.89; 95% CI 1.07–3.33; $p = 0.0362$) and more intrapartum electronic fetal monitoring (94.4% vs 88.4%; OR 2.21; 95% CI 1.13–4.29; $p = 0.0255$). There were no other statistically significant differences in outcomes related to labor and delivery but there was a trend towards more cesarean sections in the AFI group (18.8% vs 13.2%), in particular cesarean sections for fetal distress (8% vs 4%). There were no perinatal deaths and no statistically significant differences in perinatal outcome between the two groups. The use of AFI, compared with maximum pool depth, is likely to increase the number of obstetric interventions with, as yet, an uncertain impact on perinatal mortality and morbidity. **Ib A**

10 Johnson JM, Harman CR, Lange IR *et al.* (1984) Biophysical profile scoring in the management of post-term pregnancy: an analysis of 307 patients. *Am J Obstet Gynecol* **154**, 269–273. Observational study of 307 pregnancies with a gestational age of 294 days or more, assessed with twice-weekly biophysical profiles (BPP). Fetuses monitored until either spontaneous labor, or until labor was induced when the cervix was favorable, had a low incidence of perinatal morbidity and a cesarean section rate (14.7%) similar to the overall hospital rate (16.5%). Fetuses delivered because of an abnormal BPP had a high rate of cesarean section (37.5%), low 5 min Apgar score (12.5%) and admission to special care for meconium aspiration (19%). If there was intervention despite a normal BPP when the cervix was unfavorable, there was a higher rate of cesarean section for fetal distress (14%) than in cases with a normal BPP when labor was spontaneous, or induced with a favorable cervix. Induction with an unfavorable cervix and normal BPP was also associated with a very high overall cesarean section rate (42%). **IIb B**

11 Clark SL, Sabey P, Jolley K (1989) Nonstress testing with acoustic stimulation and amniotic fluid volume assessment: 5973 tests without unexpected fetal death. *Am J Obstet Gynecol* **160**, 694–697. Observational study of antepartum monitoring in 2628 high-risk pregnancies between 28 and 44 weeks gestation, 279 of these pregnancies were post-dates. The study was carried out over a 3-year period and testing was performed once or twice weekly. The testing scheme involved a nonstress test (NST), with sound stimulation if accelerations did not occur in the first 5 min of the test, and amniotic fluid volume assessment. Only 2% of NSTs were nonreactive. 17% of nonreactive NSTs were followed by abnormal contraction stress tests or biophysical profiles. The overall intervention rate was 3%. There were no unexpected antepartum fetal deaths. **III B**

12 Arabin B, Becker R, Mohnhaupt A *et al.* (1994) Prediction of fetal distress and poor outcome in prolonged pregnancy using doppler ultrasound and fetal heart rate monitoring combined with stress tests (II). *Fetal Diagn Ther* **9**,1–6. Observational study of 110 pregnancies from 290 days gestation who were monitored with nonstress tests (NST), contraction stress tests (CST), vibroacoustic stimulation tests (VAST) and Doppler tests of the common carotid and umbilical arteries until either spontaneous labor or induction. Clinicians were blinded to the results of all the tests except the NST, which was performed twice daily. The rate of delivery for fetal distress was high, with a 21% operative vaginal delivery rate and 14% cesarean section rate. NSTs and fetal Doppler measurements were more predictive of later fetal distress than VAST and CST. There were very few low 5 min Apgar scores in this study, so predictive values for these tests could not be determined. NST was the only significant test for predicting low umbilical artery pH at delivery. **III B**

13 Hofmeyr GJ (2000) Amnioinfusion for umbilical cord compression in labour. (Cochrane Review). In: *The Cochrane library*, issue 2. Oxford: Update Software. This review assesses the effects of amnioinfusion on maternal and perinatal outcome for potential or suspected umbilical cord compression or potential amnionitis. 12 studies were included. Amnioinfusion for potential or suspected umbilical cord compression was associated with the following reductions: fetal heart rate decelerations (RR 0.54, 95% CI 0.43–0.68); cesarean section for suspected fetal distress (RR 0.35, 95% CI 0.24–0.52); neonatal hospital stay greater than 3 days (RR 0.40, 95% CI 0.26–0.62); maternal hospital stay greater than 3 days (RR 0.46, 95% 0.29–0.74). The studies were, however, carried out in settings where fetal distress was not confirmed by fetal blood sampling. The results may therefore only be relevant where cesarean sections are commonly done for abnormal fetal heart rate alone. The trials reviewed are too small to address the possibility of rare but serious maternal adverse effects of amnioinfusion. **Ia A**

14 Campbell MK, Ostbye T, Irgens LM *et al.* (1997) Post-term birth: risk factors and outcomes in a 10-year cohort of Norwegian births. *Obstet Gynecol* **89**, 543–548. 10-year cohort (1978–87) of term ($n = 379445$) and postterm ($n = 65796$) births from the Medical Birth Registry of Norway. Gestational age was based on mothers' recall of the last menstrual period. After controlling for covariates, there was only a slightly increased risk of perinatal mortality in postterm as compared with term births (adjusted RR 1.11; 95% CI 0.97–1.27). For postterm births, risk factors for perinatal mortality were small size for gestational age (SGA; adjusted RR 5.68; 95% CI 4.37–7.38) and maternal age 35 years or older (adjusted RR 1.88; 95% CI 1.22–2.89), whereas large size for gestational age (LGA) was a protective factor (adjusted RR 0.51; 95% CI 0.26–1.00). Similar risk factor RRs were found for perinatal mortality in term births. Fetal distress was associated with both SGA and postterm birth; labor dysfunction and obstetric trauma were associated with both LGA and postterm birth; shoulder dystocia and maternal hemorrhage were associated with LGA only. Thus maternal complications were generally associated with larger fetal size, and fetal complications were associated with smaller fetal size. The evidence for an adverse impact on perinatal mortality of postterm birth is weak once other factors are taken into account. **III B**

47.4 Induction of labor and termination for fetal abnormality

Jane Thomas

Management option		Quality of evidence	Strength of recommendation	References
Prenatal – induction, general	Women should be allowed to make an informed choice regarding their care	IV	C	1
	Bishop score is still the most reliable indicator of success of induction	IV	C	2
Prenatal – indications for induction	Women with uncomplicated pregnancy should be offered induction beyond 41 weeks	Ia	A	3
	Women with insulin-dependent diabetes should be offered induction before 40 weeks	IV	C	2
	Women with premature rupture of membranes at term should be offered choice of immediate induction or expectant management but this should not exceed 96 h	Ia	A	4,5
	There is no evidence that induction of labor for suspected fetal macrosomia not associated with diabetes will reduce any morbidity	Ib	A	6
	There is no evidence to advocate induction of labor with history of precipitate labor or for social reasons	IIa	B	2
	Indications should be such that mother or fetus will benefit from a higher probability of a healthy outcome than if birth is delayed	IV	C	2
	Vaginal delivery should be considered an appropriate mode of delivery	IV	C	3
	Validity of specific indication for induction of labor – see specific chapters			
Labor – methods	Sweeping and stretching membranes at term reduces the need for formal induction without increasing sepsis	Ia	A	7
	In women with intact membranes, vaginal prostaglandin $(PG)E_2$ is superior to oxytocin	Ia	A	4,5
	In women with ruptured membranes, oxytocin and prostaglandin are both effective, although PG is slightly more effective	Ia	A	4,5
	Although both routes are equally effective, intravaginal PGE_2 is preferable to intracervical as it is less invasive	Ia	A	7
	PG tablets 3 mg are equally effective as PG gel 1–2 mg 6-hourly but tablets offer financial savings	Ia	A	8

Management option		Quality of evidence	Strength of recommendation	References
Labor – methods (cont'd)	Oxytocin used in women with intact membranes should be used in combination with amniotomy	Ia	A	2
	Oxytocin should not be started for 6h following PG administration	IV	C	2
	Oxytocin starting dose is 1–2mU/min, increased at intervals of 30min	IV	C	2
	Misoprostol appears to be a cheap effective induction agent. Safety issues are probably related to dose or route and are being assessed	Ia	A	9,10
	Other methods such as mechanical methods, estrogens, relaxin, hyaluronidase, castor oil, bath and enema and breast stimulation have varying efficacy	IV	C	2
Labor – monitoring	Fetal wellbeing should be established prior to induction of labor	IV	C	2
	Following insertion of PG, fetal wellbeing should be established once contractions begin	IV	C	2
	When oxytocin is being used for induction continuous electronic monitoring should be used	IV	C	2
	If there is uterine hypercontractility tocolysis should be considered	Ia	A	11
Termination of pregnancy for fetal abnormality	200 mg mifepristone followed by PG 48h later, either vaginally or orally. This regimen may need to be supplemented by an oxytocin infusion	Ib	A	12
	Vaginal misoprostol seems to be very effective, followed by gemeprost or oral misoprostol	Ib	A	12,13
	Dilatation and evacuation has not been compared to contemporary methods of midtrimester medical abortion but in comparison to older medical methods it appears to be safer	III	B	14

References

1 Royal College of Obstetricians and Gynaecologists (2001) *Induction of labour*. Evidence-based Clinical Guideline no. 9. London: RCOG Press. A multiprofessional national evidence-based guideline commissioned by the Department of Health and the National Institute for Clinical Excellence. The guideline used strict methodology with precise clinical question setting and appraisal processes. Where no evidence was available, consensus methods were used. **IV C**

2 Edwards RK, Richards DS (2000) Preinduction cervical assessment. *Clin Obstet Gynecol* **43**, 440–446. Systems of quantifying and scoring cervical factors have been sought for years to predict the duration of labor and to determine which patients may successfully and safely undergo induction of labor. The scoring system that has become most prevalent is the Bishop score. This system and its modifications take into account the dilation, effacement, consistency and position of the cervix in addition to the station of the presenting part. Many have evaluated and confirmed the validity of the Bishop score. Among the factors considered in assigning the score, the strongest association with successful labor seems to be with cervical dilation. The Bishop score has been criticized for not attributing more significance to cervical dilation. However, despite this criticism, none of the modifications to the original scoring system have been shown to improve predictability. The Bishop score would seem to be the best and most cost-effective method currently available to assess the cervix and predict the likelihood of success of labor induction and the duration of such an induction. **IV C**

3 Crowley P (2001) Interventions for preventing or improving the outcome of delivery at or beyond term. In: *Cochrane database of systematic reviews*, issue 3. Oxford: Update Software. Cochrane review of 26 trials of variable quality, showing that routine early pregnancy ultrasound reduces the incidence of postterm pregnancy (OR 0.68, 95% CI 0.57–0.82). Routine induction of labor at 41 weeks reduced perinatal mortality (OR 0.20, 95% CI 0.06–0.70) without any effect on cesarean section. **Ia A**

4 Tan BP, Hannah ME (2001) Prostaglandins versus oxytocin for prelabour rupture of membranes at term. In: *Cochrane database of systematic reviews*, issue 3. Oxford: Update Software. Systematic review of eight RCTs. On the basis of three trials, prostaglandins compared to oxytocin were associated with increased chorioamnionitis (OR 1.51, 95% CI 1.07–2.12) and neonatal infections (OR 1.63, 95% CI 1.00–2.66). On the basis of four trials, prostaglandins were associated with a decrease in epidural analgesia (OR 0.86, 95% CI 0.73–1.00) and internal fetal heart rate monitoring (based on one trial). Cesarean section, endometritis and perinatal mortality were not significantly different between the groups. **Ia A**

5 Tan BP, Hannah ME (2001) Prostaglandins for prelabour rupture of membranes at or near term. In: *Cochrane database of systematic reviews*, issue 3. Oxford: Update Software. Review of 15 trials of moderate to good quality. Induction of labor by prostaglandins was associated with a decreased risk of chorioamnionitis (OR 0.77, 95% CI 0.61–0.97), based on eight trials, and admission to neonatal intensive care (OR 0.79, 95% CI 0.66–0.94), based on seven trials. No difference was detected for rate of cesarean section, although induction by prostaglandins was associated with more frequent maternal diarrhea and use of anesthesia and/or analgesia. From the results of one trial, women were more likely to view their care positively if labor was induced with prostaglandins. **Ia A**

6 Irion O, Boulvain M (2001) Induction of labour for suspected fetal macrosomia (Cochrane Review). In: *The Cochrane library*, issue 3. Oxford, Update Software. This review of two trials including 313 women showed that, compared with expectant management, induction of labor for suspected macrosomia did not reduce the risk of cesarean section or instrumental delivery. Perinatal morbidity was similar between groups. **Ib A**

7 Bolivian M, Kelly A, Loose C *et al.* (2001) Membrane sweeping for induction of labour (Cochrane Review). In: *The Cochrane library*, issue 3. Oxford, Update Software. Cochrane review assessing a standardized methodology of sweeping of the membranes, also commonly called stripping of the membranes, usually performed without admission to hospital. This intervention has the potential to initiate labor by increasing local production of prostaglandins and thus to reduce pregnancy duration or preempt formal induction of labor with oxytocin, prostaglandins or amniotomy. 19 trials were included, 17 comparing sweeping of membranes with no treatment, three comparing sweeping with prostaglandins and one comparing sweeping with oxytocin (two studies reported more than one comparison). Risk of cesarean section was similar between groups (RR 0.97, 95% CI 0.73–1.28). Sweeping of the membranes, performed as a general policy in women at term, was associated with reduced duration of pregnancy and reduced frequency of pregnancy continuing beyond 41 weeks (RR 0.62, 95% CI 0.49–0.79) and 42 weeks (RR 0.28, 95% CI 0.15–0.50). There was no evidence of a difference in the risk of maternal or neonatal infection. Discomfort during vaginal examination and other adverse effects (bleeding, irregular contractions) were more frequently reported by women allocated to sweeping. **Ia A**

8 Kelly AJ, Kavanagh J, Thomas J (2001) Vaginal prostaglandin (PGE_2 and $PGF_{2\alpha}$) for induction of labour at term. In: *Cochrane database of systematic reviews*, issue 3. Oxford: Update Software. Systematic review of 94 studies; 42 were excluded and 52 examined a total of 9402 women. Vaginal prostaglandin $(PG)E_2$ compared with placebo or no treatment reduced the likelihood of vaginal delivery not being achieved within 24h (18% vs 99%, RR 0.19, 95% CI 0.14–0.25); the cesarean section rates were not different between groups although the risk of uterine hyperstimulation with fetal heart rate changes was increased (4.6% vs 0.51%, RR 4.14, 95% CI 1.93–8.90). Comparison of vaginal $PGF_{2\alpha}$ with placebo showed no increase in cesarean section rates but the cervical score was more likely to be improved (15% vs 60%, RR 0.25, 95% CI 0.13–0.49), and the risk of oxytocin augmentation reduced (53.9% vs 89.1%, RR 0.60, 95% CI 0.43–0.84) with the use of vaginal $PGF_{2\alpha}$. Vaginal PGE_2 tablets increased successful vaginal delivery rates in 24h; no increase in operative delivery rates and significant improvements in cervical favorability within 24–48h. **Ia A**

9 Hofmeyr GJ, Gulmezoglu AM (2001) Vaginal misoprostol for cervical ripening and induction of labour. In: *Cochrane database of systematic reviews*, issue 3. Oxford: Update Software. Compared to placebo, misoprostol was associated with increased cervical ripening (RR of unfavorable or unchanged cervix after 12–24h with misoprostol 0.09, 95% CI 0.03–0.24). It was also associated with a reduced need for oxytocin (RR 0.52, 95% CI 0.41–0.68). Misoprostol was more effective than prostaglandin $(PG)E_2$ vaginally for labor induction (RR of failure to achieve vaginal delivery in 24h 0.70, 95% CI 0.61–0.81). Oxytocin augmentation was used less often with misoprostol than with PGE_2 vaginally (RR 0.65, 95% CI 0.60–0.71). Uterine hyperstimulation and meconium-stained liquor were more common with misoprostol than with PGE_2. Lower doses of misoprostol compared to higher doses did not show significant differences except for more need for oxytocin augmentation and less uterine hyperstimulation without fetal heart rate changes. Information on women's views is conspicuously lacking. **Ia A**

10 Alfirevic Z (2001) Oral misoprostol for induction of labour. In: *Cochrane database of systematic reviews*, issue 3. Oxford: Update Software. One trial with 80 randomized women with prelabor rupture of membranes at term showed that, compared with placebo, oral misoprostol reduces the need for oxytocin infusion from 51% to 13% (RR 0.25, 95% CI 0.1–0.6) and shortens delivery time by 8.7h (95% CI 6.0–11.3). Compared with vaginal or intracervical prostaglandins, oral misoprostol showed no beneficial or harmful effects. However, only two trials with 962 randomized women in total compared oral misoprostol with vaginal dinoprostone and one trial with 200 women compared oral misoprostol with intracervical dinoprostone. Two small trials with 188 women in total compared oral misoprostol and oxytocin in women with term-ruptured membranes and found no significant differences in prespecified outcomes. In seven trials with 1278 randomized women that compared oral with vaginal misoprostol, oral misoprostol appeared to be less effective. More women in the oral misoprostol group did not achieve vaginal delivery within 24h of randomization (50%) compared with 39.7% in the vaginal misoprostol group (RR 1.27, 95% CI 1.09–1.47). The cesarean section rate was lower in the oral misoprostol group (16.7%) compared with 21.7% in the vaginal misoprostol group (RR 0.77, 95% CI 0.61–0.97). There was no difference in uterine hyperstimulation with fetal heart rate changes (8.5% vs 7.4%; RR 1.11, 95% CI 0.78–1.59). There were no reported cases of severe neonatal and maternal morbidity. **Ia A**

11 Kulier R, Hofmeyr GJ (2001) Tocolytics for suspected intrapartum fetal distress. In: *Cochrane database of systematic reviews*, issue 3. Oxford: Update Software. Three studies were included. Compared with no treatment, there were fewer failed improvements in fetal heart rate abnormalities with tocolytic therapy (RR 0.26, 95% 0.13–0.53). Beta-mimetic therapy compared with magnesium sulfate showed a nonsignificant trend towards reduced uterine activity (RR 0.07, 95% CI 0.00–1.10). **Ia A**

12 Rodger MW, Baird DT (1990) Pretreatment with mifepristone (RU 486) reduces interval between prostaglandin administration and expulsion in second trimester abortion. *Br J Obstet Gynaecol* **97**, 41–45. The effect of pretreatment with mifepristone on prostaglandin-induced abortion was investigated in a double-blind randomized trial involving 100 women in the second trimester of pregnancy. The women were randomly allocated to receive either 600mg oral mifepristone or placebo tablets 36h before the administration of gemeprost pessaries. The median interval between administration of prostaglandin and abortion was significantly shorter in the mifepristone group (6.8h) compared with the placebo group (15.8h). The women pretreated with mifepristone required significantly fewer gemeprost pessaries to induce abortion and experienced significantly less pain than the women who had received placebo. **Ib A**

13 Frydman R, Fernandez H, Pons JC *et al.* (1988) Mifepristone (RU486) and therapeutic late pregnancy termination: a double-blind study of two different doses. *Hum Reprod* **3**, 803–806. An antiprogesterone, mifepristone (RU486), was administered to 35 patients undergoing a therapeutic interruption of pregnancy during the second and third trimester for maternal or fetal indications. A randomized double-blind study test was performed using 150 and 450mg of mifepristone as pretreatment prior to prostaglandins. No toxicity or maternal morbidity were recorded. In 3 patients the onset of labor occurred spontaneously before prostaglandin administration. Mifepristone produced a modification in the consistency of the cervix with a statistical improvement in cervical calibration in the two groups, but the cervical effect was independent of the dose. **Ib A**

14 Peterson WF, Berry FN, Grace MR *et al.* (1983) Second-trimester abortion by dilatation and evacuation: an analysis of 11,747 cases. *Obstet Gynecol* **62**, 185–190. The dilatation and evacuation procedure was explored in 1971 as an alternative method of second-trimester abortion. The results in 11747 cases from 1972–81 are presented. Although complications did occur – most notably hemorrhage, cervical laceration, fever and perforation – the overall complication rate was lower than that reported for saline or prostaglandin in other large series. Further study and refinement of technique may help bring this shorter, safer and more convenient procedure within the reach of larger numbers of women seeking second-trimester abortion. **III B**

47.5 Poor progress in labor

Harry Gee

Poor progress in labor

Management option		Quality of evidence	Strength of recommendation	References
Conduct of normal labor	Use of partogram helps to detect abnormality of labor and poor progress early and thus allow timely intervention	III	B	1
	Use of partogram with an agreed protocol for management improves maternal morbidity and fetal morbidity and mortality	IIb	B	2

Management option		Quality of evidence	Strength of recommendation	References
Conduct of normal labor (cont'd)	The package of precise diagnosis of labor (active phase), early amniotomy, regular monitoring of cervical dilatation rate and correction with the empirical augmentation of uterine activity reduces the incidence of prolonged labor	III	B	3
	Compared to active management, a policy of no routine amniotomy and selective use of oxytocin does not adversely affect cesarean section rate or neonatal outcome	Ib Ia	A A	4,5 6
	Social support in labor reduces operative delivery rate	Ia	A	7
Poor progress in latent phase of first stage	Expectant management with careful watch of the fetal heart rate	–	✔	–
	Augmentation may increase cesarean section rate	–	✔	–
Poor progress in active phase of first stage	Allowing 2h of grace after crossing alert line reduces need for augmentation	III	B	8
	Judicious augmentation with oxytocin will reduce labor duration	Ib	A	4
	Studies favor 30min incremental intervals with oxytocin	Ib	A	9,10
	Obstetric outcome for most cases is no better with use of intrauterine pressure catheters compared with external tocography	Ib	A	11
	Epidural analgesia is associated with prolongation of the first and second stages of labor, malposition and increased operative vaginal delivery	Ia	A	12
Poor progress in the second stage of labor	Flexibility in the duration of the second stage is permissible	–	✔	–
	Upright posture of the mother reduces the duration of the second stage and operative delivery. There are also reductions in performance of episiotomy, perception of pain and fetal heart rate abnormalities	Ia	A	13
	Use of episiotomy should be limited and selective	Ia	A	14

References

1 Phillpott RH, Castle WM (1972) Cervicographs in the management of labour in primigravidae. II. The action line and treatment of abnormal labour. *J Obstet Gynaecol Br Commonw* **79**, 599–602. Descriptive, uncontrolled, prospective study documenting the value of a cervicogram to determine delivery. It took place in an appropriate setting in a Third World health system. 624 primigravid patients were reported. The cervicogram consisted of an Alert Line with a rate of active cervical dilatation set at 1 cm/h followed by an Action Line 4 h later. 22% women crossed the Alert Line. 50% of these delivered normally. Thus, 11% of the total experienced complications requiring intervention. **III B**

2 Anonymous (1994) World Health Organization partograph in management of labour. *Lancet* **343**, 1399–1404. Multicenter, multinational program to explore the benefits of using a standardized policy for managing labor. Precise definition of when to apply cervicography (active phase of labor), use of a standard partogram to monitor labor and a standard augmentation regimen. The incidence of prolonged labor was reduced and oxytocin augmentation was used less frequently. These features are almost certainly due to correct and consistent identification of the active phase at a later time than had formerly been the case. A slight but statistically significant improvement in spontaneous vaginal delivery was seen but cesarean section rates were not statistically different. **IIb B**

3 O'Driscoll K, Jackson RJ, Gallagher JT (1969) Prevention of prolonged labour. *Br Med J* **2**, 477–480. Report of a package of labor management employed prospectively in a cohort of 1000 nulliparous women at the National Maternity Hospital, Dublin. The package was applied only to spontaneous labor and was uncontrolled. The cohort included 10 cases of multiple pregnancy. If cervical dilatation was not progressive, amniotomy was performed and, if this failed, oxytocin was infused. There had to be a 'show', rupture of the membranes or evidence of cervical dilatation in addition to contractions to permit a diagnosis of labor. The aim of the study was to limit the duration of labor, not to influence operative intervention. The authors also wished to dispel three fallacies: that disproportion is a significant cause for delay in progress in labor; that oxytocin may rupture the primigravid uterus; that there is valid reason to differentiate between hypo- and hypertonic uterine activity. Only one labor lasted more than 24 h. Oxytocin was used in 55% of labors. The cesarean section rate was 4% and the operative vaginal delivery rate 18.9%. 3/1010 babies died in labor, 4 in the neonatal period and 4 babies were considered to have central nervous system damage. Not all of these complications were associated with oxytocin. The authors considered that their aims were achieved. **III B**

4 Frigoletto FD Jr, Lieberman E, Lang JM *et al.* (1995) A clinical trial of active management of labor. *N Engl J Med* **333**, 745–750. RCT of active management of labor in nulliparous women without medical or obstetric complications – perhaps the definitive one. Good design and adequate power. Attention was paid in active management to preparation of the patient and one-to-one care, diagnosis of labor (contractions and show, rupture of the membranes or 80% effacement of the cervix), amniotomy within 1 h of the diagnosis of labor and oxytocin augmentation if progress less than 1 cm/h. Analysis was on an 'intention to treat' basis. 3028 patients were eligible and 1934 agreed to participate – 1017 in the actively managed arm and 917 controls (care according to attendant clinician's wish). Both groups had similar clinical characteristics. Delivery and outcomes were similar in both, although labor was shorter in active management groups. Only postnatal pyrexia was less frequent in association with active management. **Ib A**

5 Cammu H, Van Eeckhout E (1996) A randomised controlled trial of early versus delayed use of amniotomy and oxytocin infusion in nulliparous labour. *Br J Obstet Gynaecol* **103**, 313–318. Small, prospective RCT. The originality of this study lies in the fact that the investigators were concerned about the high usage of oxytocin following the introduction of active management to their practice in 1986. Only uncomplicated nulliparous labors were included. Attention was paid to the diagnosis of labor. Randomization was by sealed envelope. Active management consisted of amniotomy within 1 h of admission in labor, or on evidence of delay (< 1 cm/h cervical dilatation). Oxytocin was used if progress less than 1 cm/h cervical dilatation with ruptured membranes. This was the control arm of the study. The 'study' group did not have routine amniotomy. Amniotomy was only performed on total cessation of progress. Oxytocin was used only when progress fell more than 2 h behind 0.5 cm/h cervical dilatation rate prior to 4 cm dilatation and 1 cm/h dilatation rate after 4 cm dilatation. All had one-to-one care and epidural on demand. Sample size was calculated on the assumption that cesarean section rates would be the same in both arms but that augmentation would fall by 25%. 298 women would have to be recruited to achieve a 95% significance at a power of 80%. 306 women were randomized and both groups were comparable. Oxytocin was used twice as often under active management (53% vs 27%) without significant shortening of labor. Surgical interventions were similar. **Ib A**

6 Fraser WD, Turcot L, Krauss I *et al.* (2002) Amniotomy for shortening spontaneous labour (Cochrane Review). In: *The Cochrane library*, issue 1. Oxford: Update Software. Meta-analysis of good quality. Tests of homogeneity were satisfactory with the exception of oxytocin usage. Early amniotomy reduces the duration of the first stage of labor by between 60 and 120 min. This represents a reduction of between 7% and 40%. There was no reduction in the length of the second stage. These effects were unaffected by parity. Early amniotomy did not affect heart rate but there was a trend towards increased cesarean section, although this did not reach statistical significance. The proportion of cesarean sections attributed to fetal distress was greater in the early amniotomy group. Of the neonatal outcomes, only 5 min Apgar score less than 7 showed a statistically significant difference in favor of early amniotomy, all others being nonsignificant. **Ia A**

7 Hodnett ED (2001) Caregiver support for women during childbirth. In: *Cochrane database of systematic reviews*, issue 3. Oxford: Update Software. 14 trials, involving more than 5000 women, are included in the review. The continuous presence of a support person reduced the likelihood of medication for pain relief, operative vaginal delivery, cesarean delivery and a 5 min Apgar score less than 7. Continuous support was also associated with a slight reduction in the length of labor. Six trials evaluated the effects of support on mothers' views of their childbirth experiences; while the trials used different measures (overall satisfaction, failure to cope well during labor, finding labor to be worse than expected, and level of personal control during childbirth), in each trial the results favored the group that had received continuous support. **Ia A**

8 Arulkumaran S, Koh CH, Ingemarsson I *et al.* (1987) Augmentation of labour-mode of delivery related to cervimetric progress. *Aust N Z J Obstet Gynaecol* **7**, 304–308 Study designed to investigate the possible benefits, in terms of obstetric and neonatal outcome, of a prolonged augmentation period with oxytocin in patients with dysfunctional first stage of labor. The majority of patients (65.5% of nulliparas and 83.8% of multiparas) responded with satisfactory progress within the first 4 h of augmentation and the cesarean section rate was low in this group (1.3%). In those with unsatisfactory progress during the first 4 h of augmentation a further 4 h period of augmentation resulted in vaginal delivery for 50.7% of nulliparas with primary dysfunctional labor and 33.3% of those with secondary arrest in labor. Corresponding figures for multiparas were 41.7% and 25.0% respectively. The neonatal outcome was uniformly good. It is concluded that the management protocol presented for augmentation of labor seems to be a safe procedure and might reduce the rising cesarean section rate for dystocia. **III B**

9 Blakemore KJ, Qin NG, Petrie RH *et al.* (1990) A prospective comparison of hourly and quarter-hourly oxytocin dose increase intervals for the induction of labor at term. *Obstet Gynecol* **75**, 757–761. RCT in 52 women (16 multiparas and 10 nulliparas in each arm) undergoing induction of labor using intravenous oxytocin to compare 15 min vs 60 min increments. The method of randomization is poorly specified and the power calculations appear to have been performed in retrospect. These numbers would have required a 55% difference in clinical parameters to achieved statistical significance at 0.05 level with a confidence of 80%. Statistically significant differences were not reached by any clinical parameter (duration of any stage of labor, uterine activity, perinatal outcome and operative intervention) nor for total oxytocin use. However, average dosages for the first and second stages, maximum dosage and final maintenance dose of oxytocin were lower in the 60 min incremental group. **Ib A**

10 Chua S, Arulkumaran S, Kurup A *et al.* (1991) Does prostaglandin confer significant advantage over oxytocin infusion for nulliparas with pre-labor rupture of membranes at term? *Aust N Z J Obstet Gynaecol* **31**, 134–137. Prospective RCT comparing 15 min and 30 min incremental intervals for oxytocin titration against uterine activity for the induction of labor in 224 women. The two groups were comparable for clinical features following randomization. Differences in duration of labor, oxytocin dosages, medical interventions and clinical outcomes did not reach statistical significance. **Ib A**

11 Chua S, Kurup A, Arulkumaran S *et al.* (1990) Augmentation of labor: does internal tocography result in better obstetric outcome than external tocography? *Obstet Gynecol* **76**, 164–167. Prospective RCT compares external guard ring tocodynamometry with intrauterine pressure measurement to judge uterine activity in augmented labor. 250 patients at term with a vertex presentation and progressing 2 h behind a 1 cm/h action line were given a standard intervenous oxytocin titration regimen and randomized (method not specified) to achieve 6–7 painful contractions per 15 min as judged by midwife and guard ring tocodynamometer or adequate uterine activity as computed from intrauterine pressure monitoring (Sonicaid Ltd, Chichester, UK). The two groups were comparable regarding clinical characteristics. No differences were found in oxytocin dosage, duration of labor after augmentation, operative intervention or neonatal outcome. **Ib A**

12 Howell CJ (2000) Epidural versus non-epidural analgesia for pain relief in labour (Cochrane Review). In: *The Cochrane library*, issue 4. Oxford: Update Software. Systematic review of the effects of conventional epidural analgesia on labor compared with other forms of pain relief. 11 studies are included with a total of 3157 women (nulliparas and multiparas). Medical and obstetric complications were excluded. In five studies, the method of randomization was unclear. Epidurals give better pain relief but give rise to longer first and second stages of labor. There was no increase in cesarean section rate but malposition, use of oxytocin and instrumental vaginal delivery were all increased. The effects on the fetus and neonate were inconsistent. Observational data suggest increased maternal backache, headaches and bladder problems. **Ia A**

13 Gupta JK, Nikodem VC (2001) Woman's position during second stage of labour. In: *Cochrane database of systematic reviews*, issue 3. Oxford: Update Software. Review of 18 trials of variable quality with heterogeneity; therefore, caution should be taken in interpreting results. Positions were categorized into neutral (lateral, lithotomy, Trendelenburg or knee–elbow) or upright (sitting, semirecumbent, kneeling or squatting). Upright posture reduced the duration of the second stage (5.4 min 95% CI 3.9–6.9 min), reduced operative deliveries (OR 0.82, 95% CI 0.69–0.98), reduced episiotomy (OR 0.73, 95% CI 0.64–0.84), increased second-degree tears (OR 1.30, 95% CI 1.09–1.54), increased estimated blood loss less than 500 ml (OR 1.76, 95% CI 1.34–3.32), reduced perception of pain (OR 0.59, 95% CI 0.41–0.83) and reduced fetal heart rate abnormalities (OR 0.31, 95% CI 0.11–0.91). No significant differences were found for analgesia requirements, cesarean section, third- or fourth-degree tears, need for blood transfusion, manual removal of the placenta, unpleasant experience, dissatisfaction with conduct of the second stage, persistent occiput posterior position, admission to neonatal intensive care, birth injury and perinatal death. **Ia A**

14 Carroli G, Belizan J (2001) Episiotomy for vaginal birth. In: *Cochrane database of systematic reviews*, issue 3. Oxford: Update Software. Review of six clinical trials of good quality, the aim being to compare the clinical benefit of routine episiotomy (73% incidence) with restrictive use (28%). Restrictive use reduces the risk of posterior perineal trauma (RR 0.88, 95% CI 0.84–0.92), need for perineal suturing (RR 0.74, 95% CI 0.71–0.77), healing complications at 7 days (RR 0.69, 95% CI 0.56–0.85). There was no difference in perineal pain, dyspareunia nor urinary incontinence. The only disadvantage to restrictive use is an increase in anterior perineal trauma (RR 1.79, 95% CI 1.55–2.07). **Ia A**

Malposition and malpresentations

Management option		Quality of evidence	Strength of recommendation	References
Malposition	Maternal posture does not appear to affect malposition	Ib	A	1
	Augmentation is acceptable for poor progress in first stage	Ib	A	2,3
	Assisted delivery with the vacuum extractor results in less perineal trauma for the mother	Ia	A	4
	Assisted delivery may be required	–	✔	–
	Manual correction of malposition is a safe alternative to instrumental correction	III	B	5
Brow presentation	If early in first stage – may observe to see if it converts into flexed vertex	–	✔	–
	If in established labor cesarean section safest option unless preterm	–	✔	–
Face presentation	If mentoanterior, vaginal delivery likely	–	✔	–
	Mentoposterior usually requires cesarean section	–	✔	–

References

1 Hofmeyr GJ, Kulier R (2001) Hands/knees posture in late pregnancy or labour for fetal malposition. In: *Cochrane database of systematic reviews*, issue 3. Oxford: Update Software. Review of one paper only and this of poor quality. The paper is a trial of 100 patients randomized to five arms: four different variations of the hands and knees position and one control (sitting) with 20 patients in each arm. The method of randomization is not specified. Estimation of the fetal position is by palpation. Lateral or posterior position of the presenting part was less likely to persist after 10 min in the hands and knees posture compared to sitting (RR 0.25, 95% CI 0.17–0.37). **Ib A**

2 Frigoletto FD Jr, Lieberman E, Lang JM *et al.* (1995) A clinical trial of active management of labor. *N Engl J Med* **333**, 745–750. RCT of active management of labor in nulliparous women without medical or obstetric complications – perhaps the definitive one. Good design and adequate power. Attention was paid in active management to preparation of the patient and one-to-one care, diagnosis of labor (contractions and show, rupture of the membranes or 80% effacement of the cervix), amniotomy within 1 h of the diagnosis of labor and oxytocin augmentation if progress less than 1 cm/h. Analysis was on an 'intention to treat' basis. 3028 patients were eligible and 1934 agreed to participate – 1017 in the actively managed arm and 917 controls (care according to attendant clinician's wish). Both groups had similar clinical characteristics. Delivery and outcomes were similar in both, although labor was shorter in active management groups. Only postnatal pyrexia was less frequent in association with active management. **Ib A**

3 Cammu H, Van Eeckhout E (1996) A randomised controlled trial of early versus delayed use of amniotomy and oxytocin infusion in nulliparous labour. *Br J Obstet Gynaecol* **103**, 313–318. Small, prospective RCT. The originality of this study lies in the fact that the investigators were concerned about the high usage of oxytocin following the introduction of active management to their practice in 1986. Only uncomplicated nulliparous labors were included. Attention was paid to the diagnosis of labor. Randomization was by sealed envelope. Active management consisted of amniotomy within 1 h of admission in labor, or on evidence of delay (< 1 cm/h cervical dilatation). Oxytocin was used if progress less than 1 cm/h cervical dilatation with ruptured membranes. This was the control arm of the study. The 'study' group did not have routine amniotomy. Amniotomy was only performed on total cessation of progress. Oxytocin was used only when progress fell more than 2 h behind 0.5 cm/h cervical dilatation rate prior to 4 cm dilatation and 1 cm/h dilatation rate after 4 cm dilatation. All had one-to-one care and epidural on demand. Sample size was calculated on the assumption that cesarean section rates would be the same in both arms but that augmentation would fall by 25%. 298 women would have to be recruited to achieve a 95% significance at a power of 80%. 306 women were randomized and both groups were comparable. Oxytocin was used twice as often under active management (53% vs 27%) without significant shortening of labor. Surgical interventions were similar. **Ib A**

4 Johanson RB, Menon BKV (2001) Vacuum extraction versus forceps for assisted vaginal delivery. In: *The Cochrane library*, issue 3. Oxford: Update Software. Systematic review and meta-analysis of 10 trials comparing

vacuum extraction with forceps for assisted vaginal delivery. Studies included nulliparas and multiparas. There was less maternal perineal trauma with vacuum extraction (OR 0.41, 95% CI 0.33–0.50). The vacuum extractor was, however, associated with increased cephalhematoma and retinal hemorrhages in the neonate. Serious injury with either instrument was rare and there was no evidence to suggest long-term sequelae. A higher incidence of failure was seen with the vacuum extractor but cesarean section rates were no different between the two methods. **Ia A**

5 Jain V, Guleria K, Gopalan S *et al.* (1993) Mode of delivery in deep transverse arrest. *Int J Gynaecol Obstet* **43**, 129–135. Review of the changing practice regarding method delivery for 'deep transverse arrest' in the years 1970, 1980 and 1990. In 1970 44% employed Kjelland's forceps, 44% manual rotation, virtually none vacuum and 10% cesarean section. In 1980 these modes of delivery had become 18% Kjelland's, 63% manual, 8% vacuum and 10% cesarean and by 1990, no Kjelland's, 31% manual, 27% vacuum and 42% cesarean section. Thus Kjelland's forceps are falling out of grace because of perceived risk. The requirement for skill in their use and, perhaps, in the use of manual rotation may also be contributory to these changes. The rising cesarean section rate does not appear to confer any gain in perinatal outcome. **III B**

47.6 Fetal distress in labor

Tony Kelly

Electronic fetal heart rate monitoring

Management option		Quality of evidence	Strength of recommendation	References
Care of women	Women must be able to make informed choices regarding their care or treatment via access to evidence-based information. These choices should be recognized as an integral part of the decision-making process	IV	C	1
	Women should have the same level of care and support regardless of the mode of intrapartum fetal monitoring (Reference is a systematic review but this recommendation was an indirect conclusion)	IV (Ia)	C (A)	2 2
Appropriate monitoring in an uncomplicated pregnancy	For a woman who is healthy and has had an otherwise uncomplicated pregnancy, intermittent auscultation (IA) should be offered and recommended in labor to monitor fetal wellbeing	Ia	A	3
	In the active stages of labor, IA should occur after a contraction, for a minimum of 60 s, and at least: ❑ Every 15 min in the first stage ❑ Every 5 min in second stage	Ia	A	3
	Continuous EFM should be offered and recommended in pregnancies previously monitored with intermittent auscultation: ❑ If there is evidence on auscultation of a baseline less than 110 or greater than 160 bpm ❑ If there is evidence on auscultation of any decelerations ❑ If any intrapartum risk factors develop	Ia	A	3
	Current evidence does not support the use of the admission cardiotocogram in low-risk pregnancy and it is therefore not recommended	Ib IIa	A B	4 5

➡

Management option		Quality of evidence	Strength of recommendation	References
Indications for the use of continuous EFM	Should be offered and recommended for high-risk pregnancies where there is an increased risk of perinatal death, cerebral palsy or neonatal encephalopathy Examples include: ❑ Maternal problems: – Previous cesarean section – Preeclampsia – Postterm pregnancy – Prolonged membrane rupture – Induced labor – Diabetes ❑ Fetal problems: – Fetal growth restriction – Prematurity – Oligohydramnios – Abnormal Doppler artery velocimetry – Multiple pregnancies – Meconium-stained liquor – Breech presentation	IIa	B	6
	Should be used where oxytocin is used for induction or augmentation of labor	IV	C	7
Interpretation	A grading system for fetal heart rate (FHR) patterns is recommended. This incorporates both the proposed definitions of FHR patterns and categorization schemes	IV	C	1

Categorization of fetal heart rate traces

Category	Definition
Normal	A cardiotocogram (CTG) where *all four* features fall into the reassuring category
Suspicious	A CTG whose features fall into one of the nonreassuring categories and the remainder of the features are reassuring
Pathological	A CTG whose features fall into two or more nonreassuring categories or one or more abnormal categories

Categorization of fetal heart rate features

Feature	Baseline (bpm)	Variability (bpm)	Decelerations	Accelerations
Reassuring	110–160	≥5	None	Present
Nonreassuring	100–109 161–180	<5 for >40 to <90 min	Early deceleration Variable deceleration Single prolonged deceleration up to 3 min	The absence of accelerations with an otherwise normal cardiotocogram is of uncertain significance
Abnormal	<100 >180 Sinusoidal pattern ≥10 min	<5 for ≥90 min	Atypical variable decelerations Late decelerations Single prolonged deceleration >3 min	

- ❑ In cases where the cardiotocogram falls into the suspicious category, conservative measures should be used (e.g. left lateral position, stopping oxytocic infusion)
- ❑ In cases where the cardiotocogram falls into the pathological category, conservative measures should be used and fetal blood sampling should be undertaken where appropriate/feasible. In situations where fetal blood sampling is not possible or appropriate, delivery should be expedited

References

1 Royal College of Obstetricians and Gynaecologists (2001) *The use of electronic fetal monitoring*. Evidence-based Clinical Guideline no. 8. London: RCOG Press. A multiprofessional national evidence-based guideline commissioned by the Department of Health and the National Institute for Clinical Excellence. The guideline used strict methodology with precise clinical question setting and appraisal processes. Where no evidence was available, consensus methods were used. **IV C**

2 Hodnett ED (2001) Caregiver support for women during childbirth. In: *The Cochrane library*, issue 3. Oxford, Update Software. Systematic review of 14 trials involving more than 5000 women. The continuous presence of a support person reduced the likelihood of medication for pain relief, operative vaginal delivery, cesarean delivery and a 5 min Apgar score less than 7. Continuous support was also associated with a slight reduction in the length of labor. Six trials evaluated the effects of support on mothers' views of their childbirth experiences; while the trials used different measures (overall satisfaction, failure to cope well during labor, finding labor to be worse than expected and level of personal control during childbirth), in each trial the results favored the group who had received continuous support. This review provided indirect evidence for providing the same level of care regardless of mode of monitoring. **Ia A**

3 Thacker SB, Stroup DF (2001) Continuous electronic heart rate monitoring versus intermittent auscultation for assessment during labor. In: *The Cochrane library*, issue 3. Oxford, Update Software. Systematic review of nine randomized controlled trials comparing the use of continuous electronic fetal monitoring with intermittent auscultation. Mixture of low- and high-risk labor monitored. Use of intermittent auscultation generally consistent across studies, definitions of normal and abnormal for use of electronic monitoring not as consistent. Overall no significant difference between continuous electronic monitoring and intermittent auscultation with respect to Apgar scores or perinatal mortality, although studies underpowered to detect differences in either of these. Significant reduction in neonatal seizures seen (OR 0.50, 95% CI 0.31–0.80), increase in operative delivery rates seen, both for instrumental delivery and cesarean section (lower segment cesarean section: OR 1.44, 95% CI 1.24–1.66, instrumental: OR 1.25, 95% CI 1.13–1.37). All outcomes were divided according to whether fetal blood sampling used or not. Increase in operative delivery was more marked if fetal blood sampling was not used. Two follow-up studies were included to look at outcome in relation to cerebral palsy, and no significant difference was seen between the two monitoring modalities. **Ia A**

4 Mires G, Williams F, Howie P (2001) Randomised controlled trial of cardiotocography versus Doppler auscultation of fetal heart at admission in labour in low risk obstetric population. *Br Med J* **322**, 1457–1460. RCT comparing use of cardiotocography or Doppler auscultation from admission on 3751 women admitted in spontaneous labor. The primary outcome was metabolic acidosis and no significant difference was seen. Those women who received admission cardiotocography were more likely to receive continuous electronic fetal monitoring in labor (OR 1.49, 95% CI 1.26–1.76), and require augmentation of labor (OR 1.26, 95% CI 1.02–1.56), epidural analgesia (OR 1.33, 95% CI 1.10–1.61) and operative delivery (OR 1.36, 95% CI 1.12–1.65). **Ib A**

5 Ingemarsson I, Arulkumaran S, Ingemarsson E *et al.* (1986) Admission test: a screening test for fetal distress in labor. *Obstet Gynecol* **68**, 800–806. This was a two cohort study: 130 with normal/abnormal admission tests related to acidemia; 1041 with normal/abnormal admission traces related to fetal distress. Both cohorts were classified as low-risk. Detailed classification of normal and abnormal, related to umbilical artery pH, with a cut-off of less than 7.15. The admission trace was able to identify 5% of the population at risk of increased operative delivery but was poorly predictive of acidosis. There was a significant reduced risk of cesarean section with a normal/reactive test. Results in larger proportion of women requiring continuous monitoring. **IIa B**

6 Nelson KB, Ellenberg JH (1984) Obstetric complications as risk factors for cerebral palsy or seizure disorders. *JAMA* **251**, 1843–1848. Cohort of 51 285 pregnancies examining outcome in relation to cerebral palsy and neonatal encephalopathy. Overall cerebral palsy rate 2%, no association with intrapartum care complications. No association with neonatal seizures. Association with a number of antenatal factors, especially in babies less than 2500 g. **IIa B**

7 Royal College of Obstetricians and Gynaecologists (2001) *Induction of labour*. Evidence-based Clinical Guideline no. 9. London: RCOG Press. A multiprofessional national evidence-based guideline commissioned by the Department of Health and the National Institute for Clinical Excellence. The guideline used strict methodology with precise clinical question setting and appraisal processes. Where no evidence was available, consensus methods were used. **IV C**

Additional tests and therapies used in combination with electronic fetal heart rate monitoring

Management option	Quality of evidence	Strength of recommendation	References
Units employing electronic fetal heart rate monitoring (EFM) should have ready access to fetal blood sampling (FBS) facilities	Ia	A	1

Management option	Quality of evidence	Strength of recommendation	References
Where delivery is contemplated because of an abnormal fetal heart-rate pattern and suspected fetal acidosis, FBS should be undertaken provided no technical difficulties or contraindications	Ia	A	1
FBS should be undertaken with the mother in the left lateral position	Ia	A	2
Where there is clear evidence of acute fetal compromise (e.g. prolonged deceleration greater than 3 min), FBS should not be undertaken and the baby should be delivered urgently	IV	C	3
Prolonged use of maternal facial oxygen therapy may be harmful to the fetus and should be avoided. There is no research evidence evaluating the benefits or risks associated with the short-term use of maternal facial oxygen therapy in cases of suspected fetal compromise	IV	C	3
During episodes of abnormal FHR patterns when the mother is lying supine, the mother should adopt the left lateral position	Ia	A	2
In cases of uterine hypercontractility in association with oxytocin infusion and with a suspicious or pathological CTG, the oxytocin infusion should be decreased or discontinued	IV	C	3
In the presence of abnormal FHR patterns and uterine hypercontractility not secondary to oxytocin infusion, tocolysis should be considered. A suggested regime is subcutaneous terbutaline 0.25 mg	Ia	A	4
In cases of suspected or confirmed acute fetal compromise, delivery should be accomplished as soon as possible, accounting for the severity of the FHR abnormality and relevant maternal factors. The accepted standard has been that ideally this should be accomplished within 30 min	IIa	B	5
When fetal blood sampling is undertaken the following classification should be used to guide management:	IV	C	3

Fetal blood sample result (pH)*	Subsequent action
≥7.25	FBS should be repeated if the FHR abnormality persists
7.21–7.24	Repeat FBS within 30 min or consider delivery if rapid fall since last sample
≤7.20	Delivery indicated

* All scalp pH estimations should be interpreted taking into account the previous pH measurement, the rate of progress in labor and the clinical features of the mother and baby

References

1 Thacker SB, Stroup DF (2001) Continuous electronic heart rate monitoring versus intermittent auscultation for assessment during labor. In: *The Cochrane library*, issue 3. Oxford, Update Software. Systematic review of nine randomized controlled trials comparing the use of continuous electronic fetal monitoring with intermittent auscultation. Mixture of low- and high-risk labor monitored. Use of intermittent auscultation generally consistent across studies, definitions of normal and abnormal for use of electronic monitoring not as consistent. Overall no significant difference between continuous electronic monitoring and intermittent auscultation with respect to Apgar scores or perinatal mortality, although studies underpowered to detect differences in either of these. Significant reduction in neonatal seizures seen (OR 0.50, 95% CI 0.31–0.80). increase in operative delivery rates seen, both for instrumental delivery and cesarean section (lower segment cesarean section: OR 1.44, 95% CI 1.24–1.66, instrumental:

OR 1.25, 95% CI 1.13–1.37). All outcomes were divided according to whether fetal blood sampling used or not. Increase in operative delivery was more marked if fetal blood sampling was not used. Two follow-up studies were included to look at outcome in relation to cerebral palsy, and no significant difference was seen between the two monitoring modalities. **Ia A**

2 Gupta JK, Nikodem VC (2001) Woman's position during second stage of labour. In: *The Cochrane library*, issue 3. Oxford, Update Software. Systematic review of 18 trials examining the effects of women's position in the second stage of labor. Use of any upright or lateral position, compared with supine or lithotomy positions, was associated with a reduction in abnormal fetal heart rate patterns (one trial – OR 0.31, 95% CI 0.11–0.91). There is no direct evidence relating to the use of different maternal positions in actual situations of suspected fetal distress. **Ia A.**

3 Royal College of Obstetricians and Gynaecologists (2001) *The use of electronic fetal monitoring.* Evidence-based Clinical Guideline no. 8. London: RCOG Press. A multiprofessional national evidence-based guideline commissioned by the Department of Health and the National Institute for Clinical Excellence. The guideline used strict methodology with precise clinical question setting and appraisal processes. Where no evidence was available, consensus methods were used. **IV C**

4 Kulier R, Hofmeyr GJ (2001) Tocolytics for suspected intrapartum fetal distress. In: *The Cochrane library*, issue 3. Oxford, Update Software. Systematic review of three RCTs comparing the use of a variety of tocolytics. In one study with abnormal fetal heart rate patterns and scalp pH measurements below 7.25, subcutaneous terbutaline was associated with fewer failed improvements in fetal heart rate patterns, compared to no treatment (25% vs 95%, RR 0.26, 95% CI 0.13–0.53). There was no difference in robust neonatal outcomes and the study was unblinded. **Ia A.**

5 Chauhan SP, Wilkinson K, Beresford N *et al.* (1997) Cesarean section for suspected fetal distress. Does the decision-incision time make a difference? *J Reprod Med* **42**, 347–352. 3-year cohort of all emergency cesarean sections for fetal distress. The data were divided according to whether the decision-to-incision interval was less than or greater than 30 min. Those babies delivered in less than 30 min had significantly reduced rates of umbilical artery acidosis, lower rates of pH below 7 and reduced neonatal intensive-care unit admissions. It was a small study of 117 cases and the data were not further stratified into other time groups to see if other time limits were associated with similar outcomes. **IIa B**

Meconium staining of amniotic fluid

Management option	Quality of evidence	Strength of recommendation	References
Amnioinfusion reduces the risk of cesarean section for fetal distress, fetal acidemia and meconium aspiration syndrome	Ia	A	1
Pediatrician for delivery and pharyngeal suction, but not routine endotracheal intubation in the absence of evidence of fetal hypoxia	Ia	A	2

References

1 Hofmeyr GJ (2001) Amnioinfusion for meconium-stained liquor in labour. In: *The Cochrane library*, issue 3. Oxford: Update Software. Systematic review of 10 studies, most involving small numbers of participants, giving a total of 1702 women recruited. The results were stratified depending on the degree of perinatal surveillance. Under standard perinatal surveillance, amnioinfusion was associated with a reduction in heavy meconium staining of the liquor (RR 0.03, 95% CI 0.01–0.15) and variable fetal heart rate deceleration (RR 0.47, 95% CI 0.24–0.90). No perinatal deaths were reported. Under limited perinatal surveillance, amnioinfusion was associated with a reduction in: meconium aspiration syndrome (RR 0.24, 95% CI 0.12–0.48); neonatal hypoxic ischemic encephalopathy (RR 0.07, 95% CI 0.01–0.56) and neonatal ventilation or intensive care unit admission (RR 0.56, 95% CI 0.39–0.79); there was a trend towards reduced perinatal mortality (RR 0.34, 95% CI 0.11–1.06). There was a significant reduction in cesarean sections for fetal distress (RR 0.38, 95% CI 0.23–0.61). **Ia A**

2 Halliday HL (2001) Endotracheal intubation at birth for preventing morbidity and mortality in vigorous, meconium-stained infants born at term. In: *The Cochrane library*, issue 3. Oxford: Update Software. Systematic review of four randomized controlled trials comparing policies off routine versus no (or selective) use of endotracheal intubation and aspiration in the immediate management of vigorous term meconium-stained babies at birth. Meta-analysis of these trials does not support routine use of endotracheal intubation at birth in vigorous meconium-stained babies to reduce mortality, meconium aspiration syndrome, other respiratory symptoms or disorders, pneumothorax, oxygen need, stridor, hypoxic-ischemic encephalopathy and convulsions. The event rates in these studies was low and the total included babies in the review was under 3000. the authors recommended that upper pharyngeal suction should not be abandoned. **Ia A**

Cord prolapse

Management option	Quality of evidence	Strength of recommendation	References
Cesarean section while relieving pressure on cord until delivery	III	B	1
Instrumental delivery if in the second stage and the presenting part is below the level of the ischial spines and easy prompt vaginal delivery is anticipated	III	B	1

Reference

1 Murphy DJ, MacKenzie IZ (1995) The mortality and morbidity associated with umbilical cord prolapse. *Br J Obstet Gynaecol* **102**, 826–830. Case series of 132 babies born after the identification of umbilical cord prolapse over an 8-year period. The outcomes in terms of perinatal death were lower than expected and only one was attributable to asphyxia. The majority of poor long-term outcomes were attributable to congenital abnormality and prematurity. A shorter delivery interval correlated well with Apgar scores. **III B**

Shoulder dystocia

Management option	Quality of evidence	Strength of recommendation	References
Prevention of shoulder dystocia can be achieved by a policy of elective cesarean section with confirmed macrosomia in a diabetic mother or following a previous shoulder dystocia	III IIa	B B	1–4 5
Once it has occurred: the management options are (in order): ❑ McRoberts maneuver with suprapubic pressure and extended episiotomy ❑ Wood's or similar corkscrew maneuver ❑ Deliver posterior shoulder and rotate ❑ (Zavanelli maneuver, cleidotomy, symphysiotomy)	III	B	6,7

References

1 Ecker JL, Greenberg JA, Norwitz ER *et al.* (1997) Birth weight as a predictor of brachial plexus injury. *Obstet Gynecol* **89**, 643–647. Case series. 80 cases of brachial plexus injury (n = 77616). Significant association with increasing birth weight and maternal diabetes. 919 cases of shoulder dystocia in the same period. 43 of 80 babies with brachial plexus injury had evidence of shoulder dystocia. Fewer than 5% of shoulder dystocia deliveries resulted in brachial plexus injury. Birthweight alone poorly predictive of either shoulder dystocia or brachial plexus injury. **III B**

2 Gonen R, Spiegel D, Abend M *et al.* (1996) Is macrosomia predictable, and are shoulder dystocia and birth trauma preventable? *Obstet Gynecol* **88**, 526–529. Prospective study evaluating the ability of ultrasound to detect macrosomia (>4500g) and hence prevent shoulder dystocia. Ultrasound only detected 4 of the 23 macrosomic babies. 93% of the cases of shoulder dystocia occurred in babies under 4.5kg. **III B**

3 Rouse DJ, Owen J, Goldenberg RL *et al.* (1996) The effectiveness and costs of elective cesarean delivery for fetal macrosomia diagnosed by ultrasound. *JAMA* **276**, 1480–1486. Decision analysis model to estimate the effectiveness and cost effectiveness of three decision models in the management of macrosomia and the prevention of shoulder dystocia and brachial plexus injury. Elective cesarean section for nondiabetic women with ultrasound-diagnosed macrosomic babies is not recommended but in those women with diabetes and macrosomic babies it may prevent cases of shoulder dystocia and be cost-effective. **III B**

4 Yeo GS, Lim YW, Yeong CT *et al.* (1995) An analysis of risk factors for the prediction of shoulder dystocia in 16,471 consecutive births. *Ann Acad Med Singapore* **24**, 836–840. A retrospective study of the management of 76 consecutive cases of shoulder dystocia. In most cases the McRoberts maneuver was sufficient in order to deliver the impacted shoulders. In the remainder, additional successful maneuvers included suprapubic pressure and the Woods maneuver. Based on the authors' experience, they recommend the optimal 'ABC' for the management of shoulder dystocia. It includes (A) the McRoberts maneuver, (B) suprapubic pressure, (C) the Woods maneuver, (D) delivery of posterior arm. **III B**

5 Bahar AM (1996) Risk factors and fetal outcome in cases of shoulder dystocia compared with normal deliveries of a similar birthweight. *Br J Obstet Gynaecol* **103**, 868–872. Retrospective case-control study of 69 cases of true shoulder dystocia with matched controls. Cases of shoulder dystocia had a higher incidence of previous shoulder dystocia and presence of diabetes mellitus. No significant difference in birthweight. **IIa B**

6 Gherman RB, Goodwin TM, Souter I *et al.* (1997) The McRoberts maneuver for the alleviation of shoulder dystocia: how successful is it? *Am J Obstet Gynecol* **176**, 656–661. Case series of 250 cases of shoulder dystocia (0.57%, n = 44072). McRoberts maneuver alone used in 42% and in this group there was a significantly lower birthweight than in the group requiring further maneuvers. Only 19% of the series were heavier than 4500g. **III B**

7 O'Leary JA (1993) Cephalic replacement for shoulder dystocia: present status and future role of the Zavanelli maneuver. *Obstet Gynecol* **82**, 847–850. Case series of 59 cases of Zavenelli's maneuver from a case register. 53 were successfully replaced. 40% of the infants had Apgar scores less than 7 at 5min; no cord-blood gases were available. The majority of the babies were delivered within 10min; no data were available for the total time taken to accomplish delivery including maneuvers used prior to commencement of cephalic replacement. **III B**

47.7 Pain during parturition

Tim Overton

Management option		Quality of evidence	Strength of recommendation	References
Non-pharmacological methods	Attendance at labor classes has shown little demonstrable effect on pain relief in labor	III	B	1
	Transcutaneous electrical nerve stimulation (TENS) does not relieve labor pain	Ia	A	2
	Water immersion has been advocated but there is limited evidence of benefit and it may be harmful	Ia Ib	A A	3 4,5
	Social support in labor reduces the need for pain relief	Ia	A	6
	Psychoprophylaxis – Lamaze method possible benefit (but methodological flaws in study)	IIa	B	7
Pharmacological methods	Entonox (NO/oxygen) widely used but evidence mainly observational	IV	C	8
	Systemic analgesics provide some degree of help (meperidine/pethidine most widely used) often used with phenothiazine to reduce nausea and vomiting	Ia	A	9,10
	Regional analgesia effective in reducing pain during labor but potentially adverse effects; preferred method by many for vaginal breech delivery, multiple pregnancy, low-birthweight baby, hypertension in pregnancy and prolonged labor	Ia	A	11
	Regional analgesia with vaginal delivery is associated with malposition, increased need for operative vaginal delivery	A	Ia	11
	Pudendal block is a good and safe form of analgesia for second stage	III	B	12
	Perineal infiltration with local anesthetic will reduce pain from a perineal tear and should be used for repair of tears or an episiotomy	–	✔	–

Management option		Quality of evidence	Strength of recommendation	References
Pharmacological methods (cont'd)	Diclofenac is effective in reducing postpartum pain	Ia	A	6,13
Anesthesia for cesarean section	Regional block is the preferred method of choice	IV	C	14
	Regional block using fentanyl in addition provides better analgesic effect	Ib	A	15
	Patient-controlled analgesia appears to be well tolerated	Ib	A	16
	Extradural meperidine/pethidine is good for postoperative analgesia	Ib	A	17

References

1 Lumley J, Brown S (1993) Attenders and nonattenders at childbirth education classes in Australia: how do they and their births differ? *Birth* **20**, 123–130. This study assessed the associations between attendance at childbirth preparation classes and the health behaviors, birth events, satisfaction with care and later emotional wellbeing of women having their first child. A postal survey was conducted of a population-based cohort of 1193 women who gave birth in 2 weeks in 1989 in Victoria, Australia. The response was 71.4% (790/1107). Classes were attended by 245 (83.9%) of 292 primiparous women. Those who did not attend were significantly more likely to be under age 25 years, not to have completed secondary education, to be single, to have a low family income and no health insurance, and to be public hospital clinic patients. Differences between women who attended classes and those who did not, with respect to measures of pain and to the use of procedures, interventions and pain relief, were rare and minor. No differences occurred between the groups in their satisfaction with the provision of information through pregnancy, birth, and the postnatal period. Only one of five measures of satisfaction with care was less favorable in nonattenders. Attenders were not more confident about looking after their infants at home or less likely to be depressed 8 months after birth. Significant differences occurred between the groups on four health behaviors: cigarette smoking, missed antenatal appointments, breastfeeding and alcohol consumption during pregnancy. Attendance at childbirth preparation classes in Victoria is not associated with differences in birth events, satisfaction with care or emotional wellbeing among women having their first child. **III B**

2 Carroll D, Tramer M, McQuay H *et al.* (1997) Transcutaneous electrical nerve stimulation in labour pain: a systematic review. *Br J Obstet Gynaecol* **104**, 169–175. Review of 10 randomized controlled trials involving 877 women, 436 of whom received active transcutaneous electrical nerve stimulation (TENS) and 441 who received either sham TENS or no treatment. There were no significant differences between the two groups in primary pain outcomes in any of the 10 studies. In addition, there was no difference in the use of additional analgesic interventions in the two groups. **Ia A**

3 Nikodem VC (2001) Immersion in water in pregnancy, labour and birth. In: *Cochrane Database of Systematic Reviews*, issue 3. Oxford: Update Software. Review assessing the effects of immersion in water during pregnancy, labor or birth on maternal, fetal, neonatal and caregiver outcomes. Three trials involving 988 women were included. No statistically significant differences between immersion and no immersion were detected for use of pain relief, augmentation and duration of first stage of labor, meconium-stained liquor and perineal trauma. Neonatal outcomes such as Apgar scores, umbilical arterial pH values and neonatal infection rates also showed no differences. The author concluded that there was not enough evidence to evaluate the use of immersion in water during labor. **Ia A**

4 Eckert K, Turnbull D, MacLennan A (2001) Immersion in water in the first stage of labour: a randomized controlled trial. *Birth* **28**, 84–93. Prospective randomized trial. 274 pregnant women, who were free from medical and obstetric complications and expecting a singleton pregnancy at term, were randomized to an experimental group who received immersion in a bath or to a nonbath group who received routine care. The use of pharmacological analgesia was similar for both the experimental and control groups; 85% and 77%, respectively, used major analgesia. No statistical differences were observed in the proportion of women requiring induction and augmentation of labor or in rates of perineal trauma, length of labor, mode of delivery or frequency of cardiotocographic trace abnormalities. Neonatal outcomes (birthweight, Apgar score, nursery care, meconium-stained liquor, cord pH estimations) revealed no statistically significant differences. Infants of bath group women required significantly more resuscitation than routine group women. Routine group women rated their overall experience of childbirth more positively than bath group women. Psychological outcomes such as satisfaction with care or postnatal distress were the same for both groups. **Ib A**

5 Benfield RD, Herman J, Katz VL *et al.* (2001) Hydrotherapy in labour. *Res Nurs Health* **24**, 57–67. Using a randomized, pretest–posttest control group design with repeated measures, 18 term parturients were assigned to a control or an experimental group. Experimental subjects were placed in a tub of 37°C water for 1 h during early labor. At 15 min bathers' anxiety and pain scores were decreased compared to nonbathers. At 60 min bathers' pain scores were decreased compared to nonbathers. After 15 min of immersion, bathers had a significantly greater increase in plasma volume than nonbathers. No significant differences were found in urine catecholamines or maternal–fetal complications. The small sample limits conclusions, but the findings offer preliminary support for the therapeutic effects of bathing in labor for acute, short-term anxiety and pain reduction. **Ib A**

6 Hodnett ED (2001) Caregiver support for women during childbirth. In: *Cochrane database of systematic reviews*, issue 3. Oxford: Update Software. 14 trials, involving more than 5000 women, are included in the review. The continuous presence of a support person reduced the likelihood of medication for pain relief, operative vaginal delivery, cesarean delivery and a 5 min Apgar score less than 7. Continuous support was also associated with a slight reduction in the length of labor. Six trials evaluated the effects of support on mothers' views of their childbirth experiences; while the trials used different measures (overall satisfaction, failure to cope well during labor, finding labor to be worse than expected and level of personal control during childbirth), in each trial the results favored the group who had received continuous support. **Ia A**

7 Scott JR, Rose NB (1976) Effect of psychoprophylaxis (Lamaze preparation) on labor and delivery in primiparas. *N Engl J Med* **294**, 1205–1207. This study compared labors of 129 women who had attended antenatal classes in the third trimester with matched controls that received no such education. The antenatal classes gave specific training in complex breathing techniques that coincided with uterine contractions (Lamaze technique). The group that had received the training required less analgesia in labor and had a higher frequency of spontaneous delivery. There were no differences in the length of labor, incidence of maternal complications, frequency of fetal distress, mean Apgar scores or neonatal problems. However, the women who attended the Lamaze classes were self-selected, which may have introduced significant bias. **IIa B**

8 Rosen M (1971) Recent advances in pain relief in childbirth: inhalation and systemic analgesia. *Br J Anaesth* **43**, 837–848. This review details the techniques available to women in the 1970s for pain relief in labor. Inhalational analgesia, using methoxyflurane or nitrous oxide, are discussed as well as parenteral opioid analgesics such as pentazocine. **IV C**

9 Howell CJ, Chalmers I (1992) A review of prospectively controlled comparisons of epidural with no-epidural forms of pain relief during labor. *Int J Obstet Anesth* **1**, 93–110. In this meta-analysis of studies where an attempt had been made to randomly allocate women to receive either epidural or nonepidural anesthesia, data from nine controlled trials involving 600 women were analyzed. Evidence from these trials suggested that epidural block provides more effective pain relief than other methods but that, if the epidural is continued during the second stage, there is an association with an increase in the instrumental delivery rate. **Ia A**

10 Halpern SH, Leighton BL, Ohlsson A *et al.* (1998) Effect of epidural vs parental opioid analgesia on the progress of labor: a meta-analysis. *JAMA* **280**, 2105–2110. This meta-analysis reviewed data from 10 trials enrolling 2369 patients comparing the effect of epidural analgesia with parenteral opioid on the progress of labor. Although epidural analgesia was associated with longer labors and an increase in the risk of instrumental delivery (OR 2.19, 95% CI 1.32–7.78), they were no more likely to have an instrumental delivery for dystocia (OR 0.68, 95% CI 0.31–1.49). The risk of cesarean section did not differ between the two groups, the pain scores were significantly less in the epidural group and neonates were less likely to have low 5 min Apgar scores or to need naloxone. Patients receiving epidural analgesia have longer labors. Patient satisfaction and neonatal outcome were better after epidural than parenteral opioid analgesia. **Ia A**

11 Howell CJ (2001) Epidural versus non-epidural analgesia for pain relief in labour. In: *Cochrane database of systematic reviews*, issue 3. Oxford: Update Software. This review assessed the effects of epidural analgesia on pain relief and adverse effects in labor. 11 studies involving 3157 women were included. Epidural analgesia was associated with greater pain relief than nonepidural methods but also with longer first and second stages of labor, an increased incidence of fetal malposition and increased use of oxytocin and instrumental vaginal deliveries. No statistically significant effect on cesarean section rates could be identified. The author concluded that epidural analgesia is effective in reducing pain during labor, although there appeared to be some potentially adverse effects and further research was needed to investigate adverse effects. **Ia A**

12 Schierup L, Schmidt JF, Torp Jensen A *et al.* (1988) Pudendal block in vaginal deliveries. Mepivacaine with and without epinephrine. *Acta Obstet Gynecol Scand* **67**, 195–197. Pudendal block with 20 ml 1% mepivacaine with and without epinephrine (adrenaline) was performed in 151 patients during the second stage of labor. No differences in efficacy of the block or in Apgar scores between the two groups were found. The maternal mepivacaine concentration was higher in the plain group than in the epinephrine group ($p < 0.01$) but toxic levels were never reached. In the infants, no difference in mepivacaine concentration was found between the groups ($p > 0.05$, type II error 9%) and toxic levels were not reached. The time elapsed from the pudendal block until delivery was prolonged when epinephrine was added ($p < 0.02$). We found no effect on blood pressure in either of the groups, with or without oxytocin and/or methergin. 20 ml 1% mepivacaine (plain) is a safe choice for pudendal block without the possible disadvantages of adding epinephrine. **III B**

13 Windle ML, Booker LA, Rayburn WF et al. (1989) Postpartum pain after vaginal delivery. A review of comparative analgesic trials. *J Reprod Med* **34**, 891–895. This paper reviewed a number of studies that assessed the safety and efficacy of several oral analgesics. In general nonsteroidal analgesics (NSAIDs) were consistently more useful than placebo for postpartum uterine pain and episiotomy pain. Aspirin had a more rapid onset of action than newer NSAIDs but the duration of action was shorter. Side effects and breast milk concentrations of the drugs were negligible for this short-term therapy. Although no drug was found to be preferable to the others, aspirin and ibuprofen were the least expensive. **Ia A**

14 Dresner MR, Freeman JM (2001) Anaesthesia for caesarean section. *Best Pract Res Clin Obstet Gynaecol* **15**, 127–143. Quality and choice in anesthesia for cesarean section have significantly improved over the last two decades. During this time, general anesthesia usage has decreased to the point where, in some centers, it is an occasionally used technique for severe fetal distress. This change in practice may have been responsible for the fall in anesthetic deaths in pregnant women that has occurred over the same period. The boom in regional anesthesia has improved the esthetics of childbirth by cesarean section, women's perioperative comfort and postoperative analgesia. It has, however, introduced new problems, such as delays in inducing anesthesia in emergency situations, postoperative immobility and urinary retention. The increase in anesthetic choices has led to inconsistencies in practice between individual anesthetists, and between regions and nations. It is therefore impossible for obstetricians to make assumptions about the impact of anesthesia on their patients. Where possible, anesthetic protocols and guidelines should exist in every center, with obstetricians clearly informed of relevant features. Such an approach will prevent inconsistent advice being given to patients and dangerous mistakes occurring. With every aspect of maternity care, a multidisciplinary team approach is in patients' best interests, and anesthesia for cesarean section is no exception. **IV C**

15 Paech MJ, Westmore MD, Speirs HM *et al.* (1990) A double-blind comparison of epidural bupivacaine and bupivacaine–fentanyl for cesarean section. *Anesth Intens Care* **18**, 22–30. This study assessed the benefit of adding fentanyl 100 μg to bupivacaine 0.5% plain to establish epidural anesthesia for elective cesarean section in a randomized, double-blind study of 60 healthy women. In the fentanyl group the quality of intraoperative analgesia assessed by both patients and anesthetists was significantly improved. There were no adverse maternal effects other than a 15% incidence of mild pruritus in the fentanyl group, and neonatal outcomes in both groups were the same. Plasma fentanyl was not detected in the majority of maternal and fetal cord-blood samples. The authors concluded that the addition of fentanyl was of significant benefit for routine cesarean sections. Whilst the neonatal observations were encouraging it was recognized that further work would be required to assess the effects in the potentially compromised fetus. **Ib A**

16 Lysak SZ, Eisenach JC, Dobson CE (1990) Patient-controlled epidural analgesia during labor: a comparison of three solutions with a continuous infusion control. *Anesthesiology* **72**, 44–49. This prospective study randomly allocated women during labor to receive either physician-controlled epidural anesthesia with bupivacaine, patient-controlled epidural anesthesia with bupivacaine, patient-controlled epidural anesthesia with bupivacaine and fentanyl and patient-controlled epidural anesthesia with bupivacaine, fentanyl and epinephrine (adrenaline) once a standard epidural had been established. Quality of analgesia, patient satisfaction, duration of labor and Apgar scores did not differ between groups. Although there was no significant difference in the total dose of bupivacaine administered in each group, the hourly infusion requirements were less in those receiving fentanyl. There was also a significantly increased operative delivery rate in those groups that received fentanyl, although this was felt to reflect random variation. In conclusion, patient-controlled analgesia was felt to be safe and effective but did not reduce anesthetic requirements or improve analgesia compared with physician-controlled epidurals. **Ib A**

17 Perriss BW, Latham BV, Wilson IH (1990) Analgesia following extradural and i.m. pethidine in post-caesarean section patients. *Br J Anaesth* **64**, 355–357. This prospective randomized, double-blind study compared the onset, quality and duration of analgesia following extradural pethidine (meperidine) 50 mg and intramuscular pethidine 100 mg, assessed in 30 postoperative patients who had undergone cesarean section under extradural anesthesia. Extradural pethidine provided superior analgesia, of quicker onset but with similar duration and efficacy. Both treatments were associated with a low incidence of side effects. Correspondence that followed suggested that the 'superior' benefit of pethidine given extradurally was not as great as suggested by the authors and that the marginally faster onset may have been explained by quicker systemic absorption of pethidine when given at the extradural site rather than a locally mediated effect. **Ib A**

47.8 Assisted vaginal delivery

Mark Selinger and David James

Management option		Quality of evidence	Strength of recommendation	References
Indications	Maternal: ❑ Distress, exhaustion ❑ Certain maternal medical disorders	IV	C	1,2

Management option		Quality of evidence	Strength of recommendation	References
Indications (cont'd)	**Fetal:** ❑ Presumed fetal jeopardy ❑ Breech delivery (forceps to 'aftercoming' head)	IV	C	1,2
	Process: ❑ Malposition (OP, OT, asynclitism) ❑ Unsuccessful ventouse (forceps trial with caution and facilities for cesarean section standing-by)	IV	C	1,2
	Practitioners should be aware that no indication is absolute and be able to distinguish 'standard' from 'special' indications	IV	C	1
Contra-indications	❑ Unengaged head (two fifths of this or more palpable abdominally or at/or above ischial spines vaginally) ❑ Inability to define position ❑ Malposition (face, brow) ❑ Suspected or actual cephalopelvic disproportion (pelvic-anatomy- or macrosomia-related) ❑ Certain fetal anomalies ❑ Prematurity (? less than 34 weeks for ventouse) or less than 1500 g ❑ Repeated scalp pH estimations (ventouse) ❑ Operator inexperience or lack of training with instrument	IV Ia Ib IIa IV	C A A B C	1 3 4 5 6,7
Prerequisites	❑ Engaged head (but one fifth palpable abdominally or above +2 station is potentially hazardous) ❑ Fully dilated (some argue for 9 cm+ with ventouse), membranes ruptured ❑ Empty bladder (? not for outlet delivery) ❑ Known presentation, position and station ❑ Adequate analgesia/anesthesia ❑ Experienced operator and adequate support facilities ❑ Willingness to abandon procedure if difficult ❑ Informed and consenting patient ❑ Working, serviced equipment for ventouse and matching blades for forceps	IV	C	1,2
Occiput transverse or occiput posterior options	Manual rotation/ventouse/rotational forceps	–	✔	–
	Possible delivery as occiput posterior position	–	✔	–
	Selection by circumstances, individual experience and preferences rather than scientific guidelines	IV	C	1
	Care and skill are necessary	IV	C	1

Management option		Quality of evidence	Strength of recommendation	References
Choice of instrument	Practitioners should use the most acceptable instrument for individual circumstances	IV	C	1
	Deficient knowledge and incorrect technique contribute to increased complications. Practitioners should be aware of the potential risks and necessary safety measures	IV	C	1
	Vacuum versus forceps: ❑ Vacuum has higher rates of delivery failure, cephalhematomata, retinal hemorrhages and jaundice ❑ Forceps has higher rates of regional/ general anesthesia, maternal trauma ❑ No differences in rates of cesarean section, Apgar scores, long-term (5 years) maternal and baby follow-up	Ia	A	3
	Soft versus metal vacuum cups: ❑ Soft cup has higher rates of delivery failure (especially with occiput posterior, occiput tranverse and difficult occiput anterior positions) ❑ Metal cup has higher rates of neonatal scalp trauma	Ia	A	8

References

1 Johanson RB (2000) *Instrumental vaginal delivery*. RCOG Clinical 'Green Top' Guideline. London: Royal College of Obstetricians and Gynaecologists. Evidence-based guideline reviewing the following issues relating to instrumental vaginal delivery: indications, contraindications, instrument choice, relative merits, complications, training, risk management and audit. **IV C**

2 Gei AF, Belfort MA (1999) Forceps-assisted vaginal delivery. *Obstet Gynecol Clin North Am* **26**, 345–370. Review article of operative vaginal delivery using forceps. **IV C**

3 Johanson RB, Menon BK (2000) Vacuum extraction versus forceps for assisted vaginal delivery. In: *Cochrane database of systematic reviews*, issue 2. Oxford: Update Software. Systematic review of 10 trials. The trials were of reasonable quality. Use of the vacuum extractor for assisted vaginal delivery when compared to forceps delivery was associated with significantly less maternal trauma (OR 0.41, 95% CI 0.33–0.50) and with less general and regional anesthesia. There were more deliveries with vacuum extraction (OR 1.69, 95% CI 1.31–2.19). Fewer cesarean sections were carried out in the vacuum extractor group. However the vacuum extractor was associated with an increase in neonatal cephalhematomata and retinal hemorrhages. Serious neonatal injury was uncommon with either instrument. **Ia A**

4 Johanson R, Pusey J, Livera N *et al.* (1989) North Staffordshire/Wigan assisted delivery trial. *Br J Obstet Gynaecol* **96**, 537–544. A prospective, randomized study comparing soft-cup ventouse with an unspecified number of different types of obstetric forceps in 264 primi- and multigravidas. Computer-generated sequential envelope randomization after diagnosis of need for assisted delivery. Operator preference allowed, exclusions discussed. Selective episiotomy. The ventouse failure rate (27%) was higher than that using forceps (8%). Mid/upper vaginal and third- or fourth-degree tears were more common after forceps delivery (18.9%) than ventouse delivery (6%) but 22% of the data were missing. Episiotomy rates were not discussed. There were no significant differences in the rates of fetal trauma between the two groups. **Ib A**

5 Johanson RB, Rice C, Doyle M *et al.* (1993) A randomised prospective study comparing the new vacuum extractor policy with forceps delivery. *Br J Obstet Gynaecol* **100**, 524–530. Prospective, randomized (after elective case removal at clinician's discretion) trial purporting to assess a new ventouse cup policy but reported as a trial comparing forceps and ventouse delivery in 607 primi- and multigravidas. Unspecified episiotomy policy. Insignificant differences in instrumental failure rates (ventouse 15%, forceps 10%). Significant maternal trauma was more common after forceps (17%) than ventouse (11%) delivery. There were significantly higher fetal cephalhematoma rates after ventouse (27%) than forceps (8%) delivery. Concerns about forceps-mediated serious fetal morbidity were expressed. **IIa B**

6 Thiery M (1979) Fetal hemorrhage following blood samplings and use of vacuum extractor. *Am J Obstet Gynecol* **134**, 231. Case reports of fetal hemorrhage after use of vacuum extractor after fetal scalp sampling. **IV C**

7 Roberts IF, Stone M (1978) Fetal hemorrhage: complication of vacuum extractor after fetal blood sampling. *Am J Obstet Gynecol* **132**, 109. Case report of fetal hemorrhage after use of vacuum extractor after fetal scalp sampling. **IV C**

8 Johanson R, Menon V (2000) Soft versus rigid vacuum extractor cups for assisted vaginal delivery. In: *Cochrane database of systematic reviews*, issue 2. Oxford: Update Software. Systematic review of nine trials involving 1375 women. The trials were of average quality. Soft cups were significantly more likely to fail to achieve vaginal delivery (OR 1.65, 95% CI 1.19–2.29). However, they were associated with less scalp injury (OR 0.45, 95% CI 0.15–0.60). There was no difference between the two groups in terms of maternal injury. Metal cups appear to be more suitable for 'occipitoposterior', transverse and difficult 'occipitoanterior' position deliveries. Soft cups seem to be appropriate for straightforward deliveries **Ia A**

47.9 Previous cesarean section

Lucy Kean

Management option		Quality of evidence	Strength of recommendation	References
Eligibility for trial of labor	One previous lower uterine cesarean section with no other adverse features	III	B	1–4
	Cephalic twins, nondiabetic macrosomia are probably not adverse features	III	B	5,6
	With more than one prior cesarean section, in the absence of contraindications, trial of vaginal delivery need not be discouraged	III	B	1,3,7
	With previous low vertical uterine incision (if accurate information available to confirm this) data evidence suggests that trial of vaginal delivery need not be discouraged	III	B	8
	Generally accepted contraindications include previous classical cesarean section and diabetic macrosomic fetus	III	B	2,4,7
	Patient preference may influence choice of method	III	B	9,10
Conduct of trial of labor	Critical review of progress of labor	–	✔	–
	Cervical ripening with prostaglandins is probably safe in selected cases but numbers studied are small	III	B	11–14
	Induction with misoprostol should be performed with caution	III	B	15
	Judicious use of oxytocin is acceptable but should be discontinued if response to uterine stimulation does not occur promptly	III	B	16
	Continuous fetal heart rate monitoring	IV	C	17
	The issues of intravenous access and crossmatching of blood are controversial	–	✔	–
	Routine insertion of intrauterine pressure catheter is not justified	III	B	18
	Regional anesthesia is not contraindicated	III	B	19
	Digital palpation/examination of scar only necessary with persistent postpartum bleeding	III	B	20

References

1 Flamm BL, Goings JR, Liu Y *et al.* (1994) Elective repeat cesarean delivery versus trial of labor: a prospective multicenter study. *Obstet Gynecol* **83**, 927–932. Observational study across hospitals of Southern Carolina. 7229 patients were studied, 5022 (70%) had a trial of labor and 2207 had elective repeat cesarean operations. 3746 of the women opting for a trial of labor delivered vaginally (75%). Women were selected for trial or not by their clinicians and the trial included some women undergoing trial after two prior cesarean sections. The uterine scar rupture rate was less than 1%. **III B**

2 Rosen MG, Dickinson JC (1994) Vaginal birth after cesarean: a meta-analysis of indicators for success. *Obstet Gynecol* **84**, 255–258. Study analyzing 29 papers with data concerning outcomes in women undergoing trial of labor after previous cesarean section. None of the papers included was randomized. Most were observational studies. Vaginal delivery rates for trial ranged from 54% to 89%. Women who underwent trial after prior cesarean section for breech presentation had the highest vaginal delivery rates (85%), with women who had a previous vaginal delivery achieving vaginal delivery in 84%. Where the previous cesarean section was for poor progress in labor, vaginal delivery rates were lower (67%). Women needing oxytocin also had a lower rate of vaginal delivery (63%). Women undergoing trial of labor after two or more prior cesarean sections achieved vaginal delivery in 75%; however numbers were small (345 women). 26 women inadvertently labored with known classical cesarean section scars. The uterine rupture rate for these women was 12%. **III B**

3 Miller DA, Mullin P, Hou D *et al.* (1996) Vaginal birth after cesarean: a 10-year experience. *Am J Obstet Gynecol* **175**, 194–198. Observational study examining outcomes for women undergoing trial of labor at Los Angeles County and University of Southern California Women's Hospital over a 10-year period (1983–92). Trial of labor was used in 80% of women with one previous cesarean, in 54% with two and in 30% with three or more. The success rate was significantly higher with one previous cesarean (83%) than with two or more (75.3%). Uterine rupture was three times more common with two or more previous cesareans. Among women undergoing a trial of labor, there were three rupture-related perinatal deaths and a single rupture-related maternal death. **III B**

4 Rosen MG, Dickinson JC, Westhoff CL (1991) Vaginal birth after cesarean: a meta-analysis of morbidity and mortality. *Obstet Gynecol* **77**, 465–470. Meta-analysis of observational and comparative studies examining maternal and fetal morbidity and mortality following trial of labor compared with women undergoing repeat elective cesarean section. The combined scar rupture rate for lower segment scars was 1.8% for all trials of labor, 1.9% for women undergoing repeat cesarean section without labor (no difference) and 3.3% for women who underwent emergency cesarean section during a trial of labor. Oxytocin use was associated with a rupture rate of 2.3% versus 1.5% for women not needing oxytocin. This did not reach statistical significance ($p = 0.7$). 26 women with a classical cesarean section scar labored before planned delivery. The rate of scar rupture was 12%. Maternal febrile morbidity was significantly lower after a trial of labor than after an elective repeat cesarean section (9.6 vs. 17.4%, $p < 0.001$). After excluding antepartum deaths, fetuses weighing less than 750g and congenital anomalies incompatible with life, there was no difference in perinatal death rates. The proportion of 5min Apgar scores of 6 or less was higher after a trial of labor (2.4 vs 1.6%, $p < 0.01$) but it was not possible to exclude very-low-birthweight fetuses or those with congenital anomalies from this analysis. **III B**

5 Miller DA, Mullin P, Hou D *et al.* (1990) Vaginal birth after cesarean section in twin gestation. *Obstet Gynecol* **75**, 734. Observational study of women undergoing trial of vaginal delivery with twin pregnancies. Women with a vertical uterine scar, a previous uterine rupture, an unrepaired dehiscence or obstetric contraindications to labor were excluded from a trial of labor. Between 1985 and 1994, 210 women with previous cesarean section delivered twins; 118 (56%) underwent repeat cesarean delivery without a trial of labor. 92 (44%) undertook a trial of labor with no uterine ruptures and no increase in maternal or perinatal morbidity or mortality. **III B**

6 Flamm BL, Goings JR (1989) Vaginal birth after cesarean section: is suspected fetal macrosomia a contraindication? *Obstet Gynecol* **74**, 694–697. Comparative study of outcomes in women undergoing a trial of labor (TOL) delivering large babies compared with outcomes for women undergoing TOL, delivering smaller babies and women with no uterine scar delivering large babies. Women with diabetes, classical section or unknown uterine scars were excluded. In the birthweight range of 4000–4499g, 139 of 240 women (58%) delivered vaginally. In the group with birth weights exceeding 4500g, 26 of 61 women (43%) delivered vaginally. When compared with 1475 trials of labor with birthweights under 4000g, no significant differences in perinatal or maternal morbidity were found. Comparison with a control group of 301 women with no previous uterine surgery who delivered macrosomic infants also demonstrated no significant differences in perinatal or maternal morbidity. **III B**

7 Phelan JP, Ahn MO, Diaz F *et al.* (1989) Twice a cesarean, always a cesarean? *Obstet Gynecol* **73**, 161–165. Prospective comparative study, comparing women undergoing trial of labor with two prior cesarean sections with those delivering by planned repeat cesarean section. Women with a known classical incision or a medical or obstetric contraindication to a trial of labor were excluded from an attempted vaginal delivery. 1088 were studied; of these, 501 (46%) underwent a trial of labor and 346 (69%) delivered vaginally. The overall rate of uterine dehiscence was 3%. However the rate of dehiscence was lower in women undergoing trial of labor when compared with those who did not (1.8%, versus 4.6%). Oxytocin was used in 284 (57%) and was associated with a dehiscence rate of 2.1%, versus 1.4% in the no-oxytocin group ($p = 0.7$). Successful vaginal delivery was related significantly to the use of oxytocin and to a previous vaginal delivery. **III B**

8 Adair CD, Sanchez-Ramos L, Whitaker D *et al.* (1996) Trial of labor in patients with a previous lower uterine vertical cesarean section. *Am J Obstet Gynecol* **174**, 966–970. Retrospective review of medical records, performed at a single tertiary perinatal center, of all patients with a previous low vertical cesarean section who underwent a trial of labor during the period January 1988 to December 1993. 11/77 (14.3%) had a repeat operation compared with 14/154 patients (9.0%) in the no previous cesarean section group (not significant). No differences were noted in the incidences of operative vaginal deliveries or prolonged duration of the first or second stages of labor, or in the rate or maximum dose of oxytocin infusion between the two groups. One patient in the previous cesarean section group had uterine rupture. A trial of labor in women with previous low vertical cesarean sections results in an acceptable rate of vaginal delivery and appears safe for both mother and fetus. **III B**

9 Kline J, Arias F (1996) Analysis of factors determining the selection of repeated caesarean section or trial of labor in patients with histories of prior caesarean delivery. *Aust N Z J Obstet Gynaecol* **36**, 155–158. Comparative study of 241 women with previous cesarean section, examining the motivation behind decision to attempt trial of labor or not. 120 underwent elective repeat cesarean sections and 121 had undergone trial of labor (TOL). Patients were of similar age, gravity and parity, but significantly more patients in the repeat cesarean group had their initial surgery because of failure to progress in labor; significantly more patients in the TOL group had their initial cesarean section because of fetal distress. The main factors behind the decision to attempt TOL were patient's desire (81.0%), patient's desire and physician's advice (12.4%) and physician's advice (6.6%). The main factors behind the decision to have repeat cesarean sections were medical or obstetric indication (45.8%), patient's desire (31.6%), patient's desire and physician's advice (9.1%) and physician's advice (13.3%). **III B**

10 Lau TK, Wong SH, Li CY (1994) A study of patients' acceptance towards vaginal birth after cesarean section. *Am J Perinatol* **11**, 309–312. Comparison between women undergoing repeat cesarean section and trial of labor. Patients were recruited antenatally when booking their next pregnancy, and 49 women were interviewed following their first cesarean section. Women's attitude to trying for a vaginal delivery was strongly related to the chance of success. Only 53.3% of patients would accept vaginal birth after cesarean section (VBAC) if they were told that the chance of success was 70%. A history of vaginal delivery and a negative feeling towards previous operation were positively associated with acceptance of VBAC ($p < 0.01$), while convenience of elective cesarean section and fear of vaginal delivery were the commonest reasons for refusal. The major source of negative feelings towards the previous cesarean section were postoperative pain and a long recovery period. Reluctance to accept VBAC was not related to the reason for previous cesarean section when quoted a 70% chance for successful VBAC. Women were much more accepting of VBAC if they had a prior vaginal delivery ($p = 0.007$). **III B**

11 Williams MA, Luthy DA, Zingheim RW *et al.* (1995) Preinduction prostaglandin E2 gel prior to induction of labor in women with a previous cesarean section. *Gynecol Obstet Invest* **40**, 89–93. Retrospective cohort study design was used to compare 117 women with one previous cesarean section (VBACs) with 354 nulliparas. Both groups received preinduction cervical ripening treatment with intracervical prostaglandin (PG)E_2 gel. The mean numbers of PGE_2 gel applications were 2.4 and 2.5 for VBACs and controls respectively ($p < 0.05$). 39% of VBACs entered labor spontaneously as compared with 33% of nulliparas. Mean duration of ruptured membranes (8.2 vs 12.1 h) and length of labor (20.1 vs 28.5 h) were reduced among VBACs as compared with controls ($p < 0.05$). Overall, VBACs had a higher cesarean section rate than controls (49.6 vs 31.9%, adjusted RR = 1.6, 95% CI 1.2–2.1). There were no differences in the occurrence of maternal and fetal morbidity. Overall, the efficacy and safety of 0.5 mg PGE_2 gel administered for preinduction cervical ripening in VBACs is comparable to that observed in nulliparas. **III B**

12 Stone JL, Lockwood CJ, Berkowitz G *et al.* (1984) Use of cervical prostaglandin E2 gel in patients with previous cesarean section. *Br J Obstet Gynaecol* **91**, 7–10. Retrospective comparative study where primiparous patients ($n = 94$) with one previous cesarean section were retrospectively compared to nulliparous patients ($n = 866$). Both groups experienced induction of labor with cervical ripening with 2 mg intracervical prostaglandin (PG)E_2 gel. Logistic regression analysis was used to control for confounding factors. There were no significant differences in the duration of ruptured membranes or length of labor between the two groups. No significant differences were detected in the rate or indications for cesarean section, presence of thick meconium, epidural anesthesia use, amnionitis or maternal and neonatal morbidity. There were no cases of uterine rupture in either group. **III B**

13 MacKenzie IZ, Bradley S, Embrey MP (1997) Vaginal prostaglandins and labor induction for patients previously delivered by cesarean section. *Am J Perinatol* **14**, 157–160. Observational study of 143 women undergoing induction of labor at term using prostaglandin E_2 with prior cesarean section. 76% achieved a vaginal delivery and even when the cervix was very unfavorable at the time of prostaglandin treatment, 68% achieved vaginal delivery. There was no evidence of undue risk of lower segment scar rupture. **III B**

14 Flamm BL, Anton D, Goings JR *et al.* (1987) Prostaglandin E2 for cervical ripening: a multicenter study of patients with prior cesarean delivery. *Obstet Gynecol* **70**, 709–712. Prospective cohort study of women treated with prostaglandin (PG)E_2 gel for cervical ripening prior to trial of labor after previous cesarean delivery compared with a control group who did not receive PGE_2. The women were studied at 10 different Californian hospitals. 5022 women were studied, 453 (9%) were treated with PGE_2 gel. There was no significant difference in the incidence of uterine rupture between the PGE_2 group and the control group. Indicators of maternal and perinatal morbidity were not significantly higher in the prostaglandin-treated group. **III B**

15 Choy-Hee L, Raynor BD (2001) Misoprostol induction of labor among women with a history of cesarean delivery. *Am J Obstet Gynecol* **184**, 1115–1117. Study comparing complications of labor induction with misoprostol between women with a history of cesarean delivery and women without uterine scarring. A computerized database was used to select women with a viable fetus who underwent induction of labor with misoprostol during the period from January 1996 to December 1998. Patients were given 50 μg misoprostol every 4 h. Women with a history of cesarean delivery were retrospectively compared with those without uterine scarring. A total of 425 women were given misoprostol for induction of labor: 48 had a history of cesarean delivery and 377 did not. Women with a history of cesarean delivery were more likely to be delivered abdominally (56% vs 28%, $p < 0.04$). Among women with a history of cesarean delivery, women who had a history of vaginal birth after cesarean were more likely to be delivered vaginally (92% vs 42%, $p = 0.003$). There was no difference in the overall rate of complications (2% with scarring vs 3% without scarring). There were no uterine ruptures. However, the previous cesarean group was more likely than the unscarred group to have blood loss of more than 500 ml (38% vs 22%, $p < 0.03$). Although the incidences of fetal distress were similar, neonates born to women in the previous cesarean group were more likely to have an Apgar score less than 7 at 5 min (13% vs 5%, $p < 0.04$). Thus, misoprostol induction of labor in women with a history of cesarean resulted in a higher rate of cesarean delivery than was seen among women without uterine scarring but was not associated with a higher incidence of complications. There were no uterine ruptures in either group. **III B**

16 Flamm BL, Goings JR, Fuelberth NJ *et al.* (1987) Oxytocin during labor after previous cesarean section: results of a multicenter study. *Obstet Gynecol* **70**, 709–712. Comparative study across eight hospitals. Women undergoing vaginal birth after cesarean section who needed oxytocin in labor were compared with those who did not receive oxytocin. More than one prior cesarean section was not a contraindication to oxytocin. Breech presentations and twin pregnancies were excluded. Women whose prior cesarean section was for suspected cephalopelvic disproportion were not excluded. 1776 women were studied. 485 (27%) were treated with oxytocin. 309 (64%) women needing oxytocin achieved a vaginal delivery compared with 78% of women not requiring oxytocin ($p < 0.001$). When the subsets were analyzed lower rates of vaginal delivery with oxytocin were seen only in the group whose prior cesarean section was for failure to progress. 54% vaginal delivery rate in women whose prior cesarean section was for failure to progress who required oxytocin, compared to 70% of women whose prior cesarean section was for failure to progress but who did not require oxytocin in this labor ($p < 0.001$). Oxytocin-corrected labor patterns in all other groups, and vaginal delivery rates were similar to women not requiring oxytocin. When the patients who received oxytocin were compared with those who did not, no significant differences were found with respect to uterine rupture (1.4% vs 0.54%, $p = 0.07$), maternal morbidity (10% vs 8%), fetal morbidity or fetal mortality. **III B**

17 Royal College of Obstetricians and Gynaecologists (2001) *The use of electronic fetal monitoring*. Evidence-based Clinical Guideline no. 8. London: RCOG. Multidisciplinary guideline for fetal monitoring in labor. Consensus opinion of the expert committee recommends continuous fetal monitoring in labor for women with a uterine scar. The recommendation is based on the finding that changes in the fetal heart rate are often seen with scar rupture. There are no trials of different modalities of monitoring. **IV C**

18 Devoe LD, Croom CS, Youssef AA *et al.* (1992) The prediction of 'controlled' uterine rupture by the use of intrauterine pressure catheters. *Obstet Gynecol* **80**, 626–629. Uterine activity was recorded continuously during low transverse cesarean delivery in 10 parturients using fluid-filled pressure catheters and in 10 women with solid pressure catheters. Visual analyses were performed of the last 30 min of uterine recording before uterine incision and of the period after incision; the analyses were then compared within and between the catheter groups for mean uterine tone and contraction amplitude, frequency and duration. All obstetric endpoints were similar in both catheter groups except for a higher mean birthweight in the solid-catheter group. The mean (± SD) duration of postincision monitoring was 4.7 ± 0.94 min. After uterine incision, mean tone and contraction amplitude were unchanged whereas mean contraction frequency and duration decreased significantly. Although intrauterine monitoring was brief, this model allows a unique view of 'controlled' uterine rupture. Spontaneous uterine rupture may evolve more gradually; however, neither catheter type would be likely to aid its early recognition. **III B**

19 Flamm BL, Dunnett C, Fischermann E *et al.* (1984) Vaginal delivery following cesarean section: use of oxytocin augmentation and epidural anesthesia with internal tocodynamic and internal fetal monitoring. *Am J Obstet Gynecol* **148**, 759–763. The authors present their experience with 230 trials of labor after primary low transverse cesarean section. 181 patients (79%) were delivered vaginally, 73 patients (32%) received epidural anesthesia, and 94 patients (41%) received oxytocin augmentation of labor. Internal tocodynamic and fetal heart monitoring was used in all patients. The rationale for this controversial management is discussed. **III B**

20 Perrotin F, Marret H, Fignon A *et al.* (1999) Scarred uterus: is routine exploration of the cesarean scar after vaginal birth always necessary? *J Gynecol Obstet Biol Reprod (Paris)* **28**, 253–262. Retrospective study, over a 10-year period, of a routine palpation practice in the two units of the authors' obstetric department, then a 30-month prospective study comparing, in each unit, two different attitudes toward uterine revision (routine exploration vs symptomatic patients exploration). The retrospective part reported three uterine ruptures (0.43% of all scarred uterus) and 14 dehiscences (2%) during the 10 years. All uterine ruptures were sufficiently symptomatic to be suspected prior to scar exploration. No dehiscence needed surgical treatment. Some patients with bloodless dehiscence and no repair had subsequent vaginal deliveries with no scar separation found on uterine exploration. In the prospective study, there was a significant difference in the occurrence of fever (18.9% vs 9.9%, $p < 0.05$) and antibiotic treatment (22.8% vs 12.7%, $p < 0.05$) between the two groups based on attitude toward uterine revision. These data suggest that transcervical revision of previous cesarean uterine scar should be performed only in symptomatic patients or when risk factors are present (prolonged labor, prolonged expulsive efforts, instrumental extraction). **III B**

47.10 Cesarean section

Lucy Kean

Management option	Quality of evidence	Strength of recommendation	References
Vaginal preparation with povidone iodine does not reduce postcesarean infectious morbidity	Ib	A	1
Pfannenstiel/suprapubic incision advantageous compared to vertical abdominal incision	III	B	2
Transverse lower uterine incision is associated with less maternal morbidity	III	B	3,4
Active management using oxytocic agent is better than expectant management in vaginal deliveries and one would expect same with cesarean section	Ib	A	5
Syntocinon–oxytocin is statistically better in preventing postpartum hemorrhage (PPH) than oxytocin alone but has more side effects	Ia	A	6
Bolus oxytocin is as effective as intramyometrial prostaglandin and misoprostol in preventing PPH but the latter two were more often associated with retained placenta	Ib	A	7,8
Carbetocin may be associated with less intraoperative blood loss than oxytocin	Ib	A	9
Delivery of the placenta: manual removal is associated with increased maternal blood loss and infection	Ia	A	10
Prophylactic antibiotics are associated with reduced maternal morbidity in emergency cesarean section and with reduced incidence of endometritis in elective cesarean section	Ia	A	11
Antibiotic regimes: ampicillin and first-generation cephalosporins are equally effective in reducing postoperative endometritis. Single-dose regimens are as effective as repeat doses, with the exception of urinary tract infection	Ia	A	12
Thromboprophylaxis is recommended for all women undergoing cesarean section	IV	C	13
Other techniques:			
❑ Left lateral tilt for cesarean section reduces the incidence of low Apgar scores	Ia	A	14
❑ Absorbable staples cannot at present be recommended for routine practice	Ia	A	15
❑ A single layer uterine incision closure is not associated with increased maternal morbidity	Ia	A	16
❑ Closure of the peritoneum is not necessary in routine practice	Ia	A	17
❑ There is no evidence of increased morbidity associated with exteriorization of the uterus	Ia	A	18
❑ Subrectus suction drainage reduces the rate of wound infection	Ib	A	19

References

1 Reid VC, Hartmann KE, McMahon M *et al.* (2001) Vaginal preparation with povidone iodine and postcesarean infectious morbidity: a randomized controlled trial. *Obstet Gynecol* **97**, 147–152. RCT to determine if vaginal preparation with povidone iodine before cesarean decreased the incidence of postpartum infectious morbidity (with

247 in treatment and 251 in control group). The groups were comparable. Vaginal preparation with povidone iodine before cesarean had no effect on risk for fever (RR 1.1, 95% CI 0.8–1.6), endometritis (RR 1.6, 95% CI 0.8–3.1) or wound separation (RR 0.6, 95% CI 0.3–1.3). **Ib A**

2 Mowat J, Bonnar J (1971) Abdominal wound dehiscence after caesarean section. *Br Med J* **2**, 256–257. Single-center comparative study from 1964–69 of 1635 women undergoing vertical abdominal incisions and 540 delivered using a low transverse incision. 48 (2.94%) women in the vertical incision group had a wound dehiscence (25 partial and 23 complete). 2 (0.37%) women had dehiscence in the transverse incision group. There were no differences in the rate of dehiscence between the emergency and elective cesarean section groups. **III B**

3 Irvine DS, Haddad NG (1989) Classical versus low-segment transverse incision for preterm cesarean section: maternal complications and outcome of subsequent pregnancies. *Br J Obstet Gynaecol* **96**, 371–372. 70 women undergoing classical cesarean section were compared to 71 women having a low transverse uterine incision. Cases were matched. Antibiotic prophylaxis was not routine. Classical incision was associated with a higher rate of postpartum febrile morbidity (16 vs 6%, $p < 0.01$). **III B**

4 Lao TT, Halpern SH, Crosby ET *et al.* (1993) Uterine incision and maternal blood loss in preterm cesarean section. *Arch Gynecol Obstet* **252**, 113–117. Retrospective case controlled study comparing 31 women delivered by classical cesarean section between 25 and 34 weeks gestation with 31 women delivered by lower segment cesarean section. Patients were matched for gestational age at delivery, the type of anesthesia, and the prior use of tocolytic therapy. There was a slightly higher number of laboring women in the classical incision group – 17 (54.8%) vs 9 (29%), $p < 0.05$) – and fewer presentations were cephalic (9 vs 18, $p < 0.05$). There was a significantly greater reduction in maternal hemoglobin 9 g/dl and a higher incidence of severe bleeding in the classical cesarean section group compared to the lower segment cesarean section group ($p < 0.05$). **III B**

5 Rogers J, Wood J, McCandlish R *et al.* (1998) Active versus expectant management of third stage of labour: the Hinchingbrooke randomised controlled trial. *Lancet* **351**, 693–699. 1512 women judged to be at low risk of postpartum hemorrhage (PPH; blood loss > 500 ml) were randomly assigned active management of the third stage (prophylactic oxytocic within 2 min of baby's birth, immediate cutting and clamping of the cord, delivery of placenta by controlled cord traction or maternal effort) or expectant management (no prophylactic oxytocic, no cord clamping until pulsation ceased, delivery of placenta by maternal effort). Women were also randomly assigned upright or supine posture. Analyses were by intention to treat. The rate of PPH was significantly lower with active than with expectant management (51/748, 6.8% vs 126/764, 16.5%, RR 2.42, 95% CI 1.78–3.30, $p < 0.0001$). Posture had no effect on this risk (upright 92/755, 12% vs supine 85/757, 11%). **Ib A**

6 McDonald S, Prendiville WJ, Elbourne D (2001) Prophylactic syntometrine versus oxytocin for delivery of the placenta. In: *The Cochrane library*, issue 2. Oxford: Update Software. This review was to assess the effects of ergometrine–oxytocin (syntometrine) with oxytocin alone in reducing the risk of postpartum hemorrhage. Six trials were included. Compared with oxytocin, ergometrine–oxytocin (syntometrine) was associated with a small reduction in the risk of postpartum hemorrhage (OR 0.74, 95% CI 0.65–0.85). This advantage was smaller but still significant when 10 international units of oxytocin was used. There was no difference seen between the groups using either 5 or 10 IU for blood loss equal to or greater than 1000 ml. Adverse effects of vomiting and hypertension were associated with the use of ergometrine–oxytocin. No significant differences were found in other maternal or neonatal outcomes. **Ia A**

7 Acharya G, Al-Sammarai MT, Patel N *et al.* (2001) A randomized, controlled trial comparing effect of oral misoprostol and intravenous syntocinon on intra-operative blood loss during cesarean section. *Acta Obstet Gynecol Scand* **80**, 245–250. Small RCT comparing 60 women undergoing elective cesarean section, randomized to receive either 10 U Syntocinon or 400 mg oral misoprostol after delivery of the baby. The main outcome measures were estimated blood loss and drop in measured hemoglobin. The estimated blood loss was 545 ml (CI 476–614) in the misoprostol group and 533 ml (CI 427–639) in the Syntocinon group ($p = 0.85$). There was a trend towards the placenta needing to be manually delivered in the misoprostol group (10 vs 4 women, $p = 0.067$). **Ib A**

8 Chou MM, MacKenzie IZ (1994) A prospective, double-blind, randomized comparison of prophylactic intramyometrial 15-methyl prostaglandin F2 alpha, 125 micrograms, and intravenous oxytocin, 20 units, for the control of blood loss at elective cesarean. *Am J Obstet Gynecol* **171**, 1356–1360. Double-blind RCT randomized 60 women delivered by elective lower segment cesarean section at term compared intramyometrial 15-methyl prostaglandin (PG)$F_{2\alpha}$ with intravenous oxytocin. The mean estimated blood loss was similar in both groups, with 645 ml (SD 278, range 400–1500) in the 15-methyl $PGF_{2\alpha}$ group compared with 605 ml (SD 303, range 200–1750) in the oxytocin group. **Ib A**

9 Dansereau J, Joshi AK, Helewa ME *et al.* (1999) Double-blind comparison of Carbetocin versus oxytocin in prevention of uterine atony after cesarean section. *Am J Obstet Gynecol* **180**, 670–676. Multicenter double-blind, RCT studied 659 patients undergoing elective cesarean section comparing a single 100 µg dose of Carbetocin (a long-acting oxytocin analog) with an initial intravenous dose of 5 U oxytocin followed by an 8 h infusion of 20 U oxytocin in 1000 ml. The odds of treatment failure requiring oxytocic intervention was 2.03 (95% CI 1.1–2.8) times higher in the oxytocin group than in the Carbetocin group, respectively 32/318 (10.1%) versus 15/317 (4.7%), $p < 0.05$. There was no difference in fall in hemoglobin between the two groups. **Ib A**

10 Wilkinson C, Enkin MW (2001) Manual removal of placenta at caesarean section (Cochrane Review). In: *The Cochrane library*, issue 2. Oxford: Update Software. Three randomized and quasi-randomized trials including 224

women were reviewed. Manual removal of placenta was compared to spontaneous separation and controlled cord traction for delivery in pregnant women undergoing elective or emergency cesarean section. Manual removal of the placenta was associated with a clinically important and statistically significant increase in maternal blood loss (weighted mean difference 436.35, 95% CI 347.82–524.90). Manual removal was also associated with increased postpartum endometritis (OR 5.44, 95% CI 1.25–23.75) and a statistically nonsignificant trend towards an increase in feto-maternal hemorrhage (OR 2.19, 95% CI 0.69–6.93). The review concludes that manual removal is associated with increased maternal blood loss and increased risk of infection. **Ia A**

11 Smaill F, Hofmeyr GJ (2001) Antibiotic prophylaxis for caesarean section. In: *The Cochrane library*, issue 2. Oxford: Update Software. This systematic review of 66 RCTs showed that use of prophylactic antibiotics in women undergoing cesarean section substantially reduced the incidence of episodes of fever, endometritis (RR 0.39, 95% CI 0.33–0.46), wound infection (RR 0.36, 95% CI 0.26–0.51), urinary tract infection (RR 0.4, 95% CI 0.28–0.57) and serious infection after emergency cesarean section (RR 0.28, 95% CI 0.13–0.61). The differences for elective cesarean section were less marked but reached statistical significance for endometritis (RR 0.4, 95% CI 0.2–0.79). **Ia A**

12 Hofmeyr GJ, Smaill F (2001) Antibiotic prophylaxis regimens and drugs for caesarean section. In: *The Cochrane library*, issue 2. Oxford: Update Software. This systematic review of 51 RCTs showed that no drug regimen was superior to any other and that ampicillin and first-generation cephalosporins are equally effective in reducing postoperative endometritis. Single-dose regimens are as effective as repeat doses, with the exception of urinary tract infection. **Ia A**

13 Department of Health (2000) *Why mothers die. Report on confidential enquiries into maternal deaths in the United Kingdom 1994–1996*. London: The Stationery Office. The advice that thromboembolism deterrent therapy is recommended for all women undergoing cesarean section does not derive from any randomized studies in pregnancy. This report recognizes that pregnancy is a time of hypercoagulability. Thromboembolism is the leading cause of maternal deaths in the UK, with 48 deaths reported. The report encompasses the guidance issued in the report of the Royal College of Obstetricians and Gynaecologists working party on thromboprophylaxis against thromboembolism in gynecology and obstetrics, which divides women into low, moderate and high risk with differing levels of prophylaxis for each group. Evidence from multiple trials of nonpregnant subjects suggests that peri- and postoperative thromboprophylaxis is effective in reducing thromboembolic morbidity. **IV C**

14 Wilkinson C, Enkin MW (2001) Lateral tilt for caesarean section. In: *The Cochrane library*, issue 2. Oxford: Update Software. Three trials are included, assessing 193 women, but they are all methodologically poor. Two of the three assess only elective cesarean section. All trials were pre-1974 and given the good observational data available it is unlikely that further trials will ever be undertaken. Only minimal data could be obtained from these studies. Low Apgar scores (as defined by the authors) were fewer with the use of a lateral tilt (OR 0.53, 95% CI 0.25–1.16). In general, pH measurements and oxygen saturation appeared to be somewhat better in the groups with the lateral tilt. **Ia A**

15 Wilkinson C, Enkin MW (2001) Absorbable staples for uterine incision at caesarean section. In: *The Cochrane library*, issue 2. Oxford: Update Software. Review of four trials on the use of absorbable staples to close the uterine incision showed that staples had no obvious benefit or harm in terms of time, measurable blood loss, drop in hemoglobin, need for transfusion or hemoglobin below 10g/dl. **Ia A**

16 Enkin MW, Wilkinson C (2001) Single versus two layer suturing for closing the uterine incision at caesarean section. In: *The Cochrane library*, issue 2, Oxford: Update Software. Only two trials are included, but these are both sizable and include 1066 women. One trial examined only the single outcome of radiographic scar appearance. Although allocation was unbiased in the other trial, analysis was not by intention to treat and almost 9% of the participants were excluded from analysis because of failure of compliance or missing data. Operating time was shorter by 5.6min in the single layer closure group. There were fewer radiographically determined scar defects at 3 months in the single closure group (OR 0.19, 95% CI 0.07–0.51); however, the methodology of this trial is suspect and, even if this is a true finding, its significance in clinical practice is unclear. There were no statistically significant differences in use of extra hemostatic sutures (OR 0.88, 95% CI 0.67–1.14), incidence of endometritis (OR 1.28, 95% CI 0.89–1.82), decrease in postoperative hematocrit by more than 8% (OR 1.12, 95% CI 0.82–1.52) or use of blood transfusion (OR 0.8, 95% CI 0.33–1.94). **Ia A**

17 Wilkinson CS, Enkin MW (2001) Peritoneal non-closure at caesarean section. In: *The Cochrane library*, issue 2. Oxford: Update Software. Four trials including 1194 women were assessed. Only one of the trials had good methodological quality in terms of good concealment of treatment allocation. Trials compared leaving the visceral and/or parietal peritoneum unsutured at cesarean section with suturing the peritoneum. Overall nonclosure of visceral and/or parietal peritoneum was associated with a reduced postoperative stay (WMD −0.21, CI −0.37 to −0.05) and a trend toward reduced postoperative fever and wound infection that did not quite reach statistical significance. **Ia A**

18 Wilkinson C, Enkin MW (2001) Uterine exteriorization versus intraperitoneal repair at caesarean section. In: *The Cochrane library*, issue 2. Oxford: Update Software. Two trials were included in this review, randomizing 486 women. Neither trial is methodologically strong and, as one trial excluded 20% of women from analysis, there is potential for bias. Only one of the trials assessed postoperative morbidity; however this is a large trial, including 208 women. The main outcome measures were estimated blood loss, postoperative drop in hematocrit, fever for more than 3 days, endometritis and intraoperative vomiting. There is at present insufficient data to evaluate routine use of exteriorization but it is not associated in this analysis with increased morbidity. **Ia A**

19 Loong RLC, Rogers MS, Chang AM (1988) A controlled trial on wound drainage in caesarean section. *Aust NZ J Obstet Gynaecol* **28**, 266–269. RCT of 262 women aimed to assess the effect of subrectus and subcutaneous wound drainage on the incidence of wound infection. Wound infection was less frequent in women who had a subrectus drain (5/127 vs 19/135, $p < 0.01$, standardized morbidity 0.40). **Ib A**

POSTNATAL

Chapter 48

Postnatal problems

48.1 Postpartum hemorrhage

Sunita Sharma and Hazem El-Refaey

Comments

- Randomized controlled trials in the treatment of life-threatening conditions such as postpartum hemorrhage are difficult to organize and justify. Therefore, assessment of efficacy cannot be generated from an RCT alone and there are obvious gaps in knowledge using this approach.
- Many RCTs use 'estimated blood loss' as an endpoint; however, this is poorly reproducible. Hemoglobin level has not been used as widely. Its reproducibility is beyond doubt and it is clinically relevant because it is used in assessing the need for blood transfusion. Thus, hemoglobin levels should be the outcome measure in future studies.
- There is lack of information about specific aspects of the use of uterotonic agents (e.g. intravenous versus intramuscular oxytocics or the use of bolus injections versus infusions of oxytocin).

Prevention of postpartum hemorrhage

Management option	Quality of evidence	Strength of recommendation	References
Intravenous access for women at risk	–	✔	–
Save serum for rapid cross-match if needed or actually cross-match two units for women at risk	–	✔	–
Active management of third stage for all women: ❑ Oxytocic agent ❑ Controlled cord traction ❑ Clamp and cut cord	Ia III	A B	1 2

References

Comment: There has never been a large trial to study the magnitude of effect of each single individual component of the active management package. Studies so far support the use of the entire package of active management of third stage of labor.

1 Prendiville WJ, Elbourne D, McDonald S (2001) Active versus expectant management in the third stage of labour. In: *The Cochrane library*, issue 4. Oxford: Update Software. This meta-analysis included five RCTs. Of these, four trials were of good quality. Compared to expectant management, active management (in the setting of a maternity hospital) was associated with the following reduced risks: maternal blood loss (weighted mean difference −79.33 ml, 95% CI −94.29 to −64.37); postpartum hemorrhage of more than 500 ml (RR 0.38, 95% CI 0.32–0.46); prolonged third stage of labor (weighted mean difference −9.77 min, 95% CI −10.00 to −9.53). Active management was associated with an increased risk of maternal nausea (RR 1.83, 95% CI 1.51–2.23), vomiting and raised blood pressure (probably due to the use of ergometrine). No advantages or disadvantages were apparent for the baby. The implications of this meta-analysis are less clear for other settings, including domiciliary practice (in developing and industrialized countries). **Ia A**

2 Spencer PM (1962) Controlled cord traction in the management of the third stage of labour. *Br Med J* **1** 1728–1732. A prospective uncontrolled clinical trial of 1000 consecutive deliveries in women at low risk of obstetric hemorrhage. At the delivery of anterior shoulder, intravenous ergometrine 0.5 mg was given. Following delivery of the baby, the cord was clamped and cut and the placenta was delivered by controlled cord traction. The mean blood loss and duration of the third stage was 90 ml and 6.3 min respectively. Retained placenta occurred in 2.1% of patients. **III B**

Management of primary postpartum hemorrhage

Management option		Quality of evidence	Strength of recommendation	References
Initial emergency measures	Rub-up contraction	–	✔	–
	Intravenous oxytocin (5–10IU; ergometrine 0.25–0.5mg i.m. is an alternative but should be avoided in hypertensive patients)	–	✔	–
	Establish intravenous access	–	✔	–
	Cross-match blood	–	✔	–
	General management of major obstetric hemorrhage, see Section 44.1			
Specific measures	Examine uterus to confirm atony is cause	–	✔	–
	Confirm that placenta appears intact, or uterine exploration and removal of placental fragments if suspicion of incomplete third stage	–	✔	–
	Bimanual compression is a temporary measure	–	✔	–
	Commence intravenous oxytocin infusion	III	B	1
	Give further intravenous bolus of oxytocin	–	✔	–
	Rule out trauma to vagina, cervix or uterus	–	✔	–
	Uterine packing or balloon tamponade	III	B	2,3
	Prostaglandin (PG) options: ❑ $PGF_{2\alpha}$ (0.5–1.0mg) into uterine muscle ❑ 15-methyl-PGF_{α} (0.25mg) intramuscularly or into uterine muscle ❑ Rectal misoprostol	III III Ib	B B A	4,5 6 7
	B-Lynch sutures	III	B	8,9
	Arterial embolization if units have resources and experience	III	B	10,11
	Bilateral uterine artery ligation	III	B	12,13
	Bilateral internal iliac artery ligation	III	B	14,15
	Bilateral ovarian artery ligation	III	B	16
	Hysterectomy	III	B	17,18

References

1 Daro AF, Gollin HA, Lavieri V (1952) A management of postpartum hemorrhage by prolonged administration of oxytocics. *Am J Obstet Gynecol* **64**, 1163–1166. An observational study of four patients. **III B**

2 Maier RC (1993) Control of postpartum hemorrhage with uterine packing. *Am J Obstet Gynecol* **169**, 317–323. A retrospective review of postpartum records of 10 women who underwent uterine packing during 1985–91. In one woman the instrument (Torpin packer) did not work and therefore packing was abandoned. Review of the remaining nine notes showed that seven women did not need a hysterectomy. The time interval until the pack is removed varied from 5–96h. **III B**

3 Hester JD (1975) Postpartum hemorrhage and re-evaluation of uterine packing. *Obstet Gynecol* **45**, 501–505. This study is a retrospective review of a 10-year period, during which 33 women underwent uterine packing to control postpartum hemorrhage. Of these, 29 did not require hysterectomy, although one was readmitted to the hospital with a hemoglobin value of 7.6g/dl and was managed conservatively. **III B**

4 Hayashi RH, Castillo MS, Noah ML (1984) Management of severe postpartum hemorrhage with a prostaglandin F2 alpha analogue. *Obstet Gynecol* **63**, 806–809. Prospective observational trial where 54 women with severe postpartum hemorrhage (PPH), due to uterine atony, unresponsive to conventional therapy were treated with intramuscular injection of (15-S)-15-methyl prostaglandin analog $F_{2\alpha}$-tromethamine. Successful control of PPH occurred in 86% and 7 women required surgical therapy. 6 subjects were given the prostaglandin analog intramyometrially, with dramatic success in 5 of them. **III B**

5 Bruce SL, Paul RH, Van Dorsten JP (1982) Control of postpartum uterine atony by intramyometrial prostaglandin. *Obstet Gynecol* **59**, 47S–50S. Prospective observational trial where five patients with severe PPH due to uterine atony and unresponsive to conventional treatment were treated with intramyometrial $PGF_{2\alpha}$. 60% of these women responded successfully with an increase in uterine tone. The other two women had a hysterectomy to control their blood loss. **III B**

6 O'Brien P, El-Refaey H, Gordon A *et al.* (1998) Rectally administered misoprostol for the treatment of postpartum hemorrhage unresponsive to oxytocin and ergometrine: a descriptive study. *Obstet Gynecol* **92**, 212–214. A prospective observational trial involving the use of rectally administered misoprostol (1000 μg) in 14 women with postpartum hemorrhage. The hemorrhage was controlled in all patients and a sustained uterine contraction was noted within 3 min of administration of misoprostol. **III B**

7 Lokugamage AU, Sullivan KR, Niculescu I *et al.* (2001) A randomized study comparing rectally administered misoprostol versus Syntometrine combined with an oxytocin infusion for the cessation of primary post partum hemorrhage. *Acta Obstet Gynecol Scand* **80**, 835–839. Randomized single-blinded study done to compare intramuscular Syntometrine (1 ampoule) plus Syntocinon (10 IU oxytocin diluted in 500 ml normal saline) infusion with 800 μg misoprostol administered rectally for the treatment of primary postpartum hemorrhage (PPH) in a developing country. 64 women with primary PPH due to an atonic uterus were recruited. The primary outcome was whether the hemorrhage ceased within 20 min of administering the first-line treatment, once hemorrhage was clinically recognized. A 28.1% difference between the misoprostol arm and the Syntometrine and Syntocinon arm ($p = 0.01$) was noted. Misoprostol performed better. **Ib A**

8 B-Lynch C, Coker A, Lawal AH *et al.* (1997) The B-Lynch surgical technique for the control of massive postpartum haemorrhage: an alternative to hysterectomy. Five cases reported. *Br J Obstet Gynaecol* **104**, 372–375. Report of five cases. **III B**

9 Goddard R (1998) The B-Lynch surgical technique for the control of massive postpartum haemorrhage: an alternative to hysterectomy? Five cases reported. *Br J Obstet Gynaecol* **105**, 126. Report of five cases. **III B**

10 Yamashita Y, Harada M, Yamamoto H *et al.* (1994) Transcatheter arterial embolisation of obstetric and gynaecological bleeding: efficacy and clinical outcome. *Br J Radiol* **67**, 530–534. Retrospective review of 32 patients with uncontrollable genital bleeding who were treated by arterial embolization therapy on an emergency basis. Of these, 15 women had postpartum hemorrhage (PPH). On angiography, the bleeding arteries were identified as the internal pudendal artery in 8 patients, the uterine artery in 6 and the obturator artery in 2. The site of embolized arteries included 5 anterior of the internal iliac artery, 6 internal pudendal arteries, 5 uterine arteries and 2 obturator arteries. Of the15 women with PPH, 13 did not require a hysterectomy. Postembolization ultrasound follow-up showed hematomas in the pelvic extraperitoneal space in 12 patients. 2 of these women required laparotomy for the pelvic mass while spontaneous drainage or absorption of the hematoma occurred within a month in patients with small hematomas. Menstruation resumed within 4–8 months of embolization in those who did not undergo hysterectomy. **III B**

11 Pelage JP, Le Dref O, Mateo J *et al.* (1998) Life-threatening primary postpartum hemorrhage: treatment with emergency selective arterial embolisation. *Radiology* **208**, 359–362. Prospective study of 27 consecutive women with life-threatening postpartum hemorrhage who underwent uterine embolization. Hysterectomy was performed in 2 patients before embolization failed to stop their bleeding. 2 women required repeat embolization the next day. No major complication was noted in these patients and normal menstruation returned in all women except for the 2 women who needed a hysterectomy. **III B**

12 O'Leary JL, O'Leary JA (1966) Uterine artery ligation in the control of intractable postpartum hemorrhage. *Am J Obstet Gynecol* **94**, 920–924. Retrospective reviews of 10 cases treated by the authors are reviewed. 8 were successfully managed by bilateral uterine artery ligation; 2 women required further therapy (hysterectomy and ligation of placenta site respectively). **III B**

13 O'Leary JA (1995) Uterine artery ligation in the control of postcesarean hemorrhage. *J Reprod Med* **40**, 189–193. Retrospective review of a center's experience with 265 patients with postpartum hemorrhage, where the technique of devascularizing the post-cesarean-section uterus with bilateral mass ligation of the ascending branches of the uterine arteries and veins was used. 10 patients required additional therapy. **III B**

14 Das BN, Biswas AK (1998) Ligation of internal iliac arteries in pelvic haemorrhage. *J Obstet Gynaecol Res* **24**, 251–254. A prospective observational study over 5 years to assess the value of ligation of bilateral internal iliac arteries in 15 women with postpartum hemorrhage (PPH). The method controlled PPH in all cases except one, who required hysterectomy. The method was effective in 75% of atonic PPHs and in the majority of PPHs due to other causes, including cesarean section. The surgeons felt that the procedure did not involve any hazard. **III B**

15 Fernandez H, Pons JC, Chambon G *et al.* (1988) Internal iliac artery ligation in post-partum hemorrhage. *Eur J Obstet Gynecol Reprod Biol* **28**, 213–220. Retrospective review of this procedure done in 8 patients with severe postpartum hemorrhage. Disseminated intravascular coagulation combined with causal pathology was noted in 5 patients. No patient required a hysterectomy, although one woman developed postoperative occlusion and another renal failure following secondary cortical renal necrosis. **III B**

16 Thavarasah AS, Sivalingam N, Almohdzar SA (1989) Internal iliac and ovarian artery ligation in the control of pelvic haemorrhage. *Aust N Z J Obstet Gynaecol* **29**, 22–25. Retrospective review of this procedure undertaken in 14 patients with severe postpartum hemorrhage in two hospitals during 1983–86. Bilateral internal iliac artery ligation was initially done in all patients. If the bleeding persisted, bilateral ovarian artery ligation was performed (2 patients). 4 patients required hysterectomy. 3 of these had placenta accreta and one ruptured uterus. Of the 14 patients, 2 died – one with disseminated intravascular coagulation on the third day and one 12h following cardiac arrest on the operating table. No complications of the procedure were noted. **III B**

17 Zelop CM, Harlow BL, Frigoletto FD Jr *et al.* (1993) Emergency peripartum hysterectomy. *Am J Obstet Gynecol* **168**, 1443–1448. Retrospective review of the obstetric records of women who underwent emergency postpartum hysterectomy over an 8-year period. In total 117 women were identified and despite high morbidity (postoperative infection 50%, intraoperative urological injuries 9%, blood transfusion 87%) there were no maternal deaths. **III B**

18 Castaneda S, Karrison T, Cibils LA (2000) Peripartum hysterectomy. *J Perinat Med* **28**, 472–481. Retrospective review of the hospital records of women undergoing peripartum hysterectomy during 1965–95. Of the 207 notes found, total hysterectomy was done in 94% and the procedure was planned in about 60% of these women. Blood transfusion rate was 57% and 84% in the planned and emergency procedures respectively. 12 patients needed another surgical operation to deal with surgical complications. No women died during the study period. **III B**

Management of secondary postpartum hemorrhage

Management option	Quality of evidence	Strength of recommendation	References
Clinical features important in making diagnosis. Ultrasonography of uterine contents does not distinguish blood clot from placenta; echogenic masses are found in asymptomatic women. Empty uterus on scan may allow a conservative approach	III	B	1,2
Antibiotics for 12–24h prior to surgical evacuation	–	✔	–
Uterotonics and antibiotics may reduce need for curettage	III	B	2
Surgical/suction evacuation of uterus	III	B	3,4

References

1 Edwards A, Ellwood DA (2000) Ultrasonographic evaluation of the postpartum uterus. *Ultrasound Obstet Gynecol* **16**, 640–643. Prospective study to define the ultrasonographic appearance of the uterus and the uterine cavity, in normal women making an uncomplicated postpartum recovery. The ultrasound scan revealed an echogenic mass in 51% of women with normal postpartum bleeding at 7 days, 21% at 14 days and 6% at 21 days post-partum. **III B**

2 Lee CY, Madrazo B, Drukker BH (1981) Ultrasonic evaluation of the postpartum uterus in the management of postpartum bleeding. *Obstet Gynecol* **58**, 227–232. 56 patients with postpartum bleeding underwent ultrasonic evaluation of postpartum uterus. Retained placental tissue was found in 9 patients and large blood clots in 5. 42 patients who were found to have an empty uterus were treated conservatively with intravenous oxytocin infusion. The ultrasonic diagnosis correlated well with the clinical findings and with response to treatment. **III B**

3 King PA, Duthie SJ, Dong ZG *et al.* (1989) Secondary postpartum haemorrhage. *Aust N Z J Obstet Gynaecol* **29**, 394–398. Retrospective review of 83 cases of secondary postpartum hemorrhage managed over a 3-year period. Suction evacuation was performed in 72 patients and was successful in arresting hemorrhage. There was histological confirmation of retained gestational products in only 30 (42%) of the patients treated surgically. **III B**

4 Thorsteinsson VT, Kempers RD (1970) Delayed postpartum bleeding. *Am J Obstet Gynecol* **107**, 565–571. Retrospective review of 148 patients treated with delayed postpartum hemorrhage during 1957–66. Uterotonic agents alone were successful in the management of 35.2% of patients. The remaining 94 patients (64.8%) required surgical treatment in addition to uterotonic agents. Curettage was done once in 87 patients and twice in 3 patients, while hysterectomy was carried out in 3 patients and one patient underwent myomectomy. **III B**

48.2 Other problems of the third stage

Sunita Sharma and Hazem El-Refaey

Placenta accreta

Management option	Quality of evidence	Strength of recommendation	References
Diagnosis of problem is difficult	III	B	1–3
Intravenous access and resuscitation	–	✔	–
Options for treatment: ❑ Curettage ❑ Manual removal ❑ Hysterectomy ❑ Others include overseeing implantation site, resection of implantation site, stepwise uterine devascularization	III	B	4
Treat any associated uterine atony as described above under **Treatment of primary postpartum hemorrhage**	–	✔	–

References

1 Finberg HJ, Williams JW (1992) Placenta accreta: prospective sonographic diagnosis in patients with placenta previa and prior cesarean section. *J Ultrasound Med* **11**, 333–343. A prospective evaluation for possible placenta accreta was performed in 34 patients with placenta previa and a history of one or more cesarean sections. Of 18 patients with positive sonographic results, 14 had proof of placenta accreta and 16 of the patients underwent hysterectomy. Of 16 patients with negative sonographic results, only one had placenta accreta and 2 patients required hysterectomy. Presence of numerous intraplacental vascular lacunae appears to be an additional risk criterion for placenta accreta, separate from the other criteria listed above. **III B**

2 Guy GP, Peisner DB, Timor-Tritsch IE (1990) Ultrasonographic evaluation of uteroplacental flow patterns of abnormally located and adherent placentas. *Am J Obstet Gynecol* **163**, 723–727. The study patients (76 in total) were referred to the ultrasound department with antepartum bleeding and suspected placenta previa. Of these, 10 patients were found to have persistent placenta previa with lacunar blood flow pattern on transvaginal ultrasound scan. 2 patients were lost to follow up. Retrospective analysis of clinical outcome was done on the remaining 8 patients: 7 required a cesarean hysterectomy and pathology confirmed placenta accreta/increta. Also identified were 6 patients with persistent placenta previa and no lacunar blood flow who underwent cesarean section. None of the patients in this group had placenta accreta or hemorrhagic course requiring hysterectomy or arterial ligation. **III B**

3 Levine D, Hulka CA, Ludmir J *et al.* (1997) Placenta accreta: evaluation with color Doppler US, power Doppler US, and MR imaging. *Radiology* **205**, 773–776. A study of 19 patients clinically identified to be at high risk of placenta accreta, who underwent color Doppler and power Doppler ultrasound; of these, 18 also had magnetic resonance imaging (MRI). Two reviewers interpreted images prospectively for signs of placenta accreta and their level of confidence in the diagnosis was noted. 5 cases of lower uterine segment placenta accreta were diagnosed with a high level of confidence with vaginal and power Doppler ultrasound. In one patient with posterior placenta who had undergone previous myomectomy, only MRI enabled the diagnosis of placenta accreta. Clinical outcomes showed that 7 patients had placenta accreta and 4 women underwent hysterectomy. The sensitivity and specificity of ultrasound in this diagnosis was 86% and 92% respectively. Ultrasound had 100% sensitivity for diagnosis of anterior placenta accreta. **III B**

4 Read JA, Cotton DB, Miller FC (1980) Placenta accreta: changing clinical aspects and outcome. *Obstet Gynecol* **56**, 31–34. Retrospective review of 22 women with placenta accreta diagnosed over a 4-year period. Among those delivered by cesarean section (16), hysterectomy was done in 14 cases, suture of the bleeding site alone or in combination with uterine artery ligation (3 cases) and curettage (1 case). In 2 of the 6 vaginal deliveries, hysterectomy was needed in 2 patients while curettage and manual removal were successful in the other 4. **III B**

Uterine inversion

Management option	Quality of evidence	Strength of recommendation	References
Prompt recognition and treatment are keys to successful outcome	III	B	1
Intravenous access and resuscitation	III	B	1
Options for treatment:			
❑ Manual replacement (with/without a general anesthetic and/or tocolytics)	III	B	2
❑ Hydrostatic replacement	III	B	3,4
❑ Laparotomy and correction 'from above'	III	B	3,4

References

1 Das P (1940) Inversion of the uterus. *Br J Obstet Gynaecol* **47**, 525–547. Retrospective review of 391 cases reported in the literature. Management conclusions had been drawn from analysis of the outcomes in these cases. **III B**

2 Brar HS, Greenspoon JS, Platt LD *et al.* (1989) Acute puerperal uterine inversion. New approaches to management. *J Reprod Med* **34**, 173–177. A retrospective review of 56 patients with uterine inversion during the period July 1977 to June 1986. **III B**

3 Shah-Hosseini R, Evrard JR (1989) Puerperal uterine inversion. *Obstet Gynecol* **57**, 567–570. A 10-year retrospective review of acute puerperal inversion of the uterus. There were 11 inversions in 70481 deliveries. Vaginal replacement was successful in 9 patients. One patient had a placenta accreta necessitating a supracervical hysterectomy and one patient required a laparotomy and Huntington procedure for replacement. There were no maternal deaths. **III B**

4 Dali SM, Rajbhandari S, Shrestha S (1997) Puerperal inversion of the uterus in Nepal: case reports and review of literature. *J Obstet Gynaecol Res* **23**: 319–325. Retrospective study of 6 cases of puerperal inversion of the uterus managed over 20 years. One patient with acute puerperal inversion of uterus was treated by manual reposition, 2 with chronic puerperal inversion were treated surgically by Kustner's vaginal approach. 2 patients with subacute puerperal inversion and one with chronic puerperal inversion were treated by the Haultain and Huntington method. **III B**

Uterine rupture

Management option	Quality of evidence	Strength of recommendation	References
Diagnosis confirmed by EUA or laparotomy	–	✔	–
Surgical options:			
❑ Hysterectomy	III	B	1
❑ Repair	III	B	1,2
In subsequent pregnancies, elective cesarean section is advocated by most	III	B	1

References

1 Ritchie EH (1971) Pregnancy after rupture of the pregnant uterus. *J Obstet Gynaecol Br Commonw* **78**, 642–648. A retrospective review of the literature for the outcome of pregnancies following a suture repair of ruptured uterus. Since 1923, there had been 253 pregnancies reported in 194 women following uterine rupture. The incidence of repeat rupture was 13%. In subsequent pregnancies, the rupture rate was 6.4% for lower segment scars, 46% for classical scars and 20% for other upper segment scars. Maternal mortality was 1/100 patients and perinatal mortality was 59/1000 births. **III B**

2. O'Connor RA, Gaughan B (1989) Pregnancy following simple repair of the ruptures gravid uterus. *Br J Obstet Gynaecol* **96**, 942–944. Review of 15 women who had a total of 18 pregnancies following a simple repair for a previous rupture of the uterus in pregnancy. 17 of the women had a successful outcome and there was no case of repeat rupture. 13 of the 15 women had had a previous lower segment uterine rupture. **III B**

Amniotic fluid embolism

Management option	Quality of evidence	Strength of recommendation	References
If diagnosed before death, management is largely directed toward general, resuscitative and supportive measures: ❑ Oxygen ❑ Maintain circulation (e.g. dopamine, digoxin) ❑ Intensive care unit ❑ Treat any disseminated intravascular coagulation	III IV	B C	1 2

References

1 Clark SL, Hankins GD, Dudley DA *et al.* (1995) Amniotic fluid embolism: analysis of the national registry. *Am J Obstet Gynecol* **172**, 1158–1162. A retrospective review of the medical records of 46 women diagnosed to have amniotic fluid embolism based on set criteria. Overall maternal mortality rate was 61%. Death occurred from 30min to 2 months after the initial event. Only 15% of patients survived neurologically intact. **III B**

2 Davies S (2001) Amniotic fluid embolus: a review of the literature. *Can J Anaesth* **48**, 88–98. Review article. **IV C**

48.3 Resuscitation and immediate care of the newborn

Janet Rennie

Deliveries where staff experienced in neonatal resuscitation should be informed and present

Management option		Quality of evidence	Strength of recommendation	References
Factors related to labor/ delivery	Cesarean section	III	B	1
	Breech delivery/other malpresentation	III	B	1
	Forceps/ventouse delivery (not 'lift-outs')	III	B	1
	Delivery after significant antepartum hemorrhage	III	B	1
	Prolapsed cord	III	B	1
Maternal factors	Medical disorder that may affect fetus	–	✔	–
	History of current drug or alcohol abuse	IIa	B	2
	Delivery under heavy sedation/general anesthesia	Ia III	A B	3 4,5
	Fever	IIa	B	6
Fetal factors	Multiple pregnancy (one pediatrician for each baby)	III	B	7
	Preterm delivery (<37 weeks)	IIa	B	8
	Prolonged membrane rupture or suspected chorioamnionitis	–	✔	–
	Hydramnios	–	✔	–
	Fetal distress	III	B	1
	Fetal abnormality (known/suspected)	–	✔	–
	Isoimmunization	IV	C	9

References

1 Primhak RA, Herber SM, Whincup G *et al.* (1984) Which deliveries require paediatricians in attendance? *Br Med J* **289**, 16–18. Retrospective descriptive study on the relationship between obstetric and fetal factors and low Apgar scores in 2086 full-term infants. 120/1794 deliveries had an Apgar of less than 7 at 1 min. In spontaneous vaginal vertex deliveries with fetal distress the frequency of a 1 min Apgar score below 7 was 10.2%. In operative and instrumental deliveries for fetal distress the frequency of a 1 min Apgar score below 7 was 15.6% after nonrotational forceps delivery, 13.9% after rotational forceps delivery and 45.8% after cesarean section. In the absence of fetal distress the frequency of an Apgar score below 7 was 2.4% after spontaneous deliveries, 7.1% after nonrotational forceps delivery, 13.2% after cesarean section and 18.4% after rotational forceps delivery. Attending the six categories at greatest risk (excluding preterms) led to attendance at 20% of deliveries at a yield of just over 50% of all deliveries with low to medium Apgar scores. It was concluded that neonatology services to an obstetric unit may be organized rationally with the help of these findings. **III B**

2 Eyler FD, Behnke M, Conlon M *et al.* (1994) Prenatal cocaine use: a comparison of neonates matched on maternal risk factors. *Neurotoxicol Teratol* **16**, 81–87. Case-control study on 172 cocaine users and 168 controls matched for race, age, parity, prenatal care and alcohol and nicotine use. Cocaine-exposed neonates experienced significantly more adverse events than the matched controls and were more likely to be preterm, have a low birthweight, be resuscitated at birth and remain in the hospital after their mothers were discharged. **IIa B**

3 Kolatat T, Somboonnanonda A, Lertakyamanee J *et al.* (1999) Effects of general and regional anesthesia on the neonate (a prospective, randomized trial). *J Med Assoc Thai* **82**, 40–45. Prospective randomized trial on the effects of general and regional anesthesia on the neonates of 341 women with uncomplicated pregnancies who were to be delivered at term by cesarean section and received either general anesthesia (GA; 103); epidural anesthesia (EA; 120) or spinal anesthesia (SA; 118). Outcomes were cord-blood gas analysis and Apgar scores. The Apgar scores at 1 min and 5 min were 8.3 ± 1.9 and 8.2 ± 1.6; 6.7 ± 2.8 and 9.7 ± 0.9; 9.8 ± 0.7 and 9.2 ± 1.6 in the EA, SA and GA groups respectively. It was concluded that the Apgar scores of the infants whose mothers received general anesthesia were lower than infants whose mothers received regional anesthesia. **Ia A**

4 Ong BY, Cohen MM, Palahniuk RJ (1989) Anesthesia for cesarean section: effects on neonates. *Anesth Analg* **68**, 270–275. Retrospective study on the effects of general and regional anesthesia on 3940 neonates after elective cesarean section, urgent cesarean section for failure to progress and emergency cesarean section for fetal distress. Outcomes were 1 min and 5 min Apgar scores, need for positive pressure oxygen by mask or intubation, and neonatal death. Overall, 12.5% had 1 min Apgar scores of 4 or less and 1.4% had 5 min Apgar scores of 4 or less. General anesthesia cases had worse outcomes than those with regional anesthesia. After elective section, general anesthesia was associated with a higher incidence of low Apgar scores at 1 min. In nonelective sections, general anesthesia was associated with higher rates of low Apgar scores at 1 min and 5 min and need for intubation and ventilation. There were no differences in neonatal death rates with general and regional anesthesia in the three groups. **III B**

5 Levine EM, Ghai V, Barton JJ *et al.* (1999) Pediatrician attendance at cesarean delivery: necessary or not? *Obstet Gynecol* **93**, 338–340. Retrospective study on 17 867 consecutive deliveries to determine the rates of low Apgar scores in vaginal deliveries, cesarean sections without a fetal indication using regional anesthesia, and cesarean deliveries for fetal indications, or using general anesthesia. 35 (5.8%) of 596 cesarean sections for fetal heart rate abnormality or using general anesthesia had 1 min Apgar scores under 4 in contrast to 115/10 270 (1.1%) vaginal deliveries. There was no significantly increased risk for low Apgar scores in the group of cesareans using regional anesthesia for nonfetal indications (33/2057, 1.6%). The results were similar for Apgar scores under 7 at 5 min. It was concluded that there is no convincing need for pediatrician attendance at cesarean sections using regional anesthesia for nonfetal indications. **III B**

6 Lieberman E, Eichenwald E, Mathur G *et al.* (2000) Intrapartum fever and unexplained seizures in term infants. *Pediatrics* **106**, 983–988. Case-control study on 38 term infants and 152 controls to investigate the association of noninfectious intrapartum fever (38°C or greater) with neonatal seizures in term infants. Infants with seizures were more likely to be born to mothers who were febrile during labor (31.6% vs 9.2%). Logistic regression analysis showed a 3.4 increase in the risk of unexplained neonatal seizures with intrapartum fever (OR 3.4, 95% CI 1.03–10.9). There was no evidence that the maternal fevers were due to infection. Some may have been related to epidural analgesia. **IIa B**

7 Prins RP (1994) The second-born twin: can we improve outcomes? *Am J Obstet Gynecol* **170**, 1649–1656. Retrospective study on 200 twin pairs to compare outcome between first- and second-born. The second-born twin was more likely to be intubated, have respiratory distress syndrome, a need for resuscitation and lower 5 min Apgar scores. In the under-1500 g group there were more second-born twin neonatal deaths and higher rates of intubation and resuscitation. Nonvertex presentation in the second-born twin increased chances of resuscitation, intubation and respiratory distress syndrome. These outcomes in the second-born were not affected by cesarean delivery. **III B**

8 Rogers JF, Graves WL (1993) Risk factors associated with low Apgar scores in a low-income population. *Paediatr Perinat Epidemiol* **7**, 205–216. Case-control study on 939 newborns with Apgar scores of less than 7 at 5 min compared with 2817 controls with Apgar scores of 7 or higher at 5 min to identify risk factors for these low Apgar scores. Birthweight below 2500 g and prematurity, pregnancy-induced hypertension, prolonged rupture of membranes, method of delivery and male sex were each significantly associated with Apgar scores of less than 7. Race was not found to be a significant risk factor. **IIa B**

9 Bowman J (1997) The management of hemolytic disease in the fetus and newborn. *Semin Perinatol* **21**, 39–44. Review on alloimmunization and hemolytic disease of the newborn, stating that, unless treated, hemolytic disease will result in kernicterus or fetal hydrops in 25% of cases. Neonatal exchange transfusion has eradicated kernicterus. The management of the severely affected fetus consists of early delivery, with or without fetal transfusions, depending on the gestation of the fetus. **IV C**

Resuscitation and immediate care of the newborn

Management option	Quality of evidence	Strength of recommendation	References
Thermal control: dry and wrap baby, then ABCD as below	III	B	1,2
Airway: suction as necessary	IV	C	3
Meconium-stained liquor: tracheal suction when indicated	IV Ib III	C A B	3 4 5
Breathing: consider commencing facemask ventilation or endotracheal intubation and ventilation as appropriate	IV IIb	C B	3 6
Chest compressions: consider drugs and/or other volume replacement if poor response	IV	C	3
Consider epinephrine (adrenaline) by endotracheal tube/ intravenously when no effect of ventilation on a heart rate of less than 60 bpm for over 30 s	IV	C	3
Consider naloxone to reverse possible opioid effects on respiratory efforts	Ib	A	7
No difference in resuscitation between room air and 100% oxygen	Ib	A	8
Maintain adequate levels of humidity	Ib	A	9

References

1 MacDonald HM, Mulligan JC, Allen AC *et al.* (1980) Neonatal asphyxia. I. Relationship of obstetric and neonatal complications to neonatal mortality in 38,405 consecutive deliveries. *J Pediatr* **96**, 898–902. Retrospective descriptive study to determine high-risk factors associated with birth asphyxia. Multivariate analysis showed that asphyxia occurred in 62.3% of infants of less than 27 weeks gestation and in 0.4% in infants of more than 38 weeks gestation. Among the asphyxiated neonates, growth retardation, hypothermia, hyaline membrane disease and seizures were significantly associated with an increased risk of death. **III B**

2 Blackfan KD, Yaglou CP (1933) The premature infant: a study of the effects of atmospheric conditions on growth and on development. *Am J Dis Child* **46**, 1175. Retrospective descriptive study of the effects of installing a central air-conditioning unit into nurseries on survival of premature infants. The period 1923–25 was compared to 1926–29. The body temperature of babies nursed in the heated room (after 1925) was much more stable than that of those nursed without air conditioning (before 1926). These babies gained weight faster, particularly when the humidity was high, and regained birth weight in an average of 15 days compared to 26 days. In the first period 64/123 (52%) died; in the second 97/229 (42%). For infants between 2 and 3 lb in weight the reduction in mortality was from 19/23 (82%) to 35/61 (61%). The ideal temperature was considered to be 75–100°F with 65% humidity. **III B**

3 Kattwinkel J, Niermeyer S, Nadkarni V *et al.* for the American Academy of Pediatrics (1999) Resuscitation of the newly born infant: an advisory statement from the Pediatric Working Group of the International Liaison Committee on Resuscitation. *Resuscitation* **40**, 71–88. Consensus document of the International Liaison Committee on Resuscitation (representation from North America, Europe, Australia, New Zealand, Africa, and South America) on neonatal resuscitation. It calls for the attendance of skilled personnel at every delivery, suctioning at the perineum in case of meconium-stained liquor, tracheal suction of meconium when indicated, assisted ventilation when spontaneous breathing is absent or the heart rate is less than 100 bpm, chest compression (120/min) if the heart rate is less than 60 bpm despite adequate assisted ventilation for 30 s (3:1 ratio), intratracheal or intravenous epinephrine (adrenaline; 0.01–0.03 mg/kg – 0.1–0.3 ml/kg of a 1:10000 solution) if no effect after 30 s effective assisted ventilation and chest compression. There was consensus on the insufficiency of data to recommend 100% rather than 21% oxygen, neuroprotective interventions such as cerebral hypothermia, use of a laryngeal mask versus endotracheal tube, and use of high-dose epinephrine. **IV C**

4 Wiswell TE, Gannon CM, Jacob J *et al.* (2000) Delivery room management of the apparently vigorous meconium-stained neonate: results of the multicenter, international collaborative trial. *Pediatrics* **105**, 1–7. Multicenter randomized trial comparing intubation and suction with expectant management in 2094 term newborns with vigorous meconium staining at birth. Of the 149 (7.1%) infants with respiratory distress, 62 (3.0%) developed meconium aspiration syndrome and 87 (4.2%) had findings attributed to other disorders. There were no significant differences between groups in the occurrence of meconium aspiration syndrome (3.2% vs 2.7%) or in the development of other respiratory disorders (3.8% vs 4.5%). Of 1098 successfully intubated infants, 42 (3.8%) had a total of 51 mild and transient complications. It was concluded that intubation and suctioning of the vigorous meconium-stained infant does not reduce meconium aspiration syndrome or other respiratory disorders. **Ib A**

5 Wiswell TE, Tuggle JM, Turner BS (1990) Meconium aspiration – have we made a difference? *Pediatrics* **85**, 715–721. Retrospective study on the incidence of meconium aspiration syndrome (MAS) in 176 790 neonates and its associated complications before and after the introduction of routine intubation and suctioning between 1973 and 1988. The incidence of MAS significantly decreased during the 15 years ($p = 0.043$) and the death rate from MAS also significantly declined ($p = 0.041$). Although the incidence of MAS and the related death rate have declined since the advent of combined obstetric and pediatric suctioning of the oropharynx and trachea, it was concluded that these declines were likely to have been influenced by other improvements in perinatal care during the study period. **III B**

6 Milner AD, Vyas H, Hopkin IE (1984) Efficacy of facemask resuscitation at birth. *Br Med J* **289**, 1563–1565. Experimental study comparing the expiratory tidal volume using a facemask with endotracheal intubation during the first three inflations in 18 babies with birth asphyxia. The tidal exchange in the facemask group was less than one third of that in the intubation group and rarely sufficient to produce adequate alveolar ventilation. It is concluded that in the facemask group successful resuscitation depended on the baby's own respiratory efforts. **IIb B**

7 Wiener PC, Hogg MI, Rosen M (1977) Effects of naloxone on pethidine-induced neonatal depression. *Br Med J* **2**, 228–231. Randomized controlled trial in 30 full-term infants whose mothers had had pethidine during labor. Within 1 min of birth they were given either naloxone 200 μg or normal saline intramuscularly. In the naloxone group a significant reduction in mean alveolar carbon dioxide tension and an increase in carbon dioxide excretion and mean alveolar ventilation was seen up to 48 h after birth. Consumption of milk and habituation to repeated auditory stimuli were significantly higher in the naloxone group in the first 48 h after birth. It was concluded that intramuscular naloxone reverses undesirable effects of pethidine (meperidine). **Ib A**

8 Saugstad OD, Rootwelt T, Aalen O (1998) Resuscitation of asphyxiated newborn infants with room air or oxygen: an international controlled trial: the Resair 2 study. *Pediatrics* **102**, e1. Prospective controlled multicenter trial comparing resuscitation with room air with 100% oxygen in 609 asphyxiated newborns over 999 g. Mortality in the first 7 days of life was 12.2% and 15.0% (NS), neonatal mortality was 13.9% and 19.0% (NS), death within 7 days of life and/or hypoxic–ischemic encephalopathy II and III was seen in 21.2% and 23.7% (NS) in the room air and oxygen groups respectively. It was concluded that 100% oxygen and room air are equally adequate for resuscitation of the asphyxiated newborn. **Ib A**

9 Silverman WA, Blanc WA (1957) The effect of humidity on survival of newly born premature infants. *Pediatrics* **20**, 477–487. Prospective randomized trial of nursing premature babies born between 1954 and 1956 in 30–60% humidity compared to 80–90% humidity. 166 were assigned to 30–60% and 164 to 80–90%. The rate of fall of body temperature was faster in the 30–60% group, who maintained their body temperature at a lower level thereafter. The mortality was higher in the 30–60% group. 56/160 (35%) died compared to 36/164 (22%). There was no difference in respiratory distress between the groups or of abnormal pulmonary findings at autopsy. **Ib A**

48.4 Counseling about neonatal problems

Janet Rennie

Management option		Quality of evidence	Strength of recommendation	References
General	Do not give contradictory information	–	✔	–
	Cover all reasonable outcomes	–	✔	–
	Be clear	–	✔	–
	Provide documentation	–	✔	–
	Provide addresses of support groups	–	✔	–
	Counseling is a process	–	✔	–
	Document counseling and information given	–	✔	–

➡

➡

Management option		Quality of evidence	Strength of recommendation	References
Specific	**Prepregnancy:** discuss foreseeable problems	–	✔	–
	During pregnancy: discuss as problem arises	–	✔	–
	Postnatal: discuss as problem presents	–	✔	–
Common problems where obstetricians can provide interim counseling	**The small-for-gestational-age baby:** ❑ Increased mortality and morbidity ❑ Hypoglycemia ❑ Hypoxic ischemic encephalopathy	 III III IIa IIa III	 B B B B B	 1 2,3 4 5 6
	❑ Hypothermia ❑ Polycythemia	III IIa	B B	7 4,8
	The preterm baby: ❑ Survival ❑ Necrotizing enterocolitis (animal study) ❑ Respiratory distress syndrome ❑ Hypoxic ischemic encephalopathy	 III (IIb) III IIa	 B (B) B B	 9 10 11 5,6,
	Birth trauma	–	✔	–
	Congenital abnormalities	III	B	12
	Cardiac problems	IV	C	13
	Infection	IV	C	14
	Jaundice	III	B	15
	Infant of a diabetic mother	III	B	16
	Drug withdrawal	III	B	17

References

1 Makhseed M, Jirous J, Ahmed MA *et al.* (2000) Middle cerebral artery to umbilical artery resistance index ratio in the prediction of neonatal outcome. *Int J Gynaecol Obstet* **71**, 119–125. Prospective study on the middle cerebral artery/umbilical artery resistance index ratio (C/U ratio) as a predictor of adverse perinatal outcome in 70 small-for-gestational-age singleton pregnancies between 29 and 42 weeks of gestation. It is concluded that an abnormal C/U ratio with intrauterine growth restriction is associated with high perinatal morbidity and mortality. **III B**

2 Lucas A, Moreley R, Cole TJ (1988) Adverse neurodevelopmental outcome of moderate neonatal hypoglycaemia. *Br Med J* **297**, 1304–1306. Prospective descriptive multicenter study of 661 preterm infants on the incidence of hypoglycemia. A plasma glucose concentration less than 2.6 mmol/l occurred in 433 of the infants and in 104 this was found on 3–30 separate days. When hypoglycemia was recorded on 5 or more separate days, mental and motor developmental scores at 18 months (corrected age) were significantly reduced by 14 and 13 points respectively, and the incidence of neurodevelopmental impairment (cerebral palsy or developmental delay) was increased by a factor of 3.5 (95% CI 1.3–9.4). These data suggest that moderate hypoglycemia may have serious neurodevelopmental consequences. **III B**

3 Menni F, de Lonlay P, Sevin C *et al.* (2001) Neurologic outcomes of 90 neonates and infants with persistent hyperinsulinemic hypoglycemia. *Pediatrics* **107**, 476–479. Retrospective study on the neurological development of 36 infants and 54 neonates treated medically or surgically for persistent hyperinsulinemic hypoglycemia of infancy. Severe psychomotor retardation was found in one infant and in 6 neonates. Intermediate psychomotor disability existed in 12 patients; epilepsy existed in 16. Neonatal onset was the main risk factor for severe retardation or epilepsy. Medically treated patients were less severely affected than those treated by surgery. It was concluded that neonatal hyperinsulinemic hypoglycemia may cause rapidly developing severe mental retardation and epilepsy. **III B**

4 Tenovuo A (1988) Neonatal complications in small-for-gestational age neonates. *J Perinat Med* **16**, 197–203. Prospective case-control study on neonatal complications in 118 severely small-for-gestational age (SGA) infants and 118 controls. Matching was for gestational age and mode of delivery. SGA infants had a birthweight below the 2.5th percentile. Neonatal complications (e.g. hypoglycemia, polycythemia and abnormal neurological symptoms) were found in 42% of SGA neonates and in 18% of the controls. Asphyxia was found in 16% of SGA infants and in 8.5% of control infants. A fivefold risk for hypoglycemia and an eightfold risk for abnormal neonatal neurological signs in SGA infants were found. SGA boys more often had asphyxia (22% vs 12%) and hypoglycemia (25% vs 5%) than SGA girls. Antenatal diagnosis of SGA did not decrease the neonatal complication rate. **IIa B**

5 Sung IK, Vor B, Oh W (1993) Growth and neurodevelopmental outcome of very low birth weight infants with intrauterine growth retardation: comparison with control subjects matched by birth weight and gestational age. *J Pediatr* **123**, 618–624. Case-controlled cohort study on outcome of 27 small-for-gestational-age (SGA) infants (29 ± 2 weeks and 821 ± 178 g), 27 infants gestation-matched with appropriate-size-for-gestational-age (AGA–GA; 29 ± 1 weeks, 1124 ± 85 g) and 27 birthweight-matched AGA infants (AGA–BW; 26 ± 2 weeks, 848 ± 141 g). It was found that the SGA infants did not differ from the AGA infants in neonatal course but that AGA weight-matched infants had lower Apgar scores, more days of assisted ventilation and an increased incidence of bronchopulmonary dysplasia, intraventricular hemorrhage and seizures. At 3 years of age the SGA very-low-birthweight infants had lower weight and height than both comparison groups ($p < 0.05$). Neurological outcome in SGA infants did not differ from that in AGA–GA infants. The AGA–BW infants had an increased incidence of suspect or abnormal neurological findings at 2 and 3 years of age ($p < 0.05$). **IIa B**

6 Thornberg E, Thiringer K, Odeback A *et al.* (1995) Birth asphyxia: incidence, clinical course and outcome in a Swedish population. *Acta Paediatr* **84**, 927–932. A retrospective study on 42 203 live infants. Small-for-gestational-age infants were overrepresented in the birth asphyxia group but not in the birth asphyxia–hypoxic–ischemic-encephalopathy (HIE) group. All infants with severe HIE died or developed neurological damage. Half of the infants with moderate, and all of the infants with mild HIE were reported to be normal at 18 months of age. A total of 0.3/1000 live-born infants died and 0.2/1000 developed a neurological disability related to birth asphyxia. **III B**

7 Wennergren M, Wennergren G, Vilbergsson G (1988) Obstetric characteristics and neonatal performance in a four-year small for gestational age population. *Obstet Gynecol* **72**, 615–620. Retrospective descriptive study on 160 small-for-gestational-age infants. 30% were born preterm. The cesarean section rate was 40%. Perinatal mortality was 10 times higher than in the total population, malformations excluded. Hypoglycemia and hypothermia occurred frequently. Most of the perinatal mortality occurred among SGA infants not identified before birth. **III B**

8 Merchant RH, Phadke SD, Sakhalkar VS *et al.* (1992) Hematocrit and whole blood viscosity in newborns: analysis of 100 cases. *Indian Pediatr* **29**, 555–561. Prospective study on the hematocrit and whole-blood viscosity in 25 full-term, 25 preterm, 20 term small-for-gestational-age (SGA) and 30 infants with perinatal asphyxia, at a mean age of 10 h. Polycythemia was found in 17 cases (17%) of which 8 (47.5%) were SGA. 12% of preterms were polycythemic. **III B**

9 Draper ES, Manktelow B, Field DJ *et al.* (1999) Prediction of survival for preterm births by weight and gestational age: retrospective population based study. *Br Med J* **319**, 1093–1097. Retrospective study on birth weight and gestational-age-specific survival of 3760 preterm European and Asian infants born between 22 and 32 weeks gestation, known to be alive at the onset of labor and admitted for neonatal care. Major congenital malformations were excluded. Survival by birth weight from 24 weeks gestation ranged from 9% (95% CI 7–13%) for infants with a birthweight of 250–499 g to 21% (95% CI 16–28%) for those of 1000–1249 g. At 27 weeks gestation, survival ranged from 55% (95% CI 49–61%) for infants with a birthweight of 500–749 g to 80% (95% CI 76–85%) for those of 1250–1499 g. Survival rates were similar for both ethnic groups. The odds ratio for the survival of infants from a multiple birth compared with singleton infants was 1.4 (95% CI 1.1–1.8). It is concluded that birthweight- and gestational-age-specific survival graphs for preterm infants facilitate decision-making for clinicians and parents. **III B**

10 Thornbury JC, Sibbons PD, van Velzen D *et al.* (1993) Histological investigations into the relationship between low birth weight and spontaneous bowel damage in the neonatal piglet. *Pediatr Pathol* **13**, 59–69. Animal experiment to study neonatal necrotizing enterocolitis (NEC) in small-for-gestational-age (SGA) and appropriate for gestation age, viable, term-delivered piglets. The animals were subjected to hypoxia and hyperviscosity known to induce NEC-like lesions. All lethally and sublethally runted SGA animals, but none of the controls, showed mucosal and submucosal necrosis of the distal ileum suggestive of ischemic injury. **IIa B**

11 Meirowitz NB, Ananth CV, Smulian JC *et al.* (2001) Effect of labor on infant morbidity and mortality with preterm premature rupture of membranes: United States population-based study. *Obstet Gynecol* **97**, 494–498. Retrospective cohort study on 34 594 women between 23 and 32 weeks gestation who had preterm premature rupture of the membranes by more than 12 h. Infant death occurred in 11.6%, respiratory distress syndrome (RDS) in 15.1%, assisted ventilation in 25.9% and neonatal seizures in 0.2% of cases. In small-for-gestational-age infants (below 10th centile), labor was found to be associated with early neonatal death (RR 1.24, 95%CI 1.11–1.38). In normally grown infants labor was not associated with infant death but was associated with higher rates of RDS (RR 1.15, 95% CI 1.08–1.22) and assisted ventilation (RR 1.16, 95% CI 1.08–1.24). The authors conclude that recommendations regarding clinical treatment should await future clinical trials. **III B**

12 Bhat BV, Babu L (1998) Congenital malformations at birth: a prospective study from south India. *Indian J Pediatr* **65**, 873–881. A prospective study on congenital malformations in 12 797 neonates born consecutively over 3 years. The overall incidence of malformations was 3.2% in live births and 15.7% in stillbirths. There were significantly more malformations in males ($p < 0.001$), still births ($p < 0.001$), low birthweight babies ($p < 0.001$) and preterm babies

($p < 0.001$). Consanguinity was more common among parents of malformed babies ($p < 0.001$). Musculoskeletal malformations were the commonest (9.69/1000), followed by cutaneous (6.33/1000), genitourinary (5.47/1000), gastrointestinal (5.47/1000), central nervous system (3.99/1000) and cardiac anomalies (2.03/1000). Antenatal infections and ingestion of drugs were not found to be significant factors in the causation of birth defects. **III B**

13 Kluckow M, Evans N (2001) Low systemic blood flow in the preterm infant. *Semin Neonatol* **6**, 75–84. Review on often unrecognized low systemic blood flow in the first 6–12h after birth, often to less than half of normal, before a gradual return to normal values by 24–48h. The author suggests that awareness of this problem may assist in preventing some of the complications of prematurity. **IV C**

14 Cartlidge P (2000) The epidermal barrier. *Semin Neonatol* **5**, 273–280. Review on the development of the stratum corneum during fetal life. The stratum corneum starts to develop after 24 weeks gestation and has completely developed by 24 weeks. Before 30 weeks the epidermal barrier is therefore not fully developed. It takes approximately 2–3 weeks after birth before it is. **IV C**

15 Newman TB, Klebanoff MA (1993) Neonatal hyperbilirubinemia and long term outcome: another look at the collaborative perinatal project. *Pediatrics* **92**, 651–657. Prospective multicenter cohort study on neonatal bilirubin levels and subsequent neurodevelopmental outcome in 41 324 white or black singletons with a birth weight of 2500g or more. All children had an IQ test and a neurological examination at age 7 years and a sensorineural hearing test at age 8 years. No association was found between IQ and bilirubin levels. No difference was seen in abnormal neurological examination results and sensorineural hearing loss with bilirubin levels over and below 342µmol/l. The frequency of abnormal or suspicious neurological examination results increased with increasing bilirubin levels (14.9% < 171µmol/l and 22.4% > 341µmol/l; $p < 0.001$). The authors state that the clinical importance of this finding is limited by the weakness of the association, the mild nature of the abnormalities and the lack of evidence that they are prevented by treatment. **III B**

16 Zhu L, Nakabayashi M, Takeda Y (1997) Statistical analysis of perinatal outcomes in pregnancy complicated with diabetes mellitus. *J Obstet Gynaecol Res* **23**, 555–563. Retrospective study on the outcomes of 482 pregnancies complicated by diabetes mellitus (DM). The prevalence of such pregnancies was 5.1%. Preeclampsia developed in 25.8%. The incidence of preterm delivery was 16.6% and cesarean sections were performed in 36.7%. There were significant differences in cesarean section rates between subgroups with and without diabetic complications (i.e. retinopathy and nephropathy) (69.5% vs 30.5%, $p < 0.0001$), and between preterm and term deliveries (60.0% vs 32.1%, $p < 0.0001$). The incidence of infants who were large for gestational age was 21%. There were 3 perinatal deaths (perinatal mortality rate of 6.1/1000 births). These figures did not differ from the local incidence of cesarean section and perinatal mortality rate in non-DM pregnancies of 16.3% and 7.7/1000 births respectively during the same study. It was concluded that, with accurate perinatal management, the perinatal mortality rate of DM pregnancies can be almost the same as that in the normal population. **III B**

17 Fricker HS, Segal S (1978) Narcotic addiction, pregnancy, and the newborn. *Am J Dis Child* **132**, 360–366. A retrospective study on 149 babies of 101 heroin-addicted mothers. Two thirds were born prematurely and 68% had withdrawal symptoms. The neonatal mortality rate was 6.7% and the stillbirth rate was 4%. **III B**

48.5 Puerperal problems

Doris Campbell

Postpartum psychiatric illness

Management option		Quality of evidence	Strength of recommendation	References
Postpartum blues	Reassurance, education, support by workers specifically trained to counsel for postnatal depression	Ia Ib	A A	1,2 3
Postpartum depression	Hospitalize with infant if possible	IIb	B	4
	Behavioral counseling and antidepressants provide significant improvement	Ib	A	3,5,6
	Synthetic progestogens have no place in prevention and long-acting norethisterone may increase risk	Ib	A	7
	Weigh risks/benefits of breastfeeding when prescribing antidepressants	III	B	8

Management option		Quality of evidence	Strength of recommendation	References
Postpartum psychosis	Hospitalize for safety of mother and newborn	III	B	4
	Antipsychotic medications, including electroconvulsive therapy	IV	C	9
	May also need antidepressants, lithium, benzodiazepines	–	✓	–
	Long-term support programs should be available	III	B	10

References

1 Ray KL, Hodnett ED (2000) Care giver support for postpartum depression. In: *Cochrane database of systematic reviews*, issue 4. Oxford: Update Software. Review of two studies of 137 women. One of the studies had a potential for bias due to refusal to participate and losses to follow-up. Professional and/or social report was associated with a significant reduction in depression at 25 weeks after birth. **Ia A**

2 Barlow G, Coren E (2000) Parent training programmes for improving maternal psychosocial health. In: *Cochrane database of systematic reviews*, issue 4. Oxford: Update Software. This review concluded that parenting programs can make a significant contribution to the improvement of psychosocial health in mothers with a variety of outcomes. Not all studies included related to the immediate postnatal period however. **Ia A**

3 Holden JM, Sagovsky R, Cox JL (1989) Counselling in a general practice setting: controlled study of health visitor intervention and treatment of postnatal depression. *Br Med J* **298**, 223–226. Controlled random ordered trial of 60 women identified by screening at 6 weeks and interview at 13 weeks postpartum. The intervention was eight weekly visits by health visitors specifically trained to counsel for postnatal depression. All women were reviewed by a psychiatrist who was not aware to which group the women were allocated. The difference between the groups in terms of full recovery was 32%, 69% compared with 38% in the control group. **Ib A**

4 Boath E, Cox J, Lewis M *et al.* (1999) When the cradle falls: the treatment of postnatal depression in a psychiatric day hospital compared with routine primary care. *J Affect Dis* **53**, 143–151. Study comparing 30 women treated in a specialized psychiatric day hospital with 30 women treated using routine primary care. There were no significant differences between the two groups on a variety of assessments at baseline but there were differences in outcome at 3 and 6 months. The authors concluded that a specialized day hospital was a more effective treatment setting for postnatal depression than routine primary care but commented that systematic bias was possible in their study. **IIb B**

5 Hoffbrand S, Howard L, Crawley H (2001) Antidepressant drug treatment for postnatal depression. In: *Cochrane database of systematic reviews*, issue 2. Oxford: Update Software. This review found only one trial that could be included. Fluoxetine was significantly better than a placebo and as effective as a full course of counseling. **Ib A**

6 Appleby L, Warner R, Whitton A *et al.* (1997) A controlled study of fluoxetine and cognitive–behavioural counselling in the treatment of postnatal depression. *Br Med J* **314**, 932–936. RCT with four treatment cells, fluoxetine or placebo plus one or six sessions of counseling. 87 women with postnatal depression 6–8 weeks postpartum were included. The results suggested improvement in all four treatment groups; fluoxetine was significantly better than placebo and six sessions of counseling was better than a single session. The authors concluded that both fluoxetine and behavioral counseling were effective treatments for nonpsychotic depression in postnatal women and suggested that the choice of treatment might therefore be made by the women themselves. **Ib A**

7 Lawrie TA, Herxheimer A, Dalton K (2000) Oestrogen and progesterones for preventing and treating postnatal depression. In: *Cochrane database of systematic reviews*, issue 4. Oxford: Update Software. Review of two published randomized, placebo-controlled trials; however, one was excluded. The authors concluded that synthetic progestogens had no place in the prevention of treatment of postnatal depression. Long-acting norethisterone was associated with an increased risk of depression and should therefore be used with caution in the postnatal period. Progesterone itself has not been evaluated in this context. Estrogen therapy, they concluded, may be of modest value at a late stage of severe depression. Estrogen's role in the prevention of recurrent postnatal depression has not been evaluated. **Ib A**

8 Wisner KL, Perel JM, Findling RL (1996) Antidepressant treatment during breastfeeding. *Am J Psychiatry* **153**, 1132–1137. Review of 15 published reports for finding information about antidepressants in which serum levels of drugs were obtained from nursing infants. Included were 9 antidepressants, 6 of which were not found in measurable amounts in the infants and no adverse effects were reported. There were adverse effects with 2 others. The suggested prescription of an antidepressant drug for a breastfeeding woman is a case-specific risk–benefit decision. **III B**

9 Tabbane K, Charfi F, Dellagi L *et al.* (1999) Acute postpartum psychoses. *Encephale* **3**, 12–17. Review article. The frequency of postpartum psychoses is evaluated at 1–2/1000 births. Postpartum psychosis includes major affective disorders, which is the most frequent diagnosis. The clinical pictures have specific characteristics: rapid change of symptomatology, liability of mood and frequent confusional signs. The short-term prognosis is generally good but the risk of recurrence of the mental disorder, in or outside the puerperal context, is high. At clinical, evolutionary and genetic levels, the studies do not provide arguments for the nosological autonomy of postpartum psychosis. At therapeutic level, electroconvulsive therapy is particularly efficient in this indication. **IV C**

10 Milgrom J, Burrows GD, Snellen M *et al.* (1998) Psychiatric illness in women: a review of the function of a specialist mother–baby unit. *Aust N Z J Psychiatry* **32**, 680–686. Descriptive paper of a specialist program in a psychiatric mother–baby unit. The majority of women admitted suffered from schizophrenia or other psychotic disorders, the second largest diagnostic criteria being depression. For 20 mothers, this was the first psychiatric admission and most admissions were voluntary. The mean length of stay was 21.7 days, representing a highly significant decrease in stay compared to the past 10 years in the same unit. Mothering skills were found to be incompetent or only passable in 57% of women. A small improvement occurred by the time of discharge and the majority of women were not separated from their infants. The critical need to support these women and their infants in the long term was highlighted, with recommendations for outpatient and day programs as well as supported accommodation. **III B**

Infection and thromboembolic disease

Management option		Quality of evidence	Strength of recommendation	References
Endomyometritis	**Prevention:**			
	❏ Limit vaginal examinations, intrauterine monitoring, exteriorizing the uterus at cesarean section (CS) and manual removal of placenta at CS	–	✔	–
	❏ Prophylactic antibiotics at time of CS	Ia	A	1
	Management:			
	❏ Gentamicin and clindamycin or extended-spectrum beta-lactam (e.g. imipenem/cilastatin)	Ia	A	2
	❏ Continue until afebrile for at least 24 h	–	✔	–
	❏ Imaging if patient not responding (for retained products of conception, abscess, hematoma, ovarian vein thrombosis, etc.)	III	B	3
Septic pelvic vein thrombophlebitis	Diagnosis of exclusion; no localizing symptoms	–	✔	–
	At least 7 days of therapeutic heparin	III Ib	B A	4 5
	Broad-spectrum antibiotics	Ib	A	5
	No outpatient medications needed after treatment	–	✔	–
Ovarian vein thrombosis	At least 7 days of therapeutic heparin	III	B	3
	Broad-spectrum antibiotics	III	B	3
	Coumadin, especially if extends to inferior vena cava	III	B	3
Puerperal hematomas	Expectant management and compression if less than 5 cm and not expanding	IV	C	6
	If large, evacuation, hemostasis, restoration of anatomy, closed drainage	IV III	C B	6 7
	Large hematomas above the levators require imaging for detection and surgical correction	IV	C	8

Management option		Quality of evidence	Strength of recommendation	References
Mastitis and breast abscesses	Continued pumping/expressing and feeding (unless abscess)	–	✔	–
	Oral dicloxacillin (erythromycin if allergic)	IV	C	9
	Intravenous oxacillin for treatment failures	–	✔	–
	Ultrasonography to rule out abscess if there is poor response or fluctuant mass	III	B	10
	Open or ultrasound-guided drainage for abscess	IV	C	9
	Culture milk with complicated mastitis or abscess	–	✔	–

References

1 Smaill F, Hofmeyer G (2000) Antibiotic prophylactics for caesarean section. In: *Cochrane database of systematic reviews*, issue 2. Oxford: Update Software. Review of selected randomized trials comparing antibiotic prophylactics or no treatment for both elective and nonelective cesarean section. 66 trials were included. The use of prophylactic antibiotics substantially reduced the incidence of fever, endometritis, wound infection, urinary tract infection and serious infection after cesarean section. The reduction of endometritis by two thirds to three quarters therefore justifies a policy of administering prophylactic antibiotics to women undergoing cesarean section. **Ia A**

2 French LM, Smaill F (2000) Antibiotic regimens for endometritis after delivery. In: *Cochrane database of systematic reviews*, issue 4. Oxford: Update Software. Review of selected randomized trials of different antibiotic regimens for postpartum endometritis either after cesarean section or vaginal delivery. 41 trials were included but the reviewers commented that the studies were methodologically poor. The combination of gentamicin and clindamycin was appropriate for the treatment of endometritis, with a relative risk of 1.37 compared with other regimes. Regimens whose activity included penicillin-resistant anaerobic bacteria were better than those without (RR 1.73). Continued antibiotic therapy after intravenous therapy confers no further benefit and is not needed. **Ia A**

3 Simons GR, Piwnica-Worms DR, Goldhaber SZ (1993) Ovarian vein thrombosis. *Am Heart J* **126**, 641–647. Review of five cases of ovarian vein thrombosis and a review of the literature. The conclusion is that more widespread use of computed tomography scanning and magnetic resonance imaging may lead to a more frequent diagnosis of ovarian vein thrombosis. **III B**

4 Witlin AG, Mercer BM, Sibai BM (1996) Septic pelvic thrombophlebitis or refractory postpartum fever of undetermined etiology. *J Matern Fetal Med* **5**, 355–358. Retrospective case review of 31 women with the final diagnosis of septic pelvic thrombophlebitis over an 8-year period. Cases of ovarian vein thrombosis were excluded. All had refractory febrile morbidity. All had heparin therapy but not all responded immediately. **III B**

5 Brown CE, Stettler RW, Twickler D *et al.* (1999) Puerperal septic pelvic thrombophlebitis: incidence and response to heparin therapy. *Am J Obstet Gynecol* **181**, 143–148. Women who had persistent pyrexia and pelvic infection despite adequate antibiotic therapy were included. All underwent abdominal pelvic computed tomography imaging. Those with pelvic thrombophlebitis were then randomly assigned to either continuation of antimicrobial therapy or antimicrobial therapy with the addition of heparin. 69 women met their criteria and 15 (22%) had septic pelvic thrombophlebitis. Intention to treat analysis revealed no significant difference between the responses. The incidence in this large study over a 3-year period of septic pelvic thrombophlebitis was 1/3000. **Ib A**

6 Ridgway LE (1995) Puerperal emergency. Vaginal and vulvar hematomas. *Obstet Gynecol Clin North Am* **22**, 275–282. Review article. Prevention, using good surgical technique with attention to hemostasis in the repair of lacerations and episiotomies, should limit the occurrence of this complication. Puerperal hematomas, however, are not unavoidable. Thus, one must be alert to the possibility so that the hematoma can be diagnosed early and treated aggressively. This includes correcting hypovolemia and intervening with active surgical management if the hematoma is large or expanding. **IV C**

7 Benrubi G, Neuman C, Nuss RC *et al.* (1987) Vulvar and vaginal hematomas: a retrospective study of conservative versus operative management. *South Med J* **80**, 991–994. Retrospective case study of 32 cases of vulvar and vaginal hematomas over a 10-year period. Conservative management of such hematomas resulted in more complications, more operative intervention and a longer hospital stay. **III B**

8 Chin HG, Scott DR, Resnik R *et al.* (1989) Angiographic embolization of intractable puerperal hematomas. *Am J Obstet Gynecol* **160**, 434–438. Puerperal hematomas may not respond to conventional therapy, including vaginal packing, drainage, and hypogastric artery ligation. Two cases are presented in which selective angiographic arterial embolization was used to manage this potentially lethal complication. **IV C**

9 Benson EA (1989) Management of breast abscesses. *World J Surg* **13**, 753–756. Review article. Hospital experience of breast abscess is changing as nonpuerperal abscess associated with periductal mastitis assumes increasing importance. Clinical presentation, bacteriology and management differ notably from acute puerperal abscess but the latter can still cause severe morbidity. The standard management of puerperal abscess by incision, breaking down loculi and dependent drainage may still be used but the author has shown that an alternative approach – curettage and primary obliteration of the cavity under antibiotic cover – can give equally good results with reduced morbidity. **IV C**

10 Karstrup S, Solvig J, Nolsoe CP *et al.* (1993) Acute puerperal breast abscesses: US-guided drainage. *Radiology* **188**, 807–809. Breast abscesses typically develop in lactating women. The recommended treatment is surgical incision and drainage with the patient under general anesthesia. Ultrasonically guided percutaneous drainage with local anesthesia was performed in 19 consecutive patients referred for treatment because of clinical signs of acute puerperal breast abscess. 18 of the 19 patients (95%) were successfully treated. Long-term follow-up (median, 12 months) did not show any recurrences, and the cosmetic results were excellent. 8 of the 19 patients (42%) continued nursing during and after treatment. 10 (53%) were treated on an outpatient basis. On the basis of these results, the authors recommend ultrasonically guided percutaneous treatment for use in patients with acute puerperal breast abscesses. **III B**

Other puerperal problems

Management option		Quality of evidence	Strength of recommendation	References
Pubic symphysis separation	Most resolve with rest, trochanter belts, analgesics, weightbearing assistance and time	IV	C	1
	Consider injection of symphysis with mixture of hydrocortisone and lidocaine/lignocaine (chymotrypsin)	III	B	2
	Orthopedic treatment reserved for severe cases	–	✔	–
Obstetrical paralysis	**Prevention:** ❑ Avoid prolonged, obstructed labor ❑ Proper lithotomy and pushing positions ❑ Avoid regional anesthesia when coagulopathy or infection is present (systemic or local)	–	✔	–
	Management: ❑ Splinting, physical therapy, electrical nerve stimulation ❑ Paraplegia warrants immediate magnetic resonance imaging ❑ Emergency surgery for epidural abscess or hematoma	–	✔	–
Urinary retention	12–24 h continuous drainage if more than 400 ml	–	✔	–
	Rarely, intermittent self-catheterization required	IV	C	3
	Exclude infection	–	✔	–

References

1 Snow RE, Neubert AG (1997) Peripartum pubic symphysis separation: a case series and review of the literature. *Obstet Gynecol Surv* **52**, 438–443. Review article. Conservative therapy, including bedrest, pelvic binders, ambulation devices, and mild analgesics, usually results in a complete recovery in 4–6 weeks. The occurrence of a symphyseal separation should not significantly alter the management of subsequent pregnancies and conservative therapy is recommended for any recurrence of symptoms. A retrospective review of the authors' experience with 5121 deliveries from 1994–95 found 9 cases of peripartum symphyseal separation, resulting in an incidence of 1/569 deliveries. Details regarding this case series and a review of the literature are presented. **IV C**

2 Schwartz Z, Katz Z, Lancet M (1985) Management of puerperal separation of the symphysis pubis. *Int J Gynaecol Obstet* **23**, 125–128. Uncontrolled study of 13 postpartum patients with separation of the symphysis pubis, treated by intrasymphysial injection of a combination of hydrocortisone, chymotrypsin and lidocaine (lignocaine). The authors claim that this treatment, when compared with other modes of treatment, shortened the time of morbidity and effected complete recovery. **III B**

3 Watson WJ (1991) Prolonged postpartum urinary retention. *Mil Med* **156**, 502–503. Report of two patients with prolonged postpartum urinary retention who were treated with self-intermittent catheterization rather than the use of an indwelling catheter. It was suggested that this intermittent catheterization might be advantageous. **IV C**

48.6 Postnatal contraception and sterilization

Ronnie Lamont and Paul Adinkra

Puerperal contraception

Management option	Quality of evidence	Strength of recommendation	References
Breastfeeding is a very effective contraceptive provided the mother remains amenorrheic, is not supplementing feeds and the infant is less than 6 months old	III	B	1–5
Breastfeeding is a less reliable contraceptive once the mother has had her first period, she supplements feeds with more than 150ml/day or the infant is aged over 6 months	III	B	1–5
The most popular contraceptive method in the puerperium is the use of condoms	III	B	5
Diaphragms or cervical caps should be fitted at the postnatal check	III	B	5
Intrauterine contraceptive devices are more reliable, and expelled less frequently, if fitted after involution of the uterus rather than the immediate postplacental insertion	III	B	1,4,5
The success of immediate postplacental insertion depends on correct operator placement of the device rather than the type of device	Ib IIb III	A B B	6 7 8
Progesterone-only preparations are available as mini-pills, injections, implants, vaginal rings and medicated intrauterine devices; all may cause irregular and sometimes troublesome bleeding	III	B	4,9
The infant's absorption of progestogens secreted in breast milk does not affect growth or development	IIa III	B B	10 3,11,12
Natural family planning methods are difficult to use in the puerperium	III	B	5

References

1 Burkman RT (1993) Puerperium and breast-feeding. *Curr Opin Obstet Gynecol* **5**, 683–687. Review of 31 papers focusing on a number of aspects of breastfeeding, including mothers' breastfeeding skills and attitude, the risk of human immunodeficiency virus transmission in breast milk, lactational amenorrhea and its contraceptive effects, and the effects of anesthesia and analgesia on lactation. The review also covers postpartum contraception and the nutritional resources available to low-income puerperal mothers, although this mainly applies to federal funding in the USA. **III B**

2 Short RV (1993) Lactational infertility in family planning. *Ann Med* **25**, 175–180. Review of the anthropological history of lactational infertility in past times, ending with modern trends and practice. The physiological mechanisms

responsible for these contraceptive effects are discussed. An excellent effort is made to quantify the contraceptive effect of breastfeeding and the additional benefits of breastfeeding are also discussed. **III B**

3 Diaz S, Croxatto HB (1993) Contraception in lactating women. *Curr Opin Obstet Gynecol* **5**, 815–822. Review covering the subject of lactational infertility and other nonhormonal and hormonal methods of contraception in lactating women. Taking into consideration variables such as women's choice, indicators of risk of pregnancy, fertility patterns, choice of mode of contraception and programmatic considerations, discussion is made of when contraception should start post-partum. Lactational amenorrhea and the question of transference of steroids to breastfed infants is also discussed. **III B**

4 Wang IY, Fraser IS (1994) Reproductive function and contraception in the postpartum period. *Obstet Gynecol Surv* **49**, 56–63. Review of 73 papers provides an overview of reproductive function and contraception unique to the immediate postpartum period, discussing breastfeeding, birth interval and infant and maternal health. Patterns and trends in breastfeeding are discussed, together with the resumption of menstruation, ovulation and postpartum fertility. Postpartum contraception in lactating women is discussed, with particular reference to periodic abstinence, barrier methods, intrauterine contraceptive devices, progestogen-only contraception, combined oral contraception and luteinizing-hormone-releasing-hormone agonists. **III B**

5 Kennedy KI (1996) Postpartum contraception. *Baillière's Clin Obstet Gynaecol* **10**, 25–41. Review of 65 publications starting with choice of infant feeding and antenatal counseling for contraception. For non-breastfeeding postpartum women, barrier methods, combined oral contraception, progesterone-only contraception and intrauterine contraceptive devices (IUCDs) are discussed, together with postpartum tubal sterilization and natural family planning methods. For breastfeeding postpartum women, the first choice is stated to be nonhormonal methods, i.e. the lactational amenorrhea method or postpartum tubal sterilization, IUCDs, barrier methods or natural family planning, and the second choice is given as progesterone-only methods. **III B**

6 Tatum HJ, Beltran RS, Ramos R *et al.* (1996) Immediate postplacental insertion of GYNE-T 380 and GYNE-T 380 postpartum intrauterine contraceptive devices: randomized study. *Am J Obstet Gynecol* **175**, 1231–1235. Multicenter RCT of intrauterine contraceptive devices (IUCDs) in which 300 subjects used the GYNE-T 380 IUCD and 292 subjects the GYNE-T 380 postpartum IUCD. The 1-year expulsion and efficacy rates were compared. The two IUCDs were identical except that one was inserted by means of a temporary fundal suspension system and the other was placed directly into the uterine cavity; both were inserted within 10 min of expulsion of the placenta in a term pregnancy. The results indicated that both devices were safe and effective when inserted immediately after delivery of the placenta. **Ib A**

7 Xu JX, Rivera R, Dunson TR *et al.* (1996) A comparative study of two techniques used in immediate post placental insertion (IPPI) of the Copper T-380A IUD in Shanghai, People's Republic of China. *Contraception* **54**, 33–38. 910 women, mainly primiparas, had a copper intrauterine contraceptive device (IUCD) inserted within 10 min of delivery of the placenta. In 470 of these cases the IUCD was inserted by hand and in 440 cases it was inserted using ring forceps. The results suggested that the two different insertion techniques did not significantly affect discontinuation rates and that immediate postplacental vaginal insertion appeared to be a suitable method of contraception for Chinese women postpartum. **IIb B**

8 Van Kets H, Wildemeersch D, van der Pas H *et al.* (1995) IUD expulsion solved with implant technology. *Contraception* **51**, 87–92. Study of 820 women over 3 years, covering approximately 14 000 women-months. The technique of using an improved inserter that is fixed, frameless and flexible to insert a copper intrauterine contraceptive device was found to be associated with low expulsion, high efficacy and high acceptability rates. **III B**

9 Dunson TR, McLaurin VL, Grubb GS *et al.* (1993) A multicenter clinical trial of a progestin-only oral contraceptive in lactating women. *Contraception* **47**, 23–35. In 22 sites and 14 countries, 4000 women took part in the study over a 3-year period and nearly 30 000 woman-months of experience was gathered. The study was designed to evaluate the safety, contraceptive efficacy and overall acceptability of progesterone-only oral contraception in breastfeeding women. Menstrual problems were reported by nearly 60% of women but the most common reason given for discontinuation was the woman's desire for a change in contraceptive method; only 5% discontinued the pill because of menstrual problems. The authors concluded that the progesterone-only oral contraceptive was a safe, effective and acceptable contraceptive option for postpartum breastfeeding women. **III B**

10 Molland JR, Morehead DB, Baldwin DM *et al.* (1996) Immediate postpartum insertion of the Norplant contraceptive device. *Fertil Steril* **66**, 43–48. To determine safety and efficacy,14 women received Norplant immediately post-partum and were compared to 6 controls who had bilateral tubal ligation. Significant differences between Norplant and the control group included breathing irregularities, headaches, alopecia and abdominal discomfort. While serum electrolytes, metabolic markers and blood components were all within normal limits, serum estradiol, progesterone and urinary steroid biomarkers indicated that steroid secretion was severely suppressed in the Norplant group compared with controls, who exhibited normal postpartum ovarian activity. **IIa B**

11 Kelsey JK (1996) Hormonal contraception and lactation. *J Hum Lact* **12**, 315–318. This review of 35 articles discusses progestogen contraceptives administered orally, by injection, as an implant or as a progestogen-releasing intrauterine contraceptive device. The role of combined oral contraception during the period of lactation is also discussed in depth. **III B**

12 Baheiraei A, Ardsetani N, Ghazizadeh S (2001) Effects of progestogen-only contraceptives on breast feeding and infant growth. *Int J Gynaecol Obstet* **74**, 203–205. A nonrandomized study from Iran studied 140 breastfeeding women at their 6-week postpartum visit. 51 of the women were using progestogen-only methods of contraception and 89 were using nonhormonal contraception. Breast milk components were compared between the two groups at 26 weeks and infant growth was serially checked through monthly visits during the first 6 months of life in both groups. The mean milk concentrations of calcium, phosphorus, sodium, potassium and protein were statistically similar between the two groups but triglyceride level was higher in the hormonal group and magnesium was higher in the nonhormonal group. The anthropometric variables of the infants were similar in both groups, with the exception of head circumference at 10–14 weeks of age, which was higher in the infants of the hormonal contraception group. In this study, the growth of infants fed by breast milk was not affected by hormonal contraceptives as assessed by the rate of change in weight, height and head circumference. The authors concluded that neither the progesterone-only or depo medroxyprogesterone acetate pill had any adverse effects on breast milk components or infant growth and so was a suitable and safe contraceptive method in breastfeeding women. **III B**

Puerperal sterilization

Management option	Quality of evidence	Strength of recommendation	References
Undertake puerperal sterilization immediately after birth only if there has been good antenatal counseling and informed consent	III	B	1–4
Postpone sterilization until after the puerperium (interval sterilization) if there is doubt	III	B	1–4
For early procedures, regional anesthesia using the labor epidural catheter, or spinal anesthesia, is preferable for safety reasons	III	B	2,3
The Pomeroy technique of puerperal sterilization using mini-laparotomy is safe, simple and cheap but destroys/removes 3–4 cm of tube	III	B	2
Tubal clips (e.g. Filshie or Hulka–Clemens) destroy the least amount of tube but are relatively expensive	III	B	2,5
Puerperal sterilization has a higher failure rate than interval sterilization	III	B	2

References

1 Kennedy KI (1996) Postpartum contraception. *Baillière's Clin Obstet Gynaecol* **10**, 25–41. Review of 65 publications starting with choice of infant feeding and antenatal counseling for contraception. For nonbreastfeeding postpartum women, barrier methods, combined oral contraception, progesterone-only contraception and intrauterine contraceptive devices (IUCDs) are discussed, together with postpartum tubal sterilization and natural family planning methods. For breastfeeding postpartum women, the first choice is stated to be nonhormonal methods, i.e. the lactational amenorrhea method or postpartum tubal sterilization, IUCDs, barrier methods or natural family planning, and the second choice is given as progesterone-only methods. **III B**

2 Pati S, Cullins V (2000) Female sterilization evidence. *Obstet Gynecol Clin North Am* **27**, 859–899. Review of the evidence-based approach to female sterilization, containing 336 references. For each section the level of evidence and strength of recommendation is quoted. The review covers timing, personnel, pain management, laparoscopic options, mini-laparotomy, micro-laparoscopy, laparotomy and vaginal colpotomy or culdoscopy. Occlusion methods are discussed, as are ligation methods and chemical methods. Mortality and morbidity, together with long-term effects, are discussed in depth. Failure rates and reversal are also discussed. There is a large section on noncontraceptive health effects, including ovarian cancer, sexually transmitted disease and sexuality. In the references, each quoted reference carries a classification of the level of evidence in parentheses at the end. **III B**

3 Chi IC, Petta CA, McPheeters M (1995) A review of safety, efficacy, pros and cons, and issues of puerperal tubal sterilization--an update. *Adv Contracept* **11**, 187–206. Review of puerperal tubal sterilization containing 97 references that focuses on the safety, efficacy and pros and cons of tubal sterilization performed during the puerperal period while a woman is still in hospital. The review found that tubal sterilization performed while the woman is still in hospital or on the delivery table or during the early puerperium while she remains hospitalized is operationally easy and medically safe and does not adversely affect lactation. However, reported pregnancy rates are generally higher in puerperal tubal sterilization than in interval sterilization, especially when the mechanical tubal occlusion technique is used. The authors concluded that tubal sterilization performed during the puerperium has a number of advantages

over short-acting contraceptive methods which require strict compliance for postpartum use. However, they also concluded that candidates for puerperal tubal sterilization need to be carefully screened and counseled, since post-sterilization regret is more likely. **III B**

4 Rosenfeld BL, Taskin O, Kafkashli A *et al.* (1998) Sequelae of postpartum sterilization. *Arch Gynecol Obstet* **261**, 183–187. Observational study designed to investigate the menstrual, psychosexual, psychological and somatic sequelae of a group of women who were thought to be more prone to express regret following postpartum sterilization. The follow up was conducted by questionnaire at 6 months and 5 years following the procedure. Data were available from 242 patients, 76.8% of whom were below the age of 30. 21.9% of all patients expressed regrets. About one third had various menstrual disturbances. Patients rated their sex life as generally more enjoyable in many respects. The most common psychological symptoms were irritability, nervousness and depression, while the common somatic symptoms were pelvic or abdominal pain and backache and tiredness. **III B**

5 Penfield AJ (2000) The Filshie clip for female sterilization: a review of world experience. *Am J Obstet Gynecol* **182**, 485–489. Review of Filshie clip usage, using 25 references. The Filshie clip system has been used in the UK and Europe for the past 20 years and is now the method of choice in Canada; this study from the USA reports the worldwide experience from 1981 to the present day and reveals a high level of acceptance of Filshie clip because of its effective design and ease of application. A sample of world experience, together with comparative failure rates, is recorded, as well as the US Food and Drug Administration's approval of the Filshie clip. Filshie's own recommendations regarding clip application are listed and a general review is given of the Filshie clip in contrast to other methods of tubal sterilization. A small section examines whether the Filshie is appropriate for postpartum sterilization and the review concluded that it was proved to be a highly acceptable means of tubal occlusion because of its ease of application, minimal tubal destruction, maximum reversibility and extremely low failure rate. **III B**

INDEX